Dermatological Manifestations of Kidney Disease

Julia R. Nunley • Edgar V. Lerma
Editors

Dermatological Manifestations of Kidney Disease

Springer

Editors
Julia R. Nunley
Department of Dermatology
Virginia Commonwealth University Medical Center
Nelson Clinic
Richmond, VA, USA

Edgar V. Lerma
Department of Medicine
Section of Nephrology
University of Illinois at Chicago/Advocate Christ Medical Center
Oak Lawn, IL, USA

ISBN 978-1-4939-2394-6 ISBN 978-1-4939-2395-3 (eBook)
DOI 10.1007/978-1-4939-2395-3

Library of Congress Control Number: 2015932484

Springer New York Heidelberg Dordrecht London

Printed on acid-free paper

Springer Science+Business Media LLC New York is part of Springer Science+Business Media (www.springer.com)

To all my colleagues, mentors, teachers, fellows, residents, and students, I am grateful for what each of you have shown and taught me over the past many years. I am a better student, teacher, physician, and person because of each of you.

To all my friends and family, especially my parents, I am eternally indebted and thankful for the unconditional love and support you have all given to me.

Julia R. Nunley

To all my mentors, and friends, at the University of Santo Tomas Faculty of Medicine and Surgery in Manila, Philippines, and Northwestern University Feinberg School of Medicine in Chicago, IL, who have in one way or another influenced and guided me to become the physician that I am.

To all the medical students, interns, and residents at Advocate Christ Medical Center whom I have taught or learned from, especially those who eventually decided to pursue Nephrology as a career…

To my parents and my brothers, without whose unwavering love and support through the good and bad times, I would not have persevered and reached my goals in life …

Most especially, to my two lovely and precious daughters Anastasia Zofia and Isabella Ann, whose smiles and laughter constantly provide me unparalleled joy and happiness; my very loving and understanding wife Michelle, who has always been supportive of my endeavors both personally and professionally, and who sacrificed a lot of time and exhibited unwavering patience as I devoted a significant amount of time and effort to this project. Truly, they provide me with motivation and inspiration.

Edgar V. Lerma

In memory of Lisa M. Grandinetti, MD, an extraordinary dermatologist, wife, mother, and daughter. She died of ovarian cancer on February 27, 2015.

The editors would like to acknowledge Lisa M. Grandinetti, MD, Assistant Professor in the Department of Dermatology who passed away during the production of this book project. Dr. Grandinetti was a member of the Department of Dermatology of the University of Pittsburgh. An outstanding clinician, educator, and mentor, she ran the Department's Cutaneous T-cell Lymphoma Clinic, one of the largest of its kind in the country, through which she directed the care of patients across the tri-state area. She was an accomplished investigator having led several clinical trials that provided cutting-edge therapies to her patients. Importantly, she served as the Program Director of the Dermatology Residency Program. She had a passion for education and was a friend and mentor to all of the department's trainees. She was instrumental in the completion of this book project. Lisa's research, clinical and teaching contributions will be long remembered.

Julia R. Nunley
Edgar V. Lerma

Foreword

In Greek mythology Proteus was an early sea god known for representing the constantly changing nature of the oceans, and the adjective protean has come to mean "capable of assuming many forms." The manifestations of kidney disease can be described as protean, as the loss of the ability to maintain homeostasis by regulating the composition of the blood and other body fluids affects every cell and organ system in the body. Healthy kidneys protect the whole organism by maintaining constancy of the extracellular environment and by responding to signals derived from diet and from changes in the circulation. They do so by having evolved a highly complex architecture, with more different cell types than any other organ in the body. The term uremia refers to the accumulation of solutes in the blood that are normally excreted by healthy functioning kidneys, and the myriad of retention solutes contain molecular entities toxic to almost every organ system. While the term uremia is often reserved for advanced kidney failure, we are increasingly aware that lesser degrees of kidney dysfunction are also associated with more subtle but clinically significant multiorgan dysfunction. Moreover, the kidneys, as the most highly vascularized organs in the body, are highly susceptible to injury from systemic conditions, including diseases associated with inflammation and autoimmunity. Thus, a modern-day re-paraphrasing of Osler might conclude that "he or she who knows kidney disease knows medicine."

Among the many organs affected by kidney disease is the dermis. Like the kidney, the skin, or outer covering of the body, has a protective role for the whole organism, by covering the underlying soft tissue, bone, muscle, and the internal organs. The skin is the largest organ in the body and also has a complex architecture with many layers, a multitude of cell types, and a high level of both vascularization and innervation. Perhaps it is not surprising that there are many dermatological conditions associated with kidney disease and that a majority of patients living with kidney disease also have dermatological problems. Moreover, cutaneous manifestations of systemic diseases that also involve the kidney are common, and properly diagnosing the skin condition can help lead to the correct renal diagnosis as well.

This new book edited by Nunley and Lerma fills an important niche in providing bedside clinical resources for the care of patients with kidney disease who have dermatological manifestations. The handbook format and the inclusion of many high-resolution photomicrographs greatly increase bedside utility. By including coverage of complications due to immunosuppression and kidney transplantation, the book takes a comprehensive approach useful as a single source for complex diagnostic problems. While the pace of acquisition of new medical knowledge is often fast and furious, this book provides canonical information likely to stand the "test of time," within the specific domain of nephrology and within the broader context of internal medicine.

Jonathan Himmelfarb, M.D.
Division of Nephrology
Department of Medicine
University of Washington
Seattle, WA, USA

Foreword

Drs. Nunley and Lerma have put together a stellar group of colleagues interested in the cutaneous manifestations associated with renal disease. They have included diseases that are inherited, immunologic, infectious, drug-induced, and acquired in other manners. The dermatologists that they have selected are among the elite individuals within our field, and each has provided acute insight into the disorder or disease that they have been asked to write about.

This book reveals to the reader the spectrum of skin disease that can be associated with diseases of the kidneys. If the visible clues are ignored, both common manifestations and unusual disorders will be misdiagnosed. The editors and their contributing authors have provided you with substantial information that will improve your clinical acumen and offer advantages to understanding and managing patients with cutaneous diseases that reflect kidney disease.

Jeffrey P. Callen, M.D.
Division of Dermatology
University of Louisville School of Medicine
Louisville, KY, USA

Preface

The recently published KDIGO Guidelines defined chronic kidney disease (CKD) as abnormalities of kidney structure or function present for over 3 months—regardless of underlying kidney disease. CKD is further divided into stages based on the level of function as estimated by glomerular filtration rate (GFR). According to this definition, all individuals with a GFR <60 mL/min/1.73 m^2 for 3 months are classified as having CKD, irrespective of the presence or absence of kidney damage. The rationale for including these individuals is that a reduction in kidney function to this level or lower represents loss of half or more of the adult level of normal kidney function, which may be associated with a number of systemic manifestations.

Nearly 100 % of patients with CKD have at least one significant dermatologic manifestation [1]. These cutaneous manifestations occur for various reasons: (1) diseases that affect the kidney and the skin; (2) skin conditions that are common or unique to uremia per se; (3) complications due to immunosuppression from transplantation. Although some of these conditions are inconvenient, many are serious and life altering and some life threatening. This book serves as an all-inclusive reference of these conditions readily available to practitioners providing medical care to these patients. As the population of patients with CKD continues to grow at a high rate and more care falls to primary care physicians, this information needs to be readily available.

This book is divided into three parts: (1) Dermatologic conditions seen in disorders causing chronic kidney disease, (2) Dermatologic conditions associated with chronic kidney disease, and (3) Dermatologic conditions associated with kidney transplantation. There is also a chapter focusing on pharmacological aspects of the disease process.

Each chapter provides discussions in pathobiology, extensive clinical discussions and photos, as well as in-depth treatment options. Utilizing images, recommendations for workup and therapy, the reader will be able to recognize, appropriately evaluate, and treat these conditions more effectively.

Richmond, VA, USA — Julia R. Nunley
Oak Lawn, IL, USA — Edgar V. Lerma

Reference

1. Udayakumar P, et al. Cutaneous manifestations in patients with chronic renal failure on hemodialysis. Indian J Dermatol Venereol Leprol. 2006;72:119–25.

Contents

Contributors

Ali K. Abu-Alfa, M.D. Division of Nephrology and Hypertension, Department of Internal Medicine, American University of Beirut, Beirut, Lebanon

Ehsan Azimi, M.D. Cutaneous Biology Research Center, Department of Dermatology, Massachusetts General Hospital, Charlestown, MA, USA

Brandon T. Beal, B.S. Saint Louis University School of Medicine, St. Louis, MO, USA

Jeffrey P. Callen, M.D. Division of Dermatology, University of Louisville School of Medicine, Louisville, KY, USA

Mitalee P. Christman, A.B., M.D. Department of Dermatology, Massachusetts General Hospital, Harvard Medical School, Cambridge, MA, USA

Melinda B. Chu, M.D. Department of Dermatology, Anheuser-Busch Institute, Saint Louis University, St. Louis, MO, USA

Shawn E. Cowper, M.D. Yale Dermatopathology Service, Yale University School of Medicine, New Haven, CT, USA

C. Ralph Daniel III, M.D. University of Mississippi Medical Center, Jackson, MS, USA; University of Alabama, Birmingham, AL, USA

Mark Davis, M.D. Department of Dermatology, Mayo Clinic College of Medicine, Rochester, MN, USA

Kristie Lynn Slivka Delaney, M.D. Internal Medicine, University of Illinois at Chicago/ Advocate Christ Hospital, Oak Lawn, IL, USA

Christine A. DeWitt, M.D. Department of Dermatology, Georgetown University/Washington Hospital Center, Chevy Chase, MD, USA

Krista L. Donohoe, Pharm.D., B.C.P.S., C.G.P. Department of Pharmacotherapy and Outcomes Science, Virginia Commonwealth University School of Pharmacy, Richmond, VA, USA

Sarina B. Elmariah, M.D., Ph.D. Cutaneous Biology Research Center, Massachusetts General Hospital, Charlestown, MA, USA

Mieke L.F. Flour, M.D. Department of Dermatology, University Hospitals Leuven, Leuven, Belgium

Kseniya Golubets, M.D., M.H.S. Department of Dermatology, University of Pittsburgh Medical Center, Pittsburgh, PA, USA

Lisa M. Grandinetti, M.D., F.A.A.D. Department of Dermatology, University of Pittsburgh Medical Center, Pittsburgh, PA, USA

Rebat M. Halder, M.D. Department of Dermatology, Howard University College of Medicine, Washington, DC, USA

Jonathan Himmelfarb, M.D. Division of Nephrology, Department of Medicine, University of Washington, Seattle, WA, USA

Kidney Research Institute, Department of Medicine, University of Washington, Seattle, WA, USA

Harborview Medical Center, University of Washington, Seattle, WA, USA

Dan Ilkovitch, M.D., Ph.D. Department of Dermatology, University of Pittsburgh Medical Center, Pittsburgh, PA, USA

Francisco A. Kerdel, B.Sc., M.B.B.S. Florida International University, Coral Gables, FL, USA

Davida A. Kornreich, M.D. Department of Dermatology, Icahn School of Medicine at Mount Sinai, New York, NY, USA

Daniela Kroshinsky, M.D., M.P.H. Massachusetts General Hospital, Harvard Medical School, Boston, MA, USA

Dirk R.J. Kuypers, M.D., Ph.D. Department of Nephrology and Renal Transplantation, University Hospitals Leuven, Leuven, Belgium

Avery LaChance, M.D., M.P.H. Department of Internal Medicine and Dermatology, Brigham and Women's Hospital and Harvard Medical School Teaching Hospitals, Boston, MA, USA

Edgar V. Lerma, M.D. Section of Nephrology, Department of Medicine, University of Illinois at Chicago/Advocate Christ Medical Center, Oak Lawn, IL, USA

Ethan A. Lerner, M.D., Ph.D. Cutaneous Biology Research Center, Department of Dermatology, Massachusetts General Hospital, Charlestown, MA, USA

Jenna Lester, M.D. Department of Dermatology, Warren Alpert Medical School of Brown University, Providence, RI, USA

Ian A. Maher, M.D. Department of Dermatology, Saint Louis University, St. Louis, MO, USA

Calvin O. McCall, M.D. Dermatology Section, VA Medical Center, Richmond, VA, USA
Virginia Commonwealth University, Richmond, VA, USA

Mwatsveruka N. Munhutu, M.D., M.P.H. Department of Dermatology, Howard University Hospital, Washington, DC, USA

Melissa A. Muszynski, M.D. Department of Dermatology, Georgetown University Hospital/Washington Hospital Center, Washington, DC, USA

Ivy I. Norris, B.S. University of Louisville School of Medicine, Louisville, KY, USA

Julia R. Nunley, M.D. Department of Dermatology, Virginia Commonwealth University Medical Center, Richmond, VA, USA

Ali J. Olyaei, Pharm.D. Nephrology and Hypertension, Oregon State University/Oregon Health and Sciences University, Portland, OR, USA

Cindy England Owen, M.S., M.D. Division of Dermatology, University of Louisville, Louisville, KY, USA

Punam H. Patel, Pharm.D., B.C.P.S. Department of Pharmacy, Euclid Hospital, a Cleveland Clinic Hospital, Euclid, OH, USA

Erin L. Reese, M.D. Department of Dermatology, Virginia Commonwealth University, Richmond, VA, USA

Leslie Robinson-Bostom, M.D. Division of Dermatopathology, Department of Dermatology, The Warren Alpert Medical School of Brown University, Providence, RI, USA

James D. Russell, M.D. Department of Dermatology, Virginia Commonwealth University Health System, Richmond, VA, USA

Nicole Sakka, M.D., Ph.D. Department of Dermatology, Sheba Medical Center, Tel-Hashomer, Tel Aviv, Israel

Kimberly Scott Salkey, M.D. Department of Dermatology, Eastern Virginia Medical School, Norfolk, VA, USA

Julio C. Sartori-Valinotti, M.D. Department of Dermatology, Mayo Clinic College of Medicine, Rochester, MN, USA

Avner Shemer, M.D. Department of Dermatology, Sheba Medical Center, Sackler School of Medicine, Tel-Aviv University, Tel Hashomer, Ramat-Gan, Israel

Kara M. Trapp, B.A. Georgetown University School of Medicine, Washington, DC, USA

Caroline Y. Winslow, M.D. Department of Dermatology and Cutaneous Surgery, University of Miami Miller School of Medicine, Miami, FL, USA

Annie M. Wu, B.A. Department of Dermatology, Warren Alpert Medical School of Brown University, Providence, RI, USA

Connie M. Wu, B.S. Department of Dermatology, Warren Alpert Medical School of Brown University, Providence, RI, USA

Genodermatoses

1

Erin L. Reese

Fabry Disease

Introduction

Fabry disease is an X-linked recessive disorder caused by a deficiency in the activity of alpha-galactosidase A, an enzyme responsible for breaking down sphingoglycolipids [1]. Downstream consequences include deposition of neutral glycosphingolipids within lysosomes of various tissues, ultimately leading to end-organ damage [2, 3]. It is a chronic, slowly progressive condition with effects on multiple organ systems; thus patients may present to many different specialists with seemingly unrelated medical concerns [4]. The most commonly reported signs and symptoms include neuropathic pain, cutaneous angiokeratomas, proteinuria, and cardiac complaints [5]. Early recognition of the disease is crucial, as long-term complications can be fatal; the primary causes of mortality include renal failure, heart disease, and stroke [3]. Fortunately, enzyme replacement therapy is available, and prompt initiation of this treatment can halt disease progression [6].

Epidemiology

The disease affects all ethnicities, and the incidence has been estimated between 1 in 40,000 and 1 in 117,000 live male births [5, 6]. Although the inheritance pattern is X-linked recessive, female carriers also manifest disease characteristics. Thus, it is thought that estimates of incidence are low, as they do not account for affected females [5–7].

E.L. Reese, M.D. (✉)
Department of Dermatology, Virginia Commonwealth University, 401 N. 11th Street Suite 520, Richmond, VA 23298, USA
e-mail: ereese@mcvh-vcu.edu

Genetics

Fabry disease results from mutations in the gene GLA encoding the lysosomal enzyme alpha-galactosidase A, and this gene is found on the long arm of chromosome X [7]. Hundreds of mutations have been described, with the majority being missense mutations leading to substitutions of single amino acids [7]. These mutations ultimately result in a decrease or absence in the enzymatic activity of alpha-galactosidase A, which in turn causes faulty degradation of neutral glycosphingolipids, namely globotriaosylceramide (GL-3) and digalactosylceramide [2, 7]. Over time, accumulation of these compounds progresses through three phases: cellular GL-3 deposition that begins before birth, followed by tissue changes stimulated by these deposits, and finally end-organ failure and early death [4].

Attempts to correlate genotype and phenotype have not been consistent [7]. Men are generally more severely affected, given that every cell in their body containing lysosomes is affected [4]. Women, however, can have widely varying clinical phenotypes, with some being asymptomatic and others being affected to the same degree as men. The Lyon hypothesis has been called upon to explain this phenomenon. This is a physiological process wherein random inactivation of X chromosomes occurs during fetal development. The early cell lines affected by this will proliferate and carry this inactivation forward, leading to varied expression of affected X chromosomes in different tissues [5].

Most mutations in GLA are inherited, rather than spontaneous; therefore, most patients will have affected male or carrier female family members [7]. Affected males can be identified fairly easily by measurement of alpha-galactosidase activity. On the other hand, carrier females may have normal enzyme activity levels and limited clinical manifestations. In addition, if the familial mutation is not known, screening for one of the several hundred described mutations can be quite cumbersome [7].

Patients may have variable levels of enzyme activity, which can impact the degree of clinical severity. However, a fairly low level of activity (above 10 %) is generally sufficient to prevent clinical disease [7].

J.R. Nunley and E.V. Lerma (eds.), *Dermatological Manifestations of Kidney Disease*,
DOI 10.1007/978-1-4939-2395-3_1, © Springer Science+Business Media New York 2015

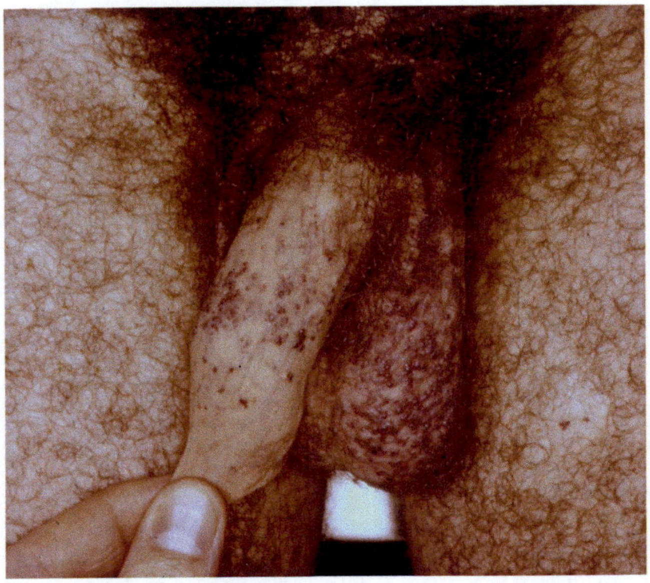

Fig. 1.1 Angiokeratomas associated with Fabry disease. Note the multiple, discrete, nonblanching, vascular papules on the penile shaft and scrotum. The differential diagnosis would also include angiokeratomas of Fordyce, which are common growths in the genital area in elderly patients and have no systemic associations. Photo courtesy of Dirk Elston, M.D.

Cutaneous Findings

Angiokeratoma corporis diffusum is the hallmark skin manifestation of Fabry disease and comprises nonblanching red to black discrete vascular papules that range in size from 1 to 10 mm and occur preferentially in a bathing trunk distribution, becoming more generalized and even involving mucosa over time [8, 9] (see Fig. 1.1). Despite their name, they are rarely hyperkeratotic [10]. Hundreds of lesions may occur. They are present in roughly 2/3 of male patients and 1/3 of female patients, and they tend to become apparent in adolescence [3]. They are thought to be caused by deposition of neutral glycosphingolipids within the endothelium of cutaneous vessels, which weakens vascular walls [9].

Angiokeratoma corporis diffusum can occur in the setting of other lysosomal storage diseases (fucosidosis, sialidosis, etc.) and sometimes in the absence of other enzymatic abnormalities, thus is not pathognomonic for Fabry disease [8, 9]. In addition, there are other variants of angiokeratoma without the systemic associations seen in Fabry patients. These include solitary angiokeratoma, angiokeratoma of Fordyce occurring in older patients on the genitals, angiokeratoma of Mibelli seen in adolescent women on the dorsal hands and feet, and angiokeratoma circumscriptum naeviformis presenting as a unilateral plaque on the trunk or extremities with a segmental distribution [8]. Isolated, solitary angiokeratomas may be misdiagnosed as cherry angiomas, warts, pyogenic granulomas, or Spitz nevi [9]. Thus skin biopsy can be important in cementing the diagnosis.

Routine histopathologic examination of an angiokeratoma fixed in formalin and stained with hematoxylin and eosin reveals a dilated, thin-walled vascular proliferation (sometimes filled with red blood cells) of the papillary dermis that is enveloped by an acanthotic epidermis with overlying hyperkeratosis of the stratum corneum [3, 8]. A standard skin biopsy will not differentiate angiokeratomas associated with Fabry from angiokeratomas of other etiologies, as the endothelial lipid inclusions characteristic of Fabry disease are destroyed with tissue processing [8]. However, electron microscopic examination of an angiokeratoma in a Fabry patient will demonstrate diagnostic "zebra bodies," which are vacuolar, electron-dense inclusions within the cytoplasm that have a lamellated appearance [3, 8].

While angiokeratomas are the most often encountered cutaneous vascular lesion in Fabry patients, telangiectasias and cherry angiomas have been reported to occur as well [11–14]. Because these lesions are quite common and can occur as multiple lesions in the general population, it is not recommended that patients presenting with these be screened for Fabry disease. However, if there is a family history of Fabry disease or personal history of other associated Fabry symptoms, further evaluation may be indicated [11, 12].

Other skin manifestations can include abnormalities of sweating, lymphedema, and characteristic facies. Hypohidrosis is reported by patients more commonly than anhidrosis or hyperhidrosis, but all have been documented to occur [3]. This is likely due to GL-3 accumulation in sweat glands [1]. In addition, the same lipid deposition that occurs in vascular endothelium has been proposed to occur in lymphatic vessels, which is thought to contribute to the development of lymphedema, seen in up to 25 % of men with Fabry disease [3, 15]. Fabry facies are seen more often in affected males, but the features can be seen to a lesser degree in females. These features include "recessed forehead, bushy eyebrows, prominent supraorbital ridges, widened nasal bridge, bulbous nasal tip, shallow midface, full lips, coarse features, posteriorly rotated ears, and prognathism" [8].

Renal Manifestations

Fabry nephropathy is caused by glomerular and renal vascular deposition of neutral glycosphingolipids, which have been demonstrated as early as in utero [16]. Thus timely diagnosis and treatment is crucial in preventing progressive decline in renal function, which can culminate in need for dialysis or kidney transplantation [4]. In fact, it is recommended that those with chronic kidney disease (men younger than age 50, women of any age) of unknown etiology be screened for Fabry disease [17], as this diagnosis may be causative in up to 0.2 % of all dialysis patients [4]. In patients with known Fabry disease, serial monitoring for albuminuria and decline in glomerular filtration rate should begin in adolescence [17]. Studies have demonstrated that enzyme replacement therapy does not appear to be effective at halting disease progression in patients with proteinuria >1 g/day or estimated glomerular filtration rate (eGFR) <60 mL/min/1.73 m^2 [17]. Therefore, initiation of enzyme replacement therapy is most beneficial in those who have not yet reached these thresholds. Chronic kidney disease stage 5 usually develops on average in patients after age 30 years, but it has been reported in a patient as young as age 16 years [17].

In patients with rapidly declining renal function, renal ultrasound should be performed to rule out other possible causes, such as renal cysts [4].

Renal biopsy can be undertaken in those with known Fabry disease and in whom it is unclear whether enzyme replacement therapy should be started. If electron microscopic examination reveals GL-3 within podocytes and vascular endothelial cells, enzyme replacement therapy may be indicated [4].

A less invasive test to assess for Fabry disease of the kidney is urine microscopy. When viewing urine sediment via polarized microscope, autofluorescent, birefringent Maltese cross lipid particles can be seen. Different morphologies of Maltese cross particles have been defined, with those having a lamellated appearance with surface protrusions being most sensitive and specific for Fabry disease [18].

Cardiovascular Manifestations

Glycosphingolipids also accumulate in various cardiac tissues, leading to dysfunction. Myocytes, valves, conduction tissue, and vascular endothelium may all be affected, and the resulting presenting symptoms include dyspnea, syncope, palpitations, or angina [19]. Over time, patients can go on to develop left ventricular hypertrophy, cardiomyopathy, dysrhythmia, ischemia, and/or valvular insufficiency [19, 20].

The cardiomyopathy of Fabry disease is classified as restrictive, due to infiltration of glycosphingolipids within the cardiac myocytes [19]. However, Fabry disease represents an unusual subset of restrictive cardiomyopathy, as there is often lack of significant left ventricular filling defects with presence of left ventricular hypertrophy (with patients meeting high voltage criteria for left ventricular hypertrophy via electrocardiogram) [21]. It was initially hypothesized that the enlargement of the ventricle was simply due to the volume of lipid deposition within the lysosomes, but it was later shown that this only accounted for 1 % of the increased left ventricular mass [21]. It is now thought that there is an increase in left ventricular muscle mass that accounts for the hypertrophy, although the etiology of this is unclear [21]. The presence of left ventricular hypertrophy can be demonstrated via echocardiography, electrocardiography, and cardiac magnetic resonance imaging [21].

Dysrhythmias occur as a result of glycosphingolipid deposition within the conduction system or by atrial dilatation and ischemia due to left ventricular hypertrophy [19, 21]. While atrial fibrillation is most commonly reported, supraventricular tachycardia, various degrees of heart block, premature ventricular beats, and nonsustained ventricular tachycardia have also been shown to occur [19, 21].

Over half of Fabry patients complain of anginal chest pain, with glycosphingolipid deposition within cardiac endothelial cells playing a role in vascular dysfunction and ultimately in myocardial injury [21]. However, the exact mechanism is unclear. Vasospasm or perhaps decreased coronary perfusion due to left ventricular hypertrophy may be causative [21]. Atherosclerotic plaques causing stenosis do occur in Fabry patients, but cardiac catheterization has not been performed routinely and thus the true incidence of this is unclear [21].

Valvular insufficiency most often manifests as mitral valve regurgitation, but patients do not generally require valve replacement [19].

Neurologic Manifestations

The peripheral, central, and autonomic nervous systems may all be affected in Fabry disease.

Fabry pain crises, occurring as attacks of neuropathic pain, may be the first manifestation of the condition. They can begin in early childhood with episodes of severe, burning pain in the distal extremities, brought on by stress, infections, or changes in temperature and lasting minutes to days [4, 22]. Deposition of GL-3 within the small vessels of the peripheral nerves leads to vascular spasm and infarction that culminates in a small-fiber peripheral neuropathy [22]. Quantitative sensory testing can be done to evaluate this and often demonstrates abnormalities in thermal sensation [23]. Punch biopsy of the skin stained for nerve fibers can also reveal a decrease in density of these fibers [24]. Involvement of large fibers (indicated by loss of vibration and pinprick sensation) generally occurs only in those with renal disease [4, 23].

Cerebrovascular disease, caused by glycosphingolipid deposition within cerebral vessels, is a common cause of morbidity and mortality in patients with Fabry disease [4, 25]. Transient ischemic attacks and ischemic strokes (preferentially affecting the vertebrobasilar territory) can occur in both men and women and often at a young age [4, 7, 25]. Half of male patients experience their first stroke before the diagnosis of Fabry disease is rendered, and it has been estimated that up to 5 % of males and 2.5 % of females with stroke of unknown cause may carry a diagnosis of Fabry disease [3, 4]. In addition to vascular disease, patients may also demonstrate white matter lesions and cortical atrophy with magnetic resonance imaging [4, 25].

Involvement of the autonomic nervous system manifests as abnormalities of sweating and gastrointestinal complaints [4].

Ophthalmologic Manifestations

Cornea verticillata, bilateral, whorl-shaped corneal opacities diagnosed by slit-lamp examination, is the characteristic eye finding in patients with Fabry disease and can be seen in nearly all patients by age 10 [25]. This clinical finding is caused by deposition of GL-3 in the limbal blood vessels of the epithelial basement membrane and does not affect vision [25]. On examination, there are yellowish lines emanating outward from the central cornea in pattern resembling a vortex. Medications and other lipid storage diseases can also cause cornea verticillata, but in Fabry disease, the deposits are lighter colored and more superficial [4, 25]. Lens opacities and tortuosity of the conjunctival vessels have also been described [25].

Other Organ Involvement

Other symptoms reported in Fabry patients are diverse and can include:

- Gastrointestinal disturbances: Nausea, vomiting, diarrhea, abdominal pain [22, 25]
- Tinnitus, hearing loss, vertigo [22]
- Obstructive and restrictive pulmonary disease: Dyspnea, cough, wheezing [17]
- Psychiatric disorders: Depression, substance abuse, suicide [22, 25]
- Sexual dysfunction: Delayed puberty, impotence, priapism, infertility [25]

Diagnosis

Signs and symptoms that suggest the diagnosis of Fabry disease are as follows: attacks of pain in distal extremities triggered by physiological or psychological stress, cutaneous angiokeratomas, proteinuria or renal failure of unknown cause, left ventricular hypertrophy, stroke, characteristic corneal opacities, and unexplained gastrointestinal complaints [7, 22].

In affected males, the diagnosis can be confirmed by measuring alpha-galactosidase A activity in plasma or peripheral leukocytes [6, 22]. Males with classic Fabry disease will have less than 1 % enzyme activity, while those with atypical forms may have higher levels of enzyme activity [22]. Some experts then suggest that GLA gene sequencing analysis be performed subsequently to identify the specific causative mutation [17]. Most families with Fabry disease have family-specific mutations, and over 300 of these have been described [6].

Female carriers have variable levels of alpha-galactosidase activity (may be normal or very low), so this test is not reliable in diagnosing women. Suspected female carriers must undergo molecular testing to confirm the diagnosis [6, 17, 22].

Other diagnostic tests can include detection of accumulating glycosphingolipids. Urinary GL-3 levels and plasma deacetylated GL-3 levels may be elevated in affected patients. In addition, analysis of urinary sediment via polarized microscopy may reveal Maltese crosses [17].

Disease Course and Prognosis

Fabry disease is chronic and slowly progressive, with premature death resulting from renal failure, heart disease, or stroke. This generally occurs at around age 50 for classically affected males, whose life span is reduced by 20–25 years compared to the general population [25]. Carrier females also experience a reduced life expectancy, with average age of death at around 70 years [3, 25].

Monitoring

The clinical effects of GL-3 accumulation are far-reaching; thus multiple disciplines are likely to be involved in the care of a patient with Fabry disease. Once a diagnosis has been established, patients should undergo complete history (including family history) and physical examination. Patients should be asked about pain and gastrointestinal symptoms, and these should be documented for longitudinal follow-up. Examination for cutaneous vascular lesions (which may occur underneath undergarments) should be done [6, 26]. Recommended laboratory evaluation can include hematology, chemistries, urinalysis, and 24 h urine collection for protein [6]. In addition, obtaining a baseline echocardiogram and electrocardiogram is advised [4, 26]. To assess for white matter lesions, a cerebral magnetic resonance imaging study may be indicated [4]. Consider referral to ophthalmology for slit-lamp examination and referral for audiologic testing as well [7].

Follow-up should occur at least annually, with many of the above tests being repeated each year [6]. However, some have recommended more frequent monitoring [17]. It is important to keep in mind that end-organ damage may occur in the absence of clinical symptoms, and the studies mentioned may help identify an early need to intervene with therapy.

Treatment

Prior to the advent of enzyme replacement therapy, treatment for Fabry disease focused primarily on supportive and symptomatic care based on the patient's complaints [6, 27]. These adjunctive therapies are still important in managing patients with Fabry disease. Pain should be controlled, although narcotics should be avoided and nonsteroidal anti-inflammatory drugs are generally ineffective [6]. Monitoring for and treatment of cardiac comorbidities such as hypertension, dysrhythmias, and hyperlipidemia should be undertaken. Providers should also consider use of antiplatelet therapy, particularly in patients with transient ischemic attacks or stroke [4, 6]. In patients with proteinuria, use of angiotensin-converting enzyme inhibitors or angiotensin receptor blockers is recommended [4, 6]. In advanced renal disease, dialysis or kidney transplantation can prolong life [6]. Given the large number of lesions, angiokeratomas are treated only when symptomatic. Different treatment modalities reported to be effective include excision, cryosurgery, and laser therapy [1].

Enzyme replacement therapy for Fabry disease in the form of recombinant alpha-galactosidase A is available in two forms. Agalsidase-alpha is produced from human fibroblasts, while agalsidase-beta is produced from Chinese hamster ovarian cells [22]. Only the latter is Food and Drug Administration (FDA) approved for use in the United States, although both forms have been approved for use outside of the United States [7]. Agalsidase-alpha is administered via intravenous infusion every 2 weeks at a dose of 0.2 mg/kg. Agalsidase-beta is also administered via intravenous infusion every 2 weeks, but the dose is higher at 1.0 mg/kg [26]. Average annual cost of enzyme replacement therapy for an adult was estimated at $250,000 in 2007 [7].

Patients generally tolerate enzyme replacement therapy well, with only a small minority of patients experiencing infusion reactions. These adverse reactions can usually be managed by premedicating patients with antihistamines or nonsteroidal anti-inflammatory drugs. Sometimes, decreasing the infusion rate is helpful. For more severe reactions, systemic corticosteroids may be needed. The reactions tend to be less severe over time [6].

Enzyme replacement therapy has been shown to decrease plasma and renal capillary endothelial levels of GL-3, with studies showing stabilization of renal function. However, some have suggested that those with advanced end-stage renal disease may not demonstrate these benefits [7]. Enzyme replacement therapy has also been demonstrated to clear glycosphingolipids from cardiac tissue, thus improving left ventricular hypertrophy and overall cardiac function [4]. Of note, cardiac disease has been reported to occur in patients actively on enzyme replacement therapy, and the effect of enzyme replacement therapy on survival has not been proven [22]. Studies have also not been able to show clearly that enzyme replacement therapy has a positive impact on cerebrovascular complications of Fabry disease [7]. Enzyme replacement therapy has been shown to improve neuropathic pain and autonomic dysfunction, but patients may require additional pain management depending on their symptoms [4, 7]. Enzyme replacement therapy has also been demonstrated to improve quality of life, improve peripheral nerve function, improve hearing and vestibular function, and relieve gastrointestinal complaints.

It is recommended that enzyme replacement therapy commence as soon as possible after a diagnosis of Fabry disease is rendered. Symptomatic carriers should also be strongly considered for enzyme replacement therapy [22].

Genetic Counseling

Fabry disease is inherited in an X-linked recessive fashion. An affected father will not pass on the mutation to his sons, as they inherit his Y chromosome, which does not contain the mutation. An affected father will pass on his faulty X chromosome to his daughters, making them carriers of Fabry disease. In the offspring of a carrier mother (who has one normal X chromosome and one affected X chromosome), 50 % of females will inherit the mutation (making them carriers as well) and 50 % of males will inherit the mutation (giving them Fabry disease) [25]. Specific recommendations for testing are shown under the diagnosis heading.

Tuberous Sclerosis

Introduction

Tuberous sclerosis is an autosomal dominant disorder caused by inactivating mutations of either of the tumor suppressor genes, TSC-1 or TSC-2, encoding for hamartin and tuberin respectively [28]. Downstream effects include activation of the mammalian target of rapamycin (mTOR) pathway with subsequent disordered cellular proliferation and differentiation, producing hamartomatous lesions in multiple organ systems including brain, skin, lungs, kidneys, heart, retina, and liver [28, 29]. The triad of seizures, mental retardation, and facial angiofibromas described by Vogt in 1908 are only present in about 30 % of patients. As reflected in this diagnostic triad, neurological and dermatological findings are the most common disease manifestations experienced by tuberous sclerosis patients, occurring in up to 90 % [28, 30]. Neurologic manifestations, namely seizures, are the leading cause of morbidity and mortality in patients with tuberous sclerosis [29]. Causes of death in affected patients vary by age, with status epilepticus and brain tumors being most common in younger patients and renal failure predominating in older patients [31]. Thus, early recognition and intervention is crucial, with both medical and surgical management playing a role. In the past several years, pharmacotherapy for tuberous sclerosis in the form of mTOR inhibitors has shown promise at causing regression of the hamartomatous lesions [32].

Epidemiology

The disease affects all ethnicities and both genders [31], and the incidence has been estimated at 1 in 6,000 live births [28]. Population-based studies have estimated an overall prevalence of 1 in 14,000 to 1 in 25,000. As most patients are diagnosed before age 15 months, prevalence decreases with age [33]. Of note, these numbers may represent underestimates of the prevalence because they do not account for undiagnosed cases in patients who have only mild disease or are asymptomatic [29].

Genetics

Tuberous sclerosis results from inactivating mutations in either the TSC-1 or TSC-2 tumor suppressor genes encoding for proteins hamartin and tuberin respectively. Although tuberous sclerosis is autosomal dominantly inherited, up to 2/3 of patients have sporadic mutations [30]. Mutations in TSC-1 are more commonly reported (15–30 % of affected families) whereas mutations in TSC-2 are slightly less common (10–20 % of affected families) [30]. Over 1,200 allelic variants have been discovered in both the TSC-1 and TSC-2 genes, accounting for the widely varying phenotypes [29]. However, it is important to note that even family members with the same genetic mutation may have differing degrees of clinical manifestations. While attempts to correlate genotype and phenotype have not been consistent, studies have demonstrated that patients with the TSC-2 mutation have more severe disease [30].

The molecular pathway affected by tuberous sclerosis gene mutations has been elucidated. In unaffected patients, hamartin and tuberin form an intracellular heterodimer that, through cell signaling pathways, ultimately inhibits the protein kinase mTOR, a regulator of cellular proliferation, differentiation, and growth [28, 29]. In patients with TSC mutations, there is constitutive activation of mTOR leading to abnormalities in cell cycle progression, cellular metabolism, gene transcription, and protein translation [28, 33]. The resulting effect is the overgrowth of widespread benign tumors called hamartomas in multiple organ systems.

Mucocutaneous Findings

Characteristic skin findings comprise a number of the diagnostic criteria for tuberous sclerosis, so a complete cutaneous examination is important in establishing the diagnosis. Clinicians should be aware that patients present with differing skin manifestations based on their age, so serial follow-up over time is also essential.

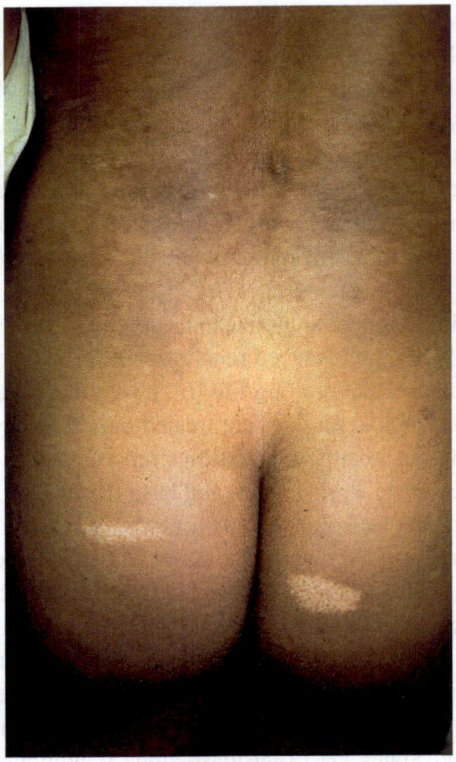

Fig. 1.2 Ash leaf macules associated with tuberous sclerosis. These hypopigmented macules and patches are often the first cutaneous manifestation of tuberous sclerosis. There are also confetti-like macules on the lower trunk. Photo courtesy of Dirk Elston, M.D.

The earliest skin finding in tuberous sclerosis patients is the ash leaf spot, an ovoid, hypopigmented macule or patch measuring 1.0–12 cm in diameter [29] (see Fig. 1.2). Ash leaf spots are one of the most common cutaneous manifestations of tuberous sclerosis, occurring in over 90 % of patients [29]. Some have described the shape of the lesion as having a sharper tip at one pole and a rounded tip at the other, while others have likened it to a thumbprint shape [29]. The lesions are generally present at birth, although they may be difficult to appreciate without the use of a Wood lamp that accentuates the pigment change. The ash leaf spots become more apparent with age and are usually obvious by age 2 [34]. At least three hypomelanotic macules must be present as part of the major diagnostic criteria for tuberous sclerosis [35]. Hypomelanotic lesions are common in the general population, with 5 % having one lesion, 1 % having two lesions, and 0.1 % having three lesions [29]. The differential diagnosis for ash leaf spots includes vitiligo, which is classically depigmented rather than hypopigmented; nevus depigmentosus, which occurs in the absence of other systemic findings; and nevus anemicus, a vascular anomaly wherein a localized hyperreactivity to catecholamines causes vasoconstriction that can be confused for hypopigmentation.

Confetti-like hypopigmented macules also occur in patients with tuberous sclerosis, with the onset being later in

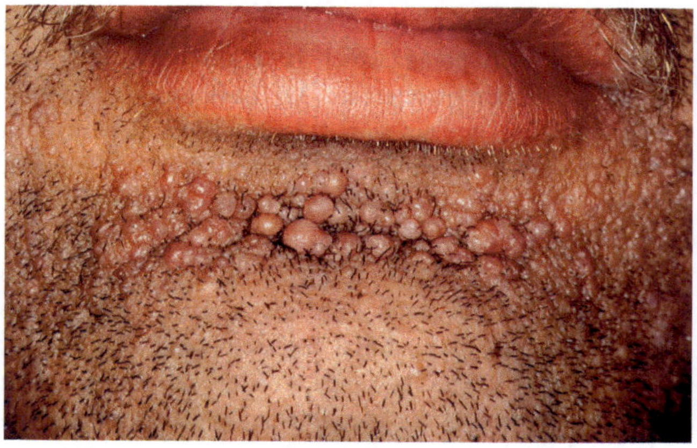

Fig. 1.3 Angiofibromas associated with tuberous sclerosis. The multiple, smooth, pink papules of the mental crease are characteristic of the condition. Photo courtesy of Dirk Elston, M.D.

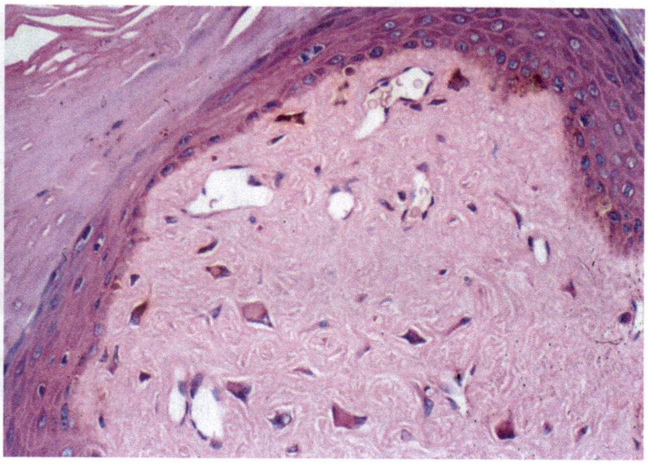

Fig. 1.4 Angiofibroma histopathology. There are stellate fibroblasts within the fibrotic dermis, which also demonstrates increased vasculature. Photo courtesy of Dirk Elston, M.D.

life [29]. They have been reported less commonly than ash leaf spots, with studies reporting presence in 3–30 % of patients [29]. These lesions are smaller than ash leaf spots, occur symmetrically over extremities, and are numerous [29]. They are one of the minor diagnostic criteria for tuberous sclerosis [35]. The confetti-like hypopigmentation may clinically mimic idiopathic guttate hypomelanosis, a benign dermatosis which is seen in middle-aged patients and has no associated systemic features [29].

Facial angiofibromas (previously labeled inaccurately as adenoma sebaceum) were a part of the initial diagnostic triad described by Vogt and remain a part of the major diagnostic criteria for tuberous sclerosis [35]. They typically appear in childhood but not before age 3 [36]. They become more prominent with puberty and can be mistaken for acne vulgaris. However, acne lesions also include comedones and pustules, which are not associated with tuberous sclerosis. Angiofibromas are skin colored to erythematous smooth papules that measure a few millimeters in diameter and occur in multiple over the central face, particularly within the nasolabial folds and sparing the central upper cutaneous lip [29]. They may be found in over 70 % of patients with tuberous sclerosis [34] (see Fig. 1.3). As the name suggests, histopathology demonstrates a fibrotic dermis containing large and stellate fibroblasts with prominent, dilated capillaries [29] (see Fig. 1.4). Facial angiofibromas are not pathognomonic for tuberous sclerosis and can be seen as an isolated finding in the general population [35]. In addition, most patients with multiple endocrine neoplasia type I will also have facial angiofibromas. Multiple facial angiofibromas can also resemble the facial adnexal neoplasms seen in other genodermatoses, such as the tricholemmomas of Cowden disease, the fibrofolliculomas and trichodiscomas of Birt-Hogg-Dubé (BHD) disease, and the cylindromas of Brooke-Spiegler disease. These lesions can be differentiated by their histopathology.

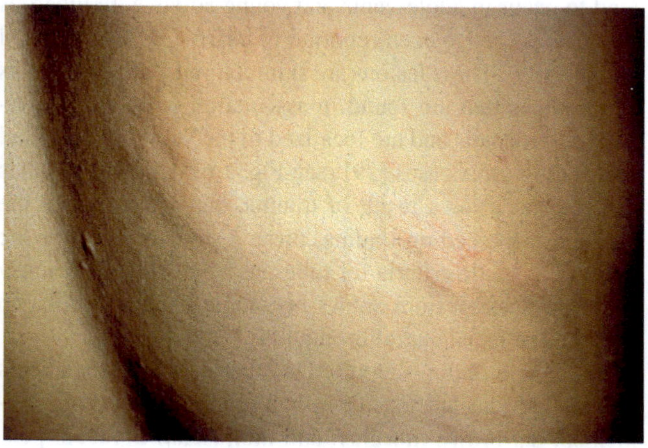

Fig. 1.5 Shagreen patch associated with tuberous sclerosis. This ill-defined, subtle, skin colored to pink plaque on the trunk has a slightly cobblestoned surface. Photo courtesy of Dirk Elston, M.D.

A forehead plaque, which is a type of angiofibroma, is present in roughly 20 % of tuberous sclerosis patients and appears in childhood, enlarging over time [34]. They are indurated, elevated plaques measuring a few centimeters in diameter that are skin colored to slightly yellow in color. It shares histologic features with facial angiofibromas [29].

Shagreen patches are connective tissue hamartomas that appear in over 30 % of young children with tuberous sclerosis [34]. The lumbosacral area is the most common site of involvement for these benign tumors, which are described as skin colored to slightly brown in color, irregularly shaped raised plaques with ill-defined borders and a cobblestoned surface [34] (see Fig. 1.5). The shagreen patch comprises one of the major diagnostic criteria for tuberous sclerosis [35]. Biopsy of this connective tissue nevus often shows dense bands of collagen with accompanying increases in

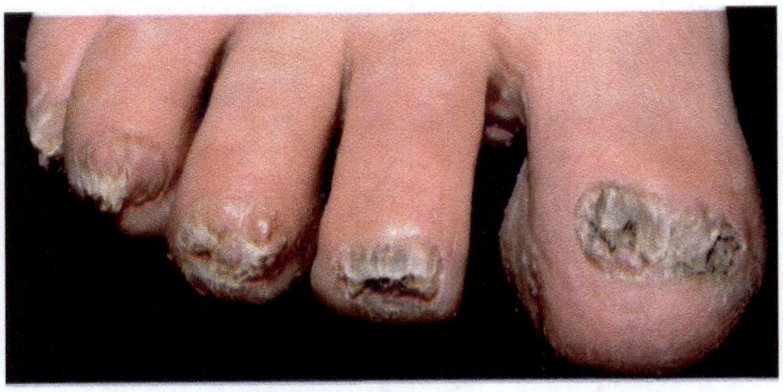

Fig. 1.6 Ungual fibromas associated with tuberous sclerosis. This patient has multiple skin colored to pink smooth nodules surrounding the nail plate with associated nail dystrophy. Photo courtesy of Dirk Elston, M.D.

connective tissue elements such as vasculature, elastic tissue, adipose tissue, and smooth muscle [29].

Fibromas of the nail unit, also known as Koenen tumors, tend to occur in adolescents and young adults with tuberous sclerosis and have been reported in nearly 70 % of affected patients [29]. These lesions are skin-colored, smooth papules and nodules that are found in association with both fingernails and toenails and are localized to the lateral or proximal nail fold in most cases [29] (see Fig. 1.6). Ungual fibromas can also occur as a result of trauma, but when seen in the absence of preceding trauma, these lesions are part of the major diagnostic criteria for tuberous sclerosis [35]. Biopsy of one of these lesions shows histologic features similar to those of the facial angiofibroma [29].

Other skin findings reported in tuberous sclerosis patients include café au lait macules (well-marginated, evenly pigmented, tan-brown macules) and molluscum fibrosum pendulum (fleshy, pedunculated papules resembling skin tags), which are quite common in the general population. Their significance in tuberous sclerosis is unclear, and these clinical findings are not included in the diagnostic criteria for tuberous sclerosis [29].

Oral examination is important in patients with suspected tuberous sclerosis, as dental enamel pitting and gingival fibromas comprise two of the minor diagnostic criteria for the condition [35]. Dental enamel pitting has been described in 50–100 % of patients with tuberous sclerosis, usually apparent at the labial surfaces of the canine and incisor teeth [29]. Gingival fibromas are most often seen on the anterior segment of the upper jaw but have been described elsewhere in the mucosa [29].

Renal Manifestations

Just as hamartomas form in the skin as a result of hyperactivation of the mTOR pathway, renal hamartomas also occur in patients with tuberous sclerosis.

The most commonly encountered renal tumor is the benign angiomyolipoma, which is seen in up to 80 % of patients with tuberous sclerosis [32]. Lesions are often multiple and bilateral and are seen up to four times more often in female patients [34]. Renal involvement begins in infancy, with size and number of lesions increasing with age [34]. Lesions are usually asymptomatic, but they may cause abdominal pain, nausea, vomiting, hematuria, and palpable masses [31]. As the name suggests, angiomyolipomas are tumors composed of abnormal vasculature, smooth muscle, and fatty tissue [30]. While they are considered benign, the most serious and common complication is spontaneous hemorrhage of the abnormal vessels (often aneurysms) contained within [32]. The risk of hemorrhage in tuberous sclerosis patients is estimated at 25–50 % (with up to 20 % of these patients presenting with hypovolemic shock), with lesions greater than 5 cm in diameter having the highest risk [28]. Surgical resection is discouraged in order to preserve renal function, and lesions are preferably treated with embolization [32]. With growth, these lesions may also encroach upon normal renal tissue, leading to dysfunction and potentially to renal failure [28]. It is important to note that these lesions can occur independently of tuberous sclerosis, as only 20 % of patients with angiomyolipomas have tuberous sclerosis [31]. However, angiomyolipomas do comprise one of the major diagnostic criteria for tuberous sclerosis [35].

Renal cysts are the second most common kidney manifestation of tuberous sclerosis, occurring in about 50 % of patients [28]. These lesions are generally asymptomatic but can lead to development of hypertension [28]. When symptomatic, lesions are usually larger than 4 cm in diameter and can cause flank pain and hematuria [34]. In 2–3 % of patients with tuberous sclerosis, their gene mutation may involve contiguous deletions in TSC-2 and the adjacent gene for polycystic kidney disease, PKD-1 [30]. These patients develop multiple, large cysts with onset of renal failure in early adulthood [30]. The presence of multiple renal cysts is one of the minor diagnostic criteria for tuberous sclerosis [35].

Renal cell carcinoma has also been reported in patients with tuberous sclerosis, but notably the overall incidence of 2–3 % is similar to that of the general population [32]. Patients with tuberous sclerosis tend to develop malignancy at an earlier age, with some studies showing an average age at diagnosis of 28 years (25 years younger than in the general population) [28]. Varied subtypes of renal cell carcinoma have been demonstrated, including clear cell, papillary, and chromophobe [31]. Benign oncocytomas have also been reported [37]. It is important to note that the true incidence of renal cell carcinoma in tuberous sclerosis may be incorrect because some cases of angiomyolipomas (particularly the epithelioid variant) may be misdiagnosed as renal cell carcinoma [37]. Immunohistochemistry can be helpful in making this distinction.

Neurologic Manifestations

As noted by Vogt in his descriptive triad of tuberous sclerosis, two of the three findings (seizures and mental retardation) result from neurologic involvement of characteristic hamartomatous lesions. However, the degree to which patients manifest these two findings is highly variable, with some having no seizures and normal intellect and others having severe, intractable seizures with profound mental retardation [34]. It has also been recognized that patients with tuberous sclerosis have impairments in cognition and behavior, with 25 % carrying a diagnosis of autism [37]. The four common central nervous system manifestations include cortical tubers, subependymal nodules, subependymal giant cell astrocytomas, and white matter abnormalities [31], with the first three lesions each accounting for major diagnostic criteria and the last accounting for a minor diagnostic criterion for tuberous sclerosis [35].

Cortical tubers are the hallmark lesion of tuberous sclerosis [37] and are thought to be responsible for causing many of the neurologic symptoms in affected patients [31]. Tubers are histologically comprised of disorganization of the six-layered structure of the cerebral cortex with proliferation of both glial and neuronal cells [30, 38]. They have been identified in patients as young as 20 weeks gestational age [32], and they are usually diagnosed by magnetic resonance imaging [38]. Cortical tubers vary in size, number, and anatomic location, and these factors likely account for the variation in clinical manifestations [38]. Foci of seizure activity map to areas where tubers are present [38], and patients with numerous (>7) tubers tend to have seizures that are more difficult to control [32]. Improvement in seizure activity with resection of the tubers has been well documented [38]. Tubers in the frontal and parietotemporal regions have been associated with autism [31]. These lesions remain present throughout life, although malignant transformation has not been reported [38].

Subependymal nodules are benign hamartomas that grow on the surface of the cerebral ventricles [38]. They are present in utero and may enlarge or calcify over time, but in most patients they are asymptomatic [30]. Subependymal nodules that are larger than 5 mm and are located near the foramen of Munro are at risk for transforming into subependymal giant cell astrocytomas (which also have benign biological features [31]), and this process occurs slowly over time [30]. The tumors pose a risk when they enlarge to sufficient size to impede the flow of cerebrospinal fluid through the foramen of Munro, leading to increased intracranial pressure [30, 38].

White matter abnormalities include radial white matter bands (this particular finding is considered a minor diagnostic criterion for tuberous sclerosis), cyst-like white matter lesions, and superficial white matter abnormalities seen with cortical tubers [31]. These can be diagnosed radiologically [31].

The most common neurological symptom in affected patients is epilepsy, which has been reported in up to 90 % of patients [38]. In addition, seizures are the leading cause of morbidity and poor quality of life in patients with tuberous sclerosis [34, 37]. The types of seizures reported include complex partial, generalized tonic-clonic, myoclonic, and infantile spasms [38]. Over time, the epilepsy progressively worsens and becomes more resistant to medical therapy; developmental delay is strongly associated with poor control of seizure activity [38]. Therefore, aggressive control of seizures either medically or surgically is recommended [37]. Specific therapies are discussed later. A majority of patients have their first epileptic event in the first 2 years of life [29], presenting with either infantile spasms or partial seizures that may progress to generalized seizures [37].

In patients with autism spectrum disorder, tuberous sclerosis is present in 1–4 %. The prevalence is equal in males and females, unlike in the general population where males outnumber females. The risk of developing autism is higher in patients with a TSC-2 mutation and in those who have early-onset infantile spasms that are refractory to therapy [38].

Cardiac Manifestations

Cardiac rhabdomyomas are intracavitary or intramural [32] benign striated muscle tumors [31] seen in 50–60 % of patients with tuberous sclerosis [29]. They are the most common primary cardiac tumor in children, and it has been reported that nearly 95 % of patients with these tumors will go on to be diagnosed with tuberous sclerosis [29]. Cardiac involvement may be the presenting sign of tuberous sclerosis, as rhabdomyomas may be diagnosed in utero [28]. In patients with tuberous sclerosis, they are often found in multiple and are usually asymptomatic [31]. When they do cause symptoms, the most common are cardiac outflow obstruction, valvular dysfunction, and dysrhythmias [34]. Over time, these growths tend to shrink in size, with only a few reports of growth around puberty [29]. Surgical removal is indicated only in those with life-threatening hemodynamic compromise. Cardiac rhabdomyomas, as single or multiple, are one of the major diagnostic criteria for tuberous sclerosis [35].

Pulmonary Manifestations

Clinically apparent lung involvement is uncommon in those with tuberous sclerosis, occurring in 1–5 % of patients [29, 31]. However, radiologic evidence of involvement may be seen in up to 50 % of women with tuberous sclerosis [31, 37]. Lymphangioleiomyomatosis is characterized by proliferation of smooth muscle cells in the lung with subsequent cystic changes of the parenchyma and is the most common pulmonary manifestation in tuberous sclerosis [37]. It is seen nearly exclusively in female patients and is usually diagnosed in women of child-bearing age [37]. Many patients are asymptomatic, but the most common symptoms in those affected are dyspnea on exertion and recurrent pneumothorax [31, 37]. Worsening of symptoms has been reported with pregnancy and use of estrogen supplements [29]. These lesions often become generalized and progressive and may lead to respiratory failure; the 10-year survival rate has been reported at nearly 80 % [30, 31]. Lymphangioleiomyomatosis has been cited as the third leading cause of death in tuberous sclerosis patients, after renal and neurologic lesions [32]. These lesions are counted as a major diagnostic criterion for tuberous sclerosis, but it should be noted that if the only two major diagnostic criteria are lymphangioleiomyomatosis and renal angiomyolipoma, patients should have other features of tuberous sclerosis in order to render a definitive diagnosis [35].

Ophthalmologic Manifestations

Retinal hamartomas are present in nearly half of affected patients [30]. They may be present at any age, but the incidence tends to increase with age [29, 30]. These hamartomas may be bilateral in a third of patients. Although usually asymptomatic, some patients do experience visual impairment [34]. Several types of retinal lesions have been described, and presence of multiple retinal hamartomas is another major diagnostic criterion for tuberous sclerosis [35].

Other Organ Involvement

Other findings reported in patients with tuberous sclerosis include:

Hamartomatous polyps of the gastrointestinal tract [34]
Hepatobiliary angiomyolipomas [30]
Bone cysts, sclerotic changes of the calvaria, periosteal new bone formation, and scoliosis [31, 34]

Diagnosis

Diagnostic criteria for tuberous sclerosis were last revised and published in 1998 and are based solely on clinical findings. They are divided into major and minor criteria, with major criteria being those features that are highly specific for tuberous sclerosis. Definite tuberous sclerosis comprises either two major features or one major feature plus two minor features. Probable tuberous sclerosis comprises one major plus one minor feature. Possible tuberous sclerosis comprises either one major or two minor features [35] (Table 1.1).

Given the large number of cutaneous findings in the diagnostic criteria, a thorough skin examination can be helpful in establishing a diagnosis. When patients have other symptoms that suggest the diagnosis, additional studies may be undertaken according to symptoms (i.e., brain magnetic resonance imaging, electroencephalography, echocardiography). In addition, molecular genetic testing for TSC-1 and TSC-2 mutations is also available to confirm the diagnosis, which is particularly helpful in young patients who may not yet manifest many of the clinical features of the condition [30].

Disease Course and Prognosis

Patients with tuberous sclerosis have widely varied clinical presentations, with some more severely affected than others. In the early 1990s, one study noted that nearly 40 % of patients with tuberous sclerosis were dead by the age of 35 usually due to uncontrolled seizure activity, infectious complications, renal disease, or pulmonary disease [31, 39]. With advances in understanding of the disease process and improvement in imaging studies and management with early intervention for complications, life expectancy has improved [34].

Monitoring

The Tuberous Sclerosis Alliance provides a summary of the recommendations for monitoring and management on its web site, and these are based on the International Tuberous Sclerosis Complex Clinical Consensus Conference (http://www.tsalliance.org/pages.aspx?content=731). At the time of diagnosis, thorough evaluation through physical examination and various imaging and diagnostic studies is indicated to determine extent of disease. Regular follow-up with appropriate subspecialists is needed to monitor disease progression and to determine need for intervention.

Treatment

Therapy for tuberous sclerosis is largely symptomatic and depends on the organ system involved. As the pathogenesis of the condition involves hyperactivation of mTOR, the use of mTOR inhibitors sirolimus and everolimus has been studied as a viable treatment option for the manifestations of tuberous sclerosis. Everolimus is the only mTOR inhibitor approved in the United States for this indication, and its use is reserved for treatment of patients over age 3 years with subependymal giant cell astrocytomas not amenable to surgical resection [33]. Both sirolimus and everolimus have shown promise in treating the various clinical manifestations of tuberous

Table 1.1 Diagnostic criteria for tuberous sclerosis

Major features
• Facial angiofibromas or forehead plaque
• Nontraumatic ungual or periungual fibroma
• Hypomelanotic macules (3 or more)
• Shagreen patch (connective tissue nevus)
• Multiple retinal nodular hamartomas
• Cortical tuber
– When cerebral cortical dysplasia and cerebral white matter migration tracts occur together, they should be counted as one rather than two features of tuberous sclerosis
• Subependymal nodule
• Subependymal giant cell astrocytoma
• Cardiac rhabdomyoma, single or multiple
• Lymphangiomyomatosis
• Renal angiomyolipoma
– When both lymphangiomyomatosis and renal angiomyolipomas are present, other features of tuberous sclerosis should be present before a definite diagnosis is assigned
Minor features
• Multiple, randomly distributed pits in dental enamel
• Hamartomatous rectal polyps
– Histologic confirmation is suggested
• Bone cysts
– Radiographic confirmation is sufficient
• Cerebral white matter radial migration lines
– Radiographic confirmation is sufficient
• Gingival fibromas
• Nonrenal hamartoma
– Histologic confirmation is suggested
• Retinal achromic patch
• "Confetti" skin lesions
• Multiple renal cysts
– Histologic confirmation is suggested

Adapted and reprinted from Roach et al., Journal of Child Neurology (13: 624–628, 1998 by SAGE Publications). Reprinted by Permission of SAGE Publications

sclerosis, in particular subependymal giant cell astrocytomas, lymphangioleiomyomatosis, and angiomyolipomas. However, larger studies with long-term follow-up are needed to determine the patient populations in which these medications are best utilized, with a focus on safety and efficacy [33].

In patients with disfiguring facial angiofibromas, the treatment is destructive with cryosurgery, curettage, dermabrasion, chemical peels, laser, and excision being utilized [29, 40]. These methods can be painful, and lesions often recur, thus requiring multiple procedures over time to maintain cosmesis [29]. Topical rapamycin has also been reported to improve the appearance of facial angiofibromas [40]. Large or symptomatic periungual fibromas are most often treated by excision, but the recurrence rate is high [29].

Renal angiomyolipomas should be serially imaged to evaluate for enlargement. Given the risk of hemorrhage with increasing size, intervention should be considered when lesions reach 3–4 cm in diameter [32]. The treatment of choice is embolization, as surgical resection may compromise renal function [32]. Patients with renal cystic disease are at risk for development of hypertension; thus aggressive control of blood pressure with angiotensin receptor blockers and angiotensin-converting enzyme inhibitors is indicated [37].

Epilepsy is often resistant to medical therapy, requiring multiple antiepileptic agents to achieve control. If a cortical tuber is recognized as an epileptogenic focus, resection can be helpful. In patients with infantile spasms, the treatment of choice is vigabatrin, an inhibitor of gamma-aminobutyric acid transaminase [32]. Use of mTOR inhibitors may be helpful in managing epilepsy as well [37]. Control of seizure activity also has a positive impact on neurocognition [37]. When subependymal giant cell astrocytomas grow to a size that may obstruct flow of cerebrospinal fluid through the foramen of Monro, resection is indicated. However, recurrence is common if residual tissue remains. In the event that one of these lesions requires surgical resection but is not amenable to this treatment modality, use of mTOR inhibitors can be helpful in shrinking tumor size [37].

Cardiac rhabdomyomas are usually asymptomatic. However, complications can include heart failure, dysrhythmias, and embolic disease. Lesions usually regress, but surgical resection is indicated for those causing hemodynamic compromise [29, 30].

There is no effective therapy for pulmonary lymphangioleiomyomatosis; thus supportive care is indicated. There is a relationship between increased estrogen and worsening of pulmonary function, so some argue for the use of estrogen-lowering agents in treatment. Lung transplant should be considered in those with FEV1 <30 % or those with disabling shortness of breath [37].

Genetic Counseling

If a patient has sufficient clinical findings to render a diagnosis of tuberous sclerosis, genetic testing can then be undertaken not only to confirm the diagnosis but also to enable the patient to know the specific mutation that caused the condition [30]. Given the autosomal dominant inheritance pattern, risk of transmission to offspring with one affected parent is 50 %. If both parents are seemingly unaffected and have one child born with tuberous sclerosis, the risk of another child having the condition is 1 in 22. If those same parents have two children born with tuberous sclerosis, the risk of the third child having the condition is 1 in 3 [34]. This is because 2 % of unaffected parents may have a gonadal mosaicism that accounts for the transmission to their children [30]. Keep in mind that over 60 % of patients have no known family history of tuberous sclerosis, and in family members of these patients, genetic testing can confirm that they do not have the mutation as well. Prenatal testing for tuberous sclerosis is also available [30].

Birt-Hogg-Dubé Syndrome

Introduction

BHD syndrome is an autosomal dominant disorder characterized by follicular hamartomas, pulmonary cysts, and renal cancer and is caused by inactivating mutations of the gene FLCN which encodes a protein folliculin, whose function has not been fully elucidated but is thought to act as a tumor suppressor [41]. Through cell signaling pathways, this protein may act upon the mTOR pathway, as in tuberous sclerosis [42]. Similarly to tuberous sclerosis, patients with BHD syndrome develop hamartomatous lesions in various organ systems, namely skin, kidneys, and lungs. However, the clinical and histologic findings differ from those seen in tuberous sclerosis. The classic triad of benign cutaneous tumors associated with BHD syndrome is the fibrofolliculoma, trichodiscoma, and acrochordon. Presence of pulmonary cysts places patients at risk for spontaneous pneumothorax. The renal tumors in BHD syndrome differ from other hereditary renal cancer syndromes in that the histologic subtypes are diverse [43]. Because pulmonary and cutaneous findings generally manifest earliest, recognition of these is important so that patients can be monitored closely for development of renal cancer, which is usually treatable if caught early [44].

Epidemiology

BHD syndrome is rare, estimated to occur in 1 in 200,000 [45]. The syndrome is likely underdiagnosed because widely variable clinical presentations may make diagnosis difficult [42]. There is no documented gender or race predilection.

Genetics

BHD syndrome results from autosomal dominantly inherited germline mutations in the FLCN gene, which encodes for the protein folliculin. Over 100 unique mutations in this gene have been reported, with the majority causing protein truncation leading to inactivation [41]. In general, no genotype-phenotype correlations have been identified; however, patients with certain specific gene mutations may be a lower risk for renal or colon neoplasia [41]. The function of folliculin has not been definitively determined. However, many of the BHD associated renal tumors demonstrate a "second hit" somatic FLCN mutation, thus confirming that folliculin has a tumor suppressor function [41]. The interacting proteins linking folliculin to the mTOR cell signaling pathway have been described, but the mechanism by which folliculin acts as a tumor suppressor has not yet been identified [46]. Therapies that target the mTOR pathway need to be studied as potential therapeutic options in this syndrome, as some data suggest that FLCN mutations may lead to either mTOR activation or inhibition depending on context [41].

Cutaneous Findings

Benign skin hamartomas may be the presenting features of BHD syndrome, and recognition of these findings should alert the clinician to evaluate for other end-organ involvement in these patients. Cutaneous lesions generally do not appear before 20 years of age [42] and comprise fibrofolliculomas, trichodiscomas, and acrochordons. Interestingly, recent studies have suggested that these three seemingly distinct histologic lesions may all be classified as

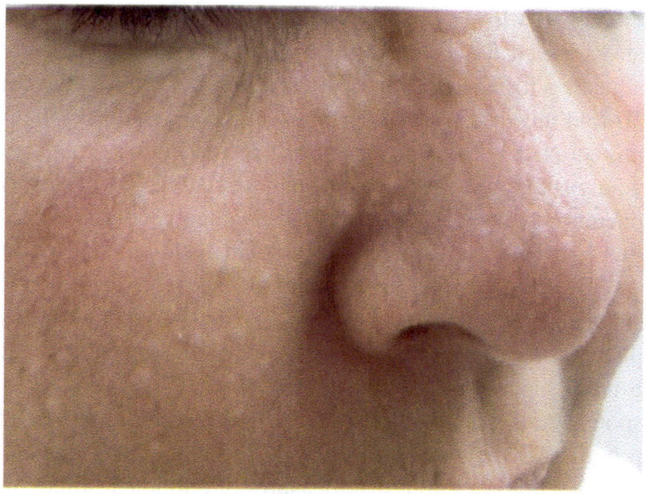

Fig. 1.7 Fibrofolliculomas of Birt-Hogg-Dubé syndrome. Note the multiple, discrete, skin colored to whitish waxy papules on the cheek and nose. Photo courtesy of Julia R. Nunley, M.D.

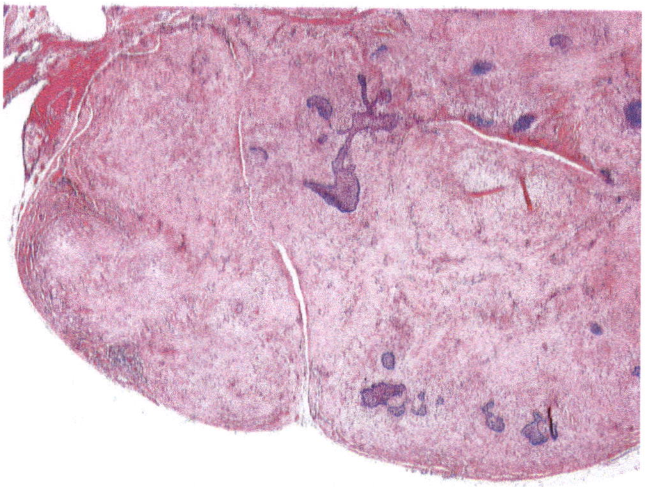

Fig. 1.8 Fibrofolliculoma histopathology. This view shows the circumscribed fibrous tissue, within which are anastomosing follicular epithelial strands. Serial sectioning through this biopsy specimen may also demonstrate features of trichodiscoma. Photo courtesy of William James, M.D.

fibrofolliculomas and were simply misdiagnosed because of sectioning and sampling error [47].

Clinically, fibrofolliculomas and trichodiscomas are indistinguishable, with patients presenting with multiple, smooth, waxy, dome-shaped, firm, whitish to skin-colored papules measuring a few millimeters in diameter, distributed most commonly over the head and neck and less commonly on the trunk [48] (see Fig. 1.7). It has been reported that up to 90 % of patients with BHD syndrome have biopsy-confirmed fibrofolliculomas [49], and this now makes up one of the major diagnostic criteria for the condition [42]. However, it is important to note that not all patients have skin findings, as some present with only renal or pulmonary manifestations [50].

The differential diagnosis for multiple facial papules includes several other genodermatoses with varying implications regarding associated internal disease. Skin biopsy is necessary to distinguish between these benign facial adnexal neoplasms. Multiple facial trichilemmomas are characteristic for Cowden syndrome, an autosomal dominant condition with increased risk of breast and thyroid cancer. The trichilemmomas are quite similar in appearance to fibrofolliculomas, but histology can distinguish these easily. Other findings in Cowden syndrome include oral cobblestoning, acral keratoses, and craniomegaly. Multiple facial trichoepitheliomas are seen in both Brooke-Spiegler syndrome and Rombo syndrome, and these lesions tend to be larger than fibrofolliculomas and are concentrated over nasolabial folds, nose, upper lip, forehead, and scalp. Both of these syndromes are autosomal dominant, with Brooke-Spiegler having no systemic associations and Rombo syndrome being associated with basal cell carcinoma and peripheral vasodilation. Again, histologic examination can easily confirm the diagnosis. Finally, tuberous sclerosis is characterized by multiple facial angiofibromas, which tend to be pinker in color than fibrofolliculomas and are concentrated around the nasolabial folds. Patients should also be examined for the other cutaneous manifestations of tuberous sclerosis, discussed earlier [47].

Skin biopsy can be done easily, as lesions are readily accessible. Histologic confirmation is recommended. Skin punch biopsy is preferred over shave biopsy to allow for deeper sampling of the follicular unit, and confirming the diagnosis often requires multiple biopsies over time with serial sectioning both horizontally and vertically through the specimen [47]. Histologically, fibrofolliculomas demonstrate a dilated follicular unit, wherein two to four cell layer thick epithelial strands extend outward from the normal follicular epithelium and anastomose with similar surrounding epithelium. Among and surrounding these interconnecting strands of epithelium is circumscribed fibrous tissue [51] (see Fig. 1.8). Trichodiscomas are characterized histologically by a stroma rich in collagen fibers and vasculature, with hair follicle units occurring in close proximity, usually at the periphery of the neoplasm. Some pathologists consider these two separate lesions. However, others argue that serial sectioning of a trichodiscoma will reveal features of fibrofolliculoma, and thus feel that these should be considered a spectrum of the same lesion [51].

There has been some debate about whether acrochordons (also known as skin tags) are truly a part of this condition, as they are so common in the general population. While these are not typically biopsied because of their classic appearance as fleshy, pedunculated, skin-colored papules occurring in body fold areas, when they are biopsied, some of these lesions demonstrate features of fibrofolliculoma [47].

Other reported benign skin findings in patients with BHD syndrome include angiolipomas, cutaneous mucinosis, leiomyomas, trichoblastomas, connective tissue nevi, lipomas, oral papules, and perifollicular fibromas. Cutaneous malignancies reported include basal cell carcinoma, squamous cell carcinoma, malignant melanoma, and dermatofibrosarcoma protuberans [42, 51].

Renal Manifestations

Up to 30 % of patients with BHD syndrome may develop renal tumors [49, 52]. It has been reported that patients with BHD syndrome have a seven times increase in the risk of renal cancer compared to the general population [42]. As in other heritable disorders where renal cancer is a feature, BHD patients tend to develop multiple, bilateral tumors at an early age (usually around the age of 50 years, but ranging from 25 to 75 years) [43]. Presence of renal tumors with these features is part of the minor diagnostic criteria for the syndrome. Typically males are at higher risk for development of renal cancer, but in this patient population, male gender puts patients only at slightly increased risk [53]. Unlike other heritable renal cancer syndromes, the renal cancers seen in BHD syndrome are diverse, with varying histologic subtypes among family members and within the same patient [43]. The predominating histologic subtype is the hybrid oncocytic tumor, with features of both oncocytoma and chromophobe renal cell carcinoma [44]. Presence of this histology comprises a minor diagnostic criterion for the syndrome. Other renal tumor histologic subtypes seen (listed from most to least common) are chromophobe, clear cell, and oncocytoma [52]. Progression to metastatic disease is uncommon, and most patients do well with monitoring and nephron-sparing surgical intervention only when tumors reach 3 cm in size [44]. Of note, benign renal cysts have also been reported in patients with BHD syndrome [42].

Pulmonary Manifestations

Patients with BHD syndrome are at risk for development of pulmonary cysts and spontaneous pneumothorax. In one study, over 80 % of patients with BHD syndrome demonstrate pulmonary cysts by imaging [49]. Cysts are often multiple, with variations in size (usually less than 1 cm), and the anatomic location is usually the basilar medial regions of the lungs, in contrast to cysts due to other etiologies [54]. Over 30 % of patients with the syndrome have been reported to have spontaneous pneumothorax [49]. Presence of multiple, bilateral, basilar lung cysts without other apparent cause is a minor diagnostic criterion for the condition [42]. Lung cysts are thought to be a precursor lesion for development of pneumothorax, with larger cyst volume and diameter conferring an increased risk of pneumothorax [49]. In one study, after adjusting for age, affected patients were reported to have a 50-fold increased risk of development of spontaneous pneumothorax; the risk decreases with increasing age (patients younger than 40 years were four times as likely to develop pneumothorax) [53]. In this same study, no gender predilection was reported, which is important in distinguishing cystic disease from lymphangioleiomyomatosis seen in tuberous sclerosis. Patients may have a single episode of spontaneous pneumothorax, but recurrences are more common [42]. Studies have not demonstrated that cystic lung disease or spontaneous pneumothorax causes increased mortality or progressive lung deterioration in these patients [49]. In addition, one study showed that measures of pulmonary function in affected patients were within the normal range [54]. Interestingly, an association with smoking and development of cysts and pneumothorax has not been clearly delineated in BHD patients [54, 55].

Other reported pulmonary manifestations seen in the syndrome are adenomatous hyperplasia, pulmonary histiocytoma, and bronchoalveolar carcinoma, but the relationship between development of these tumors and FLCN mutations remains to be seen [54].

Other Organ Involvement

Early reports of BHD syndrome linked presence of fibrofolliculomas to colon cancer. However, subsequent reports have failed to demonstrate that patients with BHD syndrome are at increased risk for colorectal neoplasms. Many other benign and malignant tumors have been reported in these patients, but no clear causality between the syndrome and the development of these tumors has been established [42].

Other findings reported in patients with BHD syndrome include [42]:

- Multinodular goiter
- Parotid adenoma
- Colorectal polyposis
- Neural tissue tumor
- Breast cancer
- Colorectal cancer
- Sarcoma of the leg
- Tonsillar cancer

Diagnosis

Diagnostic criteria for BHD syndrome were published in 2009 and are divided into major and minor criteria. Patients should have one major or two minor criteria to be diagnosed with the condition [42] (Table 1.2).

Table 1.2 Diagnostic criteria for Birt-Hogg-Dubé syndrome

Major criteria
• At least five fibrofolliculomas or trichodiscomas, at least one histologically confirmed, of adult onset[a]
• Pathogenic FLCN germline mutation
Minor criteria
• Multiple lung cysts: bilateral basally locate lung cysts with no other apparent cause, with or without spontaneous primary pneumothorax
• Renal cancer: early-onset (<50 years) or multifocal or bilateral renal cancer, or renal cancer of mixed chromophobe and oncocytic histology
• A first degree relative with Birt-Hogg-Dubé syndrome

Adapted and reprinted from Menko et al., The Lancet Oncology (10:1199–206, December 2009 by Elsevier Health Science Journals). Reprinted by permission of Elsevier Health Science Journals

[a]Fibrofolliculoma and trichodiscoma are two possible presentations of the same lesion—for the differential diagnosis, angiofibroma in tuberous sclerosis should be considered. Childhood-onset multiple familial fibrofolliculoma or trichodiscoma without other syndromic features might be a distinct entity

Disease Course and Prognosis

Because of the varying degrees of internal involvement and rarity of the condition, it is difficult to make generalized statements about prognosis. The most worrisome complication is development of renal cancer. However, these tumors are usually indolent and with appropriate follow-up, patients are afforded an excellent prognosis with rare progression to metastatic disease. Notably, those with clear cell renal cell carcinoma may be at higher risk for developing metastases [44]. Those with pulmonary involvement should be reassured that cystic disease usually does not result in respiratory failure [54].

Monitoring

Any of the following clinical findings should prompt a clinician to order genetic testing for BHD syndrome: cutaneous fibrofolliculomas, pulmonary cysts, spontaneous pneumothorax, or renal tumors (particularly the histologic subtypes discussed earlier). Patients with a family history of fibrofolliculomas, pulmonary cysts, or pneumothorax should be considered for genetic testing [44]. Baseline evaluation should include thorough history and physical examination, with a focus on assessing for end-organ involvement. Dermatologic evaluation to include punch biopsy of a suspected fibrofolliculoma as well as skin cancer screening is important. In addition, abdominal imaging (preferably magnetic resonance imaging due to higher resolution images and to minimize radiation exposure from computed tomography (CT) scanning) is indicated to screen for renal tumors [44]. This should begin at around age 20 years [42]. High-resolution chest CT scanning should be done to examine for pulmonary cysts, their anatomic location, and morphology [54]. Some also recommend baseline pulmonary function testing [54]. Patients should be discouraged from smoking, as it is a risk factor for kidney cancer and pneumothorax.

It is recommended that patients undergo repeat abdominal imaging at least every 1–3 years, but this may be done more frequently depending on the size, location, and growth rate of any renal masses found [44]. Serial chest imaging is not necessarily recommended if patients are asymptomatic and have not had pneumothorax [44]. However, patients should be counseled on symptoms of pneumothorax, particularly those who are at high risk (scuba divers and patients who undergo air travel) [42]. Periodic pulmonary function testing may be indicated, and it is important for patients to have both pneumococcal vaccination and annual influenza vaccination [54]. Routine dermatologic examination can be helpful in detecting skin cancer. Since the association between BHD syndrome and colon cancer is not clear, specific guidelines regarding screening have not been established. It is recommended that patients undergo colonoscopy as per the general population, but more frequent assessment may be needed in those with a family history of colorectal cancer [42].

Treatment

The benign skin lesions associated with BHD syndrome are usually not treated unless patients are concerned about cosmesis. There are no current effective medical therapies for fibrofolliculomas; thus destructive techniques are used most commonly. It is important to counsel patients on risk of recurrence and scarring with these methods. In addition, treatment can be difficult given the large number of lesions. The following modalities have been reported to be helpful: electrodesiccation, ablative laser therapy, curettage, shave removal, and excision [42, 56].

When following patients with renal masses, it is recommended that surgery be considered when the dominant tumor reaches 3 cm in size. At that time, nephron-sparing surgery by an experienced surgeon should be undertaken with the goal of preserving renal function [44]. Rapamycin analogues can also be considered in patients with disseminated renal cancer, as it has been shown that mutations in FLCN may impact the mTOR cell signaling pathway [42].

In patients with their first spontaneous pneumothorax, conservative measures such as observation, aspiration, or thoracostomy can be considered. However, because of the high risk of recurrence, chemical pleurodesis can be helpful in preventing future hospitalizations and surgeries associated with recurrent pneumothoraces. Some experts recommend this procedure even after patients' initial pneumothorax [54].

Genetic Testing and Counseling

In patients with clinical features consistent with the diagnosis, genetic testing for the FLCN mutation is recommended to confirm the diagnosis. Testing for FLCN germline mutations is positive in over 90 % of families with BHD syndrome, with recommendations to begin screening at age 21 years [44]. Given the autosomal dominant inheritance pattern, risk of transmission to offspring with one affected parent is 50 %.

Nail Patella Syndrome

Introduction

Nail patella syndrome is an autosomal dominant disorder caused by mutations in the LMX1b gene, a transcription factor involved in development of the dorsoventral axis of the limb during embryogenesis and whose downstream effects include regulation of type IV collagen expression in the glomerular basement membrane [57]. As a result, both ectodermal and mesodermal organs are affected [58]. The classic tetrad of clinical findings includes absent or hypoplastic nails, absent or hypoplastic patellae, elbow dysplasia with radial subluxation, and iliac horns [59]. Although not part of this tetrad, patients often develop progressive nephropathy and ocular disease as well. Nail changes are often present at birth, and recognition of these changes can alert a clinician to evaluate for skeletal, renal, and ocular involvement [60].

Epidemiology

The incidence of nail patella syndrome has been estimated at 1 in 50,000 live births, and while many affected patients may go undiagnosed, it is thought that this may be an overestimate of the true incidence of the condition [59]. It is possible to make the diagnosis at birth or even prenatally, but despite consultation with multiple subspecialists, patients can escape diagnosis for many years [60]. In addition, both within and between affected families, there is significant variability in clinical presentation, which can make diagnosis challenging [57].

Genetics

Nail patella syndrome results from loss-of-function mutations in the LMX1b gene, a member of the LIM-homeodomain family of transcription factors whose function is important in limb development and renal morphogenesis [57]. The LMX1b gene product has been shown to bind to the enhancer sequence of COL4A4, in the region responsible for expression of COL4A3 and COL4A4, two of the three genes needed for producing type IV collagen (which comprises the glomerular basement membrane). Differing theories exist as to how the autosomal dominantly inherited LMX1b mutation alters gene function, with haplo-insufficiency being favored over a dominant-negative effect. There are over 130 distinct gene mutations reported, and investigators have not been able to elucidate a genotype-phenotype correlation. Although most cases are autosomal dominantly inherited, 12.5 % of cases are sporadic. In addition, no mutation is found in 10–15 % of affected patients [59].

Cutaneous Findings

As is apparent from the name of the condition and the classically described tetrad of clinical features, nail changes are the most common diagnostic finding in this condition, seen in up to 98 % of affected patients. The nail findings can be quite variable, and fingernail abnormalities are seen more commonly than toenail abnormalities. The changes can be seen at birth and are seen bilaterally and symmetrically. Thumbnails are more severely affected, while the 5th digit fingernail is least severely affected. The opposite is true for toenails, wherein the 5th digit toenail is most often affected when toenail findings are apparent. Nails may be absent, hypoplastic, or dystrophic, with clefting, discoloration, or thickening of the nail plate [60]. The lunula of the nail represents the distal portion of the nail matrix and in unaffected patients is seen clinically as a whitish, half-moon shaped area on the proximal portion of the nail plate nearest the cuticle. It is not seen in every patient or on every nail but is usually most prominent on the thumb nails. One of the pathognomonic signs of nail patella syndrome is the presence of a triangular-shaped (rather than a half-moon shaped) lunula [57].

Another reported cutaneous finding in patients with this syndrome is loss of the normal wrinkling of the skin seen over the distal interphalangeal joints in the fingers, again more prominent over the index fingers rather than the 5th digits. This was reported in over 95 % of patients in one study [60].

Renal Manifestations

Kidney findings have been estimated to occur in up to 50 % of patients with nail patella syndrome, with renal failure occurring in up to 15 % [60]. The pathogenesis of renal disease involves

Fig. 1.9 Patellar hypoplasia associated with nail patella syndrome. Image courtesy of Curtis Hayes, M.D.

dysfunction of the glomerular basement membrane, which relates to the downstream effects of LMX1b mutation on formation of type IV collagen. The earliest sign of renal involvement is proteinuria that can begin at birth or later and may worsen during pregnancy [60]. Average age of detection of renal disease has been reported at 22 years [57]. Hematuria may also be present. Some patients with proteinuria will remain asymptomatic, while others may progress to nephrotic syndrome or rarely to renal failure. This progression usually occurs slowly, but there are some reports of rapid deterioration of renal function. Studies have been unable to discern which features are responsible for progression of renal disease [60].

Light microscopic examination of renal biopsies in affected patients reveals findings related to the degree of renal dysfunction and are generally nonspecific, with focal thickening of the glomerular basement membrane seen most consistently. Ultrastructural examination of the glomerular basement membrane reveals findings more specific for nail patella syndrome, including "focal or diffuse and irregular thickening" with patchy electron-dense and electron-lucent areas giving a "moth-eaten" appearance. In addition, electron microscopy may demonstrate irregular deposition of type III collagen bundles in the lamina densa and mesangial matrix, which is highly specific for nail patella syndrome [57]. Of note, nail patella syndrome can be differentiated from type III collagen glomerulopathy, an autosomal recessive disorder because electron microscopy of the latter shows widespread deposition of collagen type III along the mesangial matrix and lamina densa [59]. Immunofluorescence microscopy is usually negative in nail patella syndrome or shows nonspecific staining for IgM, C3, C1q in sclerotic portions of the tuft [59].

Skeletal Manifestations

Three of the four findings in the diagnostic tetrad are skeletal findings, related to the effect of LMX1b mutations on the formation of the dorsoventral axis during limb development. Patellar changes are most common, occurring in up to 93 % of patients. The patella may be absent or more frequently hypoplastic [57]. Involvement may be bilateral or asymmetric (see Figs. 1.9 and 1.10). Patients present with recurrent displacement of the patella, usually laterally and superiorly. Symptoms include pain, locking, clicking, instability, and inability to straighten the knee joint [60].

Bony changes of the elbow are also common, with abnormalities occurring in over 90 % of patients [57]. Reported findings include hypoplasia of the radial head, lateral epicondyle, and capitellum resulting in recurrent dislocation of the radial head, which can be either unilateral or bilateral [57, 60]. Symptoms are usually mild and include loss of ability to extend the elbow and elbow contractures [60].

Iliac horns are pathognomonic for nail patella syndrome and are seen in 70–80 % of patients. These are bony protuberances present on the posterior ilium that are often palpable and are usually asymptomatic [57] (see Fig. 1.11).

Other reported skeletal findings include talipes, pes planus, tight Achilles tendons, back pain, scoliosis, congenital hip dislocation, and pectus excavatum [60].

Ocular Manifestations

Open angle glaucoma has been reported to occur in around 10 % of patients with nail patella syndrome, and ocular hypertension in 7 %. The average age at which glaucoma is diagnosed is 48 years, although juvenile onset can occur [61]. Because these complications are treatable and begin earlier than would be expected for the general population, screening from a young age is recommended [60].

Lester sign has been reported in 40–50 % of patients with nail patella syndrome and consists of a zone of hyperpigmentation of the iris surrounding the pupil, with a cloverleaf configuration, most obvious in patients with blue eyes. It is not seen more frequently in those with glaucoma or ocular hypertension. In addition, it can be seen in the general population, so it is not considered pathognomonic for the condition [60].

Other Organ Involvement

Other findings reported in patients with nail patella syndrome include [60]:

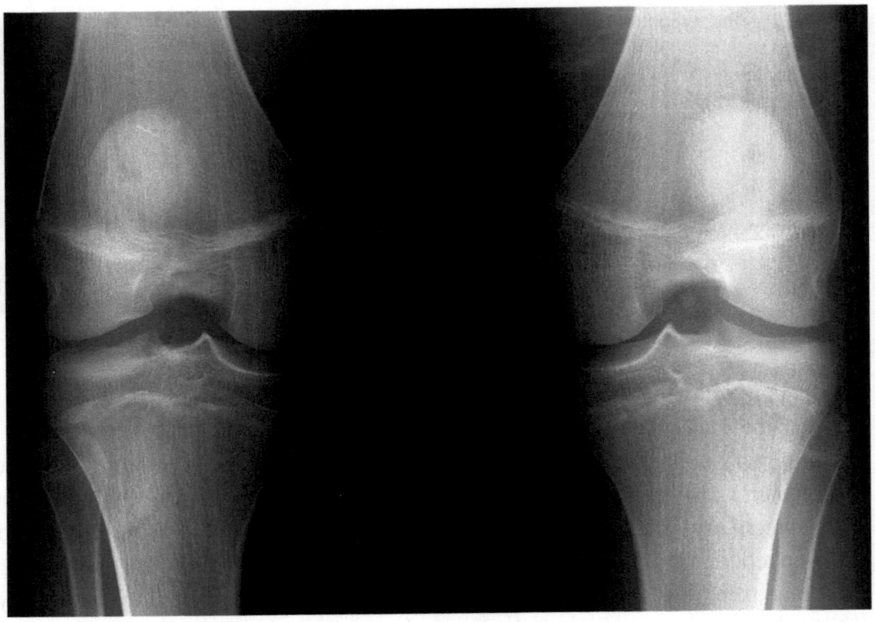

Fig. 1.10 Patellar hypoplasia associated with nail patella syndrome. Image courtesy of Curtis Hayes, M.D.

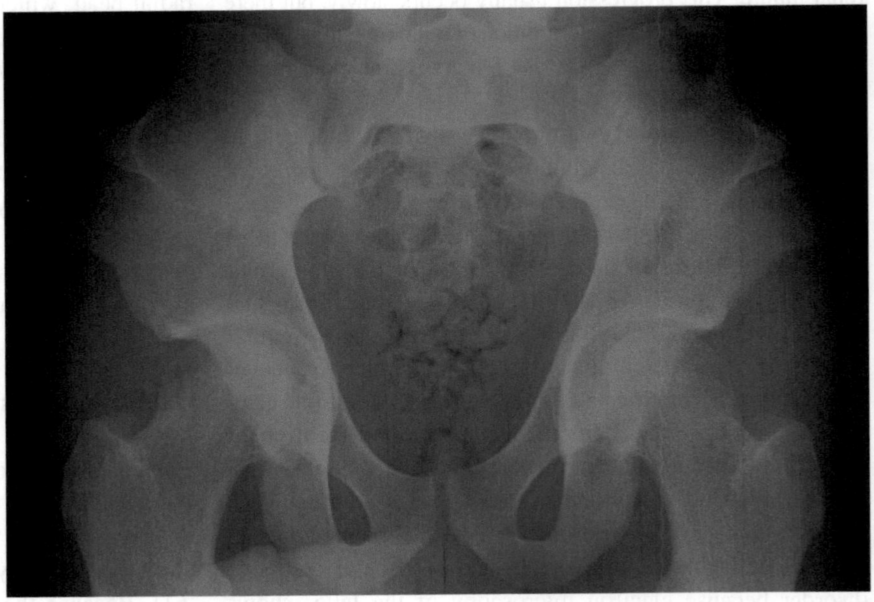

Fig. 1.11 Iliac horns associated with nail patella syndrome. Image courtesy of Curtis Hayes, M.D.

- Irritable bowel syndrome symptoms
- Acral paresthesias/peripheral neuropathy
- Epilepsy
- Attention deficit/hyperactivity disorder
- Vasomotor problems such as Raynaud syndrome
- Weak, crumbling teeth
- Depression

Diagnosis

Diagnostic criteria for nail patella syndrome have not been established, but the diagnosis should be considered in a patient with the classic clinical tetrad of absent or hypoplastic nails, absent or hypoplastic patellae, elbow dysplasia or radial subluxation, and iliac horns. The diagnosis can often be rendered at birth, but the subtle clinical findings may be missed. In patients with a known family history, prenatal diagnosis via chorionic villus sampling can be done. Keep in mind that the clinical manifestations are highly variable, even within the same family. Consultation with a geneticist to confirm the diagnosis is recommended, and molecular genetic testing for LMX1b mutations is available [59].

Disease Course and Prognosis

There are no high-quality studies estimating mortality rate or life expectancy in patients with nail patella syndrome.

However, the degree of renal involvement is the primary determinant of these variables. One study documented that 5 % of patients from 11 affected families died of renal failure, with the youngest reported at age 8 years [60]. Studies have been unable to identify clinical predictors of progression of renal disease, but fortunately, worsening renal disease affects a small number of patients with this condition. Those with nephrotic-range proteinuria may be at higher risk for loss of renal function, but this may occur quickly or over many years. In others, it may never worsen [59].

Monitoring

Once a diagnosis of nail patella syndrome has been established, patients should undergo annual screening for renal disease (measurement of blood pressure and urine albumin:creatinine ratio) beginning at birth. If abnormalities are detected, referral to a nephrologist is appropriate. Patients should be screened for glaucoma via measurement of intraocular pressure, examination of optic disc, and visual field assessment every 2 years, starting as soon as they are able to cooperate with the testing. Referral to an ophthalmologist is indicated for any abnormalities. In patients with skeletal symptoms in whom orthopedic surgery is being considered, imaging of the bone and soft tissue anatomy of the affected site should be done via magnetic resonance imaging. Genetic counseling should be offered to all patients [60].

Treatment

There are no specific treatments for kidney involvement in nail patella syndrome. It has been theorized that use of angiotensin-converting enzyme inhibitors may be renoprotective in those with proteinuria. However, since there are so few patients with nail patella syndrome who have kidney disease, there is insufficient longitudinal data to make use of these medications a universal recommendation. Cyclosporine has been shown to be beneficial in patients with Alport syndrome, another genetic disease with alterations of the glomerular basement membrane. In those patients, it has led to decreased proteinuria and stabilized renal function. There are again no high-quality studies documenting its use in nail patella syndrome, but it could be considered in patients in whom use of angiotensin-converting enzyme inhibitors may be unacceptable. There are reports of patients with nail patella syndrome improving with renal transplantation, and these patients should be considered excellent candidates for the procedure [59].

Absent or hypoplastic patellae put patients at risk for recurrent dislocations and early arthritis. Thus, surgical correction is indicated in these patients. Radial head dislocation is usually well tolerated by patients and rarely requires surgical intervention. Iliac horns are always asymptomatic and need no treatment [58].

Glaucoma can be managed by an ophthalmologist with topical ocular hypotensive agents or surgery [61].

Nail changes are asymptomatic and require no intervention.

Genetic Counseling

If a patient is diagnosed with nail patella syndrome on the basis of clinical findings, molecular genetic testing for the LMX1b mutation can be done to confirm the diagnosis. The majority of cases are inherited in an autosomal dominant fashion, meaning that the risk of transmission to offspring with one affected parent is 50 %. Prenatal testing is also available via chorionic villus sampling. There is a small proportion of patients in whom testing for LMX1b mutations is negative (10–15 %), and some may have no known family history of the condition, having a sporadic mutation (12.5 %) [59].

References

1. Mohrenschlager M, Braun-Falco M, Ring J, Abeck D. Fabry disease: recognition and management of cutaneous manifestations. Am J Clin Dermatol. 2003;4(3):189–96.
2. Brady M, Montgomery E, Brennan P, Mohindra R, Sayer JA. Diagnosing Fabry disease—delays and difficulties within discordant siblings. QJM 2013.
3. Orteu CH, Jansen T, Lidove O, Jaussaud R, Hughes DA, Pintos-Morell G, et al. Fabry disease and the skin: data from FOS, the Fabry outcome survey. Br J Dermatol. 2007;157(2):331–7.
4. Weidemann F, Sommer C, Duning T, Lanzl I, Mohrenschlager M, Naleschinski D, et al. Department-related tasks and organ-targeted therapy in Fabry disease: an interdisciplinary challenge. Am J Med. 2010;123(7):658.e1–658.e10.
5. Mehta A, Ricci R, Widmer U, Dehout F, Garcia de Lorenzo A, Kampmann C, et al. Fabry disease defined: baseline clinical manifestations of 366 patients in the Fabry Outcome Survey. Eur J Clin Invest. 2004;34(3):236–42.
6. Desnick RJ, Brady R, Barranger J, Collins AJ, Germain DP, Goldman M, et al. Fabry disease, an under-recognized multisystemic disorder: expert recommendations for diagnosis, management, and enzyme replacement therapy. Ann Intern Med. 2003;138(4):338–46.
7. Clarke JT. Narrative review: Fabry disease. Ann Intern Med. 2007;146(6):425–33.
8. Zampetti A, Orteu CH, Antuzzi D, Bongiorno MR, Manco S, Gnarra M, et al. Angiokeratoma: decision-making aid for the diagnosis of Fabry disease. Br J Dermatol. 2012;166(4):712–20.
9. Larralde M, Boggio P, Amartino H, Chamoles N. Fabry disease: a study of 6 hemizygous men and 5 heterozygous women with emphasis on dermatologic manifestations. Arch Dermatol. 2004;140(12):1440–6.
10. Choudhury S, Meehan S, Shin HT. Fabry disease: an atypical presentation. Pediatr Dermatol. 2005;22(4):334–7.
11. Hogarth V, Dhoat S, Mehta AB, Orteu CH. Late-onset Fabry disease associated with angiokeratoma of Fordyce and multiple cherry angiomas. Clin Exp Dermatol. 2011;36(5):506–8.

12. Mirceva V, Hein R, Ring J, Mohrenschlager M. A case of multiple angiomas without any angiokeratomas in a female heterozygote with Fabry disease. Australas J Dermatol. 2010;51(1):36–8.
13. Jansen T, Graue N, Dissemond J, Hillen U, Hentschke M, Grabbe S. Telangiectasias on the neck as a presenting cutaneous sign of Fabry disease. J Dermatol. 2006;33(9):652–4.
14. Nakai K, Yoneda K, Abe T, Moriue T, Matsuoka Y, Nibu N, et al. Multiple leg ulcers in a patient with Fabry disease. J Eur Acad Dermatol Venereol. 2008;22(3):382–3.
15. Amann-Vesti BR, Gitzelmann G, Widmer U, Bosshard NU, Steinmann B, Koppensteiner R. Severe lymphatic microangiopathy in Fabry disease. Lymphat Res Biol. 2003;1(3):185–9.
16. Wanner C, Oliveira JP, Ortiz A, Mauer M, Germain DP, Linthorst GE, et al. Prognostic indicators of renal disease progression in adults with Fabry disease: natural history data from the Fabry Registry. Clin J Am Soc Nephrol. 2010;5(12):2220–8.
17. Terryn W, Cochat P, Froissart R, Ortiz A, Pirson Y, Poppe B, et al. Fabry nephropathy: indications for screening and guidance for diagnosis and treatment by the European Renal Best Practice. Nephrol Dial Transplant. 2013;28(3):505–17.
18. Selvarajah M, Nicholls K, Hewitson TD, Becker GJ. Targeted urine microscopy in Anderson-Fabry disease: a cheap, sensitive and specific diagnostic technique. Nephrol Dial Transplant. 2011;26(10):3195–202.
19. Morrissey RP, Philip KJ, Schwarz ER. Cardiac abnormalities in Anderson-Fabry disease and Fabry's cardiomyopathy. Cardiovasc J Afr. 2011;22(1):38–44.
20. Patel MR, Cecchi F, Cizmarik M, Kantola I, Linhart A, Nicholls K, et al. Cardiovascular events in patients with Fabry disease natural history data from the Fabry registry. J Am Coll Cardiol. 2011;57(9):1093–9.
21. Kampmann C, Baehner F, Ries M, Beck M. Cardiac involvement in Anderson-Fabry disease. J Am Soc Nephrol. 2002;13 Suppl 2:S147–9.
22. Carubbi F, Bonilauri L. Fabry disease: raising awareness of the disease among physicians. Intern Emerg Med. 2012;7 Suppl 3:S227–31.
23. Low M, Nicholls K, Tubridy N, Hand P, Velakoulis D, Kiers L, et al. Neurology of Fabry disease. Intern Med J. 2007;37(7):436–47.
24. Laaksonen SM, Roytta M, Jaaskelainen SK, Kantola I, Penttinen M, Falck B. Neuropathic symptoms and findings in women with Fabry disease. Clin Neurophysiol. 2008;119(6):1365–72.
25. Sivley MD. Fabry disease: a review of ophthalmic and systemic manifestations. Optom Vis Sci. 2013;90(2):e63–78.
26. Mehta A, Beck M, Eyskens F, Feliciani C, Kantola I, Ramaswami U, et al. Fabry disease: a review of current management strategies. QJM. 2010;103(9):641–59.
27. Clarke JT, Iwanochko RM. Enzyme replacement therapy of Fabry disease. Mol Neurobiol. 2005;32(1):43–50.
28. Franz DN. Diagnosis and management of tuberous sclerosis complex. Semin Pediatr Neurol. 1998;5(4):253–68.
29. Schwartz RA, Fernandez G, Kotulska K, Jozwiak S. Tuberous sclerosis complex: advances in diagnosis, genetics, and management. J Am Acad Dermatol. 2007;57(2):189–202.
30. Curatolo P, Bombardieri R, Jozwiak S. Tuberous sclerosis. Lancet. 2008;372(9639):657–68.
31. Umeoka S, Koyama T, Miki Y, Akai M, Tsutsui K, Togashi K. Pictorial review of tuberous sclerosis in various organs. Radiographics. 2008;28(7):e32.
32. Crino PB, Nathanson KL, Henske EP. The tuberous sclerosis complex. N Engl J Med. 2006;355(13):1345–56.
33. Curatolo P, Moavero R. mTOR inhibitors in tuberous sclerosis complex. Curr Neuropharmacol. 2012;10(4):404–15.
34. Leung AK, Robson WL. Tuberous sclerosis complex: a review. J Pediatr Health Care. 2007;21(2):108–14.
35. Roach ES, Gomez MR, Northrup H. Tuberous sclerosis complex consensus conference: revised clinical diagnostic criteria. J Child Neurol. 1998;13(12):624–8.
36. Staley BA, Vail EA, Thiele EA. Tuberous sclerosis complex: diagnostic challenges, presenting symptoms, and commonly missed signs. Pediatrics. 2011;127(1):e117–25.
37. Franz DN, Bissler JJ, McCormack FX. Tuberous sclerosis complex: neurological, renal and pulmonary manifestations. Neuropediatrics. 2010;41(5):199–208.
38. Holmes GL, Stafstrom CE, Tuberous Sclerosis Study Group. Tuberous sclerosis complex and epilepsy: recent developments and future challenges. Epilepsia. 2007;48(4):617–30.
39. Shepherd CW, Gomez MR, Lie JT, Crowson CS. Causes of death in patients with tuberous sclerosis. Mayo Clin Proc. 1991; 66(8):792–6.
40. Koenig MK, Hebert AA, Roberson J, Samuels J, Slopis J, Woerner A, et al. Topical rapamycin therapy to alleviate the cutaneous manifestations of tuberous sclerosis complex: a double-blind, randomized, controlled trial to evaluate the safety and efficacy of topically applied rapamycin. Drugs R D. 2012;12(3):121–6.
41. Schmidt LS. Birt-Hogg-Dubé syndrome: from gene discovery to molecularly targeted therapies. Fam Cancer. 2013;12:357–64.
42. Menko FH, van Steensel MA, Giraud S, Friis-Hansen L, Richard S, Ungari S, et al. Birt-Hogg-Dubé syndrome: diagnosis and management. Lancet Oncol. 2009;10(12):1199–206.
43. Pavlovich CP, Walther MM, Eyler RA, Hewitt SM, Zbar B, Linehan WM, et al. Renal tumors in the Birt-Hogg-Dubé syndrome. Am J Surg Pathol. 2002;26(12):1542–52.
44. Stamatakis L, Metwalli AR, Middelton LA, Marston Linehan W. Diagnosis and management of BHD-associated kidney cancer. Fam Cancer. 2013;12(3):397–402.
45. Verine J, Pluvinage A, Bousquet G, Lehmann-Che J, de Bazelaire C, Soufir N, et al. Hereditary renal cancer syndromes: an update of a systematic review. Eur Urol. 2010;58(5):701–10.
46. Baba M, Hong SB, Sharma N, Warren MB, Nickerson ML, Iwamatsu A, et al. Folliculin encoded by the BHD gene interacts with a binding protein, FNIP1, and AMPK, and is involved in AMPK and mTOR signaling. Proc Natl Acad Sci U S A. 2006;103(42):15552–7.
47. Vincent A, Farley M, Chan E, James WD. Birt-Hogg-Dubé syndrome: a review of the literature and the differential diagnosis of firm facial papules. J Am Acad Dermatol. 2003;49(4):698–705.
48. Reese E, Sluzevich J, Kluijt I, Teertstra HJ, De Jong D, Horenblas S, et al. Birt-Hogg-Dubé syndrome. In: Riegert-Johnson DL, Boardman LA, Hefferon T, Roberts M, editors. Cancer syndromes. Bethesda, MD: Douglas L Riegert-Johnson; 2009.
49. Toro JR, Wei MH, Glenn GM, Weinreich M, Toure O, Vocke C, et al. BHD mutations, clinical and molecular genetic investigations of Birt-Hogg-Dubé syndrome: a new series of 50 families and a review of published reports. J Med Genet. 2008;45(6):321–31.
50. Houweling AC, Gijezen LM, Jonker MA, van Doorn MB, Oldenburg RA, van Spaendonck-Zwarts KY, et al. Renal cancer and pneumothorax risk in Birt-Hogg-Dubé syndrome; an analysis of 115 FLCN mutation carriers from 35 BHD families. Br J Cancer. 2011;105(12):1912–9.
51. Welsch MJ, Krunic A, Medenica MM. Birt-Hogg-Dubé syndrome. Int J Dermatol. 2005;44(8):668–73.
52. Pavlovich CP, Grubb III RL, Hurley K, Glenn GM, Toro J, Schmidt LS, et al. Evaluation and management of renal tumors in the Birt-Hogg-Dubé syndrome. J Urol. 2005;173(5):1482–6.
53. Zbar B, Alvord WG, Glenn G, Turner M, Pavlovich CP, Schmidt L, et al. Risk of renal and colonic neoplasms and spontaneous pneumothorax in the Birt-Hogg-Dubé syndrome. Cancer Epidemiol Biomarkers Prev. 2002;11(4):393–400.
54. Gupta N, Seyama K, McCormack FX. Pulmonary manifestations of Birt-Hogg-Dubé syndrome. Fam Cancer. 2013;12(3):387–96.

55. Tomassetti S, Carloni A, Chilosi M, Maffe A, Ungari S, Sverzellati N, et al. Pulmonary features of Birt-Hogg-Dubé syndrome: cystic lesions and pulmonary histiocytoma. Respir Med. 2011;105(5):768–74.
56. Vernooij M, Claessens T, Luijten M, van Steensel MA, Coull BJ. Birt-Hogg-Dubé syndrome and the skin. Fam Cancer. 2013;12:381–5.
57. Bongers EM, Gubler MC, Knoers NV. Nail-patella syndrome. Overview on clinical and molecular findings. Pediatr Nephrol. 2002;17(9):703–12.
58. Beguiristain JL, de Rada PD, Barriga A. Nail-patella syndrome: long term evolution. J Pediatr Orthop B. 2003;12(1):13–6.
59. Lemley KV. Kidney disease in nail-patella syndrome. Pediatr Nephrol. 2009;24(12):2345–54.
60. Sweeney E, Fryer A, Mountford R, Green A, McIntosh I. Nail patella syndrome: a review of the phenotype aided by developmental biology. J Med Genet. 2003;40(3):153–62.
61. Mimiwati Z, Mackey DA, Craig JE, Mackinnon JR, Rait JL, Liebelt JE, et al. Nail-patella syndrome and its association with glaucoma: a review of eight families. Br J Ophthalmol. 2006;90(12):1505–9.

Metabolic Disorders

2

Davida A. Kornreich

Metabolic disorders such as diabetes mellitus (DM), atherosclerosis, and amyloidosis have become increasingly prevalent in our population, and with this increased prevalence comes an increase in cases of chronic kidney disease (CKD), a common sequela of these diseases. Diabetes and atherosclerosis are in fact the two most common causes of CKD in the USA, making up two-thirds of all cases and heavily contributing to the burden of disease [1].

The systemic nature of many metabolic disorders often results in unique cutaneous findings, which can occasionally be the initial presentation of disease. Even the most obscure dermatologic manifestations are becoming increasingly prevalent in relation to the epidemiologic growth of these disorders. It, thus, is necessary for nephrologists and dermatologists to gain awareness of these cutaneous manifestations in order to diagnose and treat appropriately.

Diabetes Mellitus (DM)

DM affects the skin in approximately 60–88 % of diabetics [2]. The disease modifies the cutaneous microvasculature, keratinocytes, and fibroblasts, causing anything from mild to severe dermatologic disease. The cutaneous manifestations most often present 6–13 years after disease onset, usually correlating with microvascular disease of the kidneys, retina, and nerves. Dermatologic disorders associated with DM can be divided into two categories, common and uncommon, both of which are touched on in this chapter.

D.A. Kornreich, M.D. (✉)
Department of Dermatology, Icahn School of Medicine at Mount Sinai, 5 East 98th Street, 5th Floor, New York, NY 10029, USA

240 Central Park S., Apt 7p, New York, NY 10019, USA
e-mail: davida.kornreich@mssm.edu

Physiology/Pathogenesis

Studies indicate that an amalgamation of systemic and local factors play a role in the pathogenesis of cutaneous disease secondary to DM, with hyperglycemia being the key pathologic factor causing disease. Hyperglycemia causes inflammation, free radical production, and decreased wound healing on a local level. Systemically, it causes the microvascular changes seen with chronic disease (Fig. 2.1) [3, 4].

The mechanisms by which hyperglycemia causes these sequelae are complex. Elevated glucose levels have been found to decrease diabetics' cutaneous fibroblasts' synthetic, proliferative, and secreting abilities, thereby hindering wound healing. The fibroblasts become resistant to growth factor such as IGFR-I and epidermal growth factor (EGF), further inhibiting proliferation. Ultimately this resistance causes sensitization to ischemia, resulting in the significant ulceration and necrosis of lower extremities common in diabetics [4, 5].

Hyperglycemia further affects fibroblasts by releasing inflammatory cytokines and free radicals, causing oxidative stress, cell death and aging. Glucose produces these free radicals by altering the electron transport chain during oxidative respiration, causing auto-oxidation. Once produced, free radicals and advanced glycoxidation end products (AGEs) affect mitochondria and endothelial synthesis, resulting in protein misfolding, impaired vascular endothelial growth factor (VEGF) production, the release of tumor necrosis factor alpha (TNF-α), and upregulation of matrix metalloproteinase (MMP)-9, MMP-3, and MMP-2, causing apoptosis [4].

Hyperglycemia also affects endothelial cells, resulting in vascular damage. Similar to fibroblasts, endothelial cells are made dysfunctional by insulin resistance and free radicals. Hyperglycemia increases endothelial deoxyribonucleic acid (DNA) damage and cell death and prevents the endothelial cells from releasing nitrous oxide (N0), which under normal physiologic circumstances prevents vascular smooth muscle cell migration. The free radicals produced by hyperglycemia causes significant oxidative stress and inflammation amongst endothelial cells, which further results in vascular permeability

J.R. Nunley and E.V. Lerma (eds.), *Dermatological Manifestations of Kidney Disease*,
DOI 10.1007/978-1-4939-2395-3_2, © Springer Science+Business Media New York 2015

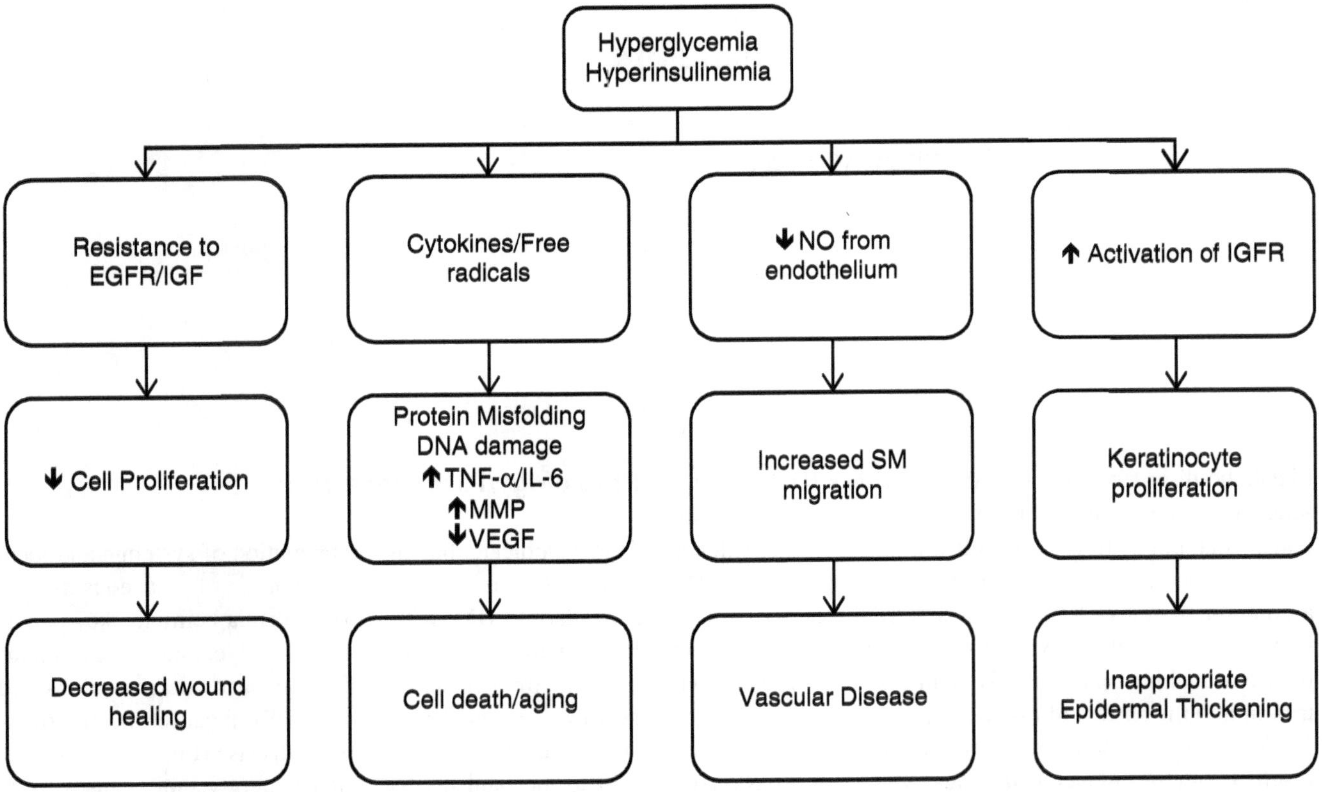

Fig. 2.1 A graph demonstrating the effects of hyperinsulinemia and hyperglycemia on the epidermis. *NO* nitric oxide, *IGFR* insulin-like growth factor receptor, *TNF-α* tumor necrosis factor alpha, *IL-6* interleukin-6, MMP matrix metalloproteinase, *VEGF* vascular endothelial growth factor

and the uncontrolled release of inflammatory cytokines, such as TNF-α and interleukin (IL)-6. Again, mitochondria are affected, impacting protein formation as well as mitochondrial DNA [4].

Keratinocytes also are affected by hyperglycemia. In vitro analysis demonstrates that glucose is directly toxic to keratinocytes, reducing proliferation and replication of these cells, hindering re-epithelialization [4]. Furthermore, hyperinsulinemia (which is widespread among type II diabetics) activates keratinocyte insulin growth factor receptors, causing inappropriate epidermal proliferation and dermatologic disease [3, 6].

Diabetics are well known for having an increased risk of cutaneous infections, and while the pathogenesis is poorly understood, the vascular changes caused by hyperglycemia play a significant role. On a macrovascular level, studies suggest that hyperglycemia increases blood viscosity and hypercoagulability (by increasing plasma fibrinogen levels), causing ischemic injury and delivering poor blood supply to affected areas [5]. Infection of this damaged tissue is made worse by microvascular disease as well as associated comorbidities such as peripheral vascular disease and diabetic neuropathy. The immune system itself is hindered by DM as well, as elevated glucose is associated with decreased phagocytosis, impaired leukocyte adherence, and delayed chemotaxis [2, 7].

Clinical Symptoms, Differential Diagnosis, Histology, and Treatment by Cutaneous Manifestation

Common conditions associated with DM include acanthosis nigricans (AN), acrochordons (skin tags), yellow skin and nails, diabetic dermopathy (shin spots), rubeosis faciei, and ulcers on the lower extremity and foot. Uncommon manifestations include diabetic bullae; diabetic thick skin; scleredema diabeticorum, eruptive xanthomas granuloma annulare, necrobiosis lipoidica (NL), and perforating dermatosis (see Table 2.1) [3]. Both the common and uncommon conditions will be discussed below.

Diabetic Dermopathy (Shin Spots)

Shin spots are the most common cutaneous manifestation of DM, found in approximately 40 % of diabetics [8]. The lesions are well demarcated, hyperpigmented, atrophic, depressions, macules, or papules that are generally located on the anterior surface of the bilateral lower extremities but can also affect the thighs, medial malleoli, and arms [6, 8–10]. Their frequency increases with duration of disease, comorbid findings (specifically microvascular disease such as nephropathy, neuropathy, and retinopathy), and male sex [6, 9]. There is no similar condition in non-diabetics [8]. Although

Table 2.1 Cutaneous manifestations of diabetes mellitus

Common	Uncommon
Acanthosis nigricans	Diabetic bullae
Acrochordons	Diabetic thick skin
Carotenoderma	Scleredema diabeticorum
Diabetic dermopathy	Eruptive xanthomas granuloma annulare
Rubeosis faciei	Necrobiosis lipoidica
Diabetic ulcers	Perforating dermatosis
Infection	

the etiology was thought to be secondary to blunt trauma given their location and association with neuropathy, this finding has not been replicated in vivo. Other studies have looked at the blood flow to these lesions and determined that they have much higher blood flow than normal appearance reference skin sites (although the reference skin of diabetics with diabetic dermopathy has much lower blood flow in general than their matched diabetic and nondiabetic controls) [8, 9]. Histologically, the most common feature observed is hemosiderin and/or melanin pigment in the superficial dermis [9]. General thickening of the blood vessels with a perivascular lymphocytic infiltrate has also been identified [3]. The lesions are asymptomatic and oftentimes resolve spontaneously (on average lasting 18–24 months) and so there is no recommended treatment [3].

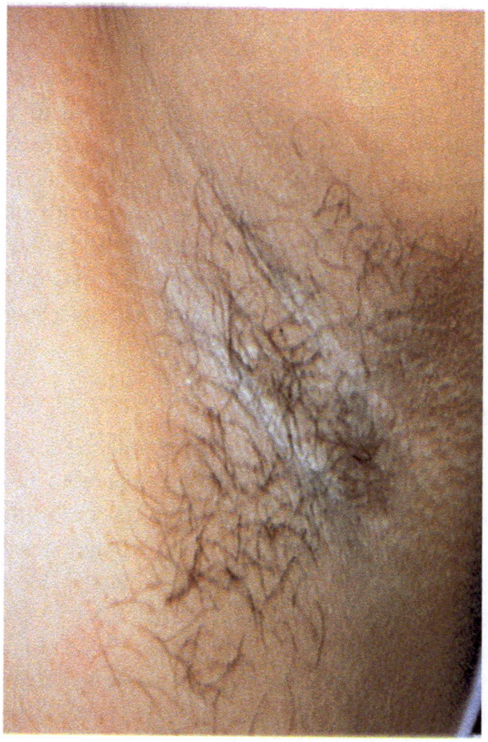

Fig. 2.2 Acanthosis nigricans within the axilla. Source: Ahmed I, Goldstein B. "Diabetes Mellitus." Clinics in Dermatology. 2006 Jan 1; 24(4):237

Acanthosis Nigricans (AN)

AN is described as a velvety thickening and hyperpigmentation of the skin most commonly located on flexural areas, such as the axilla, nape of the neck, and groin area (Fig. 2.2) [3, 11]. It is common amongst diabetics and those with obesity; those with AN have been found to have higher fasting plasma insulin levels than control subjects [3, 11, 12]. AN is less commonly found in hypothyroidism, adrenal insufficiency, genetic disorders, as a paraneoplastic syndrome, or with prolonged crutch use [6, 11]. Histologic samples demonstrate papillomatosis, hyperkeratosis, and mild acanthosis causing the hyperpigmentation [12, 13]. AN is best treated by management of the underlying disease with weight loss and diabetic control, both of which can reverse the diabetic process. Medications such as octreotide which decrease insulin secretion have also demonstrated some success in treatment, as have agents which decrease the proliferation of keratinocytes, such as topical retinoids [3, 6, 11].

Acrochordons (Skin Tags)

Acrochordons are benign pedunculated papules that occur along the neck and other major flexor surfaces such as the eyelid or axilla. They are often associated with AN and have a similar mechanism of development, with hyperinsulinemia stimulating keratinocyte proliferation [6, 10, 13]. Approximately 66–75 % of patients with acrochordons have DM [14]. Differential diagnosis could include warts, nevi, or neurofibromatosis. Histologically, it appears as a polyp with normal epidermis and a core of dermis or subcutaneous tissue. Acrochordons can be treated if desired by surgical removal, cryotherapy, or electrodissection; however, they are benign, and no treatment is necessary [3, 6, 10, 13].

Carotenodermia

Diabetics will often develop yellowing of the skin in areas of prominent sebaceous activity such as the face as well as the palms, soles, and nails; it is notably absent from the sclera. The pathogenesis of this particular condition is unclear but thought to relate to impaired metabolism of beta-carotene by the liver, thus causing its accumulation systemically [3, 15]. Beta carotene is lipophilic, and is thus attracted to the stratum corneum, which has a high lipid content. The high lipophilic state associated with DM further results in elevated beta carotene levels, as beta lipoprotein breaks down to beta carotene [15]. Another mechanism of disease is thought to be caused by glycosylation of dermal collagen, which creates a yellow hue [3, 16]. Differential diagnosis is broad, including jaundice (although in jaundice the sclera are affected), lycopenemia, riboflavinemia, and certain drugs [15]. Generally, treatment includes better glycemic control and decreasing consumption of foods high in carotene [3, 15].

Rubeosis Faciei

Rubeosis faciei is a chronic flushed appearance of the face and neck often found on diabetics (with reports as high as 60 %) [3, 6, 16]. The erythema is thought to directly correlate with dilation of vasculature and microangiopathic changes associated with the disease [3]. The differential includes erysipelas and carcinoid flush, but lacks the warmth and elevation of the former and the telangiectasias of the latter [16]. There is no real treatment except improved glycemic control and symptomatic relief by avoiding vasodilators, such as caffeine and alcohol [6].

Diabetic Foot and Ulceration

Diabetic foot is generally classified as infection, ulceration, and/or destruction of deep tissue secondary to neurologic abnormalities and peripheral vascular disease in the lower limb [17]. It is the most morbid common cutaneous manifestation of diabetes, occurring in approximately 15 % of the diabetic population and accounting for at least 70 % of lower limb amputations annually in the USA [3, 6, 18]. It is the most common cause of hospitalization amongst diabetics [3, 18]. Ulcers occur in areas of constant pressure and repeated movement; initially thick calluses form, and these break down and ulcerate [6]. Ulcer formation is directly related to the loss of protective sensation secondary to peripheral neuropathy or peripheral vascular disease, both common in diabetics [18]. Differential diagnosis includes other causes of ulceration, such as arterial or venous disease. It is imperative to treat these callouses and ulcers with aggressive debridement and offloading with devices such as a total contact cast in order to prevent secondary infection and promote healing [6, 18]. If properly cared for, the ulcers can resolve within weeks as long as vasculature is adequate. If it is inadequate, surgical intervention with revascularization procedures may be necessary, but these procedures have not been studied in large prospective analyses [6, 18].

Necrobiosis Lipoidica (NL)

NL, previously known as necrobiosis lipoidica diabeticorum, is a granulomatous disease that is characterized by red papules or plaques that grow peripherally, with a raised, active, erythematous border, ultimately causing central epidermal atrophy with telangiectasias and a yellow hue (Fig. 2.3) [3, 19]. Although the lesions can be singular, they are often multiple and bilateral, expanding to up to several centimeters in diameters [3]. The lesions develop in both type I and type II diabetics, with earlier onset in insulin dependent diabetics and with a preponderance for females [20]. While the lesions are asymptomatic and chronic, 35 % ulcerate and these can progress to squamous cell carcinoma [3, 10]. Distribution is generally on the anterior shin, but can also occur on the feet, arms, trunk, or scalp—their development is thought to relate to neuropathy, causing the distal nature of disease [3]. Histologically NL lesions are characterized by interstitial palisaded granulomas involving the dermis and subcutis with epidermal atrophy and excess lipid deposits in the dermis [10, 20]. Although 65 % of patients with NL have diabetes, the lesions have also been identified in patients with Crohn disease, ulcerative colitis, sarcoid, and granuloma annulare [20]. Because of the chronic and progressive nature of the lesions, treatment is necessary. Unfortunately, it is not very effective. Topical and intralesional steroids have been demonstrated to slow disease progression by decreasing the inflammation, however it can still take years for the lesions to resolve. For persistent disease, systemic corticosteroids, cyclosporine, ticlopidine, and TNF-α antagonists (such as etanercept and infliximab) have been used. Skin grafting remains another treatment option, although the poor wound healing and increased chance of infections associated with DM makes surgery less desirable [6, 10, 20].

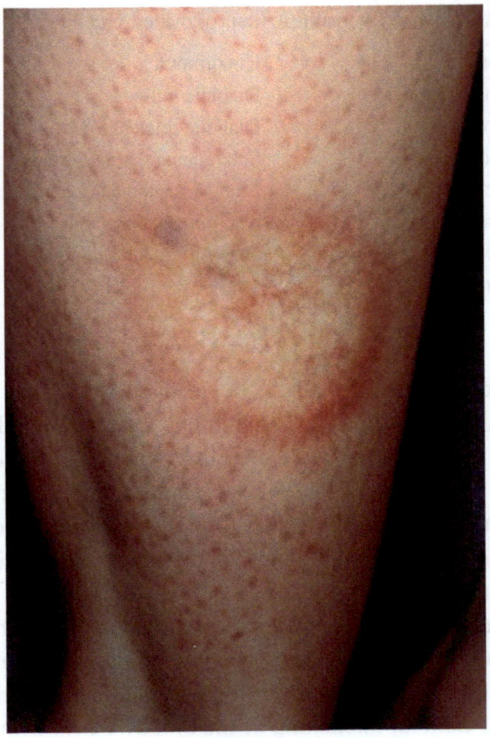

Fig. 2.3 An example of nicrobiosis lipoidica. Source: Ahmed I, Goldstein B. "Diabetes Mellitus." Clinics in Dermatology. 2006 Jan 1; 24(4):237

Bullosis Diabeticorum (Diabetic Blisters)

Blisters have been found to occur spontaneously on the hands and feet without surrounding or predisposing erythema or inflammation in approximately 0.5 % of diabetic patients (Fig. 2.4) [10, 21]. The blisters are tense and painless, containing sterile fluid and ranging from 0.5 to 3.0 cm in size [6]. Generally the bullae form abruptly and heal without scarring, as histologically they are predominately intra-epidermal; however, occasionally hemorrhagic bullae can form or the lesions can have a subepidermal cleavage site that can cause

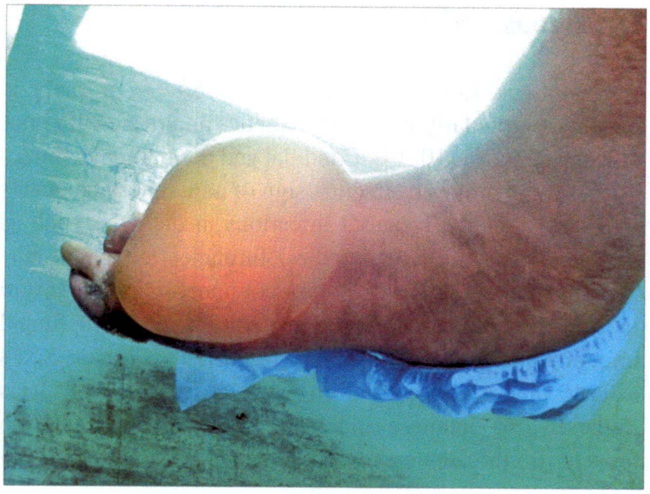

Fig. 2.4 Bullosis diabeticorum on the dorsal foot. Source: Kurdi AT. "Bullosis diabeticorum." The Lancet. 2013 Jan 1; DOI: 10.1016/S0140-6736(13)60145-2

scarring and atrophy [6, 16, 21]. The etiology of the blisters is unclear, as immunophysiologic studies have all been negative [6, 21]. Differential includes other blistering diseases such as bullous pemphigoid, epidermolysis bullosa acquisita, bullous impetigo, porphyria, bullous erythema multiforme, and allergic reactions [16, 21]. Treatment of the lesions is generally supportive, as the bullae resolve within 2–4 weeks [6]. Topical antibiotics may be used to prevent infection [6, 16].

Scleredema

Scleredema is a rare disorder involving asymptomatic, diffuse, symmetric, nonpitting indurated plaques on the neck, upper back, and shoulders (Fig. 2.5) [6, 22]. It is most common in obese males over the age of 40, and is associated with other complications such as nephropathy, retinopathy and neuropathy. It has an unpredictable course but is generally progressive, worsening with the severity of disease. Histologically the skin demonstrates thickening of the reticular dermis with mucin deposition and proliferation of mast cells between thickened collagen bundles [6, 16]. Scleredema is usually permanent, and treatment is generally ineffective, although therapies including glucocorticoids, methotrexate, and ultraviolet (UV) light therapy have demonstrated some therapeutic success [3, 6, 22]. Tight glycemic control has no effect on the condition [6].

Diabetic Thick Skin (Scleroderma-Like Skin Changes)

Compared with the general population, diabetics often develop thickened skin, which can be asymptomatic and diffuse or localized with dramatic morbidity. Approximately 20–30 % of diabetic patients develop thickening of the skin on the dorsal hand, which can progress in 8–50 % of diabetics to diabetic hand syndrome, a disease that involves stiffening of the metacarpophalangeal and proximal interphalangeal joints, limiting mobility and occasionally causing Dupuytren

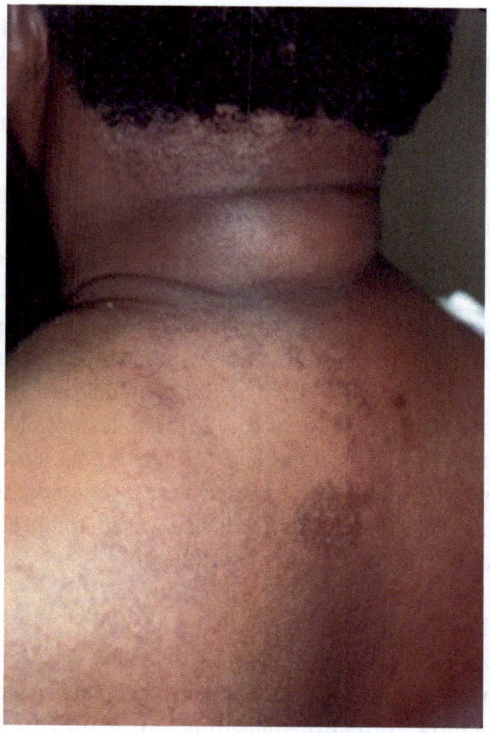

Fig. 2.5 Scleredema of the back. Source: Ahmed I, Goldstein B. "Diabetes Mellitus." Clinics in Dermatology. 2006 Jan 1; 24(4):237

contracture or sclerodactyly [3, 10, 23, 24]. When it manifests as diabetic hand syndrome, patients have limitations in extension of their hands, causing the "prayer sign" (an inability to press the palms together) [6]. Huntley papules or finger pebbles are another variant of diabetic thick skin associated with type 2 diabetics. It involves indurated thickened areas of skin localized to the extensor surfaces of the fingers, knuckles, or periungal area [6]. Although similar to scleroderma, scleroderma-like skin changes do not involve dermal atrophy, edema, pain, Raynaud phenomenon, or telangiectasias. Histologically the syndrome lacks evidence of mucin deposition (seen in scleredema diabeticorum); instead, there is a thickened dermis with accumulation of connective tissue in the reticular layer with increased cross-linkage of collagen [24]. Diabetic thick skin is a progressive condition, and is associated with double the risk of retinopathy and nephropathy. Few options are available for treatment; limited evidence exists for tight glycemic control [6].

Acquired Perforating Dermatoses (APD)

APD is a disorder characterized by hyperkeratotic papules and nodules which histologically demonstrate focal hyperkeratosis that is in contact with transepidermal, perforating, elimination of components of the dermis (such as keratin, collagen, and elastic fibers). It can be classified as four subtypes: reactive perforating collagenosis (RPC), perforating folliculitis (PF), Kyrle disease (KD), and (least commonly) elastosis perforans serpiginosa (EPS) [3, 25, 26].

Each of these subtypes has a slightly different morphology and distribution. The lesions generally appear as erythematous papules and nodules, and can sometimes have central umbilication with a keratin plug or follicular pattern of presentation, depending on the subtype. The lesions usually present on the extensor surfaces of the extremities and trunk, although EPS and RPC can also appear on the face [3, 26]. The primary symptom associated with the disease is extreme pruritus, which occurs over 70 % of the time [25]. The lesions are more common in diabetics with end-stage renal disease (ESRD) who are undergoing hemodialysis (HD), with a frequency of 5–10 % in this population [6]. APD is worsened by the Köbner effect [25]. The lesions can resolve on their own if scratching and further trauma are avoided, although steroids (topical or systemic), retinoids, allopurinol, and phototherapy have all been used for healing and symptomatic control of their pruritus [6].

Eruptive Xanthomas

Eruptive xanthomas are a collection of yellow, rapidly developing papules with an erythematous halo commonly located on the extensor surface of the extremities (Fig. 2.6) [3, 10]. Histologically they appear as well circumscribed infiltrate of foam cells, histiocytes, and fat cells within the dermis [10, 27]. They are composed entirely of triglycerides, not cholesterol esters, thus differing from most other types of xanthomas [6]. The lesions have been clearly demonstrated to be associated with hypertriglyceridemia as well as hyperglycemia, and can show rapid and complete improvement with systemic glycemic control [3, 6].

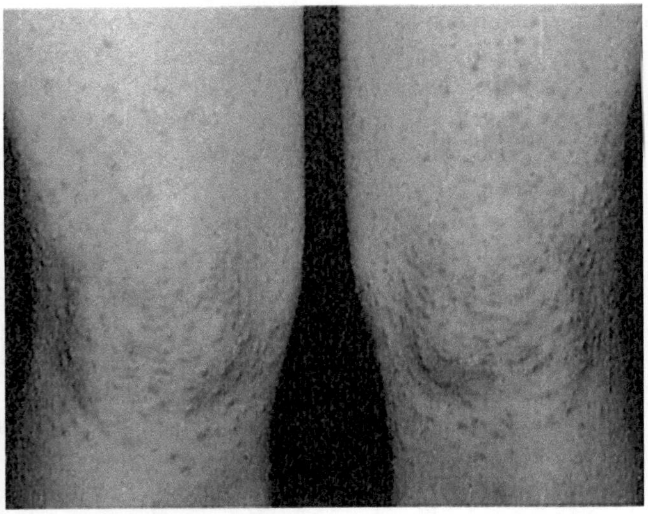

Fig. 2.6 Hundreds of small papules consistent with eruptive xanthoma. Source: Perez M, Kohn S. "Cutaneous Manifestations of Diabetes Mellitus." Journal of the American Academy of Dermatology. 1994 Apr 1; 30(4):519

Cutaneous Infections

Dermatologic infections occur in 20–50 % of diabetic patients, particularly in type II diabetics and those with poor glycemic control [10, 14]. Candidal and dermatophyte infections can oftentimes be the first sign of undiagnosed diabetes [10]. Additionally, bacterial infections in diabetics such as impetigo, folliculitis, carbuncles, furuncles, ecthyma, erythrasma, and erysipelas are more common and more severe in diabetic patients, as are more severe bacterial or fungal infections such as necrotizing fasciitis, malignant otitis externa, and rhinocerebral mucormycosis [10, 14]. It is imperative to diagnose and treat these infections early to prevent life-threatening consequences.

Amyloidosis

Amyloidosis is the syndrome of diseases caused by extracellular deposition of amyloid, a group of proteins that form characteristic fibrillary aggregates which, when deposited, interfere with normal tissue structure and function [28–30]. The clinical significance of the deposition varies considerably, ranging from asymptomatic to multiorgan failure (including CKD) [29, 30]. The nature and progression of disease partly relates to the type of protein, or amyloid, deposited—there are approximately 25 proteins currently known to cause amyloidosis, all of which are pathogenic variations of normal precursor proteins [28, 29]. Etiology is thought to be secondary to malignancy, chronic inflammation, or mutation with can occur either idiopathically, hereditarily, with advanced age, or with myeloma [28, 29, 31].

Cutaneous manifestations of the disease can be divided into two categories: primary localized cutaneous amyloidosis (PLCA) and systemic amyloidosis with cutaneous involvement [28] (Table 2.2). Both subtypes involve the deposition of amyloid into the extracellular space of the dermis; however, cutaneous amyloidosis is limited while systemic amyloidosis affects organ systems outside of the skin, resulting in an obvious discrepancy between the severity and prognostic indices of both diagnoses [28].

Physiology/Pathogenesis

Amyloidosis is a protein folding disorder resulting from the biological failure of our cells to degrade structurally abnormal proteins. These nonfunctional proteins aggregate to form insoluble amyloid fibrils [32]. The process by which amyloid fibrils form is poorly understood, but is thought to relate to abnormalities in proteolytic cleavage, the stability of a native protein (kinetic or thermodynamic), production of a conformationally altered protein, or oversecretion of a protein [32, 33].

Table 2.2 Differences between primary localized cutaneous and systemic amyloidosis

	Primary localized cutaneous amyloid	Systemic amyloid with cutaneous manifestations
Amyloid present	AK; AL with nodular amyloid	Non-AK amyloid, can be multiple
Appearance	Macular amyloidosis: Poorly delineated brownish patches or linear rippling of the skin with grayish-brown macules Lichen amyloidosis: Pruritic discrete, firm, hyperkeratotic, dome-shaped, skin colored to brownish papules	Pruritic waxy translucent papulonodular masses
Deposit location	Superficial; dermal papillae and subpapillary layers	Deep; dermal papillae, subpapillary layers, stratum reticular, subcutis, dermal appendages, blood vessels
Epidermal changes	Hyperkeratosis, irregular acanthosis with thinning of the rete ridges, and expansion of the papillae	None

The ultimate product of aggregated proteins is an amyloid fibril—a straight, nonbranching fibril that is 2–10 nm in diameter, made of a core structure composed of antiparallel beta-strands of polypeptide chains lying perpendicular to the long axis of the fibril [29, 32]. The amyloid fibrils congregate, depositing into tissues and disrupting normal architecture, causing its varied pathologic sequelae. Unfortunately, the factors that govern the anatomical distribution, rate of onset and progression, and variation amongst individuals with the same precursor proteins have not been elucidated [33].

The type of protein causing cutaneous disease in systemic verses local amyloidosis differs. The most common amyloid fibril precursor in PLCA is the amyloid keratin protein, AK, which is produced from damaged basilar keratinocytes [31, 34]. The only type of PLCA that is not the result of AK is nodular cutaneous amyloidosis, which is thought to result from a light chain protein produced by local plasma cells [34–36]. Cutaneous lesions in systemic amyloid are composed of the protein which is causing the diffuse disease [31]. For instance, in primary amyloidosis caused by amyloid light chain (AL) protein, immunoglobulin light chains are overproduced secondary to immunoglobulin dyscrasias, and the protein is deposited systemically, including within the dermis. In systemic amyloidosis, multiple types of amyloid can be present in the same lesion [31].

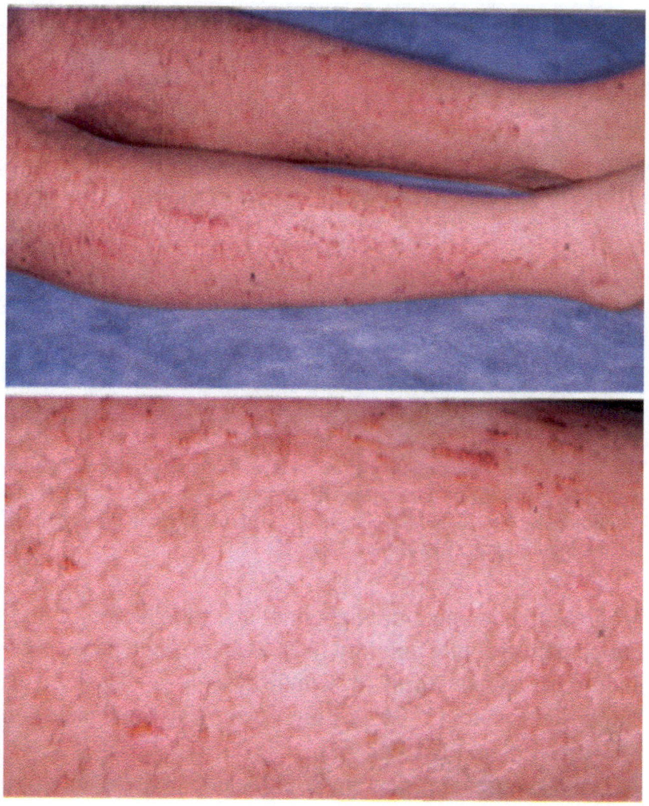

Fig. 2.7 These pruritic hyperpigmented papules/plaques on the bilateral shins demonstrate lichen amyloidosis. Source: Fernandez-Flores, A. "Cutaneous Amyloidosis: A Concept Review." The American Journal of Dermatopathology. 2012 Feb 1; 34(1):1

Clinical

Primary cutaneous amyloid is rare in the USA; it occurs most commonly in Southeast Asia and parts of South America [34, 35]. It is generally a chronic disorder, most commonly affecting the extensor tibial surface and forearms (although it has also been noted less frequently in the trunk, neck, and face) [35]. It can be primary or secondary to other cutaneous conditions such as skin tumors, nevi, seborrheic keratosis, actinic keratosis, Bowen disease, inflammation, mycosis fungoides, or psoralen plus ultraviolet A (PUVA) treatment [31]. The pathophysiology and significance of secondary cutaneous amyloid is unclear [37].

PCLA can be divided into multiple subtypes based on clinical appearance. The most common two are lichen amyloidosus (LA) and macular amyloidosis (MA), which are thought to exist on a spectrum. LA presents as discrete, firm, hyperkeratotic, dome-shaped, skin colored to brownish papules (Fig. 2.7) [35, 38]. The lesions are extremely pruritic, and can be associated with ulceration or purpura [35]. MA clinically appears as poorly delineated brownish patches or linear rippling of the skin with grayish-brown macules (Fig. 2.8) [35]. The lesions are less pruritic than in LA and can often go undetected, although later they can

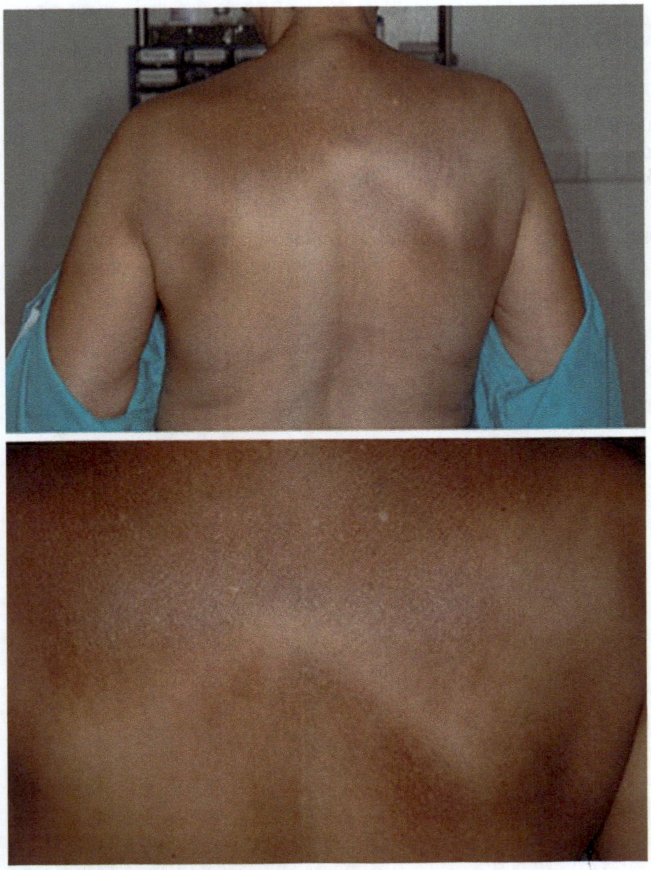

Fig. 2.8 Macular cutaneous amyloidosis on the back, which is its most common distribution. Source: Fernandez-Flores, A. "Cutaneous Amyloidosis: A Concept Review." The American Journal of Dermatopathology. 2012 Feb 1; 34(1):1

progress to become more lichenoid due to irritation or continued deposition of amyloid [35]. MA can sometimes present in a papular form, in which case it is classified as "biphasic amyloid," suggesting a clinical amalgamation between MA and LA [34, 35].

Less common types of amyloid include nodular amyloid, anosacral amyloid, bullous amyloid, poikiloderma-like amyloid, and vitilliginous amyloid [35]. Nodular amyloidosis, presenting as various colored nodules on the face, extremities, trunk, or genitalia, is unique in that it is composed of AL produced by local plasma cells. While rare, 7–50 % of cases progress to cause systemic disease, making appropriate diagnostic techniques essential [34, 35, 39].

Systemic amyloid differs significantly from cutaneous amyloidosis in its etiology and presentation. It can be associated with certain familial diseases, such as Muckle–Wells syndrome, Schnitzler syndrome, or familial Mediterranean fever. It also can be a reactive process to a systemic disorder, and has been found in such conditions as leprosy, cutaneous tuberculosis, psoriasis, discoid lupus erythematosus, hidradenitis suppurativa, dystrophic epidermolysis bullosa, and burns [31]. Patients with systemic amyloid may manifest nonspecific symptoms such as anorrhexia, weight loss, fatigue and weakness. Cutaneously the disease presents as waxy translucent papulonodular masses which are nonpruritic and localized at mucocutaneous junctions [31]. Macroglossia, alopecia, cutis laxa, or bullae can be present. Commonly there are signs of increased bleeding with purpura, periorbital ecchymosis, and petechiae, as systemic amyloid has been found to affect the clotting system [31]. One rare manifestation of systemic amyloid occurs is amyloid elastosis, when the amyloid deposits around elastic fibers causing a sclerodermatous facial appearance with pseudoxanthoma elasticum-like appearance of the neck, Raynaud phenomenon, nephrotic syndrome, and blood vessel thrombosis [31].

Differential Diagnosis

The differential diagnosis of cutaneous amyloidosis is broad, including lichen simplex chronicus, lichen planus, post inflammatory hyperpigmentation, prurigo nodularis, keratosis pilaris, papular mucinosis, colloid millium, and solar elastosis [35, 38]. The differential diagnosis for systemic amyloidosis depends on the syndrome involved.

Work Up

Work up of cutaneous amyloid should involve a full history and physical examination as well as biopsy of the lesion, with appropriate staining and immunohistochemistry. Other tests which should be performed on the serum and urine include a complete blood count, basic metabolic panel, serum protein electrophoresis, urine protein electrophoresis, 24 h urine creatinine clearance and serum immunoglobulins [40]. Biopsy of fat pads should be performed to rule out extracutaneous manifestations of disease [40].

Histology

Amyloid fibrils are visualized under light microscopy as protein aggregates. Both systemic and local forms are best known for showing apple green birefringence when stained with Congo red and viewed under polarized light (Fig. 2.9). However, some normal tissue such as collagen fibers and cytoskeletal proteins as well as certain pathologic tissues can react similarly to the dye, decreasing specificity [31, 32, 41]. Other stains that can be used include sirius red and thioflavin-T, although both have certain disadvantages, making Congo red the preferred agent [31]. To differentiate PLCA from systemic amyloid with cutaneous findings, it is important to look at the distribution of amyloid deposits within the skin. Light microscopy of PLCA demonstrates a superficial

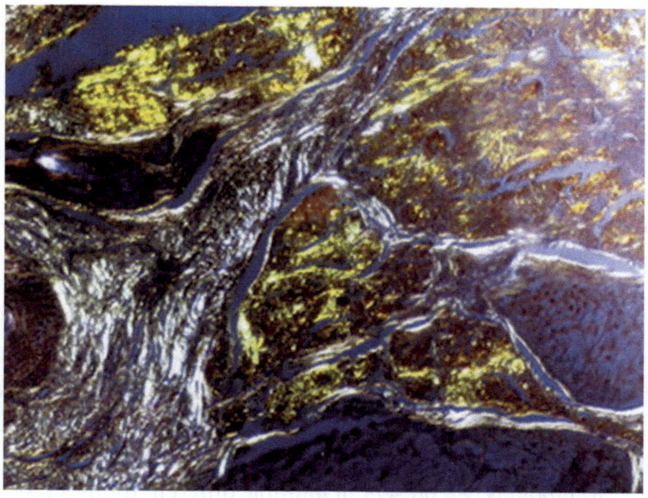

Fig. 2.9 An example of congophilia with apple-green birefringence classic for amyloidosis. Source: Fernandez-Flores, A. "Cutaneous Amyloidosis: A Concept Review." The American Journal of Dermatopathology. 2012 Feb 1; 34(1):1

infiltrate into the dermal papillae and subpapillary layers [28, 42]. The epidermis can demonstrate hyperkeratosis, irregular acanthosis with thinning of the rete ridges, and expansion of the papillae with amyloid [42]. Early lesions appear faintly eosinophilic with amorphous bundles of amyloid group in papillae, while advanced lesions showed extensive deposition [42]. In systemic amyloidosis with cutaneous involvement, deposits are distributed much deeper, in the papillae and subpapillary layers but also in the stratum reticulare, subcutis, dermal appendages, and blood vessels [28, 42]. There are rarely epidermal changes [42].

Laboratory Abnormalities

Local protein production is not detected systemically, and therefore PCLA does not demonstrate laboratory abnormalities in the serum or urine. This differs from systemic amyloidosis, where a monoclonal protein is released into the serum and a protein spike can be detected. Other laboratory abnormalities in systemic disease differ based on the distribution of amyloid deposits [34].

Imaging Studies

No imaging studies are necessary for PLCA. Specific imaging may be necessary in systemic amyloidosis; however, it must be targeted to symptomatology as it is otherwise nonspecific. While more specific methods of detecting deposits using nuclear imaging are being developed, radiotracers are only used rarely at present, specifically for amyloid associated Alzheimer disease [43].

Treatment

Treatment of cutaneous amyloid is inadequate and understudied. Initial management of PLCA includes topical steroids (under occlusion) or intralesional steroids with an oral anti-pruritic agent to combat progression of disease via rubbing. When that is ineffective, second line therapies vary. Case reports and small studies show PUVA and ultraviolet B (UVB) phototherapy to be effective, and newer studies have shown laser therapies such as pulsed dye laser treatment, carbon dioxide laser evaporation, and fractional ablative laser therapy to decrease disease burden [28, 44]. Dimethylsulfoxide (DMSO) showed promise in in vitro studies and was therefore used translationally, but in vivo analysis saw little to no effect [28, 45]. Oral retinoids have been studied in small case series', demonstrating mild to significant improvement in LA and biphasic amyloid when administered in doses of 0.5–1 mg/kg/day for 6 months [28, 46]. A case report looking at the effect of low dose oral cyclophosphamide for a similar time period also showed promising results [47]. Neither therapy has been studied in MA. Surgical therapies have also evolved to treat lesions unaffected by conservative management. Types of surgical methods used include dermabrasion, excision and skin grafting, shave excision, currettage, and cautery [28].

Treatment of systemic amyloidosis with cutaneous involvement varies based on the type of amyloid present and the etiology of disease. Management should be determined by a team of expert physicians, and therapy is geared towards prevention of disease progression by treating the potential source, such as inflammation or malignancy [28].

Atherosclerosis

Like DM, hyperlipidemia is becoming increasingly prevalent in our society. It is linked with atherosclerosis—the buildup of plaque in arteries—which in turn causes coronary artery disease, peripheral artery disease (PAD), and CKD. Hyperlipidemia can be primary (genetic, transmitted by autosomal dominant or recessive genes) or secondary (acquired, combined genetic and environmental factors), with variable types of lipoprotein affected, age of onset, and symptomatology [48, 49]. While cutaneous manifestations are less common than in DM or amyloid, they can be the first sign of disease and should be fully investigated. The two most common cutaneous findings associated with atherosclerosis and hyperlipidemia are critical leg ischemia (CLI, associated with ulceration and gangrene) and xanthomas, localized collections of lipid containing foam cells within the dermis or connective tissue [49, 50].

Table 2.3 Classification of xanthomas

	Appearance	Associated condition
Palpebrarum	Soft macules bilaterally and symmetrically on eyelid	Primary biliary cirrhosis
Planum	Yellow macules/plaques	
Palmar	Flat plaques within palmar crease	Primary biliary cirrhosis
Tendinous	Lipid within tendons, firm nodules disconnected to overlying skin	Primary familial hypercholesterolemia
Tuberous	Painless nodules over areas or pressure (knees, elbows, buttocks)	Primary familial hypercholesterolemia
Eruptive	Small rapidly developing papules	Diabetes, hypertriglyceridemia

Physiology/Pathogenesis

CLI due to PAD is a serious consequence of hyperlipidemia and atherosclerosis. It develops secondary to plaque buildup in the lower extremities, with progressive occlusive disease. Distal perfusion pressures plummet, with decreased microcirculation and nutritional distribution. Ischemic ulceration or gangrene soon develop, and can be chronic and unrelenting [51].

Xanthomas, while less morbid, can be an important harbinger of disease. The pathogenesis of xanthoma formation is similar to the mechanism by which atherosclerosis develops. Macrophages phagocytose cholesterol, forming immobile cholesterol-ester rich foam cells that are deposited in vascular endothelium (in atherosclerosis formation) or the dermis/tendons (for xanthoma formation) [50, 52]. This process occurs partly due to increased luminal osmosis of low density lipoprotein (LDL) into the subendothelial/dermal space as well as through macrophage recruitment to these areas. The LDL then undergoes oxidation, making it a recognizable target for macrophage phagocytosis [53]. Recent studies show a distinct population of normolipemic xanthomatosis thought to be linked to low high density lipoprotein and alteration in levels of specific apolipoproteins [54, 55]. Patients with histiocyte proliferation, abnormal uptake of lipoproteins by macrophages, local vascular leakage of lipoproteins, and abnormally increased tissue synthesis of lipids may also have xanthomas without dyslipidemia [49, 54]. Despite normal lipid levels, these patients are also at increased risk for atherosclerotic and cardiac disease, as xanthomas are a risk factor irrespective of lipid levels [55].

Clinical

PAD is a common and unfortunate complication of atherosclerosis, affecting up to 12 million Americans, with increased prevalence in the elderly [56]. Major risk factors include age over 40, DM, and cigarette smoking [57]. The classic symptom is intermittent claudication (pain with exertion), which progresses with severity of disease into pain at rest [51]. Ulceration occurs with worsening occlusive disease, appearing as sharply demarcated lesions with a gray or black base that can be covered with necrotic debris. The lesions are distributed in areas of pressure or distally, such as over the malleoli or toes. Surrounding skin often appears shiny with loss of hair, atrophic skin, and brittle nails [58]. Peripheral pulses are usually weak or absent [56].

Xanthomas can present in multiple different forms, classified as palpebrarum, planum, tendinous, palmar, tuberous, or eruptive [48] (Table 2.3). Planar xanthomas are the most common. They appear as yellow macules or plaques and can be further categorized into three types, xanthelasma palpebrarum (XP), xanthoma striatum palmare, and diffuse plane xanthomas. XP are the most common, appearing as soft macules that are located on the eyelid, usually bilaterally and symmetrically [49, 50, 55]. Studies indicate a significant variability in the prevalence of atherosclerotic vascular or heart disease in patients with XP, ranging from 15 % to as high as 69 % [54]. Xanthoma striatum palmare are flat lesions within the palmar crease that are closely associated with abnormal lipid levels as well as primary biliary cirrhosis, while diffuse plan xanthomas are large plaques associated with multiple myeloma [48, 49]. Tuberous and tendinous xanthomas are more commonly seen in patients with primary, familial hypercholesterolemia and are associated with an extremely high incidence of atherosclerotic disease [49, 50]. Tendinous xanthomas are characterized by diffuse infiltration of lipid within tendons, causing smooth firm nodules disconnected to the overlying skin. They are predominantly located on the Achilles tendon but also appear on extensor surfaces of the elbows, knees, and hands [48, 49]. Tuberous xanthomas are painless small, soft, yellow red or flesh colored papules that are usually located on extensor surfaces of the knees, elbows, or buttocks. Unlike tendinous xanthomas, lipid in tuberous disease deposits within the dermis itself [48]. As previously mentioned, eruptive xanthomas are small, quickly developing collections of yellow papules that are unique in their specific association with elevated triglyceride levels and DM [49, 50].

Differential Diagnosis

Arterial ulceration can be confused with other causes of leg ulceration, such as venous stasis disease, diabetic or neuropathic ulceration. They can be distinguished based on location, appearance, and comorbid symptoms [58].

Work Up

The ankle-brachial index (ABI) is the most common tool used to diagnose PAD. Claudication occurs at levels between 0.5 and 0.9 and ulceration/necrosis at levels less than 0.5 [59]. The gold standard for diagnosis is contrast arteriography, a minimally invasive procedure that is only routinely used for patients undergoing surgical or percutaneous intervention [59]. Biopsies do not routinely need to be performed; however, they may be warranted to rule out malignancy or vasculitis if there is no improvement within 3 months of treatment [58].

Xanthomas do not routinely require workup, but serum lipid panel may be recommended based on the patient and xanthoma characteristics.

Histology

Biopsies of persistent ischemic ulcers should only be performed to rule out malignant transformation [58, 60]. Histologically these ulcers are characterized by thickening of the blood vessel walls of the deep plexus due to a proliferation of endothelial cells or smooth muscle cells [60].

Xanthelomas are histologically identified by foamy histiocytes full of lipid vacuoles and cholesterol crystals located within the dermis or tendon sheath [55].

Laboratory Abnormalities

Laboratory abnormalities in patients with PAD and CLI generally relate to the potential underlying comorbidities, including DM and hyperlipidemia. Hyperlipidemia is also the predominant laboratory abnormality associated with xanthomas.

Imaging Studies

Imaging studies other than the diagnostic studies mentioned above are only necessary for PAD when there is a concern for osteomyelitis secondary to ulceration. In that case, bone scan, computed tomography (CT) scan, gallium scan, or magnetic resonance imaging (MRI) can be used to detect the level of invasion and disease [58].

Imaging studies are not necessary for diagnosis or treatment of most xanthomas, but can be used to visualize and diagnose tendinous xanthomas. CT, ultrasound, and MRI can all be performed for better visualization of tendon xanthomas [61].

Treatment

Treatment of PAD and CLI involves management of atherosclerosis to prevent progression as well as symptom control, wound healing, and possible endovascular or surgical intervention. Hyperlipidemia and diabetes should be managed appropriately with pharmacologic intervention, diet and exercise; starting a lipid-lowering agent alone can prevent progression of disease. Smoking cessation is also imperative [57, 59, 62]. Symptom management of PAD should initially involve exercise therapy, and intensive exercise programs have been demonstrated to increase maximum walking capacity [57]. Pharmacologic agents such as pentoxifylline, a methylxanthine derivative that affects red blood cell deformability and decreases fibrinogen concentrations, and cilostazol, a phosphodiesterase inhibitor, have also been used. Both agents have been demonstrated to increase walking distance when compared to a placebo (with increased efficacy of cilostazol), but neither agent has been found to be significantly disease altering [57, 59]. Once CLI has developed, there are fewer pharmacologic agents and more non-pharmacologic interventions. Wound care is a primary tenet of treatment, and debridement or vacuum assisted closure may be necessary to promote healing [57]. Pharmacologically, infused and oral prostacyclins and prostaglandins have been used; however, their effectiveness has not been adequately demonstrated, and at present they are not widely recommended [56, 63]. Some non-surgical therapies for CLI that are currently being explored include intermittent pneumatic compression, spinal cord stimulation and lumbar sympathectomy. While promising and proven better than medical management, few of these therapies are widely used [63]. Revascularization with surgical or endovascular therapy is often necessary in patients with chronic ulceration to prevent amputation. One series demonstrated an amputation rate of up to 43 % within 12 months in patients with arterial insufficiency and full thickness ulcers who did not undergo surgical revascularization. Unfortunately, one intervention is often insufficient; these patients can require multiple procedures and few will have resolution of disease [63].

Treatment of xanthomas is closely linked to cholesterol management, with diet adjustment and initiation of fibrates, statins, bile acid-binding resins, probucol, or nicotinic acid [50, 58]. While eruptive xanthomas generally resolve within weeks of systemic cholesterol treatment, tuberous xanthomas can take months and tendinous xanthomas can take years to improve, and may be permanent [49]. Xanthelasmas also tend to progress and coalesce, becoming permanent. Permanent xanthomas can be removed via topical trichloroacetic acid, laser treatment, electrodesiccation, or excision [50].

References

1. About Chronic Kidney Disease. 2013 [cited 2013 April 9th 2013]; Available from: http://www.kidney.org/kidneydisease/aboutckd.cfm
2. Timshina DK, Thappa DM, Agrawal A. A clinical study of dermatoses in diabetes to establish its markers. Indian J Dermatol. 2012;57(1):20–5.
3. Levy L, Zeichner JA. Dermatologic manifestation of diabetes. J Diabetes. 2012;4(1):68–76. Epub 2011/08/19.
4. Berlanga-Acosta JS, Schultz G, Lopez-Mola E, Guillen-Nieto G, Garcia-Siverio M, Herrera-Martinez L. Glucose toxic effects on granulation tissue productive cells: the diabetics' impaired healing. BioMed Res Int. 2013;2013:256043.
5. Levigne DT, Tobalem M, Modarressi A, Pittet-Cuenod B. Hyperglycemia increases susceptibility to ischemic necrosis. BioMed Res Int. 2013;2013:490964.
6. Namazi MR, Yosipovitch G. Diabetes mellitus. In: Callen JP, Jorizzo JL, et al., editors. Dermatological signs of internal disease. 4th ed. China: Elsevier Inc.; 2009. p. 189–209.
7. Ferringer T, Miller III F. Cutaneous manifestations of diabetes mellitus. Dermatol Clin. 2002;20(3):483–92.
8. Brugler A, Thompson S, Turner S, Ngo B, Rendell M. Skin blood flow abnormalities in diabetic dermopathy. J Am Acad Dermatol. 2011;65(3):559–63. Epub 2011/05/03.
9. McCash S, Emanuel PO. Defining diabetic dermopathy. J Dermatol. 2011;38(10):988–92. Epub 2011/07/19.
10. Van Hattem S, Bootsma AH, Thio HB. Skin manifestations of diabetes. Cleve Clin J Med. 2008;75(11):772. 4, 6–7 passim. Epub 2008/12/17.
11. Hermanns-Le T, Scheen A, Pierard GE. Acanthosis nigricans associated with insulin resistance: pathophysiology and management. Am J Clin Dermatol. 2004;5(3):199–203. Epub 2004/06/10.
12. Santoro N, Amato A, Grandone A, Brienza C, Savarese P, Tartaglione N, et al. Predicting metabolic syndrome in obese children and adolescents: look, measure and ask. Obes Facts. 2013;6(1):48–56. Epub 2013/02/23.
13. Yosipovitch G, DeVore A, Dawn A. Obesity and the skin: skin physiology and skin manifestations of obesity. J Am Acad Dermatol. 2007;56(6):901–16. quiz 17–20. Epub 2007/05/17.
14. Ahmed I, Goldstein B. Diabetes mellitus. Clin Dermatol. 2006;24(4):237–46.
15. Maharshak N, Shapiro J, Trau H. Carotenoderma—a review of the current literature. Int J Dermatol. 2003;42(3):178–81. Epub 2003/03/26.
16. Sehgal VN, Srivastava G, Aggarwal AK, Gupta M, Bhattacharya SN, Verma P. Noninsulin-dependent, type II diabetes mellitus-related dermatoses: part II. Skinmed. 2011;9(5):302–8. Epub 2011/12/15.
17. Apelqvist J. Diagnostics and treatment of the diabetic foot. Endocrine. 2012;41(3):384–97. Epub 2012/03/01.
18. Singh N, Armstrong DG, Lipsky BA. Preventing foot ulcers in patients with diabetes. JAMA. 2005;293(2):217–28. Epub 2005/01/13.
19. Bakos RM, Cartell A, Bakos L. Dermatoscopy of early-onset necrobiosis lipoidica. J Am Acad Dermatol. 2012;66(4):e143–4. Epub 2012/03/17.
20. Korber A, Dissemond J. Necrobiosis lipoidica diabeticorum. CMAJ. 2007;177(12):1498. Epub 2007/12/07.
21. Basarab T, Munn SE, McGrath J, Russell Jones R. Bullosis diabeticorum. A case report and literature review. Clin Exp Dermatol. 1995;20(3):218–20. Epub 1995/05/01.
22. Lewerenz V, Ruzicka T. Scleredema adultorum associated with type 2 diabetes mellitus: a report of three cases. J Eur Acad Dermatol Venereol. 2007;21(4):560–1. Epub 2007/03/22.
23. Pitukcheewanont P, Bali B, Somanunt S, Reiff A. Scleroderma-like skin changes not involving the hand in a prepubertal male with type I diabetes mellitus: a case report. Dermatoendocrinol. 2011;3(4):230–2. Epub 2012/01/20.
24. Yosipovitch G, Loh KC, Hock OB. Medical pearl: scleroderma-like skin changes in patients with diabetes mellitus. J Am Acad Dermatol. 2003;49(1):109–11. Epub 2003/07/02.
25. Saray Y, Seckin D, Bilezikci B. Acquired perforating dermatosis: clinicopathological features in twenty-two cases. J Eur Acad Dermatol Venereol. 2006;20(6):679–88. Epub 2006/07/14.
26. Karpouzis A, Giatromanolaki A, Sivridis E, Kouskoukis C. Acquired reactive perforating collagenosis: current status. J Dermatol. 2010; 37(7):585–92. Epub 2010/07/16.
27. Roenigk Jr HH, Fowler-Bergfeld W. Eruptive xanthoma. Arch Dermatol. 1969;99(1):125. Epub 1969/01/01.
28. Schreml S, Szeimies RM, Vogt T, Landthaler M, Schroeder J, Babilas P. Cutaneous amyloidoses and systemic amyloidoses with cutaneous involvement. Eur J Dermatol. 2010;20(2):152–60.
29. Pinney JH, Hawkins PN. Amyloidosis. Ann Clin Biochem. 2012;49(Pt 3):229–41. Epub 2012/03/10.
30. Gillmore JD, Hawkins PN, Pepys MB. Amyloidosis: a review of recent diagnostic and therapeutic developments. Br J Haematol. 1997;99(2):245–56.
31. Fernandez-Flores A. Cutaneous amyloidosis: a concept review. Am J Dermatopathol. 2012;34(1):1–14. quiz 5–7. Epub 2012/01/20.
32. Blancas-Mejia LM, Ramirez-Alvarado M. Systemic amyloidoses. Annu Rev Biochem. 2013;82:745–74. Epub 2013/03/05.
33. Gillmore JD, Hawkins PN. Drug insight: emerging therapies for amyloidosis. Nat Clin Pract Nephrol. 2006;2(5):263–70.
34. Piette WW. Dysproteinemias, plasma cell disorders, and amyloidosis. In: Callen JP, Jorizzo JL, et al., editors. Dermatological signs of internal disease. 4th ed. China: Elsevier; 2009.
35. Wang WJ. Clinical features of cutaneous amyloidoses. Clin Dermatol. 1990;8(2):13–9. Epub 1990/04/01.
36. Piette WW. Cutaneous manifestations of macrophage/dendritic cell proliferative. In: Callen JP, Jorizzo JL, et al., editors. Dermatological signs of internal disease. 4th ed. China: Elsevier Inc.; 2009. p. 149–60.
37. Wang WJ, Huang JY, Wong CK, Chang YT. A study of secondary cutaneous amyloidosis in basal cell carcinoma in Chinese patients: lack of correlation with bcl-2 or p53 protein expression. Arch Dermatol Res. 2000;292(8):379–83. Epub 2000/09/20.
38. Chuang YY, Lee DD, Lin CS, Chang YJ, Tanaka M, Chang YT, et al. Characteristic dermoscopic features of primary cutaneous amyloidosis: a study of 35 cases. Br J Dermatol. 2012;167(3):548–54. Epub 2012/05/29.
39. Lee DY, Kim YJ, Lee JY, Kim MK, Yoon TY. Primary localized cutaneous nodular amyloidosis following local trauma. Ann Dermatol. 2011;23(4):515–8. Epub 2011/12/08.
40. Borowicz J, Gillespie M, Miller R. Cutaneous amyloidosis. Skinmed. 2011;9(2):96–100. quiz 1. Epub 2011/05/10.
41. Khurana R, Uversky VN, Nielsen L, Fink AL. Is Congo red an amyloid-specific dye? J Biol Chem. 2001;276(25):22715–21. Epub 2001/06/19.
42. Li WM. Histopathology of primary cutaneous amyloidoses and systemic amyloidosis. Clin Dermatol. 1990;8(2):30–5. Epub 1990/04/01.
43. Chen W, Dilsizian V. Molecular imaging of amyloidosis: will the heart be the next target after the brain? Curr Cardiol Rep. 2012;14(2):226–33. Epub 2011/12/24.
44. Anitha B, Mysore V. Lichen amyloidosis: novel treatment with fractional ablative 2,940 nm erbium: YAG laser treatment. J Cutan Aesthet Surg. 2012;5(2):141–3. Epub 2012/10/13.
45. Breathnach SM. The cutaneous amyloidoses. Pathogenesis and therapy. Arch Dermatol. 1985;121(4):470–5. Epub 1985/04/01.
46. Hernandez-Nunez A, Dauden E, Moreno de Vega MJ, Fraga J, Aragues M, Garcia-Diez A. Widespread biphasic amyloidosis:

response to acitretin. Clin Exp Dermatol. 2001;26(3):256–9. Epub 2001/06/26.
47. Das J, Gogoi RK. Treatment of primary localised cutaneous amyloidosis with cyclophosphamide. Indian J Dermatol Venereol Leprol. 2003;69(2):163–4. Epub 2007/07/24.
48. Chan HL. Cutaneous manifestations of cardiac diseases. Singapore Med J. 1990;31(5):480–5. Epub 1990/10/01.
49. Taylor SLG, Greer KE, Jorizzo JL. Lipids. In: Callen JP, Jorizzo JL, et al., editors. Dermatological manifestations of internal disease. 4th ed. China: Elsevier; 2009.
50. Dwivedi S, Jhamb R. Cutaneous markers of coronary artery disease. World J Cardiol. 2010;2(9):262–9. Epub 2010/12/17.
51. Becker F, Robert-Ebadi H, Ricco JB, Setacci C, Cao P, de Donato G, et al. Chapter I: Definitions, epidemiology, clinical presentation and prognosis. Eur J Vasc Endovasc Surg. 2011;42 Suppl 2:S4–12. Epub 2011/12/30.
52. Pietroleonardo L, Ruzicka T. Skin manifestations in familial heterozygous hypercholesterolemia. Acta Dermatovenerol Alp Panonica Adriat. 2009;18(4):183–7. Epub 2010/01/01.
53. Schwartz CJ, Valente AJ, Sprague EA, Kelley JL, Nerem RM. The pathogenesis of atherosclerosis: an overview. Clin Cardiol. 1991;14(2 Suppl 1):I1–16. Epub 1991/02/01.
54. Bergman R. Xanthelasma palpebrarum and risk of atherosclerosis. Int J Dermatol. 1998;37(5):343–5. Epub 1998/06/10.
55. Pandhi D, Gupta P, Singal A, Tondon A, Sharma S, Madhu SV. Xanthelasma palpebrarum: a marker of premature atherosclerosis (risk of atherosclerosis in xanthelasma). Postgrad Med J. 2012;88(1038):198–204. Epub 2012/03/01.
56. Federman DG, Kravetz JD. Peripheral arterial disease: diagnosis, treatment, and systemic implications. Clin Dermatol. 2007;25(1):93–100. Epub 2007/02/06.
57. Hiatt WR. Medical treatment of peripheral arterial disease and claudication. N Engl J Med. 2001;344(21):1608–21. Epub 2001/05/24.
58. Davis MDP. Leg ulceration. In: Callen JP, Jorizzo JL, et al., editors. Dermatological signs of internal disease. 4th ed. China: Elsevier Inc.; 2009. p. 381–400.
59. Ouriel K. Peripheral arterial disease. Lancet. 2001;358(9289):1257–64. Epub 2001/10/25.
60. Shai A, Maibach HI. Wound healing and ulcers of the skin: diagnosis and therapy. Berlin: Springer; 2005.
61. Liem MS, Leuven JA, Bloem JL, Schipper J. Magnetic resonance imaging of Achilles tendon xanthomas in familial hypercholesterolemia. Skeletal Radiol. 1992;21(7):453–7. Epub 1992/01/01.
62. Blankenhorn DH, Azen SP, Crawford DW, Nessim SA, Sanmarco ME, Selzer RH, et al. Effects of colestipol-niacin therapy on human femoral atherosclerosis. Circulation. 1991;83(2):438–47. Epub 1991/02/01.
63. Slovut DP, Sullivan TM. Critical limb ischemia: medical and surgical management. Vasc Med. 2008;13(3):281–91. Epub 2008/08/09.

Hepatitis Viruses

3

Ivy I. Norris and Cindy England Owen

Patients with glomerulonephritis secondary to hepatitis C virus/hepatitis B virus (HCV/HBV) infections may have dermatologic findings that are associated with the primary infections. This chapter on the cutaneous findings related to hepatitis viruses is intended to be an easily accessible reference for images, descriptions, and treatment guidelines surrounding these conditions beneficial to the primary care providers, nephrologists, and other health care providers who manage and follow these patients on a regular basis.

Dermatologic Findings in Acute Hepatitis and Chronic Hepatitis B Infection

While the majority of the skin manifestations of hepatitis infection are associated with chronic disease, there are several skin findings which have been linked more directly to acute HBV and/or HCV infection. These include urticaria, serum-sickness like syndrome, erythema nodosum, erythema multiforme, and pruritus, among others [1].

Polyarteritis Nodosa

Polyarteritis nodosa (PAN) is a systemic necrotizing vasculitis affecting small and medium-sized blood vessels. Its relation with the HBV has been well established as approximately 50 % of PAN patients are seropositive for hepatitis B surface antigen (HBsAg) with estimates as high as 65 % in hyperendemic regions [2, 3], making it one of the more common and severe extrahepatic complications of hepatitis B infection. The relationship between PAN and HCV is less salient; however, it still deserves mention as 5–13 % of PAN cases are attributable to hepatitis C infection [4].

Patients usually develop symptoms of HBV-associated PAN within weeks to months of acute HBV infection. Patients present with symptoms of weight loss, fatigue, fever, weakness, abdominal pain, and arthralgia. Clinical signs include hypertension, renal insufficiency, neurologic dysfunction, and skin disease. About 50 % of patients with PAN present with cutaneous disease. Skin manifestations may include tender erythematous nodules, palpable purpura, livedo reticularis, and ulceration, most commonly involving the lower extremities (see Fig. 3.1). Diagnosis can sometimes be made by skin biopsy but often requires a deep biopsy to sample an affected medium-sized artery. PAN is typically antineutrophil cytoplasmic antibody (ANCA) negative, unlike many other systemic vasculitides.

Traditionally, treatment of PAN aimed at inducing remission and decreasing the risk of relapse has included corticosteroids, plasma exchange, and immunosuppressant medications such as cyclophosphamide. The benefits of immunosuppressive medications must be weighed against the cost of potentially amplified hepatitis viral replication; however, since HBV therapy is more effective in the absence of PAN, it is recognized that this transient increase in viral replication during treatment for PAN is acceptable when immediately followed by interferon therapy for the HBV. Long-term survival has been shown to be highest in patients treated with a regimen of steroids, plasma exchange and cyclophosphamide rather than steroids and plasma exchange alone [3].

It is important to note that neither the severity of PAN nor prognosis in these patients is affected by the severity of the coexistent hepatitis. Instead, outcome is more closely related to the severity of the PAN itself and the status of kidney, liver, neurological, gastrointestinal system involvement [3].

I.I. Norris, B.S.
University of Louisville School of Medicine,
500 South Preston Street, Louisville, KY 40292, USA
e-mail: ivyi.norris@gmail.com; ivy.norris@louisville.edu

C.E. Owen, M.S., M.D. (✉)
Division of Dermatology, University of Louisville,
3810 Springhurst Blvd, Suite 200, Louisville, KY 40241, USA
e-mail: ceowen01@louisville.edu

J.R. Nunley and E.V. Lerma (eds.), *Dermatological Manifestations of Kidney Disease*,
DOI 10.1007/978-1-4939-2395-3_3, © Springer Science+Business Media New York 2015

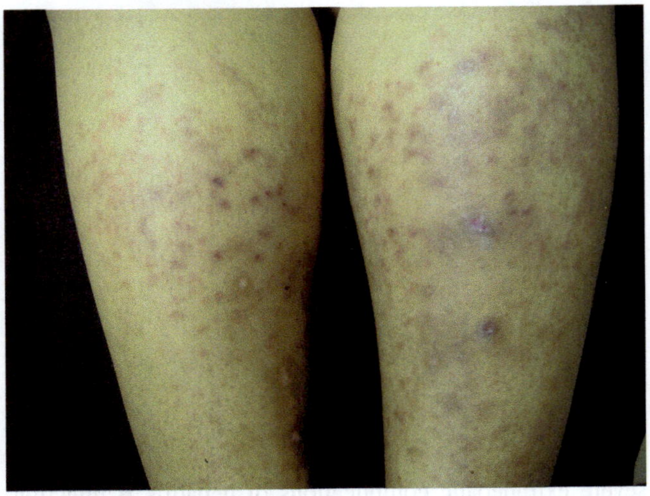

Fig. 3.1 Hyperpigmented patches in a reticulated pattern and tender nodules on the shins in a patient with polyarteritis nodosa

Gianotti–Crosti Syndrome (Papular Acrodermatitis of Childhood)

Papular acrodermatitis of childhood or Gianotti–Crosti syndrome (GCS) is seen in children between the ages of two and six who are infected with HBV. This association is strongest in endemic regions. In the USA, however, the eruption is more strongly associated with Epstein-Barr virus infection than with HBV infection. Clinically, GCS is characterized by monomorphous lightly erythematous papules or papulovesicles in an acral distribution (cheeks, buttocks, forearms, and legs); lesions erupt over the course of 2–3 days and persist for up to 3 weeks; pruritus is variable. The rash classically spares the trunk, antecubital and popliteal surfaces, and mucous membranes. Over the course of several weeks, a fine scale may form over lesions. HBV-associated Gianotti–Crosti is usually accompanied by lymphadenopathy, HBsAg positivity, and hepatitis which peaks approximately at the time of resolution of the rash [3].

Serum-Sickness Like Reaction

A serum-sickness like syndrome is the most commonly associated skin finding in patients with acute hepatitis B infection. It occurs as a prodromal syndrome in 20–30 % of infected patients and usually resolves or improves by the time the patient develops clinical jaundice. Patients commonly present with low-grade fever, malaise, polyarthralgias, lymphadenopathy, and rash. The rash is most commonly urticarial and is often pruritic.

The pathogenesis of serum-sickness-like reaction in HBV is related to circulating antigen–antibody immune complexes comprising immunoglobulin M (IgM), HBsAg, and complement which produce the anaphylatoxins 3a and 5a responsible for the urticaria and vasculitis [3].

Patients with acute hepatitis B infection may also present with other rashes such as erythema multiforme, palpable purpura, or lichenoid dermatitis.

Dermatologic Findings in Chronic Hepatitis C Infection

HCV is a single-stranded RNA flavivirus transmitted primarily through parenteral routes via contaminated blood or blood products. The virus infects and replicates in hepatocytes and peripheral monocytes. Though six different genotypes of the HCV have been identified, types 1a and 1b account for over 75 % of cases in the USA [5]. The prevalence of chronic HCV infection worldwide is estimated at 170 million, with 3–4 million people newly infected each year [6]. The major burden of disease is related to the sequelae of chronic HCV infection which results from the majority of acute HCV cases. Consequently, hepatitis C is the most common infectious cause of chronic liver disease as well as the etiologic factor in multiple systemic disorders of other organs.

The majority of dermatologic manifestations seen with HCV are observed in cases of chronic infection. It is estimated that nearly 20 % of patients with HCV infection possess at least one skin manifestation of the disease which highlights the importance of recognition. The most commonly associated skin findings with chronic HCV include mixed cryoglobulinemia syndrome (MCS), porphyria cutanea tarda (PCT), necrolytic acral erythema (NAE), and lichen planus which are discussed in this section. Properly identifying these related skin findings in patients can have important implications on the course, treatment, and disease outcome, and in some cases may be the initial presentation of the underlying viral infection.

Mixed Cryoglobulinemia Syndrome

Cryoglobulins are immunoglobulins which precipitate in cold temperature and then dissolve in warm temperatures. Type I cryoglobulinemia is commonly associated with Waldenstrom macroglobulinemia, multiple myeloma, and chronic lymphocytic leukemia. Usually the anomalous protein in type I cryoglobulinemia is monoclonal IgM. There is no association between this type and HCV. Types II and III are considered mixed cryoglobulinemia. The term "mixed cryoglobulinemia (MC)" refers to elevated serum levels of circulating cryoglobulins composed of more than one immunoglobulin component such as rheumatoid factor which are usually IgM (rarely, IgA, IgG) monoclonal or polyclonal immunoglobulin, respectively. Ninety percent of patients with this mixed-type (II or III) cryoglobulinemic vasculitis

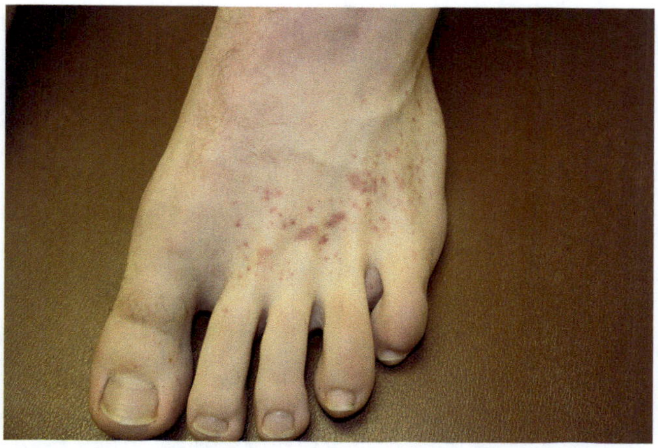

Fig. 3.2 Petechiae and palpable purpura of the feet characteristic of leukocytoclastic vasculitis associated with mixed cryoglobulinemia syndrome

have chronic HCV infection [2, 7]. Other causes of MC are HBV, human immunodeficiency virus (HIV) infection, or chronic liver disease.

Patients with mixed cryoglobulinemia syndrome (MCS) present with palpable purpura, weakness, and arthralgia. The palpable purpura typically involves the lower extremities or other dependent areas and may ulcerate (see Fig. 3.2). Purpura may be preceded by paresthesias or localized burning sensations [8]. Hyperpigmentation from hemosiderin deposition may replace the areas of purpura upon resolution. Patients with mixed essential cryoglobulinemia also may develop urticarial plaques and ulcerations, livedo reticularis, symmetric polyarthritis, myalgias, cutis marmorata, and fatigue. In more severe presentations, patients may also have hemorrhagic bullae. Raynaud phenomenon occurs in about one-third of MCS patients which, if severe, can lead to acrocyanosis, necrosis, and distal gangrene of the digits [2, 5, 7, 8].

Diagnosis of HCV-related MC relies on history, clinical manifestations (purpura), hypocomplementemia, and the presence of cryoglobulins. Testing for cryoglobulinemia can be difficult, as it requires serum drawn and maintained at constant temperature, before it is placed in ice bath for 30 min. 70 % of patients with MC will have positive rheumatoid factor [2]. Though not specific, positive titers for rheumatoid factor in patients with purpura and hypocomplementemia and in the absence of clinical signs of rheumatoid arthritis should raise suspicion for cryoglobulinemia [5]. Positive serology for HCV helps to confirm HCV-associated disease.

It is important to recognize that in addition to skin findings, patients with MCS often have renal disease. The renal disease associated with MC is highly variable and includes microscopic hematuria with or without chronic renal insufficiency, nephrotic syndrome, acute kidney failure, or acute glomerulonephritis. On renal biopsy, over 80 % of patients showed histologic evidence of membranoproliferative glomerulonephritis [9].

Histopathology of mixed cutaneous cryoglobulinemia reveals small vessel leukocytoclastic vasculitis, though this finding is not specific to MCS. Monocytic and lymphocytic inflammatory infiltrate in the vessel walls is usually appreciable histologically and responsible for associated endothelial hyperplasia, fibrinoid necrosis, and hemorrhage [2].

Treatment of MCS requires both immunosuppression and treatment of the underlying hepatitis. Depending on severity of disease, immune-directed modalities may include systemic corticosteroids, cyclophosphamide, rituximab, and plasmapheresis. In patients with HCV-associated MCS, immunosuppressive measures should be started at least 1 month before beginning antiviral therapy [10].

Mixed cryoglobulinemic vasculitis follows a benign course in about one half of affected patients. One-third of patients suffer subsequent liver or renal failure, and 15 % develop a malignancy, most commonly lymphoma due to the lymphotropic role of the HCV virus. While it does not integrate into the host deoxyribonucleic acid (DNA) of lymphocytes, proliferation and transformation of lymphocytes occurs by an indirect mechanism [11]. Rarely hepatocellular or thyroid malignancy follows MC and HCV. Prognosis for HCV-induced cryoglobulinemia is generally related to the response to therapy. Effective treatment for HCV can also be effective in managing the vasculitis associated with MC; however, a relapse of MC can be seen if HCV relapses after antiviral therapy. Poor prognostic factors include concomitant renal disease, which has 50 % mortality rate by 10 years of diagnosis [2].

Porphyria Cutanea Tarda

PCT is a photosensitivity disorder that results from decreased function of the enzyme uroporphyrinogen decarboxylase (UROD). Whether inherited or acquired, UROD dysfunction results in increased levels of circulating porphyrins and clinically identical PCT symptoms. HCV is a known etiologic agent in the sporadic/acquired type of PCT. In fact, up to 50 % of sporadic cases of PCT are associated with underlying HCV infection, though rates vary widely based on geography. PCT has been reported in 62–82 % of patients with HCV [5].

PCT is due to acquired or inherited depletion or absence of the UROD enzyme involved in the porphyrin pathway. HCV-related PCT is a result of diminished UROD activity in hepatocytes, In contrast to the inherited form of PCT which involves dysfunction of the same enzyme in both the hepatocyte and erythrocyte. While the exact pathogenesis of HCV-related PCT is unknown, it is likely that additional environmental factors must be present in the setting of liver disease to provoke a symptomatic PCT attack. These triggers

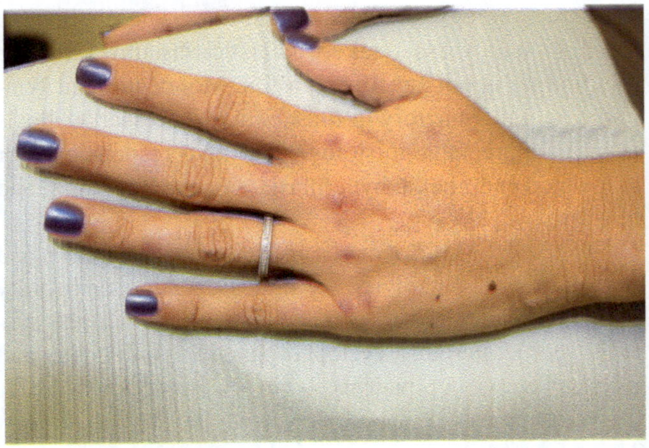

Fig. 3.3 Scarring, blisters, and milia on the dorsal hand characteristic of porphyria cutanea tarda

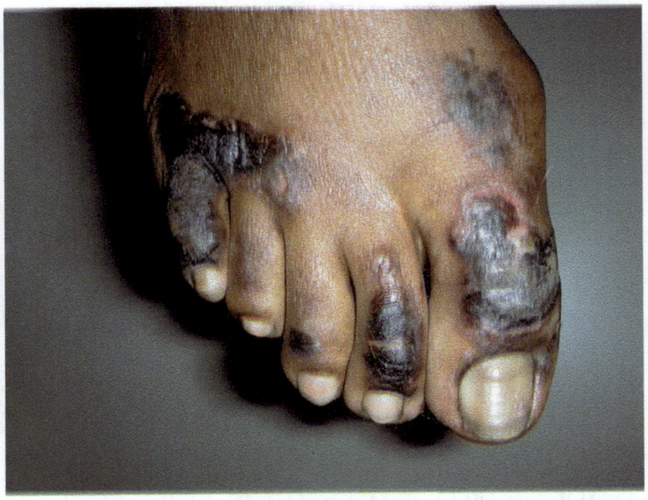

Fig. 3.4 Hyperpigmented, well-demarcated, eroded plaques of the dorsal feet in a patient with necrolytic acral erythema

may include alcohol, estrogens, or iron overload. Patients with chronic hepatitis and liver dysfunction have decreased intracellular glutathione stores and the resultant oxidative stresses are thought possibly to trigger PCT [5]. Increased levels of hepatocellular iron in HCV patients may trigger attacks of PCT. It has been proposed that patients who receive ribavirin therapy for HCV may develop symptomatic PCT as a result of high circulating iron levels from ribavirin-induced hemolysis [12].

Patients with PCT exhibit marked skin fragility and blisters in a photodistribution particularly on the dorsal surfaces of the extremities (commonly the hands) and the face (see Fig. 3.3). With time, vesicular lesions often become hemorrhagic before they scar and form milia. Hypertrichosis (especially of the zygomatic arches), hyperpigmentation, and sclerodermatous changes may be present in patients who exhibit a more chronic disease course [2, 13].

Diagnosis in a patient with clinically suspected PCT is often confirmed by testing for the presence of urinary porphyrins. Elevated urinary porphyrins >800 mcg/day in the appropriate clinical setting confirms the disease. Other lab abnormalities in patients with PCT may or may not include elevated transaminases, serum ferritin, and serum iron. In the case of a patient with confirmed PCT and no previous diagnosis of HCV or another etiologic factor, it is important to recognize the associations with the disease for prudent workup of a patient once a diagnosis of PCT has been confirmed. Patients with PCT often may present with the skin findings and have underlying undiagnosed and/or asymptomatic hepatitis C. Testing for HCV serology should be performed as well as exclusion of any other forms of chronic liver disease. It would be useful as well to test for iron overload and/or pursue genetic testing for HFE allele mutations of hereditary hemochromatosis (HH), since HH may be associated with the development of PCT with or without concomitant HCV infection [7].

Treatment of HCV-related PCT is aimed at treating the infection by suppressing viral replication. In general, the historic mainstay of treatment for PCT is routine phlebotomy and avoidance of known environmental triggers like alcohol, estrogen, and excess iron.

Necrolytic Acral Erythema

NAE was first described in 1996 and is nearly pathognomonic for HCV infection (only a few case reports of uninfected patients have been published). NAE is typically seen on the dorsum of the feet and toes as dusky, well-demarcated plaques sometimes with scale (see Fig. 3.4). Three stages of clinical disease have been described; in the acute phase, NAE is characteristically a papulosquamous or vesiculobullous eruption occurring mainly on the lower extremities. The primary skin lesion is a 2–3 mm scaly erythematous papule with or without a central erosion. The second stage marks fully developed NAE and is characterized by an increased diameter and thickness of the primary lesions as they progress to become more sharply marginated, hyperkeratotic plaques with erosion and peripheral erythema. As the disease course progresses, the erythema abates and is gradually replaced by hyperpigmentation. The plaques of NAE may remain unchanged for months or develop pustules and superficial epidermal necrosis in the central portions of the lesions. Lesions may be pruritic or may be associated with a burning pain. They are unresponsive to steroids and topical antifungals, usually prompting a biopsy that aids in the diagnosis. Histologically, NAE resembles psoriasis with its constellation of regular acanthosis, diminished granular layer, and upper dermal, perivascular, and interstitial mononuclear infiltrate extending into epidermis. However, unlike psoriasis NAE demonstrates papillomatosis as well as necrotic keratinocytes [14].

Also in contrast to psoriasis, NAE spares the nail bed and plate, distal toes, palms, and soles.

NAE is notorious for resembling other diseases clinically, though none are specifically related to HCV. In addition to psoriasis, the differential diagnosis for NAE includes necrolytic migratory erythema, pseudoglucagonoma, pellagra, and acrodermatitis enteropathica. Acrodermatitis enteropathica is caused by a zinc deficiency and can mimic NAE; however, the rash of acrodermatitis enteropathica is usually more eczematous in appearance with poorly defined lesions. Acrodermatitis enteropathica is also commonly associated with diarrhea and failure to thrive, unlike NAE. Though often acral in distribution, the dermatitis of pellagra typically erupts in photodistributed pattern and develops more rapidly than NAE. Necrolytic migratory erythema may also be confused with NAE, but it is associated uniquely with pancreatic glucagonoma and is more flexurally located than acral [14]. Patients with clinical and histopathological evidence suggestive of NAE should have a hepatitis panel as well as glucagon, zinc, and serum amino acid levels checked. In one study, only 13 % of the patients diagnosed with NAE were aware they were carriers of hepatitis C. The remaining 87 % of study patients with NAE and no known HCV diagnosis were subsequently diagnosed and confirmed by polymerase chain reaction (PCR) and enzyme-linked immunosorbent assay (ELISA) [14].

Zinc supplementation has been shown to be effective in some NAE patients with and without a demonstrated zinc deficiency. The theory is that a dysregulation in zinc metabolism within the liver plays a role in the development of NAE in HCV patients such that supplementation, regardless of the serum zinc level, may be useful if NAE is refractory to other modes of therapy [15]. Effective therapy for chronic HCV may be helpful for treating NAE as well.

Lichen Planus

Lichen planus (LP) is an inflammatory disorder affecting the skin, mucous membranes, hair, and nails. The association between lichen planus and HCV is somewhat controversial. A systematic review showed an increased prevalence of LP in patients with HCV versus controls, but the association varied geographically. Screening for HCV in patients with LP is also controversial. Many recommend screening patients in geographical locations with a known association and in patients with risk factors for HCV.

LP is characterized by flat-topped, violaceous, pruritic papules. The individual lesions are often described as having a polygonal shape and have fine white lines on the surface known as Wickham striae (see Fig. 3.5). Extremities are most commonly affected, especially the volar wrists and ankles. It is characteristic of LP to develop in sites of trauma (Köbner phenomenon). Oral lesions typically consist of a lacy white patch on the buccal mucosa or erosions. LP can also affect the nails and genital skin.

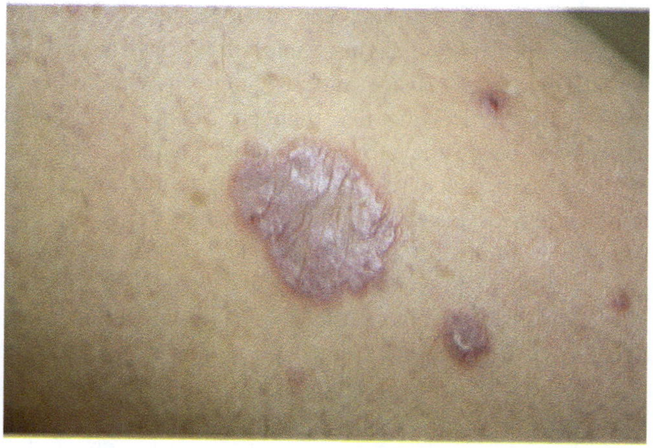

Fig. 3.5 Violaceous plaques with slight scale and Wickham stria characteristic of lichen planus

Patients with lichen planus who have an underlying HCV infection are more commonly afflicted by mucosal, erosive-type lichen planus. They generally suffer from a more chronic disease course and more generalized eruption than lichen planus seen in patients without hepatitis [5]. Treatment of lichen planus typically consists of topical or systemic corticosteroids, phototherapy, oral retinoids, or steroid-sparing immunosuppressive medications.

Therapy-Related Dermatologic Findings in HCV Patients

Distinct from the skin findings directly attributed to HCV infection are the dermatologic adverse effects (DAEs) of HCV treatment. Interferon and ribavirin have been the mainstay therapy for chronic HCV infection. Most recently, the direct-acting antiviral agents telaprevir and boceprevir have been approved for use in combination with interferon and ribavirin. Cutaneous reactions to these medications range from mild dermatitis and pruritus to more severe reactions requiring cessation of therapy.

Interferon/Ribavirin

The longstanding treatment regimen of choice for chronic HCV infection has been combination therapy with pegylated interferon alpha-2a or 2b and ribavirin. Whereas HCV infection alone is notorious for causing cutaneous disease unrelated to therapy, pegylated-interferon/ribavirin are also potential culprits, causing various cutaneous conditions in some patients receiving this regimen. While combination therapy has been shown to be more effective than interferon alone, it is also linked to a higher number of adverse dermatological effects than with interferon monotherapy [2]. The frequency and severity of dermatological adverse effects are greater still in patients receiving triple therapy (peglyated-interferon/ribavirin/telaprevir). This is discussed in more detail in the following section [16].

The onset of cutaneous reactions to interferon can be acute or delayed in onset. Cutaneous reactions have been reported as early as 5–15 days to as late as 1 year following initiation of therapy [17]. Three major cutaneous reaction types have been described. The first is an injection site reaction occurring uniquely at the injection site. These reactions may be mild consisting of only erythema, but may also be moderate to severe in nature manifesting as an abscess, ulcer, skin necrosis or as a vesiculobullous eruption.

More common than injection site reactions, affecting up to 10 % of patients, are mild, generalized, variably pruritic, rashes characterized by erythematous macules and plaques which may be morbilliform to purpuric in appearance. Spontaneous resolution despite continued use of interferon is common, often within 10–14 days of onset. Other cutaneous disorders that fall in this second category of treatment associated reactions include urticaria, pruritus, photosensitivity reactions, and dyschromias.

The third category of cutaneous disorders attributed to treatment are directly related to interferon's effects on the immune system and include psoriasis, lichen planus, erythema multiforme, erythema nodosum, granuloma annulare, and alopecia [2]. These conditions may worsen during interferon therapy, or present de novo. Although some of these may improve or resolve with cessation of therapy, psoriasis and lichen planus frequently persist. The course of alopecia is highly variable. Overall, the most common reactions include the generalized eruptions, alopecia (affecting 10 %), and psoriasis [17].

Telaprevir/Boceprevir

Two direct-acting antiviral agents, telaprevir and boceprevir, have recently been approved for use in conjunction with pegylated interferon and ribavirin for the treatment of genotype-1 hepatitis C infection. This regimen boasts higher rates of sustained virological responses and potentially reduced treatment duration, but is associated with a high rate of DAEs [16]. While traditional therapy with pegylated interferon/ribavirin has also been associated with DAEs, incidence has been 34 % of patients compared to 56 % of patients receiving telaprevir/interferon/ribavirin [18, 19].

In phase II/III telaprevir trials rashes occurring during the first 12 weeks of therapy were categorized by severity and assigned grades: grade I (mild, localized eruption), grade II (moderate), grade III (severe), or life-threatening or systemic reactions which included drug reaction with eosinophilia and systemic symptoms (DRESS), Stevens–Johnson syndrome (SJS), and toxic epidermal necrolysis (TEN) (see Fig. 3.6). 91 % (681/746) of the telaprevir-related rashes were classified as either grade I or grade II and did not require cessation of the drug. Most of the grade I/II rashes were characterized by a pruritic, eczematous dermatitis and/or xerosis and effectively managed with topical steroids, emollients, and oral antihistamines. The remaining 9 % (65/764) were classified as grade III or suspected to be a

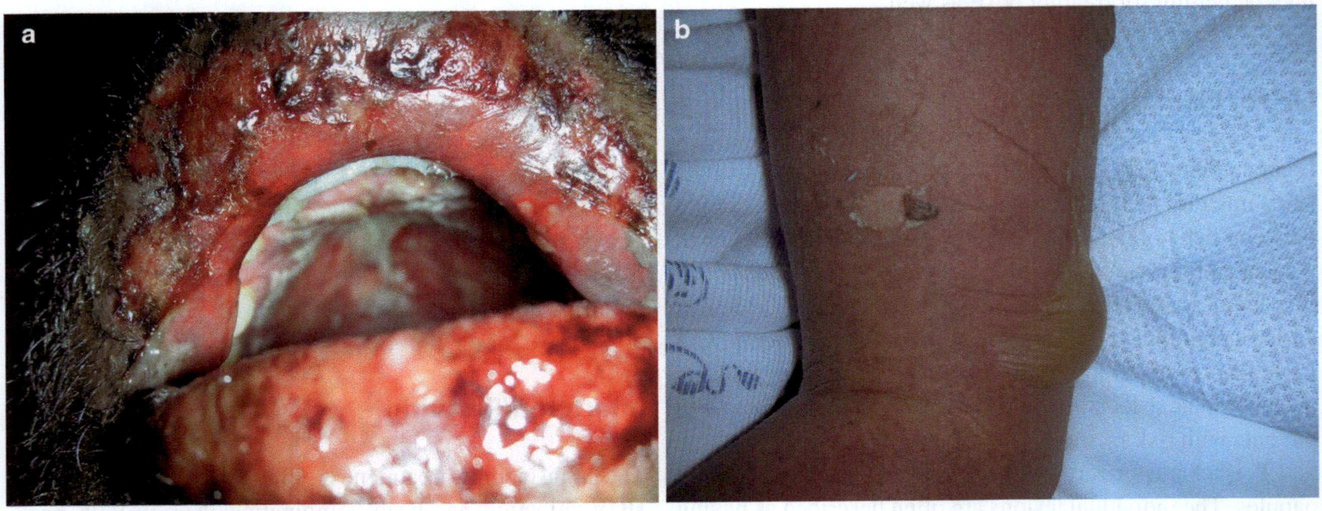

Fig. 3.6 (**a**) Severe labial and intraoral erosions in a patient with toxic epidermal necrolysis. (**b**) Sloughing skin, flaccid bullae, and erosions in toxic epidermal necrolysis

severe cutaneous adverse reaction (SCAR). It is critical to distinguish the clinical characteristics of a mild-to-moderate treatment-associated rash from those of a severe reaction such as DRESS or SJS/TEN; the latter are potentially life-threatening and warrant immediate intervention including the discontinuation of HCV treatment [16].

When choosing the appropriate HCV treatment modality for a patient, it should be emphasized that although the frequency and severity of therapy-related rashes increase with telaprevir, most adverse events were mild to moderate, effectively managed, and did not require stopping therapy. Likewise, patients who had more severe reactions typically saw gradual resolution of the dermatitis upon cessation of telaprevir.

Dermatologic Findings Related to Cirrhosis

Patients with chronic hepatitis often possess dermatologic findings associated with chronic liver disease in general. While these findings are not specific to hepatitis-related liver failure, they are important to recognize. Jaundice is the most common skin finding associated with hyperbilirubinemia and liver disease. Jaundice (icterus) appears clinically as a yellowish discoloration of the skin. It is usually most noticeable in the conjunctivae. Jaundice is typically present once serum bilirubin levels exceed 2 mg/dL, as a result of either impaired biliary excretion or obstruction. Red discoloration over the palmar surfaces of the hands is known as palmar erythema. The exact pathogenesis of palmar erythema is not known, but it is reported in about 23 % of cirrhosis patients. It is also seen in other conditions unrelated to liver disease such as pregnancy, thyrotoxicosis, and rheumatoid arthritis. Spider angiomata are another dermatologic finding in liver disease patients. These are small telangiectasias which appear on the skin as a central body (arteriole) with symmetrically radiating thin branches. They are most commonly present on the upper torso and result from excess circulating estrogen levels due to impaired hepatic detoxification [7].

References

1. Parsons ME, Russo GG, Millikan LE. Dermatologic disorders associated with viral hepatitis infections. Int J Dermatol. 1996;35(2):77–81. PubMed PMID: 8850031.
2. Rebora A. Skin diseases associated with hepatitis C virus: facts and controversies. Clin Dermatol. 2010;28(5):489–96. PubMed PMID: 20797507.
3. Jones AM, Warken K, Tyring SK. The cutaneous manifestations of viral hepatitis. Dermatol Clin. 2002;20(2):233–47. vi, PubMed PMID: 12120438.
4. Saadoun D, Terrier B, Semoun O, Sene D, Maisonobe T, Musset L, et al. Hepatitis C virus-associated polyarteritis nodosa. Arthritis Care Res. 2011;63(3):427–35. PubMed PMID: 20981809.
5. Mark J, Jackson JM. Hepatitis C and the skin. Dermatol Clin. 2002;20(3):449–58. PubMed PMID: 12170878.
6. Mohd Hanafiah K, Groeger J, Flaxman AD, Wiersma ST. Global epidemiology of hepatitis C virus infection: new estimates of age-specific antibody to HCV seroprevalence. Hepatology. 2013;57(4):1333–42. PubMed PMID: 23172780.
7. Satapathy SK, Bernstein D. Dermatologic disorders and the liver. Clin Liver Dis. 2011;15(1):165–82. PubMed PMID: 21111999.
8. Tedeschi A, Barate C, Minola E, Morra E. Cryoglobulinemia. Blood Rev. 2007;21(4):183–200. PubMed PMID: 17289231.
9. Roccatello D, Fornasieri A, Giachino O, Rossi D, Beltrame A, Banfi G, et al. Multicenter study on hepatitis C virus-related cryoglobulinemic glomerulonephritis. Am J Kidney Dis. 2007;49(1):69–82. PubMed PMID: 17185147.
10. Iannuzzella F, Vaglio A, Garini G. Management of hepatitis C virus-related mixed cryoglobulinemia. Am J Med. 2010;123(5):400–8. PubMed PMID: 20399313.
11. Hadziyannis SJ. Skin diseases associated with hepatitis C virus infection. J Eur Acad Dermatol Venereol. 1998;10(1):12–21. PubMed PMID: 9552752.
12. Cacoub P, Bourliere M, Lubbe J, Dupin N, Buggisch P, Dusheiko G, et al. Dermatological side effects of hepatitis C and its treatment: patient management in the era of direct-acting antivirals. J Hepatol. 2012;56(2):455–63. PubMed PMID: 21884670.
13. Chung CM, Nunley JR. Overview of hepatitis C and skin. Dermatol Nurs. 2006;18(5):425–30. PubMed PMID: 17131955.
14. Abdallah MA, Ghozzi MY, Monib HA, Hafez AM, Hiatt KM, Smoller BR, et al. Necrolytic acral erythema: a cutaneous sign of hepatitis C virus infection. J Am Acad Dermatol. 2005;53(2):247–51. PubMed PMID: 16021118.
15. Albeldawi M, Ebrahim V, Chiang DJ. A cutaneous marker of hepatitis C virus. Gastroenterology. 2013;144(2):275.
16. Picard O, Cacoub P. Dermatological adverse effects during genotype-1 hepatitis C treatment with the protease inhibitors telaprevir and boceprevir. Patient management. Clin Res Hepatol Gastroenterol. 2012;36(5):437–40. PubMed PMID: 22483956.
17. Stafford-Fox V, Guindon KM. Cutaneous reactions associated with alpha interferon therapy. Clin J Oncol Nurs. 2000;4(4):164–8. PubMed PMID: 11261097.
18. Rajani AK, Ravindra BK, Dkhar SA. Telaprevir: changing the standard of care of chronic hepatitis C. J Postgrad Med. 2013;59(1):42–7. PubMed PMID: 23525057.
19. Gaetano JN, Reau N. Hepatitis C: management of side effects in the era of direct-acting antivirals. Curr Gastroenterol Rep. 2013;15(1):305. PubMed PMID: 23269576.
20. Dupin N, Mallet V, Carlotti A, Vallet-Pichard A, Pol S. Severe skin rash in case of readministration of telaprevir in a patient who previously experienced a non severe rash. Hepatology. 2012;55(6):2042–3. PubMed PMID: 22234749.

Human Immunodeficiency Virus

4

Caroline Y. Winslow and Francisco A. Kerdel

Abbreviations

AIDS	Acquired immune deficiency syndrome
EF	Eosinophilic folliculitis
FTA-ABS	Fluorescent treponemal antibody-absorption
HAART	Highly active antiretroviral therapy
HIV	Human immunodeficiency virus
HLA	Human leukocyte antigen
HPV	Human papillomavirus
HSV	Herpes simplex virus
IRIS	Immune reconstitution inflammatory syndrome
KS	Kaposi sarcoma
PCR	Polymerase chain reaction
PPE	Pruritic papular eruption
PUVA	Psoralen plus ultraviolet A
RPR	Rapid plasma reagin
UVB	Ultraviolet B
VZV	Varicella zoster virus

Introduction

Approximately 34 million people worldwide are infected with the human immunodeficiency virus (HIV), with the greatest impact seen in sub-Saharan Africa [1]. Certain cutaneous infections or atypical presentations of common dermatologic diseases are suggestive of or nearly exclusive to the HIV infected population [2]. These are often correlated with CD4 T-cell count such that the astute clinician may predict a patient's immune status based on dermatologic findings and clinical presentation [3]. The advent of combination highly active antiretroviral therapy (HAART) in the 1990s has changed the face of the disease, reducing the frequency and severity of cutaneous disease associated with compromised immune status while simultaneously introducing its own complications such as medication reactions, lipodystrophy, and the immune reconstitution syndrome [4].

With the increased life expectancy in the era of HAART, non-infectious comorbidities of chronic HIV infection are garnering greater attention. Renal complications of HIV infection are common, with a relative risk of kidney disease nearly four times greater in patients with HIV than in uninfected people [5]. Etiologies of renal disease specific to the HIV-infected population include classic HIV-associated nephropathy as well as nephrotoxic effects of antiretroviral medications and antimicrobial agents used to treat opportunistic infections [6]. Furthermore, metabolic alterations associated with HAART such as hypertension, dyslipidemia and diabetes mellitus increase the risk for kidney disease in this population [7]. Other common risk factors for the development of chronic kidney disease include advanced age, female gender, African American race, low CD4 T-cell count, high HIV-ribonucleic acid (RNA) viral load, and coinfection with hepatitis C [6].

HIV-Related Cutaneous Infections

Exanthem of Acute Retroviral Syndrome

While primary infection with HIV may be entirely asymptomatic, approximately one-half to two-thirds of patients experience an acute retroviral syndrome that occurs 2–4 weeks after initial exposure to the virus [8]. The syndrome is self-limited, lasting from a few days to several

C.Y. Winslow, M.D. (✉)
Department of Dermatology and Cutaneous Surgery, University of Miami Miller School of Medicine, 1600 NW 10th Avenue, Room 2023, Miami, FL 33136, USA
e-mail: caroline.y.winslow@gmail.com

F.A. Kerdel, B.Sc., M.B.B.S.
Florida International University, 836 Ponce De Leon Blvd., Suite 204, Coral Gables, FL 33134, USA
e-mail: dr.kerdel@fadcenter.com

J.R. Nunley and E.V. Lerma (eds.), *Dermatological Manifestations of Kidney Disease*,
DOI 10.1007/978-1-4939-2395-3_4, © Springer Science+Business Media New York 2015

weeks, and is often attributed to an unspecified acute viral illness if the patient presents for medical care. Symptoms are nonspecific and may include fever, malaise, myalgias, pharyngitis, lymphadenopathy, headache, or photophobia. A morbilliform exanthem involving the face, trunk, and upper extremities is seen in 30–50 % of patients. Oral or anogenital ulcers may also be observed. Leukopenia or thrombocytopenia is sometimes seen on laboratory evaluation. HIV antibody tests are generally negative in the acute phase; diagnosis requires clinical suspicion based on recent exposure, intravenous drug use, or high-risk sexual behavior and may be confirmed with the presence of HIV deoxyribonucleic acid (DNA) or RNA via polymerase chain reaction (PCR) [8–10].

Herpes Simplex Virus

With the relative immunocompetency of early HIV infection, herpes simplex virus (HSV-1 and 2) lesions are typical in appearance, with painful grouped vesicles on an erythematous base in perioral or genital areas that erode and heal in 1–2 weeks [8] (Fig. 4.1a). Frequency of recurrence is comparable to that of the general population. Active genital ulcers increase the risk of HIV transmission to sexual partners, although this risk is decreased with HSV antiviral therapy [11]. In advanced HIV immunodeficiency, herpes ulcers may be large, widespread, chronic, verrucous, hemorrhagic, or necrotic with sometimes debilitating pain (Fig. 4.1b, c). Chronic herpetic ulcers that fail to heal after 1 month are considered by the Centers for Disease Control and Prevention to be an acquired immune deficiency syndrome (AIDS)-defining condition [2]. Diagnosis of HSV is confirmed with a swab or scraping of epithelial cells from the base of a fresh vesicle for PCR, viral culture, Tzanck smear, or direct fluorescent antibody; alternatively, a biopsy of skin lesions may be considered.

HSV is treated with a thymidine kinase inhibitor such as acyclovir, valacyclovir, or famciclovir. Primary infection is treated for 10 days with acyclovir 400 mg three times daily or valacyclovir 1 g twice daily; recurrences are treated with acyclovir 400 mg three times daily for 5 days or valacyclovir 500 mg twice daily for 3 days. Suppressive therapy, with valacyclovir 500 mg to 1 g daily or acyclovir 400 mg twice daily, may be indicated based on severity of disease or

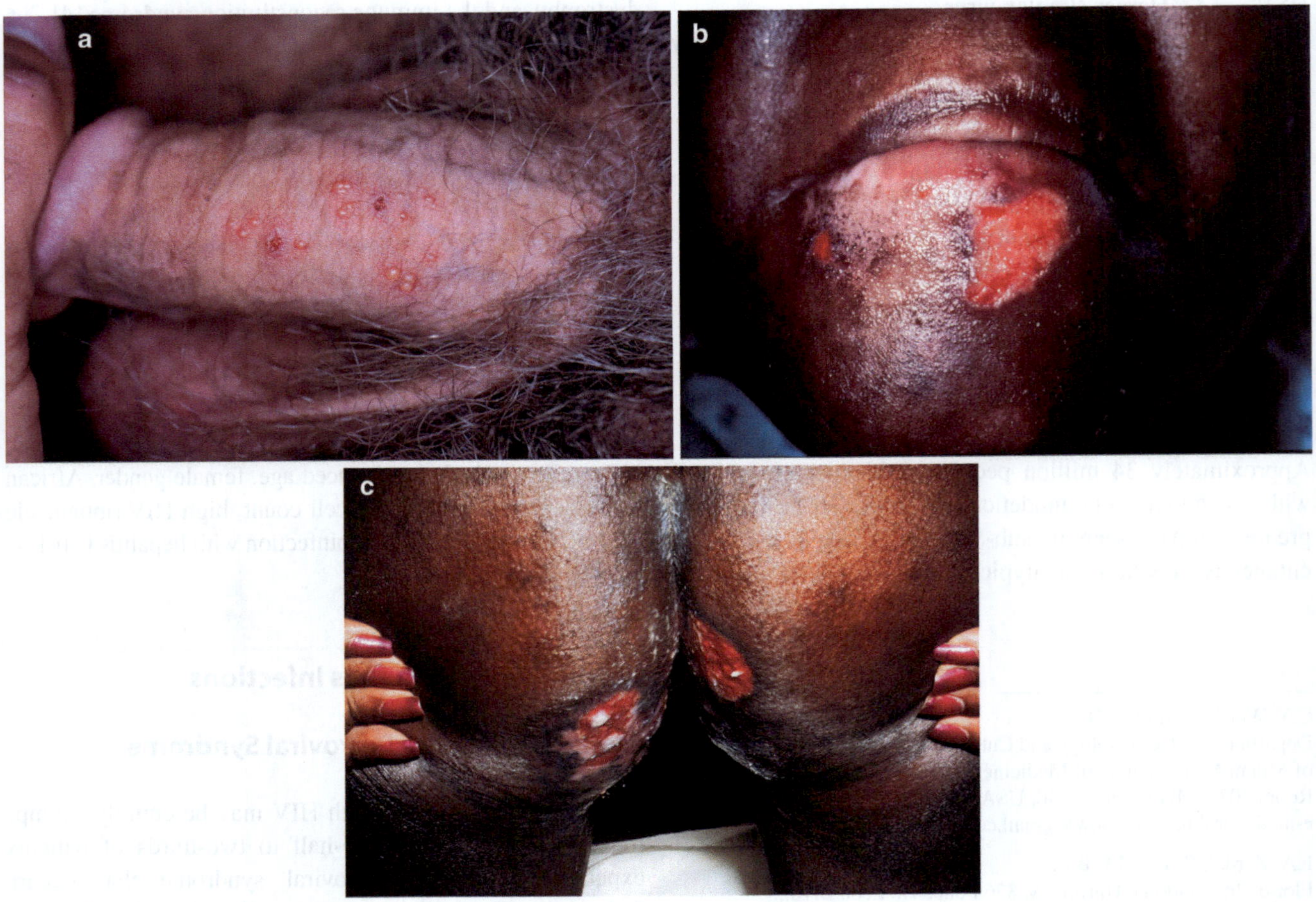

Fig. 4.1 Herpes simplex. (**a**) Grouped vesicles on an erythematous base on the penile shaft, (**b**) large chronic ulcer on the lower lip, (**c**) chronic perianal ulcers

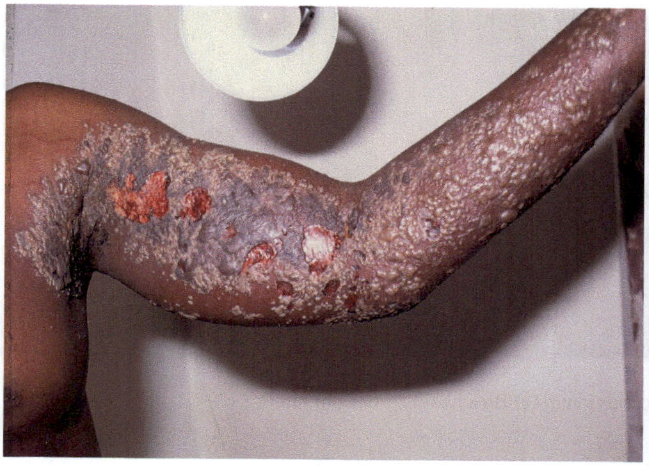

Fig. 4.2 Herpes zoster eruption in dermatomal distribution on the arm. Courtesy Dr. Ncoza Dlova

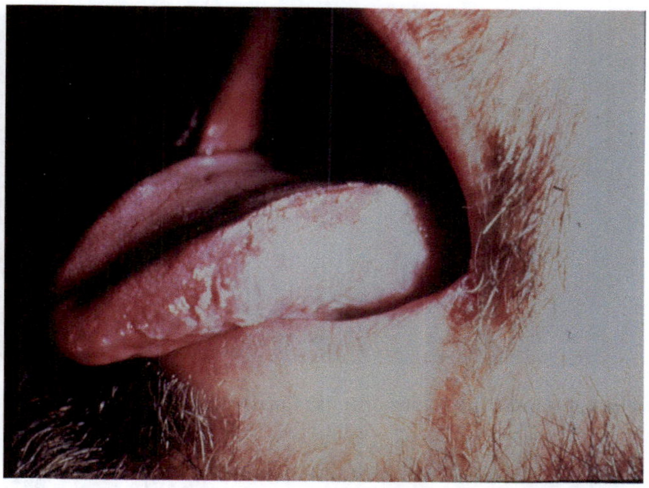

Fig. 4.3 Oral hairy leukoplakia on the lateral tongue

frequency of recurrences. Foscarnet, cidofovir, or topical trifluridine should be considered for acyclovir-resistant strains [2].

Varicella Zoster Virus

Varicella zoster virus (VZV) is common in HIV-infected patients, with increased frequency of eruptions as CD4 cell counts decrease. In the HIV-infected patient, the zoster eruption can present in the classic dermatomal distribution (Fig. 4.2), or it may be chronic, disseminated, ecthymatous, or verrucous. These severe and atypical presentations make diagnosis difficult in some cases. As in HSV, direct fluorescent antibody, viral culture, PCR, Tzanck smear, or biopsy is useful to confirm the diagnosis. Treatment is similar to HSV infections, though higher doses of medications are administered. Intravenous antiviral therapy is indicated in disseminated zoster or zoster ophthalmicus. VZV vaccine may be indicated in early-stage HIV infected adults to prevent the eruption or the ensuing postherpetic neuralgia but is not universally recommended [2].

Oral Hairy Leukoplakia

Oral hairy leukoplakia is caused by Epstein-Barr virus and is indicative of advancing immunosuppression, developing in up to 25 % of HIV infected patients. Lesions appear as adherent, corrugated white plaques with hair-like projections on the lateral tongue (Fig. 4.3). The condition is not associated with progression to malignancy. Lesions tend to regress with HAART and immune reconstitution. Treatments such as local destruction with cryotherapy, topical podophyllin or tretinoin gel, or oral antivirals such as acyclovir may be considered but are often not necessary as the condition is usually asymptomatic [2].

Human Papillomavirus

Human papillomavirus (HPV) infection is very common in HIV-positive patients, and lesions may be larger and more resistant to treatment than in immunocompetent patients. HPV is implicated in common warts, an acquired epidermodysplasia verruciformis-like syndrome, and squamous cell carcinomas of the skin. Anogenital manifestations of HPV infection include condylomata acuminata, Buschke–Lowenstein tumor (giant condyloma), Bowen disease, and intraepithelial neoplasia or invasive carcinoma of the anus, penis, vulva, or cervix (Fig. 4.4a–c). Widespread use of HAART has not decreased prevalence of genital HPV infection and has paradoxically led to an increase in cervical, anal, and vulvar malignancies because of extended life expectancy in the HIV infected population [12]. Cervical and anal Papanicolaou smear screening is advised every 6–12 months in HIV infected patients, and HPV vaccines may offer protection against reinfection or reactivation in previously exposed patients [2].

Treatment of HPV-associated condyloma is often less effective in HIV-infected patients and dependent on immune status. Surgical options include cryotherapy, usually repeated every 4–6 weeks, or excision for larger lesions. Intralesional 5-fluorouracil and interferon alpha may also be effective. Topical therapies applied by the patient include imiquimod, three times per week, or podophyllotoxin gel, 3 days on and 4 days off; in-office topical therapies applied by the clinician include podophyllotoxin solution or trichloroacetic acid.

Molluscum Contagiosum

Molluscum contagiosum lesions are commonly seen in patients with CD4 counts below 200/μL [13]. Typical skin-colored, dome-shaped umbilicated papules may be seen

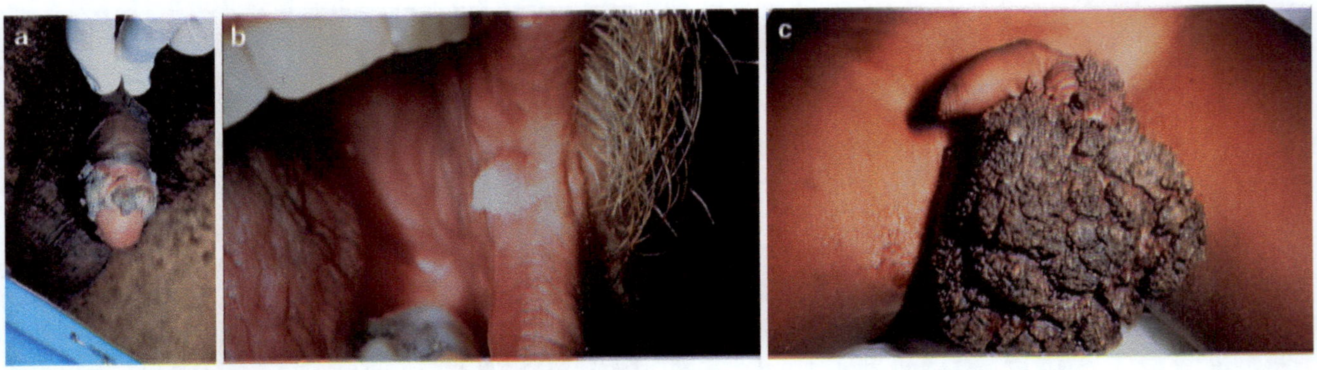

Fig. 4.4 Human papillomavirus. (**a**) Condylomata on the penis, (**b**) oral condyloma, (**c**) Buschke–Lowenstein tumor

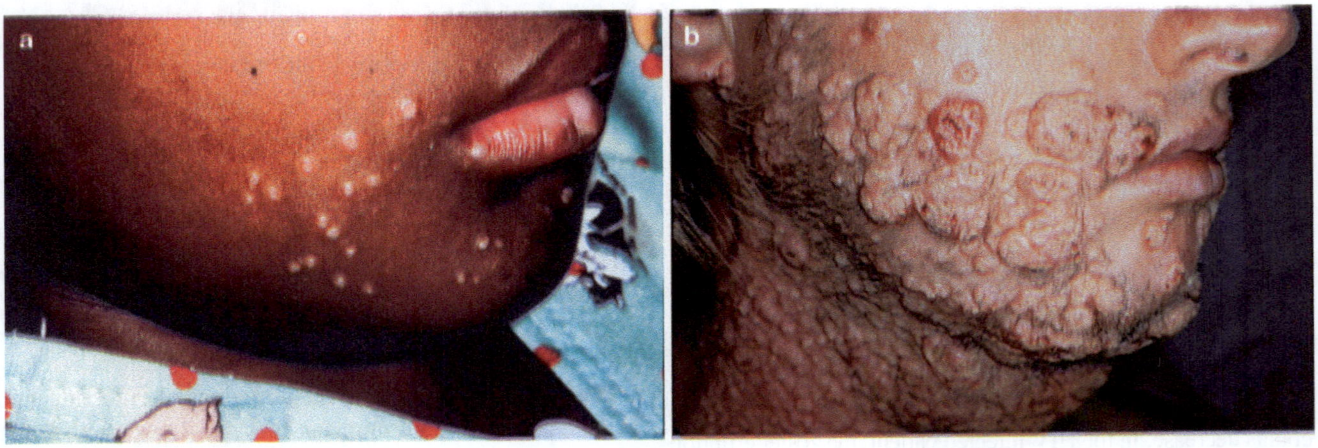

Fig. 4.5 Molluscum contagiosum. (**a**) Classic umbilicated papules on the face of a child, (**b**) giant molluscum lesions on the face

most frequently on the face, neck, groin, or intertriginous areas (Fig. 4.5a). They can progress to become large, confluent, and disfiguring (Fig. 4.5b). Lesions should be differentiated from atypical mycobacterial infections or disseminated fungal infections such as cryptococcosis, penicilliosis, or histoplamosis [2]. The diagnosis may be confirmed in office with Giemsa or toluidine blue staining of a smear of the core of the umbilicated lesions, revealing Henderson–Patterson bodies. Alternatively, a skin biopsy is diagnostic. Molluscum lesions may regress with HAART, though local destructive treatments such as cryotherapy, curettage, or electrodessication and topical therapies including imiquimod, cidofovir, cantharidin, or trichloroacetic acid are mainstays of treatment [14–16].

Staphylococcus aureus

HIV infected patients have an increased rate of *Staphylococcus aureus* colonization and resultant skin infections [11]. These commonly present as in the immunocompetent population with furuncles or carbuncles that can progress to cellulitis and abscesses (Fig. 4.6a, b). Other less frequent presentations include pyomyositis, with intramuscular abscesses, and botryomycosis, a chronic suppurative granulomatous infection with fistulae draining sulfur granules and purulent material [2]. Treatment of any abscess should include drainage. Antibiotic therapy is culture driven; oral trimethoprim-sulfamethoxazole, doxycycline, or clindamycin often have activity against methicillin-resistant strains and intravenous vancomycin is indicated for more severe infections. Eradication of colonization with intranasal mupirocin and bleach baths or chlorhexidine skin cleansers may also be helpful as a preventative measure.

Syphilis

HIV positive patients who have a history of multiple sexual partners and other sexually transmitted diseases have an increased risk of coinfection with syphilis, caused by the spirochete *Treponema pallidum*. Secondary syphilis may present with the classic papulosquamous eruption, but other atypical features may be seen in the setting of HIV coinfection such as nodulo-ulcerative lesions or palmoplantar keratoderma of syphilis [11]. HIV infection is associated with false-negative results in nontreponemal and treponemal tests such as the

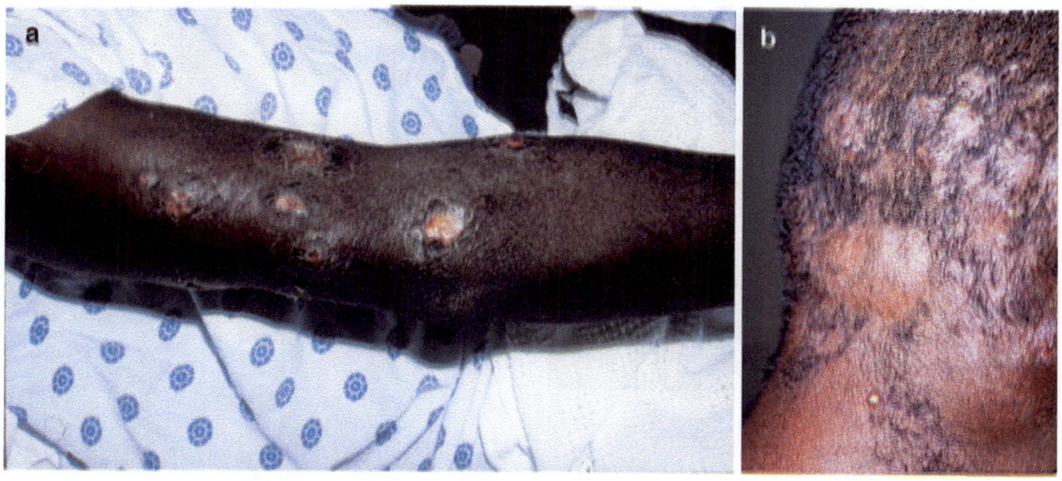

Fig. 4.6 *Staphylococcus aureus*. (**a**) Staphylococcal pyoderma, (**b**) multiple abscesses on the scalp

rapid plasma reagin (RPR) and fluorescent treponemal antibody-absorption (FTA-ABS) respectively. Furthermore, very high titers of RPR may have false-negative results that become positive with serum dilution, known as the prozone phenomenon [17]. Syphilis is treated with intramuscular benzathine penicillin, dose dependant on the stage of infection. It is controversial whether HIV patients experience an increased rate of treatment failure with standard therapy regimens or more rapid progression to secondary and tertiary syphilis [17, 18]. Lumbar puncture is indicated in any HIV positive patient with syphilis and neurologic symptoms to rule out neurosyphilis.

Bacillary Angiomatosis

Bacillary angiomatosis, due to *Bartonella henselae* or *quintana*, presents with red to violaceous papules and nodules that may resemble Kaposi sarcoma or pyogenic granuloma (Fig. 4.7). It was first described in HIV positive patients and is associated with CD4 counts lower than 100. Diagnosis may be confirmed by biopsy of skin lesions as well as bacterial culture or PCR of tissue or blood. Up to 50 % of patients with skin lesions have involvement of internal organs, often the liver and spleen [19]. Treatment is with prolonged courses of macrolides or tetracyclines for a minimum of 2 months' duration. Use of trimethoprim-sulfamethoxazole for *Pneumocystis* prophylaxis may suppress *Bartonella* and decrease the incidence of bacillary angiomatosis [2].

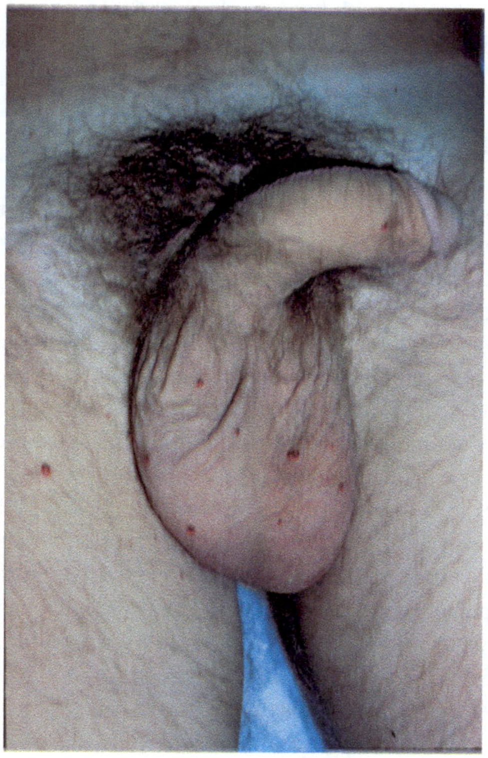

Fig. 4.7 Bacillary angiomatosis

Candidiasis

A common initial presentation of HIV infection is oral candidiasis or thrush, with white exudate on the tongue, palate, or buccal mucosa (Fig. 4.8). Other manifestations of *Candida* infections include angular cheilitis, vaginal candidiasis, chronic paronychia, or intertrigo. More severe disease is correlated with lower CD4 counts, and oropharyngeal chronic infection is a reservoir for disseminated disease and candidemia in severely immunosuppressed patients. Diagnosis may be confirmed by fungal culture or potassium hydroxide preparations of scrapings from mucous membranes. Oral candidiasis may be treated with topical nystatin "swish and swallow" preparations or clotrimazole troches. Oral fluconazole, 100 mg daily, or itraconazole, 100 mg twice daily, is indicated for chronic or recurrent disease, but prolonged use can promote

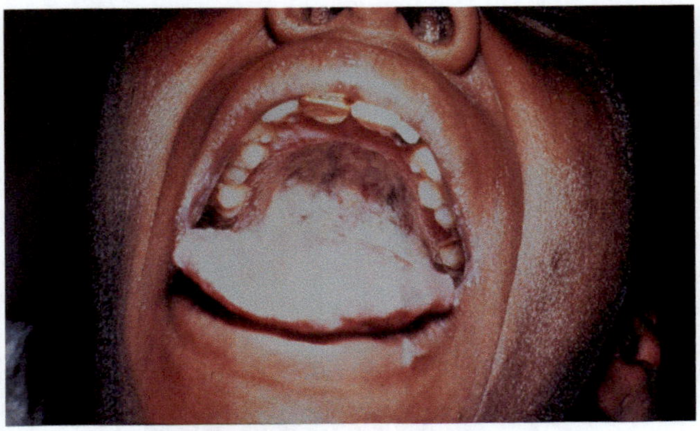

Fig. 4.8 Oral candidiasis

resistance [2]. Amphotericin, caspofungin, or voriconazole may be required for resistant organisms or disseminated infection. Prophylaxis with fluconazole, 100–200 mg weekly, may be considered in patients with severely depressed CD4 counts.

Scabies

Scabies, caused by *Sarcoptes scabiei* var. *hominis*, is the most common ectoparasitic skin infection in HIV positive patients [8]. Presentation in immunocompetent patients is similar to that of the general population, with burrows seen in interdigital web spaces, flexor aspects of the wrists, genital, periumbilical, and intertriginous areas. With more advanced HIV infection, scabies infestation may involve greater surface area of the body, including the ears, face, and scalp, or present in crusted or exaggerated papular forms with or without typical burrows (Fig. 4.9). Crusted, fissured plaques may become superinfected, in some cases leading to bacteremia. HIV-infected patients tend to have higher mite burden than immunocompetent hosts. Diagnosis is confirmed by examining scrapings of suspicious skin lesions in mineral oil for mites, ova or feces. Scabies infestation is treated with topical permethrin 5 % cream, which may require repeated applications, or oral ivermectin 200 μg/kg administered in two doses 2 weeks apart [2]. Keratolytics such as topical salicylic acid should be considered in patients with thick crust and scale to allow penetration of topical medications. Close household contacts should be treated in confirmed cases.

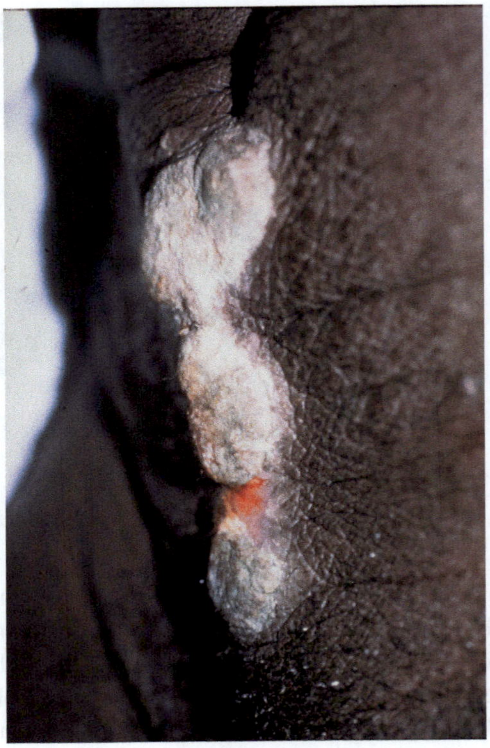

Fig. 4.9 Plaque of crusted scabies in the umbilical region

Non-infectious HIV-Related Cutaneous Disorders

Seborrheic Dermatitis

Seborrheic dermatitis is the most common cutaneous manifestation of HIV, affecting up to 85 % of patients [20]. It may be seen in all stages of disease but becomes more severe, diffuse, and resistant to therapy with more advanced immunosuppression [21]. HIV-infected patients often exhibit the typical presentation of pink plaques with greasy yellow scale on the scalp, face, and central chest (Fig. 4.10). With more advanced HIV infection, patients may present with involvement of the entire face and chest or even total body erythroderma. An abrupt onset of seborrheic dermatitis or a severe worsening of a preexisting case should prompt HIV testing.

Seborrheic dermatitis has been linked to *Malassezia* yeast, although studies investigating the amount or species of these commensal organisms have failed to demonstrate consistent differences between patients with seborrheic dermatitis and normal controls [22]. The disease responds to antifungal medications such as topical ketoconazole cream or shampoo, terbinafine cream or zinc pyrithione shampoo. Other topical treatments include selenium sulfide and sulfur or tar shampoos, low potency topical corticosteroids, or metronidazole gel. In more severe cases, oral antifungals may be considered as an adjunct to topical preparations; options include ketoconazole 200 mg daily for 4 weeks, itraconazole 200 mg daily for 7 days, or terbinafine 250 mg daily for 4 weeks [22].

Psoriasis in HIV

Psoriasis prevalence in HIV patients is slightly higher than that of the normal population, affecting approximately 2–5 % of HIV infected patients [8, 23]. Clinical manifestations in HIV patients are similar to non-infected individuals, including classic chronic plaque psoriasis (Fig. 4.11a, b), though some HIV patients are more prone to developing palmoplantar psoriasis and psoriatic arthritis. Other possible presentations include guttate psoriasis, often developing after streptococcal or staphylococcal infections; sebopsoriasis, with clinical features of both seborrheic dermatitis and psoriasis; or total body involvement (erythroderma) that may become secondarily infected. The severity of psoriasis worsens in advanced AIDS and a preexisting psoriasis is usually exacerbated with HIV infection [23]. As in seborrheic dermatitis, an acute worsening or abrupt onset of psoriasis should prompt the consideration of HIV screening.

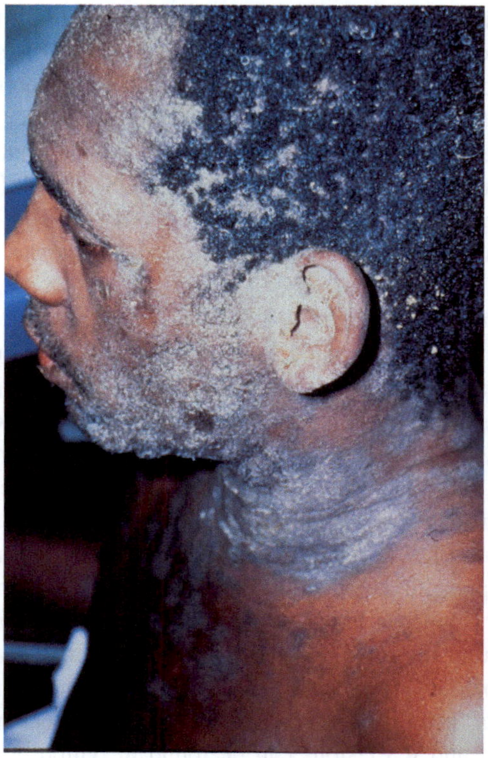

Fig. 4.10 Scaling plaques on the scalp, face, and chest in a patient with seborrheic dermatitis

Topical preparations are the first line treatment in HIV-related psoriasis, including emollients, corticosteroids, vitamin D3 analogues, and tazarotene. Phototherapy, ultraviolet B (UVB), or psoralen plus ultraviolet A (PUVA) are also useful treatments, but may pose a problem for patients with photosensitivity due to HIV or photosensitizing medications [24]. HAART may be considered the treatment of choice for moderate to severe psoriasis. Reduction in HIV viral load is associated to a subsequent decrease in tumor necrosis factor-alpha (TNF-α), an important mediator in the pathogenesis of psoriasis [25]. Oral retinoids such as acitretin, dosed at 10–25 mg daily, should be considered second line treatment for HIV-infected psoriasis patients refractory to topical therapy and may be combined with phototherapy. Systemic immunosuppressants must be reserved as the last option because of the risk of opportunistic infections. However, some studies show promise for the use of etanercept in HIV patients [26].

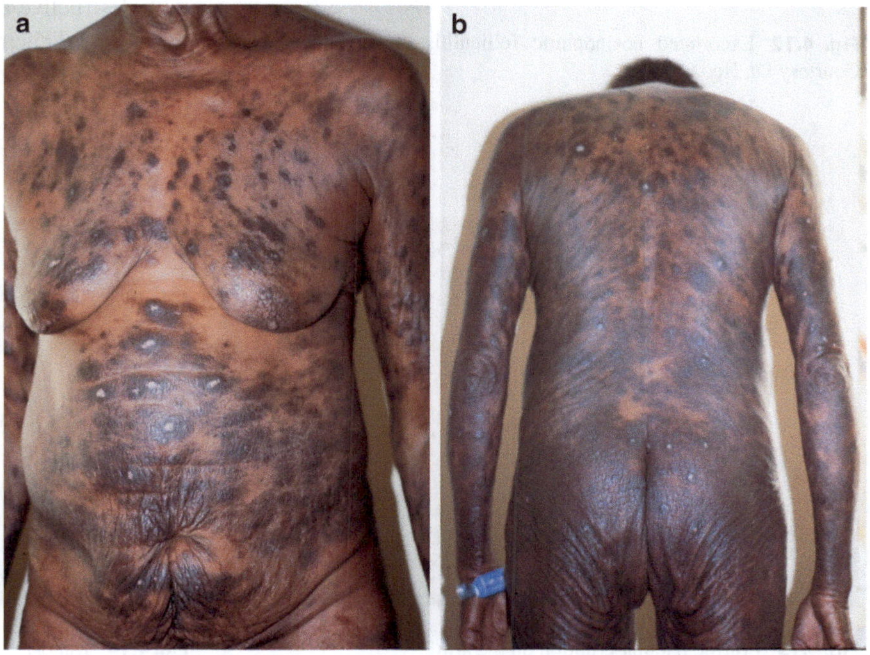

Fig. 4.11 (**a**, **b**) Psoriasis

Pruritus, Eosinophilic Folliculitis, and Pruritic Papular Eruption

Pruritus is a common complaint in HIV patients, especially with advanced disease, and may be related to metabolic disorders or specific dermatoses such as atopic dermatitis, scabies, drug reactions, pruritic papular eruption (PPE) of HIV, and eosinophilic folliculitis (EF). PPE and EF remain poorly differentiated and some authors argue that they are the same entity [27]. Both are characterized by pruritic perifollicular erythematous papules and pustules. In EF, lesions are usually distributed on the head, trunk, and upper limbs (Fig. 4.12), while PPE has a greater involvement of the extremities than the trunk or face (Fig. 4.13). Eosinophilia may be observed in both diseases. Several treatment options have shown efficacy in these entities, including phototherapy, oral and topical corticosteroids, systemic antibiotics, itraconazole, and isotretinoin [28].

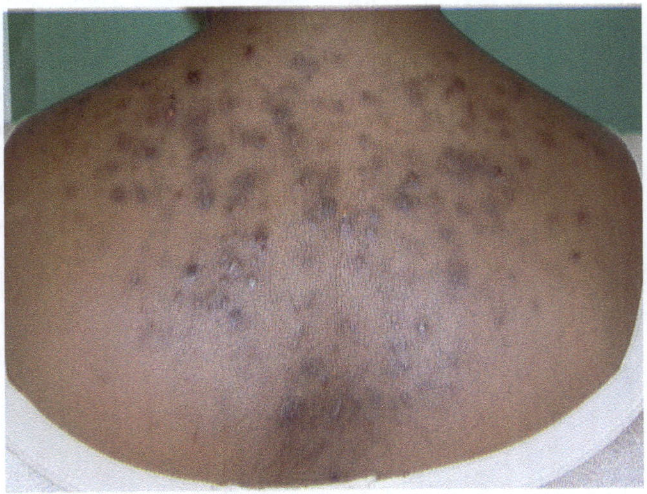

Fig. 4.12 Excoriated eosinophilic folliculitis on the upper back. Courtesy Dr. Ncoza Dlova

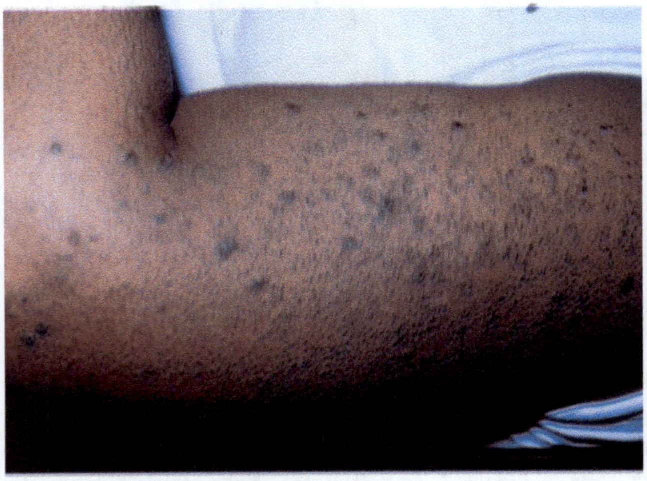

Fig. 4.13 Pruritic papular eruption on the arm

Neoplasms Associated with HIV

Kaposi Sarcoma

Kaposi sarcoma (KS) is a vascular endothelial proliferation induced by human herpesvirus type 8 (HHV-8) infection [29]. It is debatable whether this entity is a true neoplasm or a reactive proliferation. The four main subtypes of KS include classical sporadic, African endemic, iatrogenic immunosuppression-associated, and AIDS-related. In AIDS patients, HHV-8 is also implicated in other types of tumors such as non-Hodgkin lymphoma and Castleman disease [30].

Clinical presentation of KS varies from macular lesions in early stages to large and sometimes ulcerated plaques and nodules in advanced stages (Fig. 4.14). The lesions are typically asymptomatic and may vary in color from pink to red, purple, or deep blue. Chronic lesions may become deep brown secondary to postinflammatory hyperpigmentation, especially in dark skinned patients [31]. In contrast to other variants of KS, initial lesions in HIV-associated disease typically appear in the upper body, especially the head and neck. The oral mucosa is frequently involved and represents the presenting site in 10–15 % of cases. If untreated, coalescent large plaques may lead to functional impairment. In AIDS patients, involvement of extracutaneous sites occurs more rapidly, and KS lesions can be found in lymph nodes, the gastrointestinal tract and lungs.

Treatment varies depending on the extent of disease, progression pattern, and immune status. HAART itself can be very effective, but initiation of HAART can also induce flares of KS as part of the immune reconstitution inflammatory syndrome (IRIS) [32]. Localized disease may be treated with destructive methods such as cryosurgery, radiotherapy, intralesional chemotherapy with vinblastine or interferon, or topical alitretinoin gel. In more advanced or extracutaneous disease, systemic chemotherapy with doxorubicin, daunorubicin, or paclitaxel may be necessary [33].

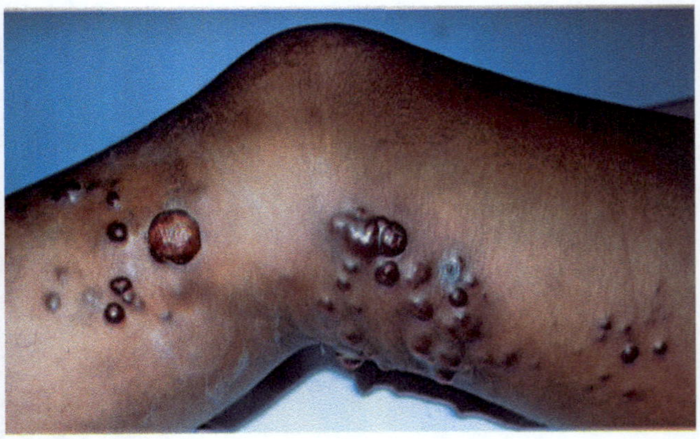

Fig. 4.14 Kaposi sarcoma

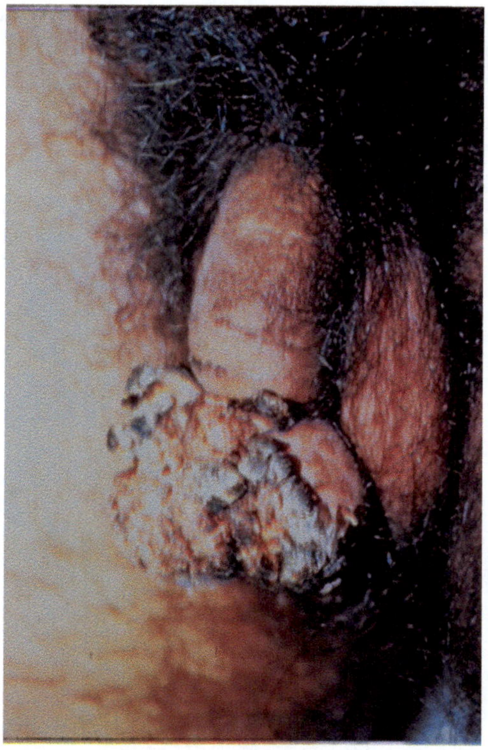

Fig. 4.15 Squamous cell carcinoma on the penis

Squamous Cell Carcinoma

Individuals with HIV infection have an increased risk of oral, cervical, penile, anal, and vulvar squamous cell carcinoma related to oncogenic subtypes of HPV, especially types 16 and 18 (Fig. 4.15). There is a high rate of coinfection with HPV and HIV, and HIV patients exhibit decreased capacity for CD4 lymphocyte-mediated clearance of HPV infections [34]. Current screening recommendations for cervical cancer have contributed to a successful decline in its incidence [35]. However, anal cancer is increasing at an alarming rate in high-risk groups, particularly in homosexual men regardless of HIV status and in HIV-positive individuals of both sexes. Guidelines for the screening and management of HPV-related anal cancer in high-risk population are still being defined, but regular anal Papanicolaou smears are advised in HIV positive patients as a screening tool.

Cutaneous Toxicities of Antiretroviral Therapy

HAART-associated cutaneous toxicities are exceedingly common, with severity ranging from mild to life-threatening. Concern about cosmetic issues may cause patients to discontinue use of medications, leading to medication resistance [36]. As multidrug therapy is standard of care in HIV infection and patients are treated with a carefully chosen cocktail of several medications, identification of the one agent responsible for a certain cutaneous side effect may be challenging but necessary to avoid unneeded discontinuation of effective treatments.

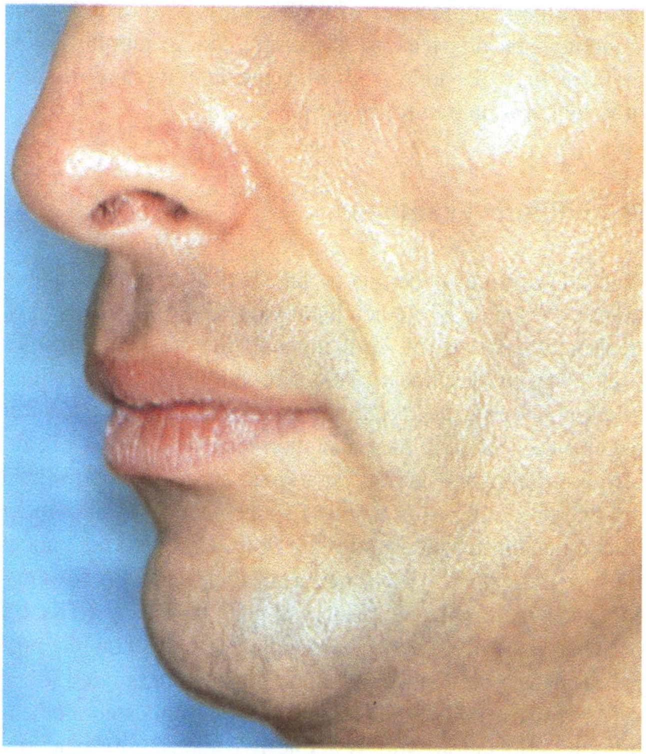

Fig. 4.16 Lipodystrophy syndrome in HIV. Loss of facial fat as seen in this image (lipoatrophy) is a common finding. Courtesy of Julia R. Nunley, M.D.

Lipodystrophy Syndrome

Lipodystrophy in HIV-positive patients is frequently associated with protease inhibitors such as indinavir as well as nucleoside reverse transcriptase inhibitors, most notably stavudine. The syndrome may develop in more than 50 % of patients treated with these medications. The risk is increased in older patients and with longer duration of therapy. Patients exhibit changes in body fat composition, most commonly loss of fat in the face (Fig. 4.16), extremities, and buttocks and accumulation of fat in the dorsocervical and abdominal areas. Gynecomastia is often present. Patients also develop metabolic abnormalities including insulin resistance, diabetes mellitus, hypertriglyceridemia, and low serum high-density lipoprotein (HDL) cholesterol levels, with an associated increased risk of pancreatitis and cardiovascular disease. Soft tissue augmentation with injectable fillers such as poly-L-lactic acid and calcium hydroxylapatite, which are both approved by the Food and Drug Administration for the treatment of HIV lipoatrophy, can help to address cosmetic concerns. Patient assistance programs may be available through the manufacturer of these products to decrease the sometimes prohibitive cost of therapy. The metabolic abnormalities may be addressed with medical therapy, dietary modifications, and exercise [36].

Morbilliform Exanthem

A morbilliform exanthem is by far the most common cutaneous manifestation of medication toxicity in HIV patients [37]. It usually consists of erythematous macules and papules coalescing into confluent plaques on the trunk and proximal limbs, although it may become generalized (Fig. 4.17). It is frequently seen after initiation of non-nucleoside reverse transcriptase inhibitors such as nevirapine and efavirenz [38]. In the majority of cases, it resolves spontaneously even without discontinuation of the responsible drug. However, the patient must be closely observed for signs of progression to Stevens–Johnson syndrome, toxic epidermal necrolysis (Fig. 4.18a, b), or hypersensitivity syndrome, which may lead to a rapidly progressive and potentially fatal multiorgan system failure [38].

Abacavir is one of the most frequently implicated medications in association with systemic hypersensitivity reaction, which usually occurs within the first 6 weeks of therapy. Patients may present with a maculopapular rash, urticaria, targetoid or erythema multiforme-like lesions, or total body erythroderma. In any suspected case, the abacavir should be discontinued immediately and the patient monitored closely for abnormalities in peripheral blood counts or liver function. The human leukocyte antigen (HLA) B*5701 allele has been associated with a higher risk of hypersensitivity reaction; screening before initiation of the medication is recommended by the manufacturer to prevent a serious adverse drug reaction [36, 39]. Patch testing for abacavir hypersensitivity is another effective screening option [36].

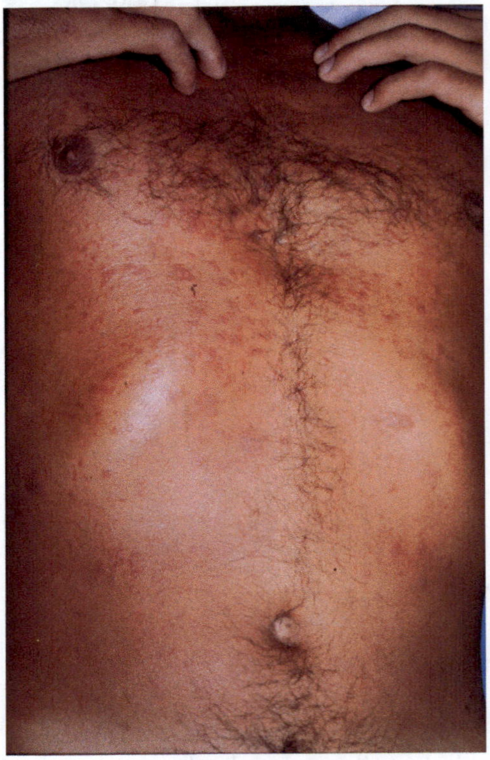

Fig. 4.17 Morbilliform drug eruption

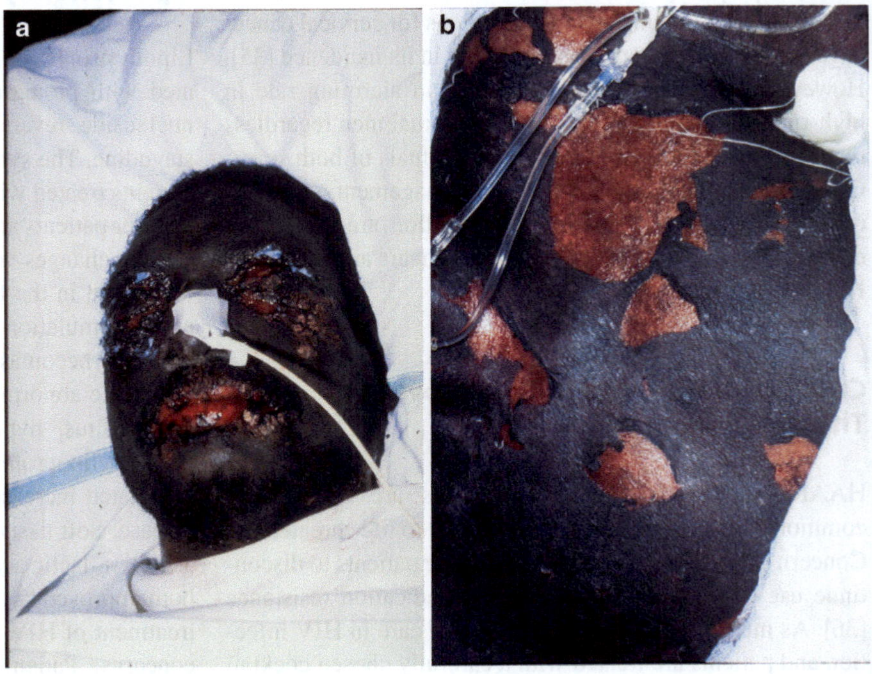

Fig. 4.18 Toxic epidermal necrolysis (**a**) Ocular and oral mucosal involvement, (**b**) epidermal detachment and sloughing on the abdomen

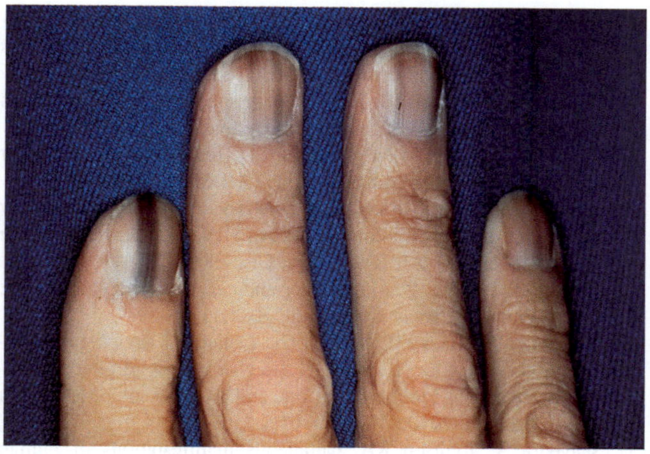

Fig. 4.19 Nail pigmentary changes due to zidovudine

Pigmentary Changes

Medication-associated pigmentary changes may be localized or generalized and may be seen in association with different processes such as psoriasiform or lichenoid drug reactions. Zidovudine, a nucleoside reverse transcriptase inhibitor, can cause brown or blue nail discoloration that may be either diffuse or in bands of longitudinal melanonychia (Fig. 4.19). Hyperpigmentation of the skin and mucous membranes is a less frequently seen associated finding. This side effect appears to be dose dependent, seen more commonly at the higher doses of zidovudine used in the 1980s and 1990s but less frequently reported today. Patients with darker skin tones are at higher risk, and the hyperpigmentation gradually resolves after discontinuation of the medication [36].

Immune Reconstitution Inflammatory Syndrome (IRIS)

Since the introduction of HAART, the prognosis of HIV has changed significantly, with fewer opportunistic infections and a slower progression to AIDS. However, upon initiating therapy, some patients, especially those with very low CD4 counts, may develop a paradoxical clinical deterioration of disease as they recover the ability to mount an inflammatory response. This is known as the IRIS, thought to be related to a deregulated immune response to subclinical infections or residual non-viable antigens [40]. Cutaneous manifestations of IRIS can be divided into two groups, infectious and inflammatory, and usually appear within the first 3 months of HAART therapy. IRIS must be differentiated from a new infection or a medication reaction, which can be challenging.

Clinical manifestations generally resemble the typical manifestations of these entities in the immunocompetent host [41]. The most common infectious diseases are HPV, VZV, molluscum contagiosum, mycobacterial and fungal infections. Among the inflammatory dermatoses, autoimmune reactions, sarcoidosis, and other granulomatous dermatoses such as tattoo reactions may be observed [41]. There is no specific treatment for IRIS and no recommended prophylaxis because of the variability and unpredictable manifestations of this entity. Prompt diagnosis of underlying infections and developing manifestations is paramount to avoid severe complications that may be life-threatening in some cases [38].

References

1. De Cock KM, Jaffe HW, Curran JW. The evolving epidemiology of HIV/AIDS. AIDS. 2012;26:1205.
2. Hogan MT. Cutaneous infections associated with HIV/AIDS. Dermatol Clin. 2006;24:473.
3. Nnoruka EN, Chukwuka JC, Anisuiba B. Correlation of mucocutaneous manifestations of HIV/AIDS infection with CD4 counts and disease progression. Int J Dermatol. 2007;46:14.
4. Cedeno-Laurent F, Gomez-Flores M, Mendez N, et al. New insights into HIV-1-primary skin disorders. J Int AIDS Soc. 2011;14:5.
5. Islam FM, Wu J, Jansson J, et al. Relative risk of renal disease among people living with HIV: a systematic review and meta-analysis. BMC Public Health. 2012;12:234.
6. Miro JM, Cofan F, Trullas JC, et al. Renal dysfunction in the setting of HIV/AIDS. Curr HIV/AIDS Rep. 2012;9:187.
7. Wyatt CM. The kidney in HIV infection: beyond HIV-associated nephropathy. Top Antiviral Med. 2012;20(3):106.
8. Khambaty MM, Hsu SS. Dermatology of the patient with HIV. Emerg Med Clin N Am. 2010;28:355.
9. Hulsebosch HJ, Claessen FA, VanGinkel CJ, et al. Human immunodeficiency virus exanthem. J Am Acad Dermatol. 1990;23:483.
10. Abrams DI. Clinical manifestations of HIV infection, including persistent generalized lymphadenopathy and AIDS-related complex. J Am Acad Dermatol. 1990;22:1217.
11. Rodgers S, Leslie KS. Skin infections in HIV-infected individuals in the era of HAART. Curr Opin Infect Dis. 2011;24:124.
12. Gormley R, Kovarik C. Dermatologic manifestations of HPV in HIV-infected individuals. Curr HIV/AIDS Rep. 2009;6:130.
13. Maurer T. Dermatologic manifestations of HIV infection. Top HIV Med. 2005;13(5):149.
14. Toro JR, Wood LV, Patel NK, et al. Topical cidofovir: a novel treatment for recalcitrant molluscum contagiosum in children infected with human immunodeficiency virus 1. Arch Dermatol. 2000;136(8):983.
15. Theiler M, Kempf W, Kerl K, et al. Disseminated molluscum contagiosum in a HIV-positive child: improvement after therapy with 5% imiquimod. J Dermatol Case Rep. 2011;5(2):19.
16. Sadick N, Sorhaindo L. A comparative split-face study of cryosurgery and trichloroacetic acid 100% peels in the treatment of HIV-associated disseminated facial molluscum contagiosum. Cutis. 2009;83(6):299.
17. Golden MR, Marra CM, Homes KK. Update on syphilis: resurgence of an old problem. JAMA. 2003;290(11):1510–4.
18. Gregory N, Sanchez M, Buchness MR. The spectrum of syphilis in patients with human immunodeficiency virus infection. J Am Acad Dermatol. 1990;22(6 Pt 1):1061–7.
19. Gasquet S, Maurin M, Brouqui P, et al. Bacillary angiomatosis by *Bartonella quintana* in an HIV-infected patient. J Am Acad Dermatol. 2000;42(2):299–301.

20. Zancanaro PC, McGirt LY, Mammelak AJ, et al. Cutaneous manifestations of HIV in the era of highly active antiretroviral therapy: an institutional urban clinic experience. J Am Acad Dermatol. 2006;54(4):581–8.
21. Smith KJ, Skelton HG, Yeager J, et al. Cutaneous findings in HIV-1 positive patients: a 42-month prospective study. J Am Acad Dermatol. 1994;31:746–54.
22. Gupta AK, Bluhm R. Seborrheic dermatitis. J Eur Acad Dermatol Venereol. 2004;18(1):13–26.
23. Mallon E, Bunker CB. HIV-associated psoriasis. AIDS Patient Care Stds. 2000;14:239–46.
24. Morar N, Willis-Owen SA, Maurer T, et al. HIV-associated psoriasis: pathogenesis, clinical features, and management. Lancet Infect Dis. 2010;10(7):470–8.
25. Menon K, Van Voorhees AS, Bebo BF, et al. Psoriasis in patients with HIV infection: from the medical board of the National Psoriasis Foundation. J Am Acad Dermatol. 2010;62(2):291–9.
26. Ting PT, Koo JY. Use of etanercept in human immunodeficiency virus (HIV) and acquired immunodeficiency syndrome (AIDS) patients. Int J Dermatol. 2006;45(6):689–92.
27. Afonso JP, Tomimori J, Michalany NS, et al. Pruritic papular eruption and eosinophilic folliculitis associated with human immunodeficiency virus (HIV) infection: a histopathological and immunohistochemical comparative study. J Am Acad Dermatol. 2012;67(2):269–75.
28. Fearfield LA, Rowe A, Francis N, et al. Itchy folliculitis and human immunodeficiency virus infection: clinicopathological and immunological features, pathogenesis and treatment. Br J Dermatol. 1999;141:3–11.
29. Chang Y, Cesarman E, Pessin MS, et al. Identification of herpesvirus-like DNA sequences in AIDS-associated Kaposi's sarcoma. Science. 1994;266:1865–9.
30. Schwartz RA, Micali G, Nasca MR, et al. Kaposi sarcoma: a continuing conundrum. J Am Acad Dermatol. 2008;59(2):179–206.
31. Friedman-Kien AE, Saltzman BR. Clinical manifestations of classical, endemic African, and epidemic AIDS-associated Kaposi's sarcoma. J Am Acad Dermatol. 1990;22(6 Pt 2):1237–50.
32. Costner M, Cockerell CJ. The changing spectrum of the cutaneous manifestations of HIV disease. Arch Dermatol. 1998;134:1290.
33. Aldenhoven M, Barlo NP, Sanders CJ. Therapeutic strategies for epidemic Kaposi's sarcoma. Int J STD AIDS. 2006;17:571–8.
34. Ng'andwe C, Lowe J, Richards P, et al. The distribution of sexually transmitted human papillomaviruses in HIV positive and negative patients in Zambia. Afr BMC Infect Dis. 2007;7:77.
35. Darragh T, Winkler B. Anal cancer and cervical cancer screening: key differences. Cancer Cytopathol. 2011;119:5–19.
36. Introcaso CE, Hines JM, Kovarik CL. Cutaneous toxicities of antiretroviral therapy for HIV. Part I. Lipodystrophy syndrome, nucleoside reverse transcriptase inhibitors, and protease inhibitors. J Am Acad Dermatol. 2010;63(4):549–61.
37. Saavedra A, Johnson RA. Cutaneous manifestations of human immunodeficiency virus disease. In: Wolff K, Goldsmith LA, Katz SI, et al., editors. Fitzpatrick's dermatology in general medicine. 7th ed. New York, NY: McGraw-Hill; 2008. p. 1927–40.
38. Introcaso CE, Hines JM, Kovarik CL. Cutaneous toxicities of antiretroviral therapy for HIV. Part II. Nonnucleoside reverse transcriptase inhibitors, entry and fusion inhibitors, integrase inhibitors, and immune reconstitution syndrome. J Am Acad Dermatol. 2010;63(4):563–9.
39. Lyher J, Glesby MJ. Dermatologic adverse effects of antiretroviral therapy: recognition and management. Am J Clin Dermatol. 2007;8:221–33.
40. Murdoch DM, Venter WDF, Van Rie A, et al. Immune reconstitution inflammatory syndrome. AIDS Res Ther. 2007;4:1–9.
41. Shelburne SA, Hamill RJ, Rodríguez-Barradas MC, et al. Immune reconstitution inflammatory syndrome: emergence of a unique syndrome during highly active antiretroviral therapy. Medicine (Baltimore). 2002;81:213–27.

Rheumatologic Conditions

5

Kseniya Golubets, Dan Ilkovitch, and Lisa M. Grandinetti

Systemic Lupus Erythematosus

Introduction

There are multiple variants of systemic lupus erythematosus (SLE), a multiorgan autoimmune disease, which vary in histopathology and the degree of associated dermatologic involvement. Cutaneous manifestations of SLE make up 4 of the 11 American College of Rheumatology (ACR) criteria (malar rash, discoid rash, photosensitivity, oral ulcers) for SLE classification—a useful tool for categorizing lupus for research purposes but less so for diagnosis in the clinical setting [1].

Specific cutaneous lupus lesions can be organized into specific and nonspecific lesions. SLE-*specific* lesions come in three major forms: acute, subacute, and chronic, and its variants [2]. These include acute cutaneous lupus erythematosus (ACLE), subacute cutaneous lupus erythematosus (SCLE), discoid lupus erythematosus (DLE), lupus erythematosus tumidus (LET), and lupus panniculitis (LP). These variants are not mutually exclusive and often coexist in the same patient [2].

Pathogenesis

The pathogenesis of lupus results from a multifactorial interplay of genetic and environmental risk factors (such as Ultraviolet A (UVA)/Ultraviolet B (UVB) exposure), that create a complex environment of immune cells and cytokines/chemokines, resulting in cytotoxic keratinocyte and tissue damage [2].

K. Golubets, M.D., M.H.S. • D. Ilkovitch, M.D., Ph.D.
L.M. Grandinetti, M.D., F.A.A.D. (✉)
Department of Dermatology, University of Pittsburgh, Presbyterian South Tower, Suite 3880, 200 Lothrop Street, Pittsburgh, PA 15213, USA
e-mail: golubetsk@upmc.edu; ilkovitchd@upmc.edu; grandinettilm@upmc.edu

Clinical

Acute cutaneous lupus erythematosus (*ACLE*) is the cutaneous phenotype with the strongest association with systemic disease. It is usually transient, resolves without scarring and can be accompanied by oral ulceration [2]. It is characterized by malar erythema ("butterfly rash"), as well as telangiectasias, erosions, dyspigmentation, and epidermal atrophy (i.e., poikiloderma) (Fig. 5.1). Other less common ACLE variants include: toxic epidermal necrolysis-like eruption of acute lupus erythematosus, also known as acute syndrome of apoptotic pan-epidermolysis (ASAP), and an entity named Rowell eruption (erythema multiforme-like lesions in lupus patients), which may be a severe variant of ACLE or SCLE.

Subacute cutaneous lupus erythematosus (*SCLE*) (Fig. 5.2) is an eruption that lasts longer than ACLE, but similar to ACLE it does not result in scarring, with a relatively good prognosis [1, 3], affecting photosensitive areas on the sides of the face, upper trunk, and extremities. Since lesions can be annular, with raised red borders and central clearing, or scaly patches, they can be confused with figurate erythemas or dermatophyte infections, and dermatomyositis can often mimic SCLE. SCLE can also be induced by a wide variety of medications including numerous antihypertensives, terbinafine, and an assortment of other medications [2, 3].

Chronic cutaneous lupus erythematosus (*CCLE*) is subdivided into four subgroups: DLE, LET, LP, and chilblain lupus. DLE (Fig. 5.3) is characterized by chronic and inflammatory discoid lesions, which can lead to permanent disfiguring scars. It frequently involves the head (i.e., ears, scalp, face) and less frequently the mucosal surfaces (i.e., ocular, nasal, oral, and genital). Active lesions are more indurated, while healing lesions are more atrophic, which can heal with hypopigmentation or hyperpigmentation. One complication of DLE is development of squamous cell carcinoma within the lesions. DLE lesions are 1 of the 11 American Rheumatism Association (ARA) criteria for SLE and may be a presenting sign of SLE [2]. Approximately 5–10 % of patients will have a DLE-SLE overlap, with a relatively benign but chronic course [3].

J.R. Nunley and E.V. Lerma (eds.), *Dermatological Manifestations of Kidney Disease*,
DOI 10.1007/978-1-4939-2395-3_5, © Springer Science+Business Media New York 2015

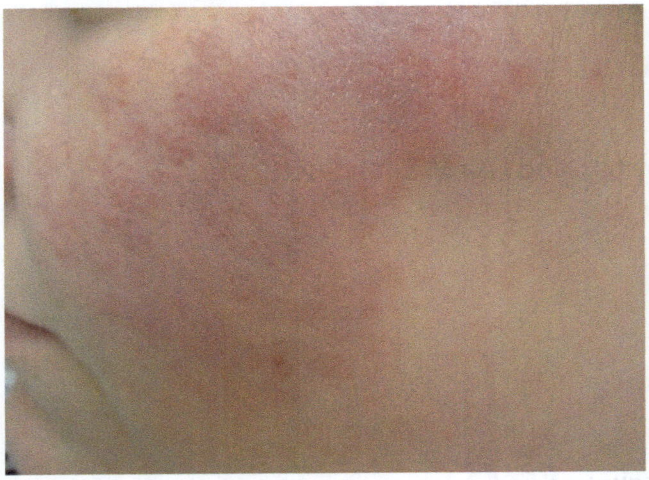

Fig. 5.1 Malar rash of acute cutaneous lupus erythematosus. Photo courtesy of Oleg Akilov, M.D., Ph.D.

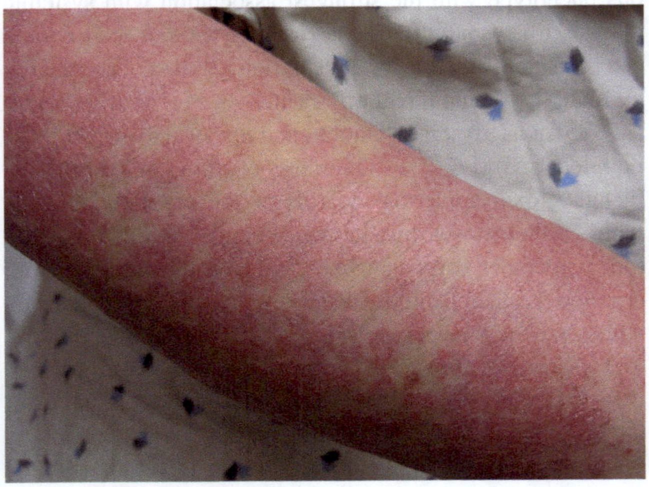

Fig. 5.2 Scaly erythematous plaques on the forearms consistent with SCLE. Photo courtesy of Joseph C. English, III, M.D.

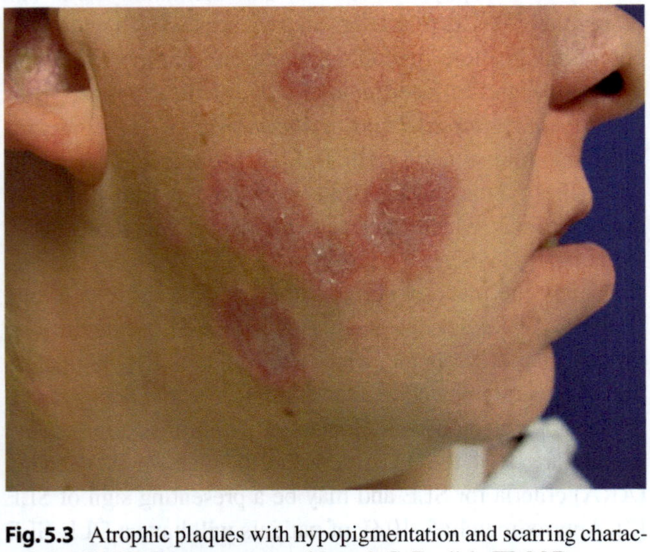

Fig. 5.3 Atrophic plaques with hypopigmentation and scarring characteristic of DLE. Photo courtesy of Joseph C. English, III, M.D.

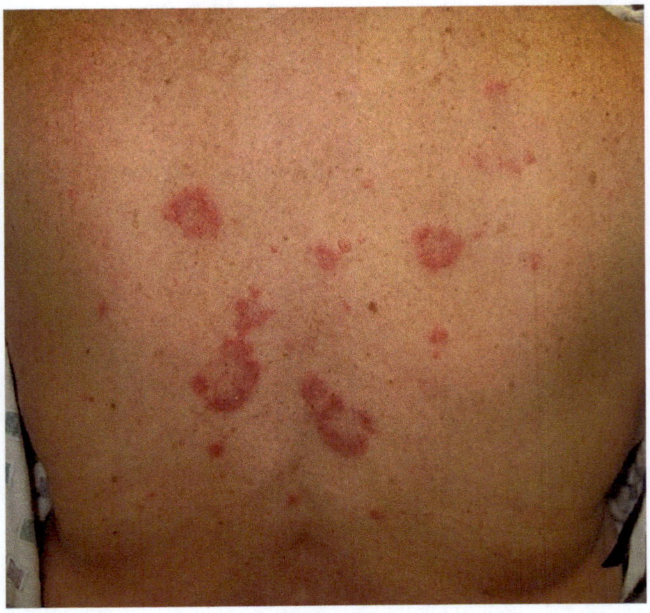

Fig. 5.4 Lupus erythematosus tumidus. Indurated erythematous plaques on the trunk. Photo courtesy of Joseph C. English, III, M.D.

A second subgroup of chronic lupus is LET (Fig. 5.4), which is seen less commonly. LET is characterized by indurated lesions, located on the sun exposed regions of the face and trunk [4]. Lesions can be reproducible with phototesting [5] and resolve without scarring or atrophy. LET is believed by some to be related to Jessner lymphocytic infiltrate [6] , which is a benign lymphocytic infiltrate of the skin with similar clinical annular plaques and central clearing.

The third subgroup of chronic lupus is *lupus panniculitis* (*LP*), an inflammation of the fat that results in erythematous indurated plaques characteristically located on the face, upper trunk, and arms, as well as thighs and buttocks [7]. Ulceration of the lesions has been reported in 6–28 % of patients in different studies, though to be caused by impaired circulation as a result of fibrin deposits or tissue hyaline necrosis of fat [7]. These lesions may result in lipoatrophy creating depressed skin regions (Fig. 5.5) [2, 7]. It is important to distinguish LP from the fatal subcutaneous panniculitis-like-T-cell lymphoma [8].

Chilblain lupus erythematosus (*CHLE*) or SLE pernio represents the fourth subgroup of chronic cutaneous lupus, with characteristic dusky purple papules and plaques on the acral surfaces (i.e., fingers, toes, nose) (Fig. 5.6). CHLE is triggered by cold, and moist or damp conditions. Compromised perfusion can result in partially necrotic and malodorous superinfected ulcerations [9]. Some lesions with time may develop into a discoid lesion [2] and approximately 18 % may progress to SLE [9]. It is also possible that a patient may have concurrent chilblains (also known as perniosis), which is a cold-sensitive disorder resulting from abnormal inflammatory response to cold thought to be vascular in origin. CHLE can

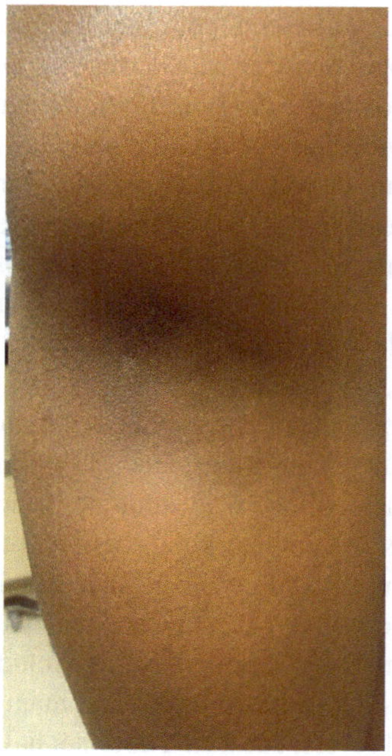

Fig. 5.5 Lupus panniculitis in the arm resulting in lipoatrophy. Photo courtesy of Oleg Akilov, M.D., Ph.D.

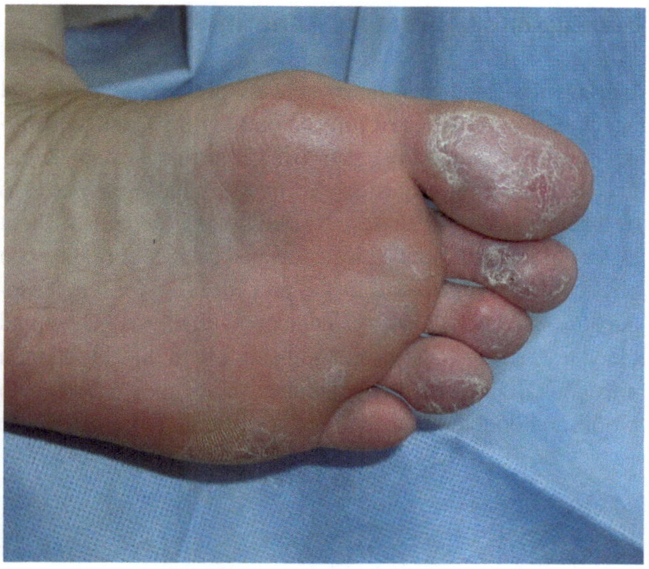

Fig. 5.6 Chilblain lupus. Without knowing the clinical history, chilblain lupus can be difficult to distinguish from simple cold-induced injury. Seen here are the dusky purple changes typical for this condition. Photo courtesy of Julia R. Nunley, M.D.

be sporadic or inherited via an autosomal dominant missense mutation. There are some reports describing tumor necrosis factor alpha (TNF-α)-antagonist-induced chilblain lupus [10].

Additional, nonspecific lesions can be associated with, but not limited to, SLE. Blisters can be seen in lupus patients, which could represent bullous lupus erythematosus (BLE) lesions (found to be associated with active LE) (Fig. 5.7) or could represent a concurrent disease process (i.e., pseudoporphyria,

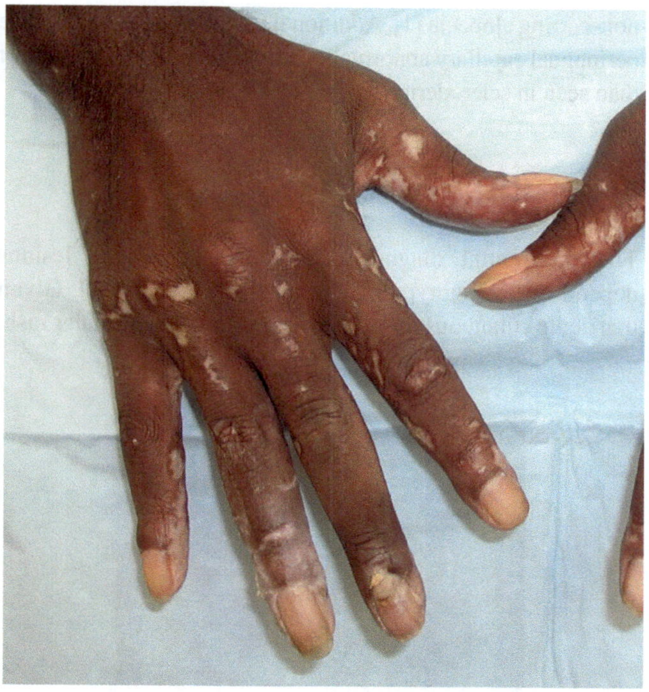

Fig. 5.7 Bullous lupus. Seen in this image are various stages of bullous lupus; some lesions are still vesicular, whereas others have resulted in a scar. Photo courtesy of Julia R. Nunley, M.D.

immunobullous diseases, etc.) [3]. Patients with BLE have a good response to treatment with oral dapsone and often have antibodies to type VII collagen. Other nonspecific lesions seen in LE patients are vascular lesions [2], and low complement levels of C3 and C4 point to connective tissue vasculitis. Systemic involvement should be considered in patients with cutaneous lupus and other associated findings, such as livedo reticularis ("lacy" vascular pattern on extremities) (Fig. 5.8), Raynaud phenomenon (cyanotic finger tips or other acral sites, due an exaggerated vascular response to cold/emotion) (Fig. 5.9a, b), erythema of the palms and periungual telangiectasias. Other clues of systemic disease are purpuric lesions, ulcers and urticarial papules, and atrophie blanche (hypopigmented atrophic scars, usually on lower extremities) (Fig. 5.10) [2]. Of note, findings of livedo reticularis, thromboses, and ulcerations are also associated with antiphospholipid antibodies. Also, keep in mind syndromes that may be associated with some of these findings, such as Sneddon syndrome (associated with livedo reticularis and ischemic central nervous system (CNS) disease) as well as Hughes syndrome (associated with antiphospholipid syndrome).

Alopecia occurs in as high as 45 % of patients with lupus [1]. Scarring alopecia is more common with discoid LE lesions, whereas diffuse nonscarring alopecia is more associated with systemic disease (Fig. 5.11). Overall, lupus patients have increased risk of alopecia areata [11]. Moreover, systemic medical therapy for lupus may be responsible for some of the nonscarring alopecia [1]. Additionally, patients with lupus have periungual capillary abnormalities, but these are less prominent than seen in scleroderma or dermatomyositis [2].

Differential Diagnosis

The differential diagnoses for cutaneous lupus lesions depend on the subtype of lupus noted on exam [2]. Given that acute cutaneous lupus often presents with the malar rash,

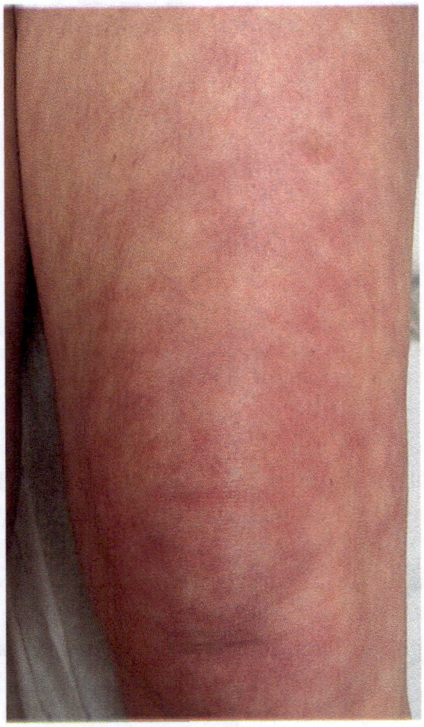

Fig. 5.8 Livedo reticularis. Lacy vascular pattern on extremities. Photo courtesy of Joseph C. English, III, M.D.

keep in mind the differential of other common entities, such as rosacea, atopic or seborrheic dermatitis, as well as phototoxic and photoallergic drug reactions, dermatomyositis, and pemphigus erythematosus. Annular scaly lesions of subacute cutaneous lupus can look like psoriasis, fungal infections, figurate erythemas (e.g., erythema annulare centrifugum), atopic or contact dermatitis, and dermatomyositis. Facial discoid lupus can look similar to tinea, lichen planus, and lichen planopilaris, Jessner lymphocytic infiltrate, polymorphous light eruption, sarcoidosis, lupus vulgaris, non-melanoma skin cancer and other lymphocytic infiltrations, granuloma faciale, and fungal infections. For the differential of LET, consider Jessner lymphocytic infiltrate, reticular erythematous mucinosis and polymorphous light eruption. When considering LP, one should consider other panniculitidies, such as erythema nodosum, subcutaneous panniculitis like T cell lymphoma. Finally, it is imperative to exclude drug-induced lupus, which is a systemic reaction that manifest with a rash, arthralgias and fevers, but which does not have CNS and kidney involvement seen with SLE, and which commonly resolves with discontinuation of the inciting drug.

Workup and Laboratory Abnormalities

Workup for cutaneous lupus includes performing a lesional punch biopsy for hematoxylin and eosin (H&E), and performing direct immunofluorescence (DIF), if histology is not definitive. If the skin biopsy is consistent with lupus, one needs to evaluate for systemic disease by questioning the patient about history of arthritis, noting any associated cutaneous findings on physical exam (discussed above) and checking for lymphadenopathy. Additional testing includes a urinalysis (UA), and blood tests such as complete blood count with diff, blood urea nitrogen (BUN), creatinine, antinuclear antibody (ANA) with profile anti-double stranded (ds) deoxyribonucleic acid (DNA)

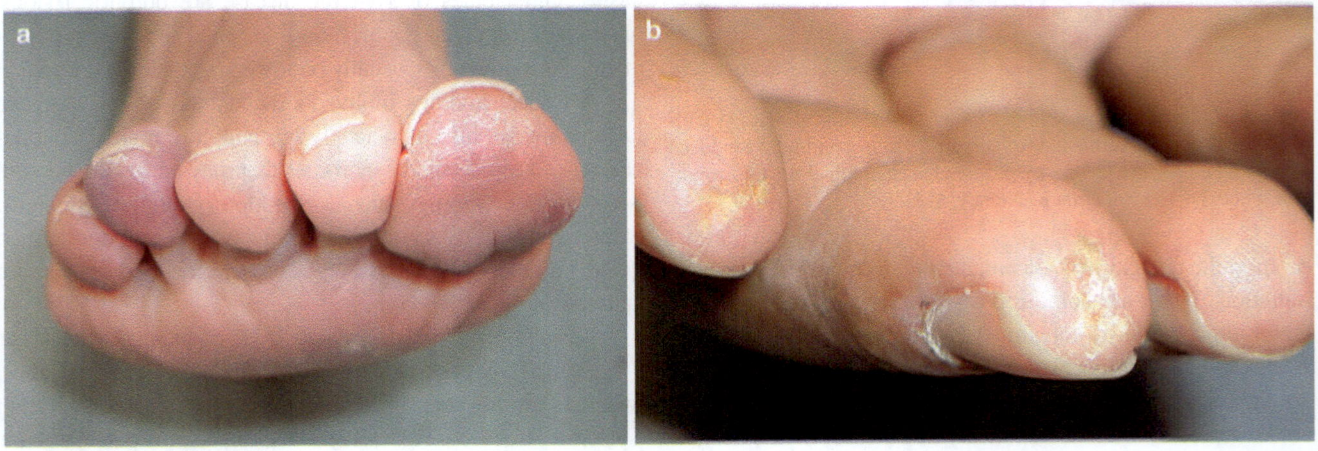

Fig. 5.9 Raynaud phenomenon is most common in patients with scleroderma. Seen here are two of the classic changes. Image **a** demonstrates the dusky blue that is transient; image **b** is a result of the chronic ischemia with skin necrosis. Photo courtesy of Julia R. Nunley, M.D.

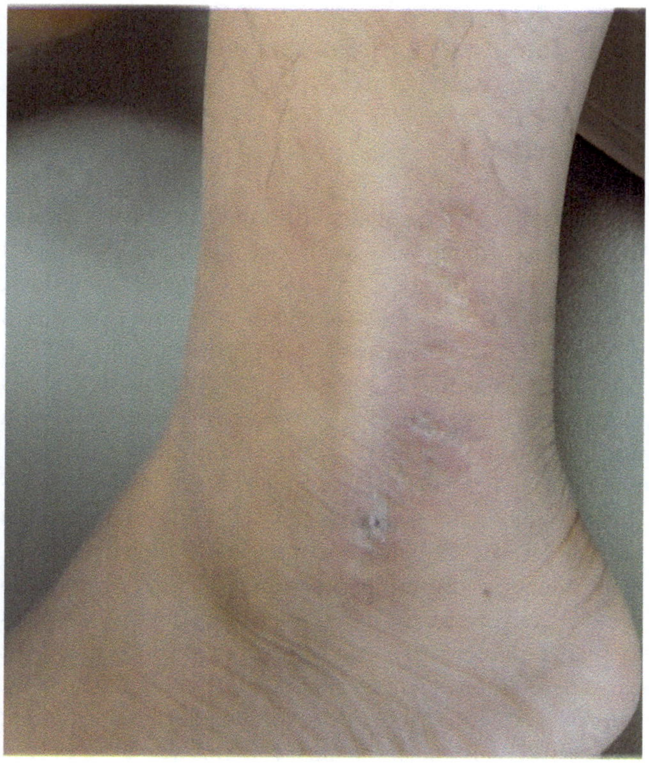

Fig. 5.10 Hypopigmented stellate scarring on the lower extremities consistent with atrophie blanche. Photo courtesy of Joseph C. English, III, M.D.

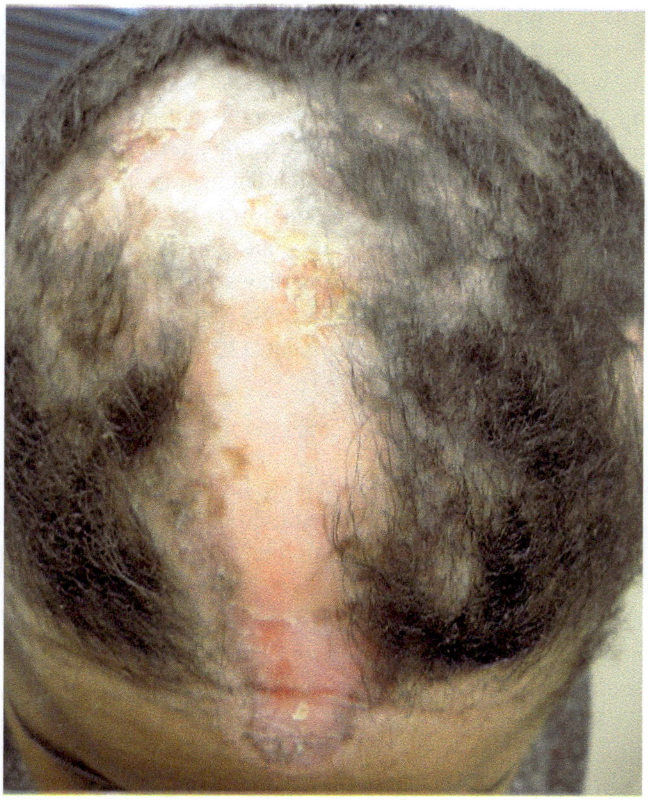

Fig. 5.11 Scarring alopecia in the setting of discoid lupus erythematosus. Photo courtesy of Joseph C. English, III, M.D.

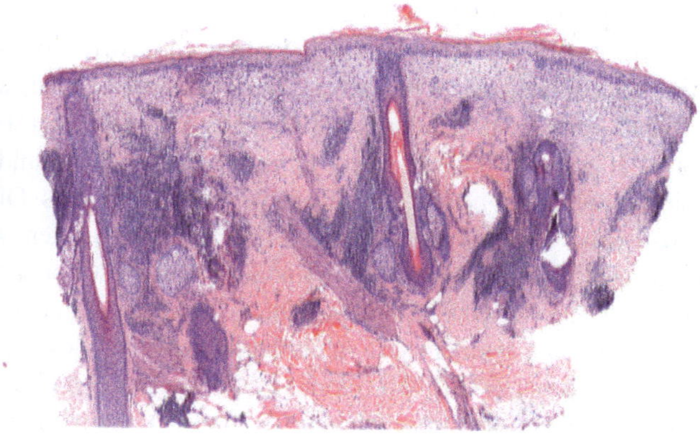

Fig. 5.12 Photomicrograph of a skin biopsy demonstrating basal layer cell damage with lymphohistiocytic inflammation and periadnexal inflammation. Photo courtesy of John Vu, M.D., Ph.D.

and anti-smooth muscle (Sm) antibodies, complement levels (C3, C4), and erythrocyte sedimentation rate (ESR). A diagnosis of SLE will be based on fulfilling the required 4 of 11 criteria [12, 13]. Of note, an inherited complement deficiency should be considered in a child with severe cutaneous disease and glomerulonephritis [14–16].

Histopathology

On histopathological evaluation there is presence of basal layer cell damage, lymphohistiocytic inflammation at the interface of dermal and epidermal junction, and periadnexal inflammation (Fig. 5.12). Overall, there is variable follicular plugging and scarring, but discoid lesions have more epidermal atrophy and follicular plugging [2, 17]. There is prominent dermal mucin deposition seen in LE tumidus, and LP has inflammation of the subcutis. Even though DIF evaluation of skin is not necessary for diagnosis, when it is performed one will see granular immunoglobulin G (IgG) and/or immunoglobulin M (IgM) antibody deposition at dermal–epidermal junction in lesional and nonlesional skin, and hair follicles.

Laboratory Abnormalities

Abnormalities may be seen in the laboratory studies listed above in section labeled workup. In addition, appropriate laboratory studies should be ordered to evaluate for the possibility of antiphospholipid syndrome.

Treatment

When choosing the appropriate treatments for cutaneous lupus, which include both topical and systemic agents, one has to weigh the benefit and the side effect profile of the medications. Topical steroids are often safe to use, from mild potency steroids such as desonide 0.05 % ointment that can be used on the face, to moderate potency steroids such as triamcinolone 0.1 % ointment that can be used on the rest of body, both applied twice a day. Intralesional steroids (such as triamcinolone in a concentration of 10 mg/mL) are safe to use for active discoid and tumid lesions, sparing the patient side effects of systemic steroids. Of note, discoid lupus may be the rare instance when high potency steroids (such as clobetasol 0.05 % ointment) can be used on the face [2]. There is anecdotal evidence for use of topical immunomodulators such as calcineurin inhibitors or topical retinoids in cutaneous lupus [18–20]. Intravenous immunoglobulin (IVIG), systemic immunosuppressant therapy (see below), and biologic therapies such as belimumab (the first Food and Drug Administration (FDA)-approved targeted therapy for SLE) have been shown to have efficacy in mild to moderate disease [21].

Treatment of cutaneous lupus and associated systemic disease is accomplished with several agents [2]. The gold standard for systemic therapy are antimalarial agents such as hydroxychloroquine (200 mg PO daily to twice a day, max 6.5 mg/kg ideal body weight/day), chloroquine (125–250 PO daily; up to 3.5–4 mg/kg ideal body weight/day), or quinacrine (100 mg PO daily). For cutaneous disease that is resistant to antimalarials, one could use oral retinoids (e.g., acitretin, isotretinoin), thalidomide (initiate at 50–100 mg PO daily; after desired response drop to maintenance dose of 25–50 mg daily or if possible, every 3–4 days), or dapsone (for bullous SLE). Immunosuppressive agents such as systemic corticosteroids, mycophenolate mofetil, azathioprine, and sulfasalazine are used as well. Finally, immune response modifier agents used for treatment of cutaneous lupus resistant to other therapies are rituximab, abatacept, belimumab, and anti-interleukin (IL)-6 antibody and anti-IL-10 antibodies.

Patients should also be educated about sun protection and avoidance, which can act as triggering and exacerbating factors in the disease. Smoking has been shown to correlate with resistance to antimalarial therapy, and thus smoking cessation should be encouraged.

Prognosis

The prognosis of cutaneous lupus depends on the subtype, the associated progression of systemic involvement, and response to treatment. Patients with CCLE or SCLE primarily have skin involvement and generally lack organ involvement, which usually indicates a benign course [3]. Patients with ACLE have the highest risk of internal disease involvement; however, patients with any type of cutaneous LE can develop systemic involvement. Cutaneous diseases that are refractory to antimalarials are likely to be refractory other treatments as well [2]. Scarring is seen more commonly in SLE and discoid lupus, whereas is not typically seen in ACLE, SCLE, tumid lupus and LP. Late-onset SLE is associated with a worse prognosis [22].

Granulomatosis with Polyangiitis (Wegener Granulomatosis)

Introduction

Granulomatosis with polyangiitis (GPA), previously known as Wegener granulomatosis, is one of the antineutrophil cytoplasmic antibody (ANCA) associated vasculitides, which also includes microscopic polyangiitis (MPA) and eosinophilic granulomatosis with polyangiitis (EGPA, previously known as Churg–Strauss syndrome). GPA is characterized by a triad of: (1) systemic vasculitis of skin and oral mucosa, (2) necrotizing granulomatous inflammation of the upper and lower respiratory tracts, and (3) pauci-immune glomerulonephritis [23–25]. GPA has a high mortality rate if untreated, and there is variation in severity, from focal involvement (i.e., only airway disease) to systemic or generalized disease (multiorgan) [25]. GPA has a predilection for white middle aged adults, affecting 5–12 cases per million and has a slight female predominance [2]. Primary systemic vasculitis is exceedingly rare in children; however, GPA is one of the most common vasculitides seen in this population [26].

Pathogenesis

The pathogenesis of GPA is thought to be multifactorial, and is influenced by the presence of ANCAs and environmental, as well as genetic factors. ANCA (particularly anti-PR3) have been shown to activate neutrophils presenting specific antigens (possibly infectious), activating alternative complement pathway and furthering an inflammatory vicious cycle that eventually leads to granuloma formation [27]. There are reports of *Staphylococcus aureus* nasal carriage correlating with disease relapse, which may play a role in nasal/pulmonary pathogenesis of GPA [28, 29]. ANCA antibodies are seen in 85–95 % of affected patients [30].

Clinical

Diagnosis of GPA can be made based on the 1990 ACR criteria, when two of the following four criteria are present: (1) nasal or oral inflammation, (2) abnormal chest radiograph, (3) abnormal urinary sediment (microhematuria >5 red blood cells per high-power field or red blood cell casts in urine sediment), and (4) granulomatous inflammation on biopsy. ACR criteria may not be appropriate for children with vasculitis; as such the European League Against Rheumatism/Pediatric Rheumatology European Society (EULAR/PRES) has proposed some additional criteria including not only nasal, but sinus inflammation, imaging studies to include

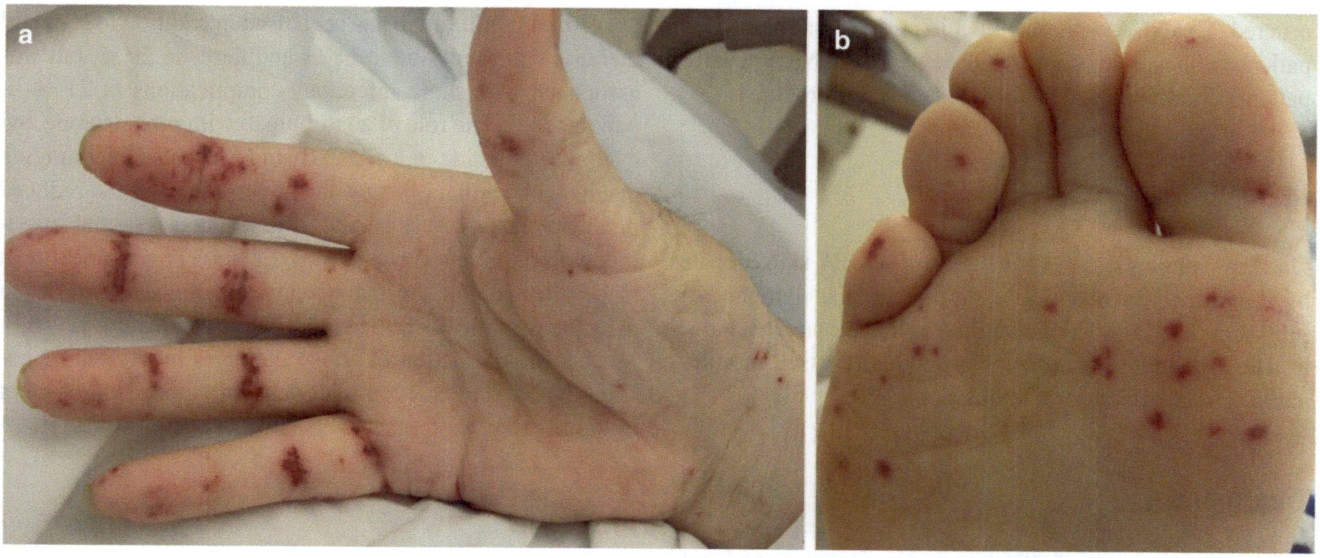

Fig. 5.13 (a, b) Palpable purpura on the extremities of a patient with granulomatosis with polyangiitis (Wegener granulomatosis)

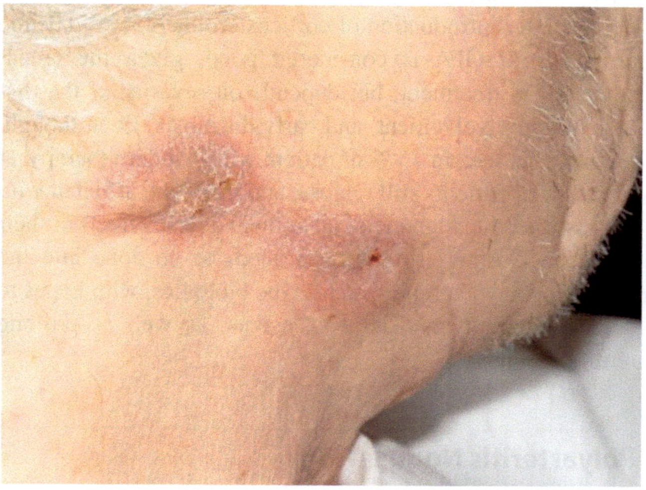

Fig. 5.14 Subcutaneous nodules on the face of a patient with granulomatosis with polyangiitis (Wegener granulomatosis)

chest computed tomography (CT), as well as other criteria. However, the new criteria have shown no improvement over the ACR criteria in disease classification [31].

Cutaneous involvement occurs in 46–66 % of GPA patients [32], but only 10 % of patients have it as a presenting feature [2]. The most common lesions are palpable purpura (Fig. 5.13a, b), followed by oral ulcers and red, friable gingival tissue and hyperplastic gums ("strawberry gums"). Oral involvement can be seen in 10–62 % of patients, but may be a presenting sign in 5–10 % of patients in GPA [32, 33]. Ten percent of patients will have painful subcutaneous nodules and ulcers found on the elbows, as well as the face and scalp, which resemble pyoderma gangrenosum. They may be mistaken for rheumatoid nodules, but GPA lesions can ulcerate unlike rheumatoid nodules (Fig. 5.14) [32].

Airway involvement of the upper or lower respiratory tracts affects between 60 and 90 % of patients [2, 32], with more than 70 % of cases presenting with nasal, sinus, tracheal, and ear symptoms. Other signs and symptoms include recurrent epistaxis, mucosal ulcerations, nasal septal perforation, and saddle nose deformity. Furthermore, pulmonary involvement includes hemoptysis, dyspnea, cough, or pleuritis, with infiltrates and nodes on chest radiograph [2, 32]. Renal disease affects 18 % of patients at presentation and 77 % of patients eventually develop glomerulonephritis [23]. Necrotizing vasculitis of GPA also affects other organs, causing musculoskeletal (70 %), ocular (30–60 %), neurologic (20–50 %), and gastrointestinal (GI) (5–10 %) disease [32].

Differential Diagnosis

The differential diagnosis of GPA includes other ANCA-associated vasculitides, especially EGPA, which is another necrotizing granulomatous vasculitis. EGPA can also present with the papulonecrotic lesions seen in GPA, but on biopsy the former has eosinophils and pink instead of blue necrobiosis as well as evident peripheral eosinophilia (>10^9/L) [32].

Workup and Laboratory Abnormalities

The workup for GPA includes inflammatory labs, such as erythrocyte sedimentation rate (ESR) and C-reactive protein (CRP), as well as CBC to check for anemia and elevated white blood cell count [2]. Fifty percent of patients have a positive rheumatoid factor. Cytoplasmic ANCA (c-ANCA) with anti-proteinase 3(anti-PR-3) specificity and antimyeloperoxidase (anti-MPO or p-ANCA) antibodies should be ordered. C-ANCA with anti-PR3 is positive in 75–80 % of patients with classic or severe GPA, whereas ANCA negative patients usually have focal disease and better prognosis [32].

Histopathology

On histopathological examination, most GPA skin biopsies have nonspecific changes with perivascular lymphocytic infiltrates, but 25–50 % of the time will demonstrate characteristic necrotizing leukocytoclastic small vessel vasculitis and/or granulomatous inflammation [2, 17].

Treatment

The goal of treatment of GPA is prompt recognition and early institution of treatment to prevent severe complications. Standard treatment of active severe GPA includes systemic glucocorticoids (1 mg/kg/day of prednisone) plus oral daily cyclophosphamide for 3–6 months. This treatment results in a remission in up to 75 % of patients, improvement in 91 % and survival in 80 %, but relapses occur 50 % of the time [2, 23]. Treatment with cyclophosphamide is associated with several serious side effects, including but not limited to transitional carcinoma of the bladder in 6–15 % of patients, myelodysplasia, and skin cancer [34]. There is evidence for intravenous cyclophosphamide pulses inducing remissions, with multiple low-dose treatments may be required to prevent relapses [35].

Alternatives to cyclophosphamide for induction or maintenance therapy for classic GPA include azathioprine, methotrexate (MTX), and mycophenolate mofetil [36, 37]. Methotrexate has been shown to have similar efficacy in inducing remission as compared to cyclophosphamide in active but not severe disease [38], and has the same rate of relapse with lower toxicity as maintenance therapy [38, 39]. Besides MTX and cyclophosphamide, maintenance therapy can also be accomplished with azathioprine or mycophenolate mofetil for 2 years or more. However, azathioprine maintenance therapy has been linked to higher relapse rate in anti-PR-3 positive patients. There are also reports of use of IVIG or plasmapheresis in severe, refractory vasculitis or when contraindications to cyclophosphamide exist [34]. Trimethoprim–sulfamethoxazole is recommended during the immunosuppressive regimen, for *Pneumocystis jiroveci pneumonia* prophylaxis, and some believe to decrease relapses associated with *S. aureus* respiratory infections and nasal carriage.

There is also promising evidence for use of biologic agents in GPA. The combination of rituximab in addition to corticosteroids may be as effective as cyclophosphamide plus corticosteroids in inducing remissions, but there are unclear effects on relapses and granulomatous manifestation [34, 40, 41]. Infliximab has been used in addition to standard therapy with remission in 88 % and flares in 20 %, but was associated with more infectious complications in 21 % of patients [42]. The role of adalimumab with prednisolone and cyclophosphamide in a phase II study revealed encouraging results with similar efficacy and adverse events, and reduced prednisolone exposure in ANCA-associated systemic vasculitis with renal involvement [43]. Etanercept was not shown to be effective for the maintenance of remission and even associated with increased risk of malignancy [2, 37]. Mechanisms of action of above therapies involve immunosuppression via depletion of B cells or suppression of other immune cells.

Prognosis

Before the 1950s, no treatment for GPA was available and patients would die from pulmonary or renal complications after a median of 5 months [44], which was increased to 12 months after introduction of corticosteroids [45]. Today, the prognosis of GPA is considered good, given the recent advances in treatment, but depends on severity of the disease, organ involvement, and early diagnosis. Even though, remission is seen in 75 % of patient with standard therapy, at least half of patients still relapse, and many are afflicted with the associated malignancies and other adverse effects of their therapies. Further investigation needs to be done into the promising new therapies such as the biologics, with hopes to decrease toxicity and adverse events, as well as prolong remission rates.

Polyarteritis Nodosa (PAN)

Introduction

Polyarteritis nodosa (PAN) is a multisystem, medium sized vessel segmental necrotizing vasculitis, with either only cutaneous (also referred to as organ limited, benign, or cutaneous PAN) or with associated extracutaneous manifestations (also referred to as classic or systemic PAN).

Pathogenesis

The pathophysiology of PAN is unknown, but immune complex deposition has been proposed as one possible mechanism of pathogenesis [46]. PAN has many associations, including infections, like the hepatitis B virus (HBV) infection (seen in 7 % of PAN, and may be associated with increased gastrointestinal symptoms and worse prognosis [47, 48]), hepatitis C virus infection [49], streptococcal (in children), parvovirus B19 and human immunodeficiency virus (HIV) infection [2]. Malignancy, such as hairy cell leukemia, is another reported association [50]. Inflammatory conditions like inflammatory bowel disease (IBD), SLE, and familial Mediterranean fever have been observed with PAN, as well as certain medications, such as minocycline [2].

Clinical

PAN is a difficult diagnosis to make, given the nonspecific clinical features, controversial diagnostic inclusion criteria and low prevalence of the disease [51]. Several authors and reports categorized PAN into subtypes [52], including classic PAN (associated with hepatitis B and with more widespread disease [53]), ANCA negative PAN [46], benign cutaneous PAN (associated with fever, neutropenia and cutaneous ulcers, with possible association with IBD), Kawasaki disease associated [54], and MPA PAN (ANCA positive PAN in 10 % cases). Some authors argue that, even though PAN is a medium vessel vasculitis, there must still be some involvement of arterioles, capillaries or venules, which makes it all that more difficult to separate from entities such as MPA which includes small and medium sized vessels [51]. Several attempts have been made to reclassify vasculitides, but due to difficulty in diagnostic testing and other factors, no ideal criteria exist [52].

Symptoms of PAN result from ischemic damage to various vital organs, such as the skin, nervous system, muscle, heart, and kidney. Approximately 10 % of all PAN cases are cutaneous PAN or organ-limited PAN [2], which is distinguished from systemic PAN by lack of visceral involvement by angiography [51]. Cutaneous manifestations include palpable purpura (pustular or ulcerative), livedo racemosa, retiform purpura, "punched out" ulcers, subcutaneous nodules, and peripheral gangrene (Fig. 5.15) [52]. Cutaneous PAN is most commonly seen in children, which rarely progresses to systemic PAN [52], and is associated with streptococcal infections [55]. Skin involvement in PAN can be associated with symptoms of joint pain and ocular disease, as seen in MPA and GPA [2].

Twenty-five percent of patients with classic, or systemic, PAN can have the above mentioned cutaneous findings. Extracutaneous manifestations of systemic PAN have been described to include fever, arthralgias, myalgias (myopathy with increased CPK levels), paresthesias ("stocking and glove distribution," mononeuritis multiplex foot drop or wrist drop), abdominal pain (sometimes from mesenteric ischemia), orchitis (associated with HBV infection), renovascular hypertension (HTN)/renal failure (not glomerulonephritis), congestive heart failure causing shortness of breath, and cerebral infarcts, but often spares the lungs [2]. A recent large single center retrospective study of pediatric PAN cases revealed most patient

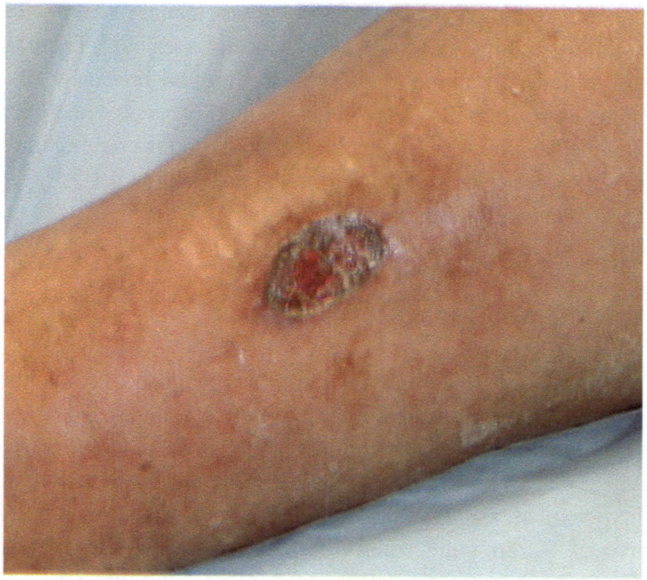

Fig. 5.15 Cutaneous polyarteritis nodosa. Histologic evaluation of this leg ulcer demonstrated changes diagnostic for polyarteritis nodosa; the systemic evaluation was negative. This lesion healed with low-dose corticosteroid therapy. Photo courtesy of Julia R. Nunley, M.D.

presented with fevers, fatigue, weight loss, and myalgias, with skin involvement in 88 %, musculoskeletal in 75 %, renal in 19 %, as well as gastrointestinal (GI) in 10 % and neurological manifestations in 10 % of patients [56]. This study also revealed possible novel link between severe GI disease and systemic PAN relapse, with relapse being lower in children than adults, pointing to the possibility that childhood PAN has a higher chance of permanent remission.

Differential Diagnosis

There is a broad differential for PAN, including cryoglobulinemic vasculitis and autoimmune connective tissue disease [2]. PAN should be a diagnosis of exclusion, after GPA, MPA and EGPA have all been excluded. Given that PAN can cause aneurysms, one needs to consider diseases with aneurysmal dilatation, such as atherosclerosis, fibromuscular dysplasia, lupus, emboli and left atrial myxoma, neurofibromatosis, and Ehlers–Danlos syndrome [2]. Also on the differential, are etiologies that cause cutaneous necrosis, such as emboli and disorders of vasculopathy. Finally, one needs to rule out nodular tuberculosis before starting immunosuppressive treatment.

Histopathology

The histology of PAN is characteristic for necrotizing vasculitis in affected skin located in the deeper dermis and subcutaneous fat, as well as leukocytoclastic vasculitis of small to medium sized vessels of visceral sites [17]. There is infiltration of neutrophils within and around arterial walls, with rare eosinophils. Vessel walls eventually become necrotic, and the development of aneurysmal dilatation is common due to vessel wall weakening. Perivascular deposits of C3, IgM, and fibrin can be seen on DIF [2].

Workup and Laboratory Findings

There is no test to definitively make the diagnosis of PAN, but rather tests are performed to rule out other conditions such as cryoglobulinemias, autoimmune connective tissue disease, MPA, GPA, and EGPA and to determine the extent of organ involvement. For example, high ANA titers are more suggestive of autoimmune connective tissue disease, and ANCA positivity is more suggestive of another condition such as GPA. Blood cultures are usually performed to exclude endovascular infections. Tissue biopsies of involved organs, including skin, muscle, nerve, kidney, and testes can be performed to support the diagnosis. Nonspecific leukocytosis, elevated ESR, and thrombocytosis can be seen on serum testing.

Imaging Studies

In addition to tissue biopsies, imaging is becoming increasingly used to aid with diagnosis. Angiography allows detection of microaneurysms in the renal, celiac, and mesenteric arteries [57], and CT or magnetic resonance imaging (MRI) can be used to visualize luminal narrowing or wall thickening, and even follow-up response to therapy [58].

Treatment

First line therapy for PAN involves systemic corticosteroids with prednisone, at a dose of 1 mg/kg/day, tapered slowly over 6–12 months [59]. Approximately half of patients are expected to have a complete response to systemic corticosteroids, while others may require additional immunosuppressants or immune-modulators [60]. Cyclophosphamide, at doses of 2 mg/kg/day PO or pulses IV of 0.5–1.0 g/m^2/month, have been used successfully in patients with internal organ involvement or patients with steroid refractory disease [60, 61]. In patients with cutaneous limited disease, MTX has also been shown to be an option for treatment [62]. While not a first line treatment, there is evidence that tumor necrosis factor (TNF) inhibitors can also provide relief in refractory disease [63, 64]. Treatment of diseases associated with PAN, such as HBV infections, is also important in the management of these patients.

Prognosis

Prognosis in PAN depends on systemic involvement of the disease, timing of initiation of treatment, and ability to control the progression of systemic involvement. Without treatment there is a less than 20 % 5-year survival, and with treatment this can be improved to 80 % 5-year survival [65].

Henoch–Schönlein Purpura (HSP)

Introduction

Henoch–Schönlein Purpura (HSP) is a small vessel vasculitis, most often presenting with a tetrad of symptoms including purpura, arthritis, abdominal pain, and hematuria. It is thought to occur secondary to immunoglobulin A (IgA) deposition in vessel walls, often following respiratory tract infections in children. In children it is the most common vasculitis, and 90 % of HSP occurs in children less than 10 years of age.

Pathogenesis

Disease pathogenesis is secondary to IgA deposition in the venules of the skin and mesangium of the kidney. HSP often presents 1–2 weeks following an upper respiratory infection in children. Approximately 50 % of children will have positive anti-streptolysin O (ASO) titers, suggestive of prior streptococcal infection. Other infections such as methicillin-resistant *Staphylococcus aureus* (MRSA) have also been associated with presentation of HSP [66], and genetic polymorphisms may predispose some children to the development of this condition. High levels of transforming growth factor (TGF)-beta secreting T cells leading to high levels of IgA anti-cardiolipin antibody production have been found in children with HSP [67]. Additionally, glycosylation of IgA may be aberrant and predispose patients to development of HSP [68].

Clinical Presentation

As the name suggests, purpura is the main finding in all patients with this disease (Figs. 5.16a, b). In addition to purpura of the skin, other cutaneous findings can include urticaria, bullae, and areas of necrosis. The cutaneous presentation is usually symmetric, localized to the buttocks and lower extremities, but has also been reported to involve the trunk and face. Extracutaneous symptoms such as abdominal pain can be found in 65 %, fever in 40 % of children and less commonly in adults, arthritis in 75 %, and nephritis in 50 % [69]. Some children will present with GI complications such as severe bleeding and intussusceptions [70]. While lesions

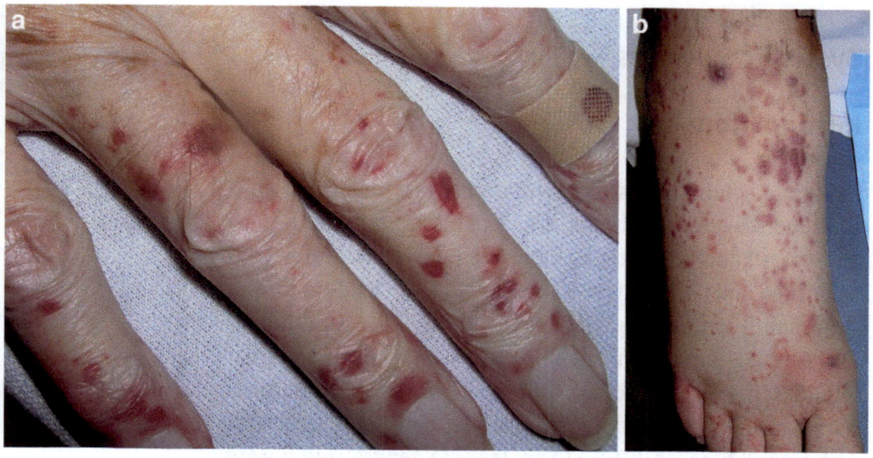

Fig. 5.16 (a, b) Henoch–Schönlein purpura. Palpable purpura commonly presents on extremities and buttocks. Photos courtesy of Joseph C. English, III, M.D.

begin to regress within 2 weeks, a third of children will have a recurrence within 4 months. Interestingly, one report associated recurrences with initial treatment with corticosteroids [71]. Adults often present with more severe cutaneous findings of necrotic cutaneous lesions, diarrhea, and leukocytosis [72]. Furthermore, there is a potential association of adult HSP with malignancies such as multiple myeloma and lung cancer [73]. The prognosis for children with HSP has been associated with the severity of renal involvement [74].

Differential Diagnosis

The differential for HSP from a cutaneous standpoint can include other small vessel vasculitides such as acute hemorrhagic edema of infancy, urticarial vasculitis, erythema elevatum diutinum, and vasculitis secondary to medications, infection, or malignancy. With the extracutaneous clinical findings of HSP one needs to consider other causes of arthritis such as lupus erythematosus, juvenile idiopathic arthritis, and pathologies that may lead to abdominal pain.

Histopathology

HSP will show evidence of vasculitis on hemotoxylin & eosin (H&E), with necrosis of small vessels in the superficial dermis and fibrin deposition. The key to diagnosis is performing a direct immunofluorescence (DIF) of tissue showing perivascular deposits of IgA, C3, and fibrin. Deposition of other immunoglobulins is also possible, but IgA is prominent.

Workup and Laboratory Findings

Skin biopsy with DIF is important for the diagnosis, as nearly all patients with HSP present with cutaneous findings. Renal biopsy can also be performed to confirm the diagnosis, and ensure that another cause of renal pathology is not ongoing. Findings in bloodwork can be nonspecific, with leukocytosis and elevated ESR. UA should be obtained in all suspected cases, and can present with red blood cell or white blood cell casts and proteinuria. Serum creatinine can also help to monitor degree of renal damage. Serum levels of IgA may be elevated and can be used to aid in diagnosis [68, 75]. Presence of IgA on immunofluorescence has been independently associated with renal involvement, however is not indicative of the severity of renal damage [76].

Treatment

Most cases of HSP are self-limited, so supportive treatment is the mainstay of therapy, and pain can be treated with nonsteroidal anti-inflammatory drugs (NSAIDs). Various diseases which involve IgA respond well to dapsone and colchicine, by reducing neutrophil chemotaxis and inflammation, and likewise in HSP can decrease duration of the skin lesions [77]. Systemic corticosteroids can provide relief and shorten duration of arthritis and abdominal pain. Corticosteroids have been used to treat severe nephritis in HSP, however the evidence is not clear whether corticosteroids can prevent long-term kidney disease [78, 79].

Prognosis

HSP has a favorable prognosis in both children and adults, with complete recovery in greater than 90 % of both populations. One third of children can have recurrences, however this is not associated with any worse long-term outcome. Rarely patients can have persistent disease leading to end-stage renal disease.

Systemic Sclerosis

Introduction

Systemic sclerosis, also known as *scleroderma*, is an autoimmune disease which can affect the skin, internal organs, and vasculature. Two types have been described, referred to as limited and diffuse types. The limited form leads to fibrotic skin mainly on the fingers, hands and the face. Additionally the limited form can include *CREST* syndrome, which includes five components: *C*alcinosis, *R*aynaud syndrome, *E*sophageal dysmotility, *S*clerodactyly, and *T*elangiectasias. The second type, or diffuse form, leads to generalized fibrotic skin changes which can involve the entire body. Women have a threefold to fourfold higher prevalence than men, with an onset in the third to fifth decade of life. The diffuse form is more prevalent among black patients, who also have a higher mortality.

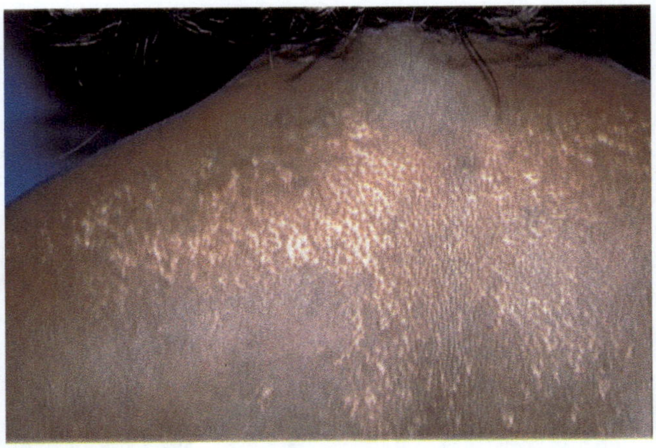

Fig. 5.17 Systemic sclerosis. "Salt and pepper" pattern of dyspigmentation in areas of sclerosis. Photo courtesy of Joseph C. English, III, M.D.

Pathogenesis

The pathogenesis of systemic sclerosis remains unknown, but a multifactorial process is thought to occur [80, 81]. One component involves the dysfunction of vasculature, secondary to impaired angiogenesis and unresponsiveness to vasodilation or constriction factors. This can lead to the various manifestations of the disease, such as large vessel dysregulation presenting as renal crisis or pulmonary hypertension (HTN), and small vessel dysregulation leading to Raynaud and skin fibrosis. A second component is immune cell activation and autoantibody production. Antibodies that stimulate monocyte activation can promote a chronic inflammatory state, and also apoptosis of endothelial cells. Furthermore, an increase in oligoclonal T cells in the skin and lungs with a Th2 and Th17 phenotype seem to be prevalent. Autoantibodies that likely play a role in the pathogenesis are often also used for diagnostic purposes, including anti-topoisomerase I (Scl-70), anticentromere, and anti-platelet-derived growth factor (PDGF). A third component is the increased fibrosis of tissue. Fibrosis may be secondary to elevated levels of TGF-β that induce connective tissue growth factor (CTGF), leading to excess collagen, proteoglycans, adhesion molecules, and other matrix components. Elevated expression of TGF-β responsive genes have also been correlated with the diffuse type of systemic sclerosis [82].

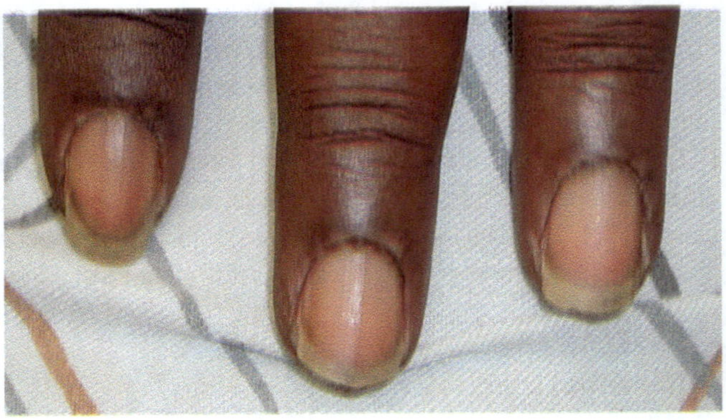

Fig. 5.18 Scleroderma. Proximal nail fold changes are common in scleroderma and lupus. Tortuous and abnormal telangiectasia are common in both conditions. Depigmentation is more common in scleroderma. Courtesy of Julia R. Nunley, M.D.

Clinical Presentation

Skin findings in systemic sclerosis can evolve from an initial presentation of edematous skin with pitting edema, to an indurated phase in which the skin hardens, and in the late phase with skin atrophy. The limited versus diffuse type of systemic sclerosis indicate the extent of skin involvement, as described above. Additionally the limited form can involve the constellation of findings grouped as CREST syndrome. The findings in CREST syndrome can also be seen in the diffuse form of the disease, but are usually more pronounced and in the setting of more extensive skin involvement [83]. Progression rates of skin thickening have also been correlated with severity of disease, and are a predictor of increased mortality [84]. Additional skin findings include a "salt and pepper" pattern of dyspigmentation in areas of sclerosis, with sparing of perifollicular skin (Fig. 5.17). Telangiectasias are another skin finding, and is also a component of the CREST syndrome. Sclerotic skin lesions on extremities, near joints, can further be complicated by dystrophic calcifications. Skin discoloration of the digits can also be noted as in Raynaud phenomenon, also a component of CREST syndrome (Fig. 5.18) [85]. As the name suggests, this is a systemic disease, and can thus present with renal crisis, pulmonary alveolitis and fibrosis, pulmonary HTN, cardiac abnormalities, and GI dysmotility.

Differential Diagnosis

The differential for systemic sclerosis includes other systemic disorders such as nephrogenic systemic fibrosis, scleredema, morphea, eosinophilic fasciitis, and scleromyxedema.

Histopathology

Skin biopsies can be helpful in the diagnosis of systemic sclerosis. H&E will show evidence of compact or hyalinized collagen, excessive collagen, loss of adipose tissue, minimal lymphocytic infiltrate, and trapping of adnexal structures. DIF is not helpful in this diagnosis.

Workup, Laboratory Findings, Imaging Studies

Diagnostic criteria have been proposed by the ACR, and indicate that the patient must fulfill either the major criteria of sclerodermatous lesions proximal to the MCP joints, or two of three minor criteria which include sclerodactyly, digital pitting scars of the fingertips, and pulmonary fibrosis. Skin biopsies and bloodwork for autoimmune markers and antibodies can aid in the diagnosis, and help rule out other conditions. Most patients will have a positive ANA, with a nucleolar and discrete speckled pattern. The diffuse form of disease will usually have anti-topoisomerase I (Scl-70), and anti-RNP antibodies, while patients with the limited form are more likely to have anti-centromere positive titers. Identification of these antibodies can help in determination of prognosis, as it may help distinguish patient that remain as a limited type or progress to the diffuse form [86]. Additionally prevalence of anti-RNP in systemic sclerosis may indicate an increased risk of associated malignancy [87]. Due to the systemic nature of the disease it is also important to work up patients by evaluating their pulmonary function, cardiac status, renal function, and GI motility.

Treatment

Treatments for systemic sclerosis are mainly focused on treating extracutaneous manifestations, as progression of cutaneous sclerosis has been difficult to halt. Lung disease can be treated with cyclophosphamide, mycophenolate mofetil, and vasodilators. Cardiac and renal disease can be controlled with angiotensin converting enzyme (ACE) inhibitors, and diuretics. GI disease can be treated with metoclopramide to improve gastric motility. Cutaneous manifestations such as Raynaud phenomenon can be treated with behavioral modifications of avoiding cold temperatures, smoking cessation, calcium channel blockers (CCB), angiotensin receptor blockers (ARB), and phosphodiesterase inhibitors. Development of ulcers is best treated by occlusive dressings and proper wound care. Several modalities have been trialed for cutaneous sclerosis but most treatments seems to have similar efficacy, including MTX, minocycline, penicillamine, psoralen plus UVA (PUVA), and UVA phototherapy [88–90]. Several mechanism specific therapeutics have also been trialed with some hope for success, such as halofuginone, an inhibitor of type I collagen synthesis and TGF-β, bosentan, an endothelin receptor antagonist, and iloprost, a suppressor of CTGF [91–93]. In cases of calcinosis cutis, low-dose warfarin can decrease inflammation and sodium thiosulfate may help decrease calcium deposits.

Prognosis

Scleroderma can have a bleak prognosis with extensive systemic involvement and lack of good treatments. The 5 year mortality rate is approximately 10 %, mainly due to pulmonary disease. As noted above, prognosis has also been correlated to extent of skin involvement.

Psoriasis

Introduction

Psoriasis is a common, chronic, systemic inflammatory disorder of the skin and joints and affects greater than 2 % of the US population [94]. While it can occur at any age, there is often a bimodal distribution with presentation occurring between 15 and 20 years of age, and a second peak at 55–60 years [94]. Numerous studies in the past decade have demonstrated a link between psoriasis, obesity, metabolic syndrome, and cardiovascular disease [95–100]. The association of renal disease in the setting of psoriasis has long been the subject of debate. Prior studies have attempted to shed light on the subject, but the results have been conflicting. A recent large population based cohort study by Wan et al. provides convincing evidence of an association between moderate (3–10 % body surface area (BSA)) to severe psoriasis(>10 % BSA) and chronic kidney disease (CKD) [101]. After adjusting for confounding variables such as sex, age, cardiovascular disease, diabetes, HTN, hyperlipidemia, NSAID use, and body mass index, the authors found that psoriasis remained an independent risk factor for the development of CKD

[101]. Consensus guidelines regarding the evaluation and monitoring of renal function in patients with psoriasis are lacking and further studies are warranted.

Pathogenesis

The pathogenesis of psoriasis remains an area of active research. Various triggers (cutaneous injury, streptococcal infection, medications, pregnancy, psychogenic stress, smoking, alcohol, etc.) have been identified that may hasten the development of the psoriatic plaque in a genetically predisposed individual [102–105]. The initiation of cutaneous lesion formation is thought to occur when a trigger causes DNA to be released from keratinocytes. The DNA then complexes with cellular proteins and activates plasmacytoid dendritic cells (PDCs). Activated PDCs release interferons, which activate myeloid dendritic cells, ultimately leading to keratinocyte proliferation [106]. A pathogenic cycle of disease is formed when activated myeloid dendritic cells release interleukins and activate naive T cells. These activated T cells are recruited to the lesions and begin producing numerous cytokines, including interferon gamma, IL-17, and IL-22. This cytokine milieu increases keratinocyte proliferation and works to maintain the pathologic cycle [106]. The pathogenesis of CKD in psoriasis is unclear. Case reports have noted an association between psoriasis and glomerulopathies, including IgA and membranous nephropathies, focal segmental glomerulosclerosis and extracapillary glomerulonephritis [107], however, the mechanism of renal injury in the setting of psoriasis is unknown.

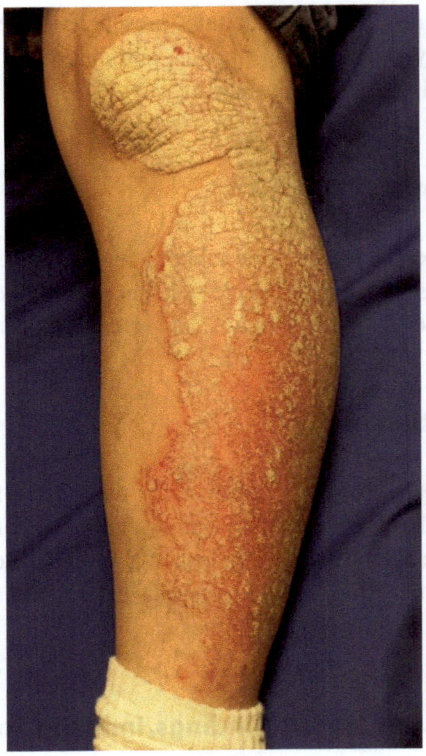

Fig. 5.19 Diffuse scaly erythematous plaques consistent with chronic plaque psoriasis

Clinical Presentation

Psoriasis is a papulosquamous disease, characterized by scaly papules and plaques [94]. While there are multiple clinical presentations of psoriasis, chronic plaque psoriasis is the most common clinical phenotype and accounts for more than 80 % of cases (Fig. 5.19). It typically presents with well-demarcated, scaly, erythematous plaques of variable sizes with a relatively symmetric distribution. Involvement of the extensor surfaces such as the elbows and knees and of the scalp, trunk, and intergluteal cleft is common (Fig. 5.20) [108].

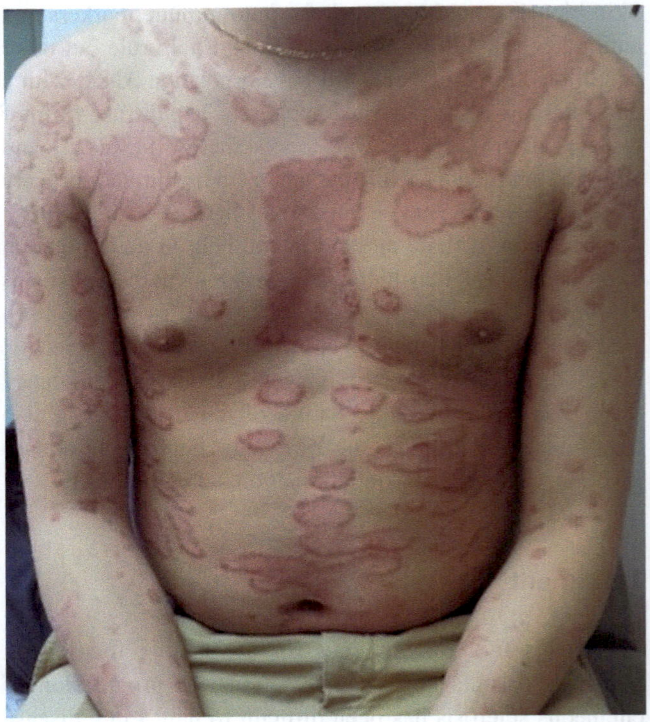

Fig. 5.20 Chronic Plaque psoriasis. Involvement of the extensor surfaces such as the elbows and knees and of the scalp, trunk, and intergluteal cleft is common

Differential Diagnosis

The differential diagnoses for psoriasis are broad and include other papulosquamous conditions, including pityriasis rosea, eczematous processes such as atopic dermatitis, nummular eczema, or contact dermatitis, neoplastic conditions such as cutaneous T-cell lymphoma, infectious processes such as superficial dermatophyte infections(tinea) and candidal intertrigo (more common for flexural or inverse psoriasis). While the diagnosis is often made clinically, punch biopsy can be very helpful in differentiating the above diagnoses.

Histopathology

The histopathology of psoriasis is dynamic and varies between early stage disease versus long standing or advanced stage. Classical, well established psoriasis demonstrates regular acanthosis (or thickening of the stratum spinosum), regular elongation of the rete ridges, parakeratosis, and thinning of the suprapapillary plates [109]. Intracorneal collections of neutrophils, termed Munro microabscesses, are also characteristic of psoriasis.

Workup, Laboratory Findings, Imaging Studies

The diagnosis of psoriasis is often made clinically; however, punch biopsy may be needed in more difficult cases and to aid in differentiating psoriasis from other dermatologic mimickers.

With regard to evaluating for renal disease in patients with psoriasis, routine screening UA for microalbuminuria, serum creatinine and blood urea nitrogen testing should be considered in patient with moderate to severe disease (affecting greater than 3 % BSA) [101]. Higher prevalence of pathologic albuminuria in patients with psoriasis has been demonstrated, suggesting subclinical glomerular damage [110].

Treatment

Treatment options for plaque psoriasis vary on the extent of disease. Limited plaque psoriasis involving 5 % or less of the BSA can be treated with topical corticosteroids as first line therapy [108]. High potency topical corticosteroids applied twice daily for 2–4 weeks, followed by the gradual addition of a steroid sparing agent, such as the vitamin D analogues calcipotriene or calcitriol, to minimize long-term topical corticosteroid side effects is considered an effective multiagent topical regimen. Phototherapy (narrow band UVB (nbUVB) and PUVA) is an effective adjunctive therapy for the treatment of psoriasis and is considered a first line therapy for diffuse involvement.

Systemic therapies including MTX, cyclosporine, and the TNF-α inhibitors are indicated for patients with greater than 5–10 % BSA and/or evidence of extracutaneous involvement, such as psoriatic arthritis.

Prognosis

Psoriasis has been documented to cause a demonstrable and significant reduction in a patient's quality of life, similar to patients with other chronic diseases such as ischemic heart disease and diabetes [111]. And while psoriasis is not a fatal illness, recent studies documenting the association between psoriasis and other comorbidities such as heart disease and metabolic syndrome suggest that these patients have greater morbidity relative to age-related peers [95, 112].

Regarding renal disease in psoriasis, Wan et al. reported a dose-dependent relationship between the severity of psoriasis and the prevalence of moderate to severe CKD [101]. This relationship remained significant, even when nephrotoxic medications such as cyclosporine and MTX were excluded [101, 113]. The authors suggest close monitoring with routine screening UA in patients with greater than 3 % BSA is advisable [101]. While additional studies are required to validate these recommendations from a clinical and cost-effectiveness standpoint, increased screening efforts will allow for the earlier detection and intervention of renal disease in patients with concurrent moderate to severe psoriasis [101].

References

1. Hochberg MC. Updating the American College of Rheumatology revised criteria for the classification of systemic lupus erythematosus. Arthritis Rheum. 1997;40(9):1725. doi:10.1002/1529-0131(199709)40:9<1725::AID-ART29>3.0.CO;2-Y. PubMed PMID: 9324032.
2. Bolognia JL, Jorizzo JL, Schaffer JV. Dermatology, vol. 1–2. 3rd ed. New York: Elsevier; 2012.
3. Callen JP. Cutaneous lupus erythematosus: a personal approach to management. Australas J Dermatol. 2006;47(1):13–27. doi:10.1111/j.1440-0960.2006.00217.x. PubMed PMID: 16405478.
4. Kuhn A, Richter-Hintz D, Oslislo C, Ruzicka T, Megahed M, Lehmann P. Lupus erythematosus tumidus—a neglected subset of cutaneous Lupus erythematosus: report of 40 cases. Arch Dermatol. 2000;136(8):1033–41. PubMed PMID: 10926740.
5. Lehmann P, Homey B. Clinic and pathophysiology of photosensitivity in lupus erythematosus. Autoimmun Rev. 2009;8(6):456–61. doi:10.1016/j.autrev.2008.12.012. PubMed PMID: 19167524.
6. Weber F, Schmuth M, Fritsch P, Sepp N. Lymphocytic infiltration of the skin is a photosensitive variant of lupus erythematosus: evidence by phototesting. Br J Dermatol. 2001;144(2):292–6. PMID: 11251561.
7. Arai S, Katsuoka K. Clinical entity of Lupus erythematosus panniculitis/lupus erythematosus profundus. Autoimmun Rev. 2009;8(6):449–52. doi:10.1016/j.autrev.2008.12.011. PubMed PMID: 19162248.
8. Ma L, Bandarchi B, Glusac EJ. Fatal subcutaneous panniculitis-like T-cell lymphoma with interface change and dermal mucin, a dead ringer for lupus erythematosus. J Cutan Pathol. 2005;32(5):360–5. doi:10.1111/j.0303-6987.2005.00331.x. PubMed PMID: 15811122.
9. Hedrich CM, Fiebig B, Hauck FH, Sallmann S, Hahn G, Pfeiffer C, et al. Chilblain lupus erythematosus—a review of literature.

Clin Rheumatol. 2008;27(10):1341. doi:10.1007/s10067-008-0975-0. PubMed PMID: 19125230.

10. Sifuentes Giraldo WA, Ahijon Lana M, Garcia Villanueva MJ, Gonzalez Garcia C, Vazquez DM. Chilblain lupus induced by TNF-alpha antagonists: a case report and literature review. Clin Rheumatol. 2012;31(3):563–8. doi:10.1007/s10067-011-1924-x. PubMed PMID: 22207249.
11. Werth VP, White WL, Sanchez MR, Franks AG. Incidence of alopecia areata in lupus erythematosus. Arch Dermatol. 1992;128(3):368–71. PMID: 1550369.
12. Tan EM, Cohen AS, Fries JF, Masi AT, McShane DJ, Rothfield NF, et al. The 1982 revised criteria for the classification of systemic lupus erythematosus. Arthritis Rheum. 1982;25(11):1271–7. PMID: 7138600.
13. Petri M, Orbai AM, Alarcon GS, Gordon C, Merrill JT, Fortin PR, et al. Derivation and validation of the Systemic Lupus International Collaborating Clinics classification criteria for systemic lupus erythematosus. Arthritis Rheum. 2012;64(8):2677–86. doi:10.1002/art.34473. PMID: 22553077.
14. Kallel-Sellami M, Baili-Klila L, Zerzeri Y, Laadhar L, Blouin J, Abdelmoula MS, et al. Pediatric systemic lupus erythematosus with C1q deficiency. Ann N Y Acad Sci. 2007;1108:193–6.
15. Welch TR, Blystone LW. Renal disease associated with inherited disorders of the complement system. Pediatr Nephrol (Berlin, Germany). 2009;24(8):1439–44. doi:10.1007/s00467-008-1027-3. PMID: 18958500.
16. Roberts JL, Schwartz MM, Lewis EJ. Hereditary C2 deficiency and systemic lupus erythematosus associated with severe glomerulonephritis. Clin Exp Immunol. 1978;31(2):328–38. PMID: 348363.
17. Barnhill RL. Textbook of dermatopathology. New York: Health Professions Division, McGraw-Hill; 2004. p. 1093.
18. Avgerinou G, Papafragkaki DK, Nasiopoulou A, Arapaki A, Katsambas A, Stavropoulos PG. Effectiveness of topical calcineurin inhibitors as monotherapy or in combination with hydroxychloroquine in cutaneous lupus erythematosus. J Eur Acad Dermatol Venereol. 2012;26(6):762–7. doi:10.1111/j.1468-3083.2011.04161.x. PubMed PMID: 21707772.
19. Sardy M, Ruzicka T, Kuhn A. Topical calcineurin inhibitors in cutaneous lupus erythematosus. Arch Dermatol Res. 2009;301(1):93–8. doi:10.1007/s00403-008-0894-6. PubMed PMID: 18797893.
20. Kuhn A, Ruland V, Bonsmann G. Cutaneous lupus erythematosus: update of therapeutic options part I. J Am Acad Dermatol. 2011;65(6):e179–93. doi:10.1016/j.jaad.2010.06.018. PubMed PMID: 20739095.
21. Rosman Z, Shoenfeld Y, Zandman-Goddard G. Biologic therapy for autoimmune diseases: an update. BMC Med. 2013;11:88. doi:10.1186/1741-7015-11-88. PubMed PMID: 23557513; PubMed Central PMCID: PMC3616818.
22. Arnaud L, Mathian A, Boddaert J, Amoura Z. Late-onset systemic lupus erythematosus: epidemiology, diagnosis and treatment. Drugs Aging. 2012;29(3):181–9. doi:10.2165/11598550-000000000-00000. PubMed PMID: 22263748.
23. Hoffman GS, Kerr GS, Leavitt RY, Hallahan CW, Lebovics RS, Travis WD, et al. Wegener granulomatosis: an analysis of 158 patients. Ann Intern Med. 1992;116(6):488–98. PMID: 1739240.
24. Mubashir E, Ahmed MM, Hayat S, Latif S, Heldmann M, Berney SM. Wegener granulomatosis: a case report and update. South Med J. 2006;99(9):977–88. PubMed PMID: 17004532.
25. Jennette JC. Nomenclature and classification of vasculitis: lessons learned from granulomatosis with polyangiitis (Wegener's granulomatosis). Clin Exp Immunol. 2011;164 Suppl 1:7–10. doi:10.1111/j.1365-2249.2011.04357.x. PubMed PMID: 21447122; PubMed Central PMCID: PMC3095856.
26. Gajic-Veljic M, Nikolic M, Peco-Antic A, Bogdanovic R, Andrejevic S, Bonaci-Nikolic B. Granulomatosis with polyangiitis (Wegener's granulomatosis) in children: report of three cases with cutaneous manifestations and literature review. Pediatr Dermatol. 2012. doi:10.1111/pde.12034. PMID: 23145989.
27. Jennette JC, Falk RJ, Hu P, Xiao H. Pathogenesis of antineutrophil cytoplasmic autoantibody-associated small-vessel vasculitis. Annu Rev Pathol. 2013;8:139–60. doi:10.1146/annurev-pathol-011811-132453. PMID: 23347350.
28. Fauci AS, Haynes BF, Katz P, Wolff SM. Wegener's granulomatosis: prospective clinical and therapeutic experience with 85 patients for 21 years. Ann Intern Med. 1983;98(1):76–85. PMID: 6336643.
29. Stegeman CA, Tervaert JW, Sluiter WJ, Manson WL, de Jong PE, Kallenberg CG. Association of chronic nasal carriage of Staphylococcus aureus and higher relapse rates in Wegener granulomatosis. Ann Intern Med. 1994;120(1):12–7. PMID: 8250451.
30. Jennette JC, Falk RJ. Small-vessel vasculitis. N Engl J Med. 1997;337(21):1512–23. doi:10.1056/NEJM199711203372106. PMID: 9366584.
31. Cabral DA, Uribe AG, Benseler S, O'Neil KM, Hashkes PJ, Higgins G, et al. Classification, presentation, and initial treatment of Wegener's granulomatosis in childhood. Arthritis Rheum. 2009;60(11):3413–24. doi:10.1002/art.24876. PMID: 19877069.
32. Fiorentino DF. Cutaneous vasculitis. J Am Acad Dermatol. 2003;48(3):311–40. doi:10.1067/mjd.2003.212. PMID: 12637912.
33. Stewart C, Cohen D, Bhattacharyya I, Scheitler L, Riley S, Calamia K, et al. Oral manifestations of Wegener's granulomatosis: a report of three cases and a literature review. J Am Dent Assoc. 2007;138(3):338–48. quiz 96, 98. PubMed PMID: 17332039.
34. Langford CA. Update on the treatment of granulomatosis with polyangiitis (Wegener's). Curr Treat Options Cardiovasc Med. 2012;14(2):164–76. doi:10.1007/s11936-012-0165-x. PubMed PMID: 22270373.
35. de Groot K, Harper L, Jayne DR, Flores Suarez LF, Gregorini G, Gross WL, et al. Pulse versus daily oral cyclophosphamide for induction of remission in antineutrophil cytoplasmic antibody-associated vasculitis: a randomized trial. Ann Intern Med. 2009;150(10):670–80. PubMed PMID: 19451574.
36. Bosch X, Guilabert A, Espinosa G, Mirapeix E. Treatment of antineutrophil cytoplasmic antibody associated vasculitis: a systematic review. JAMA. 2007;298(6):655–69. doi:10.1001/jama.298.6.655.
37. Bosch X, Guilabert A, Font J. Antineutrophil cytoplasmic antibodies. Lancet. 2006;368(9533):404–18. doi:10.1016/S0140-6736(06)69114-9. PMID: 17684188.
38. De Groot K, Rasmussen N, Bacon PA, Tervaert JW, Feighery C, Gregorini G, et al. Randomized trial of cyclophosphamide versus methotrexate for induction of remission in early systemic antineutrophil cytoplasmic antibody-associated vasculitis. Arthritis Rheum. 2005;52(8):2461–9. doi:10.1002/art.21142. PubMed PMID: 16052573.
39. Holle JU, Gross WL, Latza U, Nolle B, Ambrosch P, Heller M, et al. Improved outcome in 445 patients with Wegener's granulomatosis in a German vasculitis center over four decades. Arthritis Rheum. 2011;63(1):257–66. doi:10.1002/art.27763. PubMed PMID: 20862686.
40. Bosch X. Inflammation: rituximab in ANCA vasculitis and lupus: bittersweet results. Nat Rev Nephrol. 2010;6(3):137–9. doi:10.1038/nrneph.2010.13. PMID: 20186231.
41. Gomez-Puerta JA, Quintana LF, Stone JH, Ramos-Casals M, Bosch X. B-cell depleting agents for ANCA vasculitides: a new therapeutic approach. Autoimmun Rev. 2012;11(9):646–52. doi:10.1016/j.autrev.2011.11.007. PMID: 22146313.

42. Booth A, Harper L, Hammad T, Bacon P, Griffith M, Levy J, et al. Prospective study of TNFalpha blockade with infliximab in anti-neutrophil cytoplasmic antibody-associated systemic vasculitis. J Am Soc Nephrol. 2004;15(3):717–21. PubMed PMID: 14978174.
43. Laurino S, Chaudhry A, Booth A, Conte G, Jayne D. Prospective study of TNFalpha blockade with adalimumab in ANCA-associated systemic vasculitis with renal involvement. Nephrol Dial Transplant. 2010;25(10):3307–14. doi:10.1093/ndt/gfq187. PubMed PMID: 20368305.
44. Walton EW. Giant-cell granuloma of the respiratory tract (Wegener's granulomatosis). Br Med J. 1958;2(5091):265–70. PubMed PMID: 13560836; PubMed Central PMCID: PMC2026251.
45. Hollander D, Manning RT. The use of alkylating agents in the treatment of Wegener's granulomatosis. Ann Intern Med. 1967;67(2):393–8. PubMed PMID: 6036397.
46. Guillevin L, Mahr A, Callard P, Godmer P, Pagnoux C, Leray E, et al. Hepatitis B virus-associated polyarteritis nodosa: clinical characteristics, outcome, and impact of treatment in 115 patients. Medicine (Baltimore). 2005;84(5):313–22. PMID: 16148731.
47. Pagnoux C, Mahr A, Cohen P, Guillevin L. Presentation and outcome of gastrointestinal involvement in systemic necrotizing vasculitides: analysis of 62 patients with polyarteritis nodosa, microscopic polyangiitis, Wegener granulomatosis, Churg-Strauss syndrome, or rheumatoid arthritis-associated vasculitis. Medicine (Baltimore). 2005;84(2):115–28. PMID: 15758841.
48. Levine SM, Hellmann DB, Stone JH. Gastrointestinal involvement in polyarteritis nodosa (1986-2000): presentation and outcomes in 24 patients. Am J Med. 2002;112(5):386–91. PMID: 11904113.
49. Ramos-Casals M, Jara LJ, Medina F, Rosas J, Calvo-Alen J, Mana J, et al. Systemic autoimmune diseases co-existing with chronic hepatitis C virus infection (the HISPAMEC Registry): patterns of clinical and immunological expression in 180 cases. J Intern Med. 2005;257(6):549–57. doi:10.1111/j.1365-2796.2005.01490.x. PMID: 15910559.
50. Hasler P, Kistler H, Gerber H. Vasculitides in hairy cell leukemia. Semin Arthritis Rheum. 1995;25(2):134–42. PubMed PMID: 8578313.
51. Segelmark M, Selga D. The challenge of managing patients with polyarteritis nodosa. Curr Opin Rheumatol. 2007;19(1):33–8. doi:10.1097/BOR.0b013e328011cb6f. PMID: 17143093.
52. Ozen S, Ruperto N, Dillon MJ, Bagga A, Barron K, Davin JC, et al. EULAR/PReS endorsed consensus criteria for the classification of childhood vasculitides. Ann Rheum Dis. 2006;65(7):936–41. doi:10.1136/ard.2005.046300. PMID: 16322081.
53. Bourgarit A, Le Toumelin P, Pagnoux C, Cohen P, Mahr A, Le Guern V, et al. Deaths occurring during the first year after treatment onset for polyarteritis nodosa, microscopic polyangiitis, and Churg-Strauss syndrome: a retrospective analysis of causes and factors predictive of mortality based on 595 patients. Medicine (Baltimore). 2005;84(5):323–30. PMID: 16148732.
54. Yamazaki-Nakashimada MA, Espinosa-Lopez M, Hernandez-Bautista V, Espinosa-Padilla S, Espinosa-Rosales F. Catastrophic Kawasaki disease or juvenile polyarteritis nodosa? Semin Arthritis Rheum. 2006;35(6):349–54. doi:10.1016/j.semarthrit.2006.02.002. PubMed PMID: 16765711.
55. David J, Ansell BM, Woo P. Polyarteritis nodosa associated with streptococcus. Arch Dis Child. 1993;69(6):685–8. PMID: 7904442.
56. Eleftheriou D, Dillon M, Tullus K, Marks S, Pilkington C, Roebuck D, et al. Systemic polyarteritis nodosa in the young: a single centre experience over 32 years. Arthritis Rheum. 2013. doi:10.1002/art.38024. PubMed PMID: 23754739.
57. Schmidt WA. Use of imaging studies in the diagnosis of vasculitis. Curr Rheumatol Rep. 2004;6:203.
58. Kato T, Fujii K, Ishii E, et al. A case of polyarteritis nodosa with lesions of the superior mesenteric artery illustrating the diagnostic usefulness of three-dimensional computed tomographic angiography. Clin Rheumatol. 2005;24:628.
59. Guillevin L, Pagnoux C. When should immunosuppressants be prescribed to treat systemic vasculitides? Intern Med. 2003;42:313.
60. Ribi C, Cohen P, Pagnoux C, et al. Treatment of polyarteritis nodosa and microscopic polyangiitis without poor-prognosis factors: a prospective randomized study of one hundred twenty-four patients. Arthritis Rheum. 2010;62:1186.
61. Fauci AS, Katz P, Haynes BF, Wolff SM. Cyclophosphamide therapy of severe systemic necrotizing vasculitis. N Engl J Med. 1979;301:235.
62. Schartz NE, Alaoui S, Vignon-Pennamen MD, et al. Successful treatment in two cases of steroid-dependent cutaneous polyarteritis nodosa with low-dose methotrexate. Dermatology. 2001;203:336.
63. Al-Bishri J, le Riche N, Pope JE. Refractory polyarteritis nodosa successfully treated with infliximab. J Rheumatol. 2005;32:1371.
64. Keystone EC. The utility of tumour necrosis factor blockade in orphan diseases. Ann Rheum Dis. 2004;63 Suppl 2:ii79.
65. Gayraud M, Guillevin L, le Toumelin P, et al. Long-term followup of polyarteritis nodosa, microscopic polyangiitis, and Churg-Strauss syndrome: analysis of four prospective trials including 278 patients. Arthritis Rheum. 2001;44:666.
66. Eftychiou C, Samarkos M, Golfinopoulou S, et al. Henoch-Schonlein purpura associated with methicillin-resistant Staphylococcus aureus infection. Am J Med. 2006;119:85.
67. Yang YH, Huang MT, Lin SC, et al. Increased transforming growth factor-beta (TGF-beta)-secreting T cells and IgA anti-cardiolipin antibody levels during acute stage of childhood Henoch-Schönlein purpura. Clin Exp Immunol. 2000;122:285.
68. Lau KK, Wyatt RJ, Moldoveanu Z, et al. Serum levels of galactose-deficient IgA in children with IgA nephropathy and Henoch-Schönlein purpura. Pediatr Nephrol. 2007;22:2067.
69. Saulsbury F. Clinical update: Henoch-Schonlein purpura. Lancet. 2007;369:976–8.
70. Chang WL, Yang YH, Lin YT, Chiang BL. Gastrointestinal manifestations in Henoch-Schönlein purpura: a review of 261 patients. Acta Paediatr. 2004;93:1427.
71. Trapani S, Micheli A, Grisolia F, et al. Henoch Schonlein purpura in childhood: epidemiological and clinical analysis of 150 cases over a 5-year period and review of literature. Semin Arthritis Rheum. 2005;35:143.
72. Blanco R, Martínez-Taboada VM, Rodríguez-Valverde V, et al. Henoch-Schönlein purpura in adulthood and childhood: two different expressions of the same syndrome. Arthritis Rheum. 1997;40:859.
73. Pillebout E, Thervet E, Hill G, et al. Henoch-Schonlein purpura associated with malignancy in adults. J Am Acad Dermatol. 2006;55:s65–70.
74. Saulsbury FT. Henoch-Schönlein purpura in children. Report of 100 patients and review of the literature. Medicine (Baltimore). 1999;78:395.
75. Trygstad CW, Stiehm ER. Elevated serum IgA globulin in anaphylactoid purpura. Pediatrics. 1971;47:1023.
76. Barnadas MA, Perez E, Gich I, et al. Diagnostic, prognostic and pathogenic value of the direct immunofluorescence test in cutaneous leukocytoclastic vasculitis. Int J Dermatol. 2004;43:19–26.
77. Iqbal H, Evans A. Dapsone therapy for Henoch-Schonlein purpura: a case series. Arch Dis Child. 2005;90:985–6.
78. Chartapisak W, Opastirakul S, Hodson EM, et al. Interventions for preventing and treating kidney disease in Henoch-Schonlein purpura. Cochrane Database Syst Rev. 2009;(3):CD005128.
79. Weiss PF, Feinstein JA, Luan X, et al. Effects of corticosteroid on Henoch-Schonlein purpura: a systematic review. Pediatrics. 2007;120:1079–87.

80. Katsumoto TR, Whitfield ML, Connolly MK. The pathogenesis of systemic sclerosis. Annu Rev Pathol. 2011;6:509–37.
81. Gabrielli A, Avvedimento EV, Kreig T. Scleroderma: mechanisms of disease. N Engl J Med. 2009;360:1989–2003.
82. Sargent JL, Milano A, Bhattacharyya S. TGFb-responsive gene signature is associated with a subset of diffuse scleroderma with increased disease severity. J Invest Dermatol. 2010;130:694–705.
83. Akesson A, Wollheim FA. Organ manifestations in 100 patients with progressive systemic sclerosis: a comparison between the CREST syndrome and diffuse scleroderma. Br J Rheumatol. 1989;28(4):281.
84. Domsic RT, Rodriguez-Reyna T, Lucas M, Fertig N, Medsger Jr TA. Skin thickness progression rate: a predictor of mortality and early internal organ involvement in diffuse scleroderma. Ann Rheum Dis. 2011;70(1):104–9. Epub 2010 Aug 2.
85. Wigley FM. Raynaud phenomenon. N Engl J Med. 2002;347:1001–8.
86. Reveille JD, Solomon DH. American College of Rheumatology Ad Hoc Committee of Immunologic Testing Guidelines. Evidence-based guidelines for the use of immunologic tests: anticentromere, Scl-70, and nucleolar antibodies. Arthritis Rheum. 2003;49:399.
87. Nikpour M, Hissaria P, Byron J, et al. Prevalence, correlates and clinical usefulness of antibodies to RNA polymerase III in systemic sclerosis: a cross-sectional analysis of data from an Australian cohort. Arthritis Res Ther. 2011;13:R211.
88. Stege H, Berneburg M, Humke S, Klammer M, et al. High-dose UVA1 radiation therapy for localized scleroderma. J Am Acad Dermatol. 1997;36(6 Pt 1):938.
89. Andres C, Kollmar A, Mempel M, Hein R, Ring J, Eberlein B. Successful ultraviolet A1 phototherapy in the treatment of localized scleroderma: a retrospective and prospective study. Br J Dermatol. 2010;162(2):445–7. Epub 2009 Aug 08.
90. Su TI, Khanna D, Furst DE, Danovitch G, Burger C, Maranian P, Clements PJ. Rapamycin versus methotrexate in early diffuse systemic sclerosis: results from a randomized, single-blind pilot study. Arthritis Rheum. 2009;60(12):3821.
91. McGaha TL, Phelps RG, Spiera H, Bona C. Halofuginone, an inhibitor of type-I collagen synthesis and skin sclerosis, blocks transforming-growth-factor-beta-mediated Smad3 activation in fibroblasts. J Invest Dermatol. 2002;118(3):461.
92. Korn JH, Mayes M, Matucci Cerinic M, Rainisio M, Pope J, et al. Digital ulcers in systemic sclerosis: prevention by treatment with bosentan, an oral endothelin receptor antagonist. Arthritis Rheum. 2004;50(12):3985.
93. Stratton R, Shiwen X, Martini G, Holmes A, Leask A, Haberberger T, Martin GR, Black CM, Abraham D. Iloprost suppresses connective tissue growth factor production in fibroblasts and in the skin of scleroderma patients. J Clin Invest. 2001;108(2):241.
94. Langley RGB, Krueger GG, Griffiths CEM. Psoriasis: epidemiology, clinical features, and quality of life. Ann Rheum Dis. 2005;64:ii18–23.
95. Gelfand JM, Neimann AL, Shin DB, Wang X, Margolis DJ, Troxel AB. Risk of myocardial infarction in patients with psoriasis. JAMA. 2006;296:1735–41.
96. Abuabara K, Azfar RS, Shin DB, Neimann AL, Troxel AB, Gelfand JM. Cause-specific mortality in patients with severe psoriasis: a population-based cohort study in the U.K. Br J Dermatol. 2010;163:586–92.
97. Ahlehoff O, Gislason GH, Charlot M, et al. Psoriasis is associated with clinically significant cardiovascular risk: a Danish nationwide cohort study. J Intern Med. 2011;270:147–57.
98. Lin HW, Wang KH, Lin HC, Lin HC. Increased risk of acute myocardial infarction in patients with psoriasis: a 5-year population-based study in Taiwan. J Am Acad Dermatol. 2011;64:495–501.
99. Bremmer S, Van Voorhees AS, Hsu S, et al. National Psoriasis Foundation. Obesity and psoriasis: from the Medical Board of the National Psoriasis Foundation. J Am Acad Dermatol. 2010;63:1058–69.
100. Tobin AM, Veale DJ, Fitzgerald O, et al. Cardiovascular disease and risk factors in patients with psoriasis and psoriatic arthritis. J Rheumatol. 2010;37:1386–94. Abstract/FREE Full Text.
101. Wan J, Wang S, Haynes K, Denburg MR, Shin DB, Gelfand JM. Risk of moderate to advanced kidney disease in patients with psoriasis: population based cohort study. BMJ. 2013;347:f5961.
102. American Academy of Dermatology Work Group, Menter A, Korman NJ, Elmets CA, et al. Guidelines of care for the management of psoriasis and psoriatic arthritis: section 6 Guidelines of care for the treatment of psoriasis and psoriatic arthritis: case-based presentations and evidence-based conclusions. J Am Acad Dermatol. 2011;65:137–74.
103. Mallbris L, Larsson P, Bergqvist S, Vingård E, Granath F, Ståhle M. Psoriasis phenotype at disease onset: clinical characterization of 400 adult cases. J Invest Dermatol. 2005;124:499–504.
104. Armstrong AW, Armstrong EJ, Fuller EN, Sockolov ME, Voyles SV. Smoking and pathogenesis of psoriasis: a review of oxidative, inflammatory and genetic mechanisms. Br J Dermatol. 2011;165:1162–8.
105. Qureshi AA, Dominguez PL, Choi HK, Han J, Curhan G. Alcohol intake and risk of incident psoriasis in US women: a prospective study. Arch Dermatol. 2010;146:1364–9.
106. Nestle FO, Kaplan DH, Barker J. Psoriasis. N Engl J Med. 2009;361:496–509.
107. Singh NP, Prakash A, Kubba S, et al. Psoriatic nephropathy—does and entity exist? Ren Fail. 2005;27(1):123–7.
108. Villaseñor-Park J, Wheeler D, Grandinetti L. Psoriasis: evolving treatment for a complex disease. Cleve Clin J Med. 2012;79(6):413–23.
109. DeRosa G, Mignogna C. The histopathology of psoriasis. Reumatismo. 2007;59 Suppl 1:46–8.
110. Dervisoglu E, Akturk AS, Yildiz K, et al. The spectrum of renal abnormalities in patients with psoriasis. Int Urol Nephrol. 2012;44(2):509–14.
111. Finlay AY, Kelly SE. Psoriasis—an index of disability. Clin Exp Dermatol. 1987;12:8–112.
112. Langan SM, Seminara NM, Shin DB, et al. Prevalence of metabolic syndrome in patients with psoriasis: a population based study in the United Kingdom. J Invest Dermatol. 2012;132:556–62.
113. Farmer CK, Stevens PE. Chronic kidney disease: psoriasis—a risk factor for chronic kidney disease? Nat Rev Nephrol. 2014;10(1):12–3.

Xerosis

6

Connie M. Wu, Annie M. Wu, Jenna Lester, and Leslie Robinson-Bostom

Introduction/Overview

Xerosis cutis in chronic kidney disease (CKD) may present as either a generalized condition or as a more localized process, most commonly observed on the extremities [1]. It is one of the most common cutaneous problems associated with chronic renal failure, with an overall frequency of 75 % among renal dialysis patients [2]. A number of studies have reported uremic xerosis in 50–85 % of patients undergoing renal dialysis, with higher prevalence among peritoneal dialysis patients than hemodialysis patients [3–5]. Among renal dialysis patients, 30–40 % experience mild xerosis; 25–50 % experience moderate xerosis; and 15–30 % experience severe xerosis [5, 6]. In addition to symptoms of dryness and itch, xerosis increases risk of infection by prolonging wound healing time [7]. Whereas some studies have found a relationship between uremic xerosis and the onset and/or severity of pruritus, other studies did not find such a correlation [5, 6, 8, 9]. Thus, it appears that among patients with pruritus, xerosis may exacerbate symptoms of pruritus by lessening the threshold for itch [10].

C.M. Wu, B.S.
Department of Dermatology, Warren Alpert Medical School of Brown University, Box G-9522, Providence, RI 02903, USA
e-mail: connie_wu@brown.edu

A.M. Wu, B.A.
Department of Dermatology, Warren Alpert Medical School of Brown University, Box G-9180, Providence, RI 02903, USA
e-mail: annie_wu@brown.edu

J. Lester, M.D.
Department of Dermatology, Warren Alpert Medical School of Brown University, APC Building, 593 Eddy Street, Providence, RI 02903, USA
e-mail: JennaLester1@gmail.com

L. Robinson-Bostom, M.D. (✉)
Division of Dermatopathology, Department of Dermatology, Rhode Island Hospital, The Warren Alpert Medical School of Brown University, 593 Eddy Street, APC-10, Providence, RI 02903, USA
e-mail: lrobinson-bostom@lifespan.org

Physiology/Pathogenesis

A variety of factors have been implicated in the development of uremic xerosis. Xerosis associated with end stage renal disease is believed to be caused by shrinkage of eccrine sweat glands and atrophy of sebaceous glands, which can be correlated with increased age or the use of diuretics [3, 7]. Dehydration of the dermis resulting from fluid shifts during dialysis may contribute to the development of xerosis. Studies have also suggested that elevated pH in the stratum corneum of renal dialysis patients may disrupt the skin barrier by interfering with protease activation [11, 12]. Uremic xerosis has also been associated with hypothyroidism, zinc or essential fatty acid deficiency, altered vitamin A metabolism, neurologic disorders that decrease sweating, lymphoma, human immunodeficiency virus (HIV) infection, obstructive biliary disease, and radiation therapy [13–15].

Clinical

Xerosis primarily affects extensor surfaces of forearms, legs, and thighs [3], and can present with pruritus, although pruritus has a distinct pathophysiology (Figs. 6.1, 6.2, 6.3, 6.4, 6.5, and 6.6). Severe cases may present with scaling, desquamation, and fissures (Fig. 6.3). Chronic scratching of affected areas can result in painful excoriations and lichenified (thickened) plaques which may become infected. Additionally, uremic xerosis has been correlated with adverse psychological outcomes, indicated by significantly worse Dermatology Life Quality Index (DLQI) and Short-Form (SF-12) scale scores among patients with uremic xerosis compared to the normal population [2]. In addition to xerosis intensity, other factors such as young age and intensity of uremic pruritus may negatively affect quality of life [4].

J.R. Nunley and E.V. Lerma (eds.), *Dermatological Manifestations of Kidney Disease*,
DOI 10.1007/978-1-4939-2395-3_6, © Springer Science+Business Media New York 2015

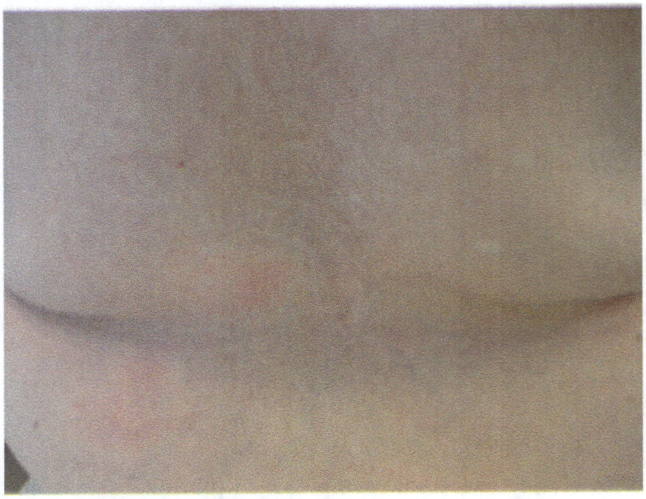

Fig. 6.1 Patient's trunk with xerosis, with fine scale and several nummular patches of mild erythema

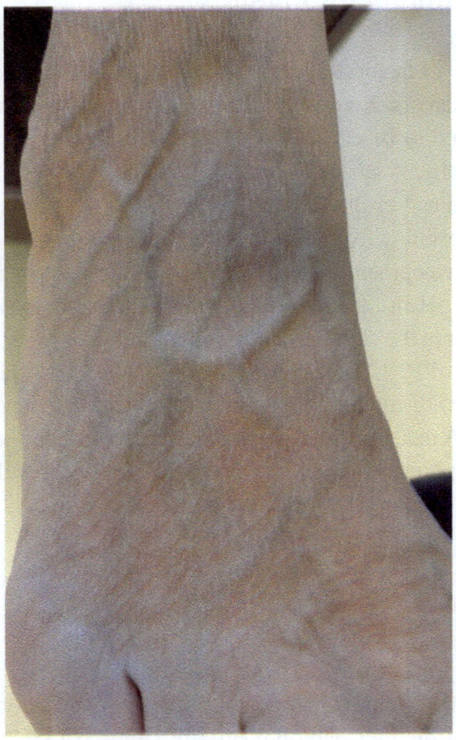

Fig. 6.2 Patient's foot with xerosis and fine scale

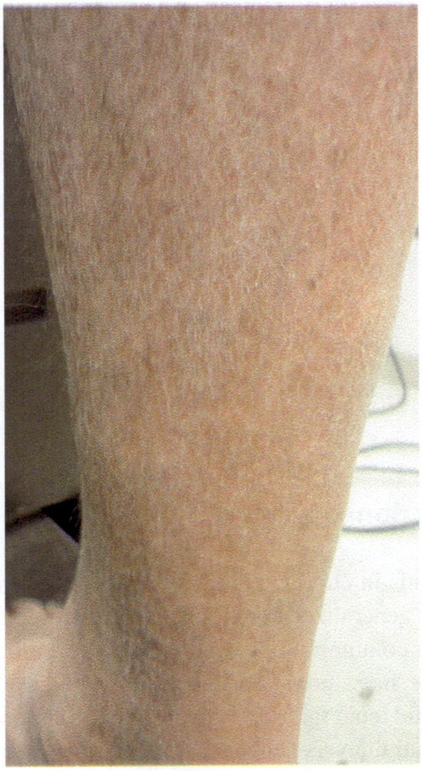

Fig. 6.3 Patient's calf with xerosis and fine scale

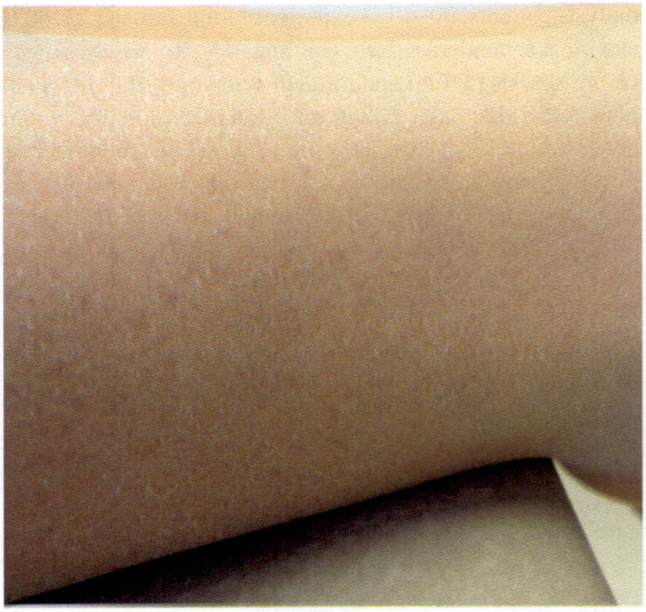

Fig. 6.4 Patient's ankle and lateral lower leg, with mild xerosis

Differential Diagnoses

The differential diagnoses includes ichthyosis, atopic dermatitis, exfoliative dermatitis, asteatotic dermatitis, or any process that causes dry skin, including inadequate use of emollients. Ichthyosis can be acquired or inherited in an autosomal dominant or recessive fashion. Ichthyosis vulgaris is the most common form of ichthyosis and presents with fish-like scale sparing flexural surfaces. Atopic dermatitis tends to be stimulated by irritants such as food or environmental allergens, leading to itchiness, redness, and scaling; skin of the anticubital fossa, popliteal fossa, feet, ankles, hands, wrists, upper chest, neck, face, and eyelids tend to be affected. Although atopic dermatitis is seen in all ages with varying symptoms correlated with age, it is most

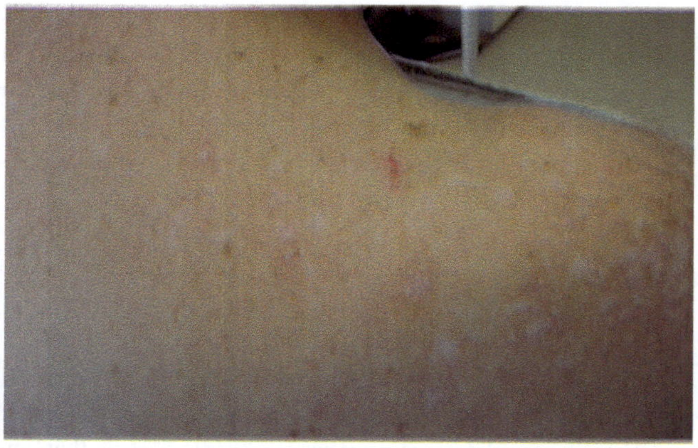

Fig. 6.5 Patient's upper back with mild xerosis, coexistent excoriations, hypopigmented scars consistent with previous trauma from pruritis

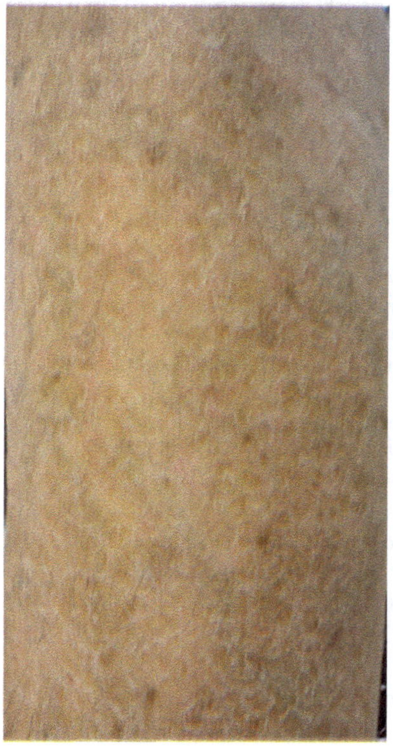

Fig. 6.6 Patient's leg with chronic photodamage and xerosis

prevalent in younger patients, particularly infants and children. Exfoliative dermatitis or erythroderma may result from drug therapy, systemic or cutaneous disease, or idiopathic causes, and manifests as generalized erythema and scaling affecting almost the entire body. Asteatotic dermatitis is most commonly seen in elderly patients, as a result of decreased sebaceous and sweat gland activity, and tends to affect the shins, hands, and trunk. It can present with pruritus and appears as "cracked porcelain" with irregular scaling and polygonal fissures.

Workup

A complete history (social, family, environmental, exposure history; past medical history, medications). Important factors to note:

- Bathing habits: frequency and method; types of soaps/cleansers used
- Emollient usage: frequency and method; types of emollients used
- Dietary: fatty acid intake; fluid intake
- Fabric contact: clothing, bedding (wool can exacerbate symptoms)
- Common complaints: scaling, tightness, chapping; exacerbation of symptoms in winter

Conduct a focused physical examination, including thyroid and full skin exam

- Can present as localized or generalized, commonly on extremities
- Extremely dry skin presents with redness, cracking, scaling
- Scratching may be evidenced by excoriations

Diagnostic Workup

- For cases of acute onset and those associated with systemic symptoms, consider complete blood count (CBC), thyroid function tests, blood urea nitrogen (BUN) and creatinine, liver function tests, human immunodeficiency virus (HIV) testing, chest X-ray, erythrocyte sedimentation rate (ESR), immunoglobulin E (IgE), antinuclear antibody (ANA), and C-reactive protein (CRP)
- If conservative therapy fails, consider age-appropriate malignancy screening

Histology

Biopsies are rarely indicated as dry skin can be easily diagnosed clinically. Histological findings include atrophy of the pilosebaceous follicles and eccrine sweat glands [16].

Treatment

Patients should apply petroleum or non-petroleum based hypoallergenic emollients to moist or wet skin daily, and should be advised to avoid excessive hand washing or showering which strip the skin of natural oils [4]. Neutral-pH products or liquid cleansers containing petrolatum should be used instead of harsh antibacterial soaps. For scaly patches without fissures, lactic acid containing moisturizers are indicated. To ensure adequate hydration, a cool mist humidifier may be used during dry winter months. The diet should include adequate water intake, appropriate for a CKD patient, and adequate intake of essential fatty acids. Cotton clothing and bedding should be used instead of wool and other irritating fabrics.

Drugs

Emollients aim to target the key abnormalities of xerosis, including inadequate water transport to the stratum corneum; poor water-binding; and barrier disturbances. Both classes of emollients, those comprising oil-in-water emulsions (light formulation) with 5 % urea and those comprising water-in-oil emulsions (rich formulation) with 10 % urea, applied twice daily over a 2-week period are effective in alleviating dryness and scaling [17, 18]. Table 6.1 includes a list of important emollient ingredients with specific roles in treatment of xerosis. Although a single emollient may not contain all of the listed ingredients, formulations combining ingredients which serve different purposes, such as humectants, physiological lipids, and natural moisturizing factors (NMF), are effective in treating xerosis [10]. A number of clinical studies have shown improvement in dryness with drugs containing urea, dexpanthenol, ammonium lactate, lactate, lactic acid, and/or pyrrolidone carboxylic acid as active substances (Table 6.2).

Prognosis

Patients with xerosis generally respond well to routine emollient usage. However, underlying conditions such as systemic and genetic complications may cause chronic xerosis that can only be controlled with rigorous treatment. New formulas of cleansers and emollients have improved prognoses.

Conflicts of Interest C.M.W., A.M.W., J.L., and L.R.B. report no conflicts of interest.

Table 6.1 Important ingredients and functions in emollients

Ingredient	Role
Non-physiological lipids (petrolatum, mineral, vegetable oil)	Replaces lost natural skin lipids, improve barrier function
Physiological lipids (ceramides, free fatty acids, cholesterol)	Repairs damaged intracellular lipid lamellae [19]; promotes epidermal differentiation through signaling (ceramides); increases lipid content of *stratum corneum*; improves barrier function
Glycerol (humectant)	Treats symptoms not due to lipid depletion: restores normal aquaporin-3 function for skin hydration and elasticity [20]
Natural moisturizing factors (urea, lactate, potassium, amino acids, PCA, sugars)	Restores epidermal ion gradient to attract and retain water in *stratum corneum* [21]
Antipruritics (glycine, NGF inhibitors, opioid receptor agonists, chamomile extracts, corticosteroids, endocannabinoids)	Glycine alleviates itching and reduce scratching by blocking histamine release from mastocytes [22]
	Inhibit nerve growth by blocking NGF [23]
	Corticosteroids relieve inflammation; may cause skin thinning [24]
	Endocannabinoids improve itch and dryness [25]
Dexpanthenol	Supports fibroblast proliferation [26] and epidermal differentiation; supports normal synthesis of lipids and proteins [27]; relieves scaling, roughness, redness, itch [17]

PCA pyrrolidone carboxylic acid, *NGF* nerve growth factor

Table 6.2 Clinical studies on the effect of moisturizers on dry skin

Condition	Active substance	Control	Effect on dryness
Xerosis	10 % urea with dexpanthenol	Untreated baseline	Improved with decreased roughness, redness, cracks [17]
Dry skin	3 and 10 % urea	Untreated	Improved [28]
Xerosis	12 % ammonium lactate	Petrolatum based cream	Improved more with active substance than with control [29]
Xerosis on legs	12 % ammonium lactate	5 % lactic acid +2.5 % PCA	Improved more with active substance than control [30]
Xerosis on legs	12 % lactate	5 % lactic acid/emollient lotion	Improved, but patients using 12 % had longer remission [31]
Xerosis	5 % lactic acid	Eucerin lotion	Improved more with active substance than control [32]
Xerosis	5 % PCA	Placebo and 10 % urea	Active more than placebo, equal to urea [33]
Xerosis	15 % glycerol and 10 % paraffin	Oil-in-water emulsion devoid of active substances	Improved more with active substance than with placebo [34]

PCA pyrrolidone carboxylic acid

References

1. Khanna D, Singal A, Kalra OP. Comparison of cutaneous manifestations in chronic kidney disease with or without dialysis. Postgrad Med J. 2010;86(1021):641–7.
2. Szepietowski JC, Reich A, Schwartz RA. Uraemic xerosis. Nephrol Dial Transplant. 2004;19:2709–12.
3. Udayakumar P, Balasubramanian S, Ramalingam KS, Lakshmi C, Srinivas CR, Mathew AC. Cutaneous manifestations in patients with chronic renal failure on hemodialysis. Indian J Dermatol Venereol Leprol. 2006;72(2):119–25.
4. Szepietowski JC, Balaskas E, Taube K, Taberly A, Dupuy P. Quality of life in patients with uraemic xerosis and pruritus. Acta Derm Venereol. 2011;91(3):313–7.
5. Balaskas EV, Chu M, Uldall RP, et al. Pruritus in continuous ambulatory peritoneal dialysis and hemodialysis patients. Perit Dial Int. 1992;13:527S–32.
6. Szepietowski JC, Sikora M, Kunsztal M, et al. Ureamic pruritus: a clinical study of maintenance haemodialysis patients. J Dermatol. 2002;29:621–7.
7. Avermaete A, Altmeyer P, Bacharach-Buhles M. Skin changes in dialysis patients: a review. Nephrol Dial Transplant. 2001;16(12):2293–6.
8. Morton CA, Lafferty M, Hau C, et al. Pruritus and skin hydration during dialysis. Nephrol Dial Transplant. 1996;11:2031–6.
9. Young Jr A, Sweeney E, David D, et al. Dermatologic evaluation of pruritus in patients on hemodialysis. N Y State J Med. 1973; 73:2670–4.
10. Zucker I, Yosipovitch G, David M, et al. Prevalence and characterization of uremic pruritus in patients undergoing hemodialysis: uremic pruritus is still a major problem for patients with end-stage renal disease. J Am Acad Dermatol. 2003;49:842–6.
11. Yosipovitch G, Reis J, Tur E, et al. Sweat secretion, stratum corneum hydration, small nerve function and pruritus in patients with advance chronic renal failure. Br J Dermatol. 1995;133:561–4.
12. Elias PM, Crumrine D, Rassner U, et al. Basis for abnormal desquamation and permeability dysfunction in RXLI. J Invest Dermatol. 2004;122:314–9.
13. Heyman WR, Gans EH, Manders SM, et al. Xerosis in hypothyroidism: a potential role for the use of topical thyroid hormone in euthyroid patients. Med Hypotheses. 2001;57:736–7399.
14. Singh F, Rudikoff D. HIV-associated pruritus: etiology and management. Am J Clin Dermatol. 2003;4:177–88.
15. Vahlquist A, Berne B, Berne C. Skin content and plasma transport of vitamin A and beta carotene in chronic renal failure. Eur J Clin Invest. 1982;12:343–50.
16. Falodun O, Ogunbiyi A, Salako B, George AK. Skin changes in patients with chronic renal failure. Saudi J Kidney Dis Transpl. 2011;22(2):268–72.
17. Castello M, Milani M. Efficacy of topical hydrating and emollient lotion containing 10 % urea ISDIN (R) plus dexpanthenol (Ureadin Rx 10) in the treatment of skin xerosis and pruritus in hemodialyzed patients: an open prospective pilot trial. G Ital Dermatol Venerol. 2011;146(5):321–5.
18. Weber TM, Kausch M, Rippke F, Schoelermann AM, Filbry AW. Treatment of xerosis with a topical formulation containing glyceryl glucoside, natural moisturizing factors, and ceramide. J Clin Aesthet Dermatol. 2012;5(8):29–39.
19. Chamlin SL, Kao J, Freiden IJ, Sheu MY, Fowler AJ, Fluhr JW, Williams ML, Elias PM. Ceramide-dominant barrier repair lipids alleviate childhood atopic dermatitis: changes in barrier function provide a sensitive indicator of disease activity. J Am Acad Dermatol. 2002;47(2):198–208.
20. El Ghalbzouri A, Lamme E, Ponec M. Crucial role of fibroblasts in regulating epidermal morphogenesis. Cell Tissue Res. 2002;310(2): 189–99.
21. Nakagawa N, Sakai S, Matusmoto M, Yamada K, Nagano M, Yuki T, Sumida Y, Uchiwa H. Relationship between NMF (lactate and potassium) content and the physical properties of the stratum corneum in healthy subjects. J Invest Dermatol. 2004;122(3):755–63.
22. Paubert-Braquet M, Lefranµois G, Picquot S. Etude in vitro du pouvoir antiprurigineux du glycocolle: effet sur la dégranulation des mastocytes. Therapeutique. 1992;95:2–3.
23. Twycross R, Greaves MW, Handwerker H, Jones EA, Libretto SE, Szepietowski JC, Zylicz Z. Itch: scratching more than the surface. Q J Med. 2003;96(1):7–26.
24. Rawlings AV. Trends in stratum corneum research and the management of dry skin conditions. Int J Cosmet Sci. 2003;25:63–95.
25. Wang H, Yosipovitch G. New insights into the pathophysiology and treatment of chronic itch in patients with end-stage renal disease, chronic liver disease, and lymphoma. Int J Dermatol. 2010;49(1):1–11.
26. Weimann BI, Hermann D. Studies on wound healing: effects of calcium D-pantothenate on the migration, proliferation and protein synthesis of human dermal fibroblasts in culture. Int J Vitam Nutr Res. 1999;69(2):113–9.
27. Lacroix B, Didier E, Grenier JF. Effects of pantothenic acid on fibroblastic cell cultures. Res Exp Med. 1988;188(5):391–6.
28. Serup J. A double-blind comparison of two creams containing urea as the active ingredient: assessment of efficacy and side-effects by non-invasive techniques and a clinical scoring scheme. Acta Derm Venereol. 1992;177:34–43.
29. Wehr R, Krochmal L, Bagatell F, et al. A controlled two-center study of lactate 12 % lotion and a petrolatum-based creme in patients with xerosis. Cutis. 1986;37:205–9.
30. Rogers RS, Callen J, Wehr R, et al. Comparative efficacy of 12 % ammonium lactate lotion and 5 % lactic acid lotion in the treatment of moderate to severe xerosis. J Am Acad Dermatol. 1989;21:714–6.
31. Dahl MV, Dahl AC. 12 % lactate lotion for the treatment of xerosis. Arch Dermatol. 1983;119:27–30.
32. Wehr RF, Kantor I, Jones EL, et al. A controlled comparative efficacy study of 5 % ammonium lactate lotion versus an emollient control lotion in the treatment of moderate xerosis. J Am Acad Dermatol. 1991;25:849–51.
33. Middleton JD, Roberts ME. Effect of a skin cream containing the sodium salt of pyrrolidone carboxylic acid on dry and flaky skin. J Soc Cosmet Chem. 1978;29:201–5.
34. Balaskas E, Szepietowski JC, Bessis D, Ioannides D, Ponticelli C, et al. Randomized, double-blind study with glycerol and paraffin in uremic xerosis. Clin J Am Soc Nephrol. 2011;6:748–53.

Pruritus in Chronic Kidney Disease

7

Ehsan Azimi, Ethan A. Lerner, and Sarina B. Elmariah

Introduction

Pruritus in chronic kidney disease (CKD), classically known as uremic pruritus or renal itch, is one of the most common complications of end-stage renal disease. According to the Dialysis Outcomes and Practice Patterns Study (DOPPS), a global cross-sectional study of 18,801 hemodialysis (HD) patients from more than 300 dialysis units across 12 countries, 42 % of HD patients experienced moderate to severe pruritus [1]. Daily itching has been reported by 84 % of HD patients enrolled in smaller longitudinal studies and up to 59 % of these patients have been reported to suffer from ongoing itch for more than a year [2]. The prevalence of chronic itch is higher in HD patients (50–90 %), as compared to patients with compromised renal function but not requiring HD (15–49 %) [1, 3]. The intensity and prevalence of itch does not depend on age, gender, ethnicity, or duration of dialysis, although it is more prevalent in those undergoing HD as compared to peritoneal dialysis [4]. CKD patients may suffer from inflammatory, neuropathic, and occasionally psychogenic forms of itch. HD patients suffering from itch have an impaired quality of life and higher rates of depression, fatigue, and poor sleep quality as compared to HD patients without itch. The DOPPS study reported a 17 % increase in mortality for HD patients with moderate to severe itch as compared to those with mild or no itch; however, this increase in mortality was no longer significant after controlling for sleep quality between the two groups [1]. A prospective study involving 321 chronic HD patients demonstrated increased overall mortality in patients with moderate to severe renal itch who had elevated high-sensitive C-reactive protein levels (hs-CRP) compared to those with no/mild renal itch and lower hs-CRP levels. These findings suggest that inflammation may contribute to increased mortality in those most severely affected by itch [5]. Overall, itch imposes a large burden on CKD patients worldwide, and renal transplant remains the only definitive treatment for renal itch [6].

Physiology/Pathogenesis

Itch may develop in the setting of primary skin or systemic diseases. The basic mechanisms underlying itch and their relation to systemic disease are under intense investigation. Specialized cutaneous somatosensory nerve endings sense different types of stimuli that result in itch, pain, light touch, and other sensations. Several different theories have been proposed to describe the afferent pathways that transmit itch signals to the brain: however, studies over the last 15 years using various methodologies including microneurography, electrophysiology, and transgenic approaches support what is known as the "labeled line" theory of itch. According to this theory, itch is initiated by activation of itch-specific receptors expressed by peripheral sensory nerves in the skin, and these signals are then relayed by sensory-specific neural pathways from the skin to the brain [7, 8].

Despite having a beneficial role in the treatment of urticarial or other histamine-related disorders, antihistamine therapy is ineffective in the management of most types of itch [9, 10]. The observation that cowhage spicules isolated from the tropical legume *Mucuna pruriens* elicit an intense itch that is not accompanied by burning, wheal, or flare provided initial evidence for the existence of a non-histaminergic itch pathway. Microneurographic studies in humans and primates demonstrate that histamine stimulates a population of mechanically insensitive unmyelinated C-fibers while cowhage stimulates a subset of mechanically sensitive, histamine-insensitive polymodal C-fibers as well as a subset of thinly myelinated Aδ fibers [11–13].

E. Azimi, M.D. • E.A. Lerner, M.D., Ph.D. (✉)
S.B. Elmariah, M.D., Ph.D.
Cutaneous Biology Research Center, Department of Dermatology, Massachusetts General Hospital, Building 149, 13th Street, Charlestown, MA 02129, USA

Harvard Medical School, Boston, MA, USA
e-mail: eazimi@partners.org; elerner@partners.org; sbelmariah@partners.org

J.R. Nunley and E.V. Lerma (eds.), *Dermatological Manifestations of Kidney Disease*,
DOI 10.1007/978-1-4939-2395-3_7, © Springer Science+Business Media New York 2015

The specific pathogenesis of renal itch remains unclear. Several of the more common hypotheses proposed to explain itch in CKD patients are summarized below. These include altered hormone and mineral metabolism, structural alterations in the skin that lead to compromised hydration, and increased systemic inflammation and immune dysregulation in the skin, all of which are thought to indirectly lead to abnormal and/or heightened activation of itch fibers. Emerging evidence from clinical therapeutic reports suggest that CKD patients may also have primary alterations in nociceptive sensory pathways in the peripheral and/or central nervous system.

Altered mineral and hormone metabolism are thought to contribute to renal itch in some CKD patients. Several studies report that risk factors for renal itch include elevated calcium and phosphate levels [14, 15], hyperparathyroidism [16, 17], elevated serum magnesium and aluminum concentrations [18, 19], and inadequate dialysis [14, 20], although the exact relation of these factors to the sensation of itch is unknown. A study performed on HD patients who underwent parathyroidectomy for the treatment of secondary hyperparathyroidism reported decreased itch after surgery. In this study, calcium phosphate levels were the only factor which correlated with decreased postsurgical itch [17]. In another recent study involving 99 HD patients, higher serum phosphorous levels correlated with higher frequency and severity of itch [21]. These authors suggested that decreased dietary intake of phosphate by HD patients is a helpful and cost-effective method to control renal itch. In contrast to these reports, a case control study evaluating the relationship between alterations in mineral metabolism and renal itch in 105 HD patients did not find any statistically significant association between itch and serum levels of calcium, phosphorus, the calcium/phosphorous ratio, or parathyroid hormone [22]. It remains unclear whether altered mineral metabolism is a causative factor for renal itch, or simply a marker of those patients with more advanced or poorly controlled disease.

Xerosis, or dry skin, is another common finding in HD patients which may precipitate or exacerbate itch [23]. Alterations in the structure of the stratum corneum (SC) and aberrant retention of corneodesmosomes within the upper layers of the SC have been proposed to alter the hydration and mechanical properties of the epidermis and thereby allow abnormal stimulation of epidermal nerve fibers [24]. Abnormalities in the structure of SC may also be associated with alterations in surface lipids, pH, water metabolism, and cytokine levels in the epidermis [25]. Aquaporin-3 (AQP-3), an integral membrane channel in keratinocytes, facilitates the transport of glycerol from the circulation into the epidermis [26]. Endogenous glycerol influences SC hydration in human skin [27]; therefore decreased AQP-3 expression, which has been demonstrated in rat models of acute [28] and chronic renal failure [29], could explain xerosis in CKD patients. Elevated skin pH in CKD patients could lead to activation of serine proteases and alteration in skin barrier integrity, both of which may be associated with increased sensation of itch [30, 31]. Despite an evolving understanding of why skin in CKD patients may have altered hydration, there is controversy over whether the symptoms of renal itch arise primarily due to these changes. While some studies have demonstrated a relationship between skin dryness and renal itch [32, 33], one study that formally assessed skin barrier function in CKD patients failed to identify any positive correlations between skin barrier integrity, glycerol content, skin pH, and renal itch [34]. While xerosis in CKD patients may be improved by regular use of emollients, aggressive hydration fails to completely alleviate renal itch in the majority of cases.

An alternate theory to explain renal itch is the immune hypothesis. This hypothesis proposes that CKD promotes a pro-inflammatory state and that itch is the result of systemic inflammation rather than a local skin disorder. Increased mast cell release of histamine has been reported in patients undergoing HD [35, 36], although antihistamines rarely improve renal itch [37]. Other studies have shown imbalanced Th1 and Th2 responses leading to higher levels of Th1 cells, CRP, interleukin (IL)-6, and IL-2 levels in CKD patients with itch compared to those without itch [38]. Consistent with observations of immune dysregulation, immunosuppressants including tacrolimus [39, 40] and thalidomide [41] have been used effectively to treat renal itch in some cases. In addition, ultraviolet B (UVB) phototherapy, which is thought to modulate Th1 and Th2 responses in the skin, has also been shown to attenuate renal itch [42].

Altered neural innervation or activity in the peripheral and/or central nervous system may play a role in the pathogenesis of many types of chronic itch. One study attempted to determine the relationship between renal itch and somatic neuropathy and/or dysautonomia. In this report, 51 CKD patients underwent basic neurological examination, nerve conduction velocity studies, itch assessment by means of a questionnaire, and autonomic nervous system testing using the R-R interval variation test in basal and profound breath conditions (RRIV) and the sympathetic skin response (SSR). Itch was found in 63 % of patients, and most of them had clinical symptoms and signs of peripheral sensorimotor neuropathy and dysautonomia. Although it did not reach significance, a trend towards a relationship between itch and abnormal or delayed SSRs was observed. No relationship was identified between renal itch and RRIV values. These findings suggest that neural dysfunction in CKD patients may play an important role in the pathogenesis of renal itch. Furthermore, renal itch may reflect somatic neuropathy rather than to autonomic dysfunction [43].

Imbalances in opioidergic tone have been proposed as a cause of renal itch. It was thought that μ-opioid receptor (μOR) activation in the brain and spinal cord were solely responsible for itch sensation and similarly that central κOR activation mediated anti-pruritic effects. Growing data now suggests that opioids may also modulate itch directly in the skin. Both μORs and κORs and their endogenous agonists are functional in different skin structures, including peripheral nerves, keratinocytes, melanocytes, hair follicles, dermal mast cells, macrophages, and other immune cells [44], suggesting that cutaneous populations directly communicate via opioid signaling. Activation of ORs in the skin may not only induce or attenuate itch, but may also regulate cutaneous inflammatory responses [45].

Clinical evidence supporting a role for opioid imbalance as a cause of itch was first published in 1979 when naltrexone, a μOR antagonist, was reported to decrease itch in a patient with cholestatic pruritus [46]. In 1984, intravenous naloxone, also a μOR antagonist, was reported to effectively reduce renal itch [47]. Placebo-controlled trials with μOR antagonists were subsequently carried out in CKD patients to assess their efficacy for treatment of renal itch, but results from different studies have not been consistent [48, 49]. In contrast, activation of κORs by their agonists has been shown to inhibit itch in both animals and humans, and has been reported to be of benefit in the treatment of renal itch as well. Nalfurafine, a selective κOR agonist, was approved in Japan in 2009 for the treatment of itch in HD patients. In 2010, a randomized double-blind placebo-controlled study performed in 337 HD patients confirmed that nalfurafine successfully alleviates severe renal itch [50].

Significant progress has been made over the last decade identifying molecular markers of itch sensory pathways, including protease activated receptors, mas-related G protein-coupled receptors, neuropeptide natriuretic polypeptide b, and gastrin-releasing peptide. Whether these mediators and specific neural pathways are altered in the skin or central nervous system of patients with renal itch is unknown. Further studies are required to better understand the relative roles of the immune and nervous system dysregulation in the pathogenesis of renal itch.

Clinical Manifestations

The clinical manifestations of renal itch are highly variable depending on the individual. Itch may be generalized or localized and may affect any area of the body including the face or scalp. Renal itch often occurs in a symmetric distribution, most commonly involving the back, abdomen, arms, and scalp (particularly vertex) [1, 51]. In the majority of patients with renal itch, symptoms are considered chronic, with 35–59 % of patients experiencing itch for at least 1 year. Only 7 % of the patients experience itch for a month or less [51]. Most patients (42–84 %) with renal itch report bouts of itch on a daily basis [2, 51]. The intensity of itch in CKD tends to fluctuate but is usually considered moderate to severe, rated by patients to be worse than a mosquito bite [51]. It is usually more intense at night and interferes with sleep [1]. Dry skin, sweat, and heat have been reported to exacerbate renal itch [51].

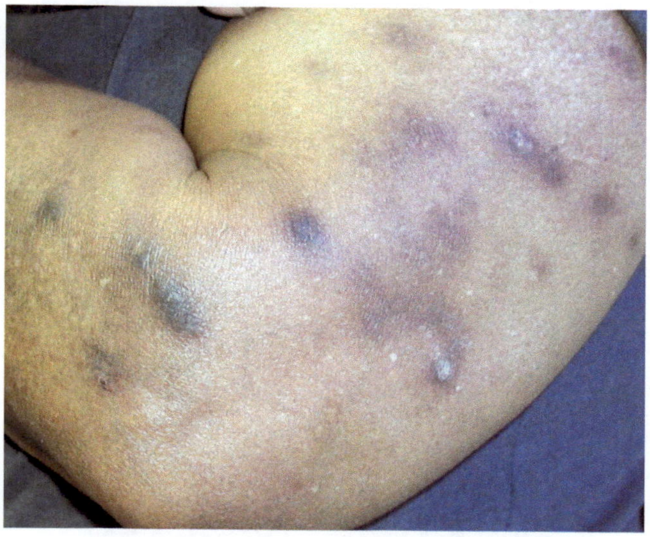

Fig. 7.1 Prurigo nodules. Courtesy of Julia R. Nunley, M.D.

Chronic scratching, associated with uremic pruritus, results in a wide variety of cutaneous changes. Figure 7.1 demonstrates the discrete hyperkeratotic, broad-based papules classic for prurigo nodularis. Figure 7.2 demonstrates acutely excoriated papules in various stages of healing, as well as depigmented scars from older lesions. Figure 7.3 also shows acutely scratched lesions with resultant scars but with more expansive lesions. How and why the itch–scratch cycle results in such varied morphology is poorly understood.

Despite potentially severe itch, there is often a marked absence of clinically apparent inflammation within the skin. Skin changes in patients with CKD may simply reflect the mechanical damage from continuous scratching including excoriations, altered skin pigmentation, secondary prurigo nodularis, and lichenification or thickening of the skin. In some cases patients may also have eczematous changes or superimposed infections such as impetigo which results from barrier disruption [52].

Differential Diagnosis

Given the high prevalence of renal itch in patients undergoing HD, this diagnosis must be considered in any CKD patient presenting with pruritus. As many patients with CKD suffer from other medical comorbidities or primary cutaneous diseases, a thorough evaluation must be undertaken for each patient to identify the cause of itch on an individual basis.

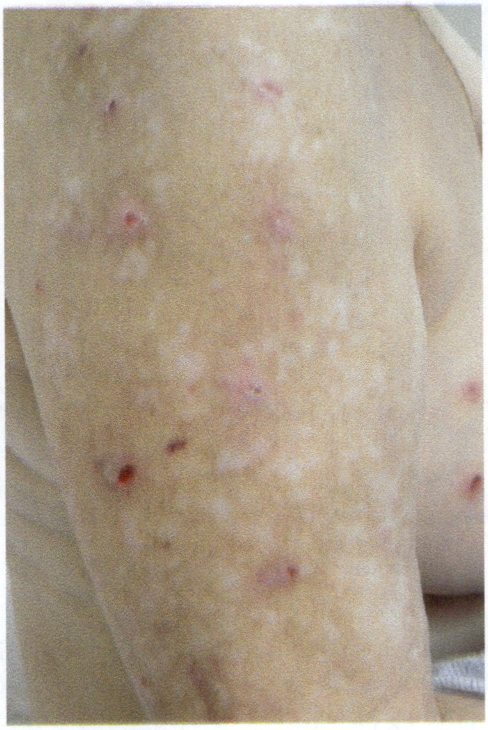

Fig. 7.2 Excoriations in various stages of healing. Courtesy of Julia R. Nunley, M.D.

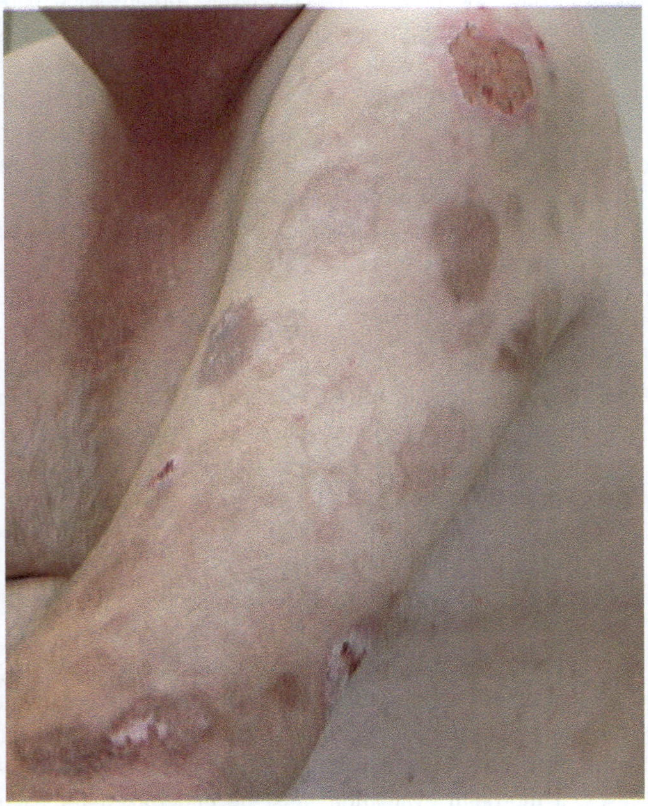

Fig. 7.3 Extensive excoriations. Courtesy of Julia R. Nunley, M.D.

Xerosis is a very common condition observed in CKD patients and may contribute to symptoms despite not being the primary cause of renal itch [51, 53, 54] in more severe cases. Xerosis alone is the cause of mild itch in the occasional CKD patient. In such cases, the itch may respond well to emollients [55].

Acquired perforating disorders such as perforating folliculitis, Kyrle disease (KD), and reactive perforating collagenosis occur in 4.5–10 % of CKD patients [56–58] and may often be confused by nondermatologists for prurigo nodularis.

Arteriovenous (AV) shunt dermatitis, which results from venous flow obstruction or flow reversal, causes hyperpigmentation and thickening of skin resembling chronic venous stasis changes. AV shunt dermatitis occurs in up to 8 % of patients on chronic dialysis (58–60) and must be distinguished from lichenification or other secondary skin changes due to renal itch as well as allergic contact dermatitis due to materials used during dialysis sessions.

Infections, infestations, and underlying systemic disorders must also be considered in the differential diagnosis of CKD patients with itch, in part due to an impaired cellular immunity that predisposes this population to such conditions [53, 59]. For example, scabies causes intractable pruritus and may often go undiagnosed or inadequately treated in CKD patients [60]. Viral infections such as hepatitis C virus (HCV) and human immunodeficiency virus (HIV) may be associated with chronic itch and should be considered in the differential of renal itch. Systemic causes of pruritus such as lymphoma, cholestasis, or hypersensitivity reactions to medications must be ruled out in CKD patients with chronic itch.

The following criteria [51] have been proposed to help in making the diagnosis of renal itch: (1) Pruritus appears shortly before the onset of dialysis, or at any time, without evidence of any other active disease that could explain the itch. (2) Patients experience episodes of itch three or more times during a period of less than 2 weeks, with the symptom appearing several times a day, lasting a minimum of a few minutes, and causing distress to the patient. (3) Appearance of an itch in a regular pattern during a period of 6 months, but less frequently than listed above.

Diagnostic Evaluation

A standard work-up to evaluate a patient with chronic itch includes basic laboratory examination to screen for systemic disorders that may be associated with itch, e.g. lymphoma and other malignancies, polycythemia vera, cholestasis, thyroid disease, diabetes, or HIV. Tests include a complete blood count with differential, serum creatinine and blood urea nitrogen values, serum bilirubin (direct and indirect), serum aminotransferases and alkaline phosphatase, thyroid-stimulating hormone and thyroxin, fasting glucose value, HIV antibody test (in high risk individuals), HCV screening and evaluation of iron stores, stool for occult blood, and serum protein electrophoresis and immunofixation. Assessment of patients in which there is a high suspicion of a diagnosis of renal itch should also include laboratory evaluation of calcium, phosphorus, and parathyroid hormone, as these values are frequently abnormal in patients with severe renal itch.

A chest X-ray may also be considered to screen for malignancy or infectious etiologies. A skin biopsy may be performed to distinguish between primary inflammatory and secondary skin changes, although is usually nondiagnostic in cases of renal itch.

Treatment (Table 7.1)

At present, other than transplantation, no therapy has proven widely effective in the management of renal itch. Most treatment recommendations for this condition are based on case series or small, uncontrolled clinical trials; therefore an individualized, stepwise approach based on response to therapy should be undertaken. Reduced itch has been reported following increases in the daily dialysate volume, time, and frequency of dialysis [20, 61], treating underlying hyperparathyroidism, hyperphosphatemia and lowering calcium phosphate levels [16, 17]. A recent 5 year prospective cohort study of HD patients found that HD with the target of Kt/V ≥ 1.5 and the use of high flux dialyzer was effective in reducing the intensity of renal itch [62]. Despite some controversy surrounding the role of these measures in renal itch, optimizing dialysis conditions and correction of electrolyte imbalance should be considered initially.

Table 7.1 Therapeutic approaches to the itch of chronic kidney disease

Treatment	Comments/recommendations
Optimize dialysate	Correct electrolyte imbalances Target KtV ≥1.5
Emollients	Creams or bland ointments 10 % urea plus dexpanthenol lotion Sericin cream
Topical analgesics	Pramoxine 1 % lotion twice daily
Antihistamines	Hydroxyzine 10–25 mg PO 2–4 times daily
Mast cell stabilizers	Cromonlyn sodium 4 % cream or 135 mg PO three times daily
Anticonvulsants	Gabapentin 100–400 mg up to three times weekly after dialysis
Antidepressants	Mirtazapine 7.5–30 mg PO daily
Opioid antagonists/antagonists	Nalfurafine 5 μg IV after dialysis
Phototherapy	Narrowband UVB phototherapy three times weekly
Renal transplant	Usually curative

PO per os, *IV* intravenous, *UVB* ultraviolet B

Patients with CKD, and in particular renal itch, often suffer from xerosis which may exacerbate their symptoms. Regular use of emollients is thus recommended to preserve the integrity of the skin barrier and to reduce water loss and exposure to environmental irritants [54]. While there are no specific studies that compare the efficacy of different types of emollients in patients with renal itch, application of a high water content emollient and an emollient containing structured lipids with endocannabinoids have been demonstrated to be beneficial in two separate small studies [55, 63]. A pilot trial performed on 15 HD patients with topical application of a lotion containing urea plus dexpanthenolim proved both skin dryness (evaluated by scoring scaling roughness, redness, and cracks on the skin) and itch. A recent double-blind trialin 50 HD patients found that application of a cream containing sericin, a water-soluble, high molecular weight biopolymer derived from silk worms, to effectively decrease skin irritation, hyperpigmentation, and itch compared to placebo [64]. Sericin contains 32 % serine, the primary amino-acid of natural moisture factor in human skin [65]. Sericin also has anti-inflammatory properties and decreases levels of tumor necrosis factor alpha (TNF-α) and IL-1β [66]. Emollients with higher lipid content such as ointments and creams are generally preferred over lotions or gels, as they provide superior occlusion and corneocyte hydration, promoting improved skin barrier function.

Topical analgesic agents, including pramoxine and capsaicin, have been used with some success in renal itch. A lotion containing 1 % pramoxine has been shown to be effective in renal itch [67]. In one study, 28 HD patients with moderate to severe renal itch applied 1 % pramoxine lotion twice daily for 4 weeks and a significant reduction in itch intensity was observed in the treatment group (61 %) compared to controls (12 %). Topical capsaicin has been reported to be successful in some patients with renal itch, but studies regarding its efficacy are conflicting. It is frequently discontinued by patients due to a burning sensation following initial applications such that it is not recommended as a first line topical agent, especially in patients with generalized itch or involvement of large skin areas [68–72].

Studies regarding the use of immunomodulators are not conclusive. Topical tacrolimus has been studied but the results are controversial and show limited benefit [39, 40]. It is not recommended for prolonged use in renal itch patients. While frequently attempted in the treatment of renal itch, no studies have formally evaluated the effectiveness of steroids for this condition.

Oral antihistamines have been classically used for the treatment of all types of chronic itch. Mast cell stabilizing effects of antihistamines have been implicated as their potential beneficial mechanism in renal itch. Both oral (135 mg three times daily) and topical (4 % cream) cromolyn sodium (CS) have been shown to effectively reduce itch in HD patients [73, 74]. It is not clear that decreased levels of specific mast cell mediators are responsible for the beneficial effects of these agents. As CS poses minimal harm and has only rare side effects, some studies recommend using it before initiating other antihistamines or neuroleptic agents for the treatment of renal itch [73]. As evidence that renal itch is histamine-mediated is lacking, the sedative properties of most antihistamines are probably responsible for itch relief in the limited number of patients responding to these agents. A trial of sedating antihistamines such as hydroxyzine (10–25 mg, 2–4 times daily by mouth) may be tried in CKD patients considering their low side effect profile.

Most patients suffer from persistent itch despite optimizing dialysis conditions and initiating regular antihistamine therapy. For these patients, low dose treatment with gabapentin and pregablin should be considered as the next therapeutic step. Although their exact mechanism in decreasing itch is unknown, these neuroleptic agents, analogs of the major inhibitory neurotransmitter γ-aminobutyric acid (GABA), are postulated to inhibit itch pathways in both the peripheral and central nervous systems, similar to their action in treating chronic pain and sensory neuropathies [75]. Different treatment regimens for gabapentin, including 300 mg after each dialysis session [76] and 400 mg twice weekly [77] have been reported to be effective. Caution is advised when starting these agents, as dizziness and somnolence are frequently encountered side effects.

Selective serotonin reuptake inhibitors (SSRIs) and selective norepinephrine reuptake inhibitors (SNRIs) have been used in the treatment of systemic itch. They are postulated to decrease itch by reducing central sensitization through alterations of both serotonin and α2 noradrenergic receptors [75]. Mirtazapine has been shown to reduce nocturnal itch and is favored by some clinicians for the treatment of renal itch [78, 79].

Systemic therapy with opioid modulators has been used in the treatment of renal itch. There are conflicting data regarding effectiveness of μ-opioid antagonists such as naltrexone in renal itch. A study performed in 15 HD patients suggested short-term efficacy of naltrexone in ameliorating renal itch [48], while a subsequent study in 23 patients did not find any statistically significant difference between naltrexone and placebo in alleviating renal itch [49]. μ-opioid antagonists must also be used with caution, as they may worsen pain caused by comorbid conditions in CKD patients. A meta-analysis of two multicenter, randomized, double-blind, placebo-controlled trials showed decreased itch and sleep disturbance in HD patients after intravenous postdialysis administration of 5 μg of nalfurafine, a selective κ-opioid agonist, compared with placebo (36 versus 14 % respectively) [50]. Butorphanol, a κ-opioid agonist and partial μ-antagonist, has shown some benefit in treating some cases of intractable itch, although not specifically renal itch [80].

UVB phototherapy has been demonstrated to be effective for renal itch and is probably vastly underutilized. Potential limitations include access to an office that provides this therapy in which case use of home phototherapy units should be considered. UVB irradiation appears to alter skin sensitivity to pruritogens and decrease the level of proinflammatory cytokines [81, 82]. In an open pilot study of 20 patients with renal itch, narrowband UVB phototherapy was performed (maximum daily dose of 1,500 mJ/cm^2) over a 6-week duration [83]. Eight of ten patients who completed the treatment duration experienced reduction in itch. Symptoms recurred in four of the eight responders after cessation of UVB treatment. UVB has a minimal risk of carcinogenesis in the therapeutic treatment of inflammatory skin conditions such as psoriasis but this risk in the CKD population has not been evaluated.

Renal transplant is the only definitive treatment for patients with refractory itch not responding to these therapeutic options [6]. Relaxation techniques and behavioral therapies may be considered as adjunctive options in patients with psychogenic itch components.

Prognosis

Renal itch has a major negative impact on the quality of life of CKD patients. Patients with moderate to severe pruritus had a 13 % higher mortality risk compared to those not affected by renal itch, in DOPPS I and a 21 % higher risk in DOPPS II and an overall higher mortality risk of 17 % [1]. The exact underlying mechanism of renal itch is still unknown and no drug specifically targets this type of itch. Several compounds, including additional κ-opioid agonists, are being evaluated for the treatment of CKD itch. Combined with advances in understanding itch signaling pathways and dysregulation of the neuro-immune axis, better treatments for patients with CKD or renal itch are on the horizon.

Acknowledgments This work has been supported by grants from the NIH, R01AR057744 and Leo Pharma to EAL and by the Dermatology Foundation to SBE.

References

1. Pisoni RL, Wikstrom B, Elder SJ, Akizawa T, Asano Y, Keen ML, et al. Pruritus in haemodialysis patients: international results from the dialysis outcomes and practice patterns study (DOPPS). Nephrol Dial Transplant. 2006;21(12):3495–505 [Research Support, Non-U.S. Gov't].
2. Mathur VS, Lindberg J, Germain M, Block G, Tumlin J, Smith M, et al. A longitudinal study of uremic pruritus in hemodialysis patients. Clin J Am Soc Nephrol. 2010;5(8):1410–9 [Comparative Study Multicenter Study].
3. Kurban MS, Boueiz A, Kibbi AG. Cutaneous manifestations of chronic kidney disease. Clin Dermatol. 2008;26(3):255–64 [Review].

4. Wang H, Yosipovitch G. New insights into the pathophysiology and treatment of chronic itch in patients with end-stage renal disease, chronic liver disease, and lymphoma. Int J Dermatol. 2010;49(1):1–11 [Research Support, N.I.H., Extramural Review].
5. Chen HY, Chiu YL, Hsu SP, Pai MF, Lai CF, Yang JY, et al. Elevated C-reactive protein level in hemodialysis patients with moderate/severe uremic pruritus: a potential mediator of high overall mortality. Q J Assoc Phys. 2010;103(11):837–46 [Research Support, Non-U.S. Gov't].
6. Altmeyer P, Kachel HG, Schafer G, Fassbinder W. Normalization of uremic skin changes following kidney transplantation. Hautarzt. 1986;37(4):217–21.
7. Dhand A, Aminoff MJ. The neurology of itch. Brain. 2013;22.
8. Schmelz M, Schmidt R, Bickel A, Handwerker HO, Torebjork HE. Specific C-receptors for itch in human skin. J Neurosci. 1997;17(20):8003–8 [Research Support, Non-U.S. Gov't].
9. Berthjones J, Grahambrown RAC. Failure of terfenadine in relieving the pruritus of atopic-dermatitis. Br J Dermatol. 1989;121(5): 635–7 [Article].
10. Krause L, Shuster S. Mechanism of action of antipruritic drugs. BMJ. 1983;287(6400):1199–200.
11. Namer B, Carr R, Johanek LM, Schmelz M, Handwerker HO, Ringkamp M. Separate peripheral pathways for pruritus in man. J Neurophysiol. 2008;100(4):2062–9 [Research Support, N.I.H., Extramural Research Support, Non-U.S. Gov't].
12. Davidson S, Zhang X, Yoon CH, Khasabov SG, Simone DA, Giesler Jr GJ. The itch-producing agents histamine and cowhage activate separate populations of primate spinothalamic tract neurons. J Neurosci. 2007;27(37):10007–14 [Comparative Study Research Support, N.I.H., Extramural].
13. Ringkamp M, Schepers RJ, Shimada SG, Johanek LM, Hartke TV, Borzan J, et al. A role for nociceptive, myelinated nerve fibers in itch sensation. J Neurosci. 2011;31(42):14841–9 [Research Support, N.I.H., Extramural].
14. Narita I, Alchi B, Omori K, Sato F, Ajiro J, Saga D, et al. Etiology and prognostic significance of severe uremic pruritus in chronic hemodialysis patients. Kidney Int. 2006;69(9):1626–32 [Research Support, Non-U.S. Gov't].
15. Duque MI, Thevarajah S, Chan YH, Tuttle AB, Freedman BI, Yosipovitch G. Uremic pruritus is associated with higher kt/V and serum calcium concentration. Clin Nephrol. 2006;66(3):184–91.
16. Massry SG, Popovtzer MM, Coburn JW, Makoff DL, Maxwell MH, Kleeman CR. Intractable pruritus as a manifestation of secondary hyperparathyroidism in uremia. Disappearance of itching after subtotal parathyroidectomy. N Engl J Med. 1968;279(13):697–700.
17. Chou FF, Ho JC, Huang SC, Sheen-Chen SM. A study on pruritus after parathyroidectomy for secondary hyperparathyroidism. J Am Coll Surg. 2000;190(1):65–70.
18. Friga V, Linos A, Linos DA. Is aluminum toxicity responsible for uremic pruritus in chronic hemodialysis patients? Nephron. 1997;75(1):48–53 [Comparative Study].
19. Navarro-Gonzalez JF, Mora-Fernandez C, Garcia-Perez J. Clinical implications of disordered magnesium homeostasis in chronic renal failure and dialysis. Semin Dial. 2009;22(1):37–44 [Review].
20. Hiroshige K, Kabashima N, Takasugi M, Kuroiwa A. Optimal dialysis improves uremic pruritus. Am J Kidney Dis. 1995;25(3):413–9 [Clinical Trial Randomized Controlled Trial].
21. Gatmiri SM, Mahdavi-Mazdeh M, Lessan-Pezeshki M, Abbasi M. Uremic pruritus and serum phosphorus level. Acta Med Iran. 2013;51(7):477–81.
22. Welter Ede Q, Frainer RH, Maldotti A, Losekann A, Weber MB. Evaluating the association between alterations in mineral metabolism and pruritus in hemodialysis patients. An Bras Dermatol. 2011;86(1):31–6.
23. Cawley EP, Hoch-Ligheti C, Bond GM. The eccrine sweat glands of patients in uremia. Arch Dermatol. 1961;84:889–97.
24. Yosipovitch G. Dry skin and impairment of barrier function associated with itch – new insights. Int J Cosmet Sci. 2004;26(1):1–7.
25. Miyamoto T, Nojima H, Shinkado T, Nakahashi T, Kuraishi Y. Itch-associated response induced by experimental dry skin in mice. Jpn J Pharmacol. 2002;88(3):285–92.
26. Hara-Chikuma M, Verkman AS. Aquaporin-3 functions as a glycerol transporter in mammalian skin. Biol Cell. 2005;97(7):479–86 [Research Support, N.I.H., Extramural Research Support, Non--U.S. Gov't Research Support, U.S. Gov't, P.H.S. Review].
27. Choi EH, Man MQ, Wang F, Zhang X, Brown BE, Feingold KR, et al. Is endogenous glycerol a determinant of stratum corneum hydration in humans? J Invest Dermatol. 2005;125(2):288–93 [Research Support, N.I.H., Extramural Research Support, Non--U.S. Gov't Research Support, U.S. Gov't, Non-P.H.S. Research Support, U.S. Gov't, P.H.S.].
28. Gong H, Wang W, Kwon TH, Jonassen T, Frokiaer J, Nielsen S. Reduced renal expression of AQP2, p-AQP2 and AQP3 in haemorrhagic shock-induced acute renal failure. Nephrol Dial Transplant. 2003;18(12):2551–9 [Research Support, Non-U.S. Gov't].
29. Kwon TH, Frokiaer J, Knepper MA, Nielsen S. Reduced AQP1, -2, and -3 levels in kidneys of rats with CRF induced by surgical reduction in renal mass. Am J Physiol. 1998;275(5 Pt 2):F724–41 [Research Support, Non-U.S. Gov't Research Support, U.S. Gov't, P.H.S.].
30. Yosipovitch G, Tur E, Morduchowicz G, Boner G. Skin surface pH, moisture, and pruritus in haemodialysis patients. Nephrol Dial Transplant. 1993;8(10):1129–32 [Comparative Study].
31. Hachem JP, Crumrine D, Fluhr J, Brown BE, Feingold KR, Elias PM. pH directly regulates epidermal permeability barrier homeostasis, and stratum corneum integrity/cohesion. J Invest Dermatol. 2003;121(2):345–53 [Research Support, U.S. Gov't, Non-P.H.S. Research Support, U.S. Gov't, P.H.S.].
32. Young Jr AW, Sweeney EW, David DS, Cheigh J, Hochgelerenl EL, Sakai S, et al. Dermatologic evaluation of pruritus in patients on hemodialysis. N Y State J Med. 1973;73(22):2670–4.
33. Balaskas EV, Chu M, Uldall RP, Gupta A, Oreopoulos DG. Pruritus in continuous ambulatory peritoneal dialysis and hemodialysis patients. Perit Dial Int. 1993;13 Suppl 2:527–32 [Research Support, Non-U.S. Gov't].
34. Yosipovitch G, Duque MI, Patel TS, Ishiuji Y, Guzman-Sanchez DA, Dawn AG, et al. Skin barrier structure and function and their relationship to pruritus in end-stage renal disease. Nephrol Dial Transplant. 2007;22(11):3268–72.
35. Yosipovitch G, Greaves MW, Schmelz M. Itch. Lancet. 2003;361(9358):690–4 [Review].
36. Andrew D, Craig AD. Spinothalamic lamina I neurons selectively sensitive to histamine: a central neural pathway for itch. Nat Neurosci. 2001;4(1):72–7 [Research Support, Non-U.S. Gov't Research Support, U.S. Gov't, P.H.S.].
37. Mettang T, Fritz P, Weber J, Machleidt C, Hubel E, Kuhlmann U. Uremic pruritus in patients on hemodialysis or continuous ambulatory peritoneal dialysis (CAPD). The role of plasma histamine and skin mast cells. Clin Nephrol. 1990;34(3):136–41 [Comparative Study Research Support, Non-U.S. Gov't].
38. Mettang T, Pauli-Magnus C, Alscher DM. Uraemic pruritus – new perspectives and insights from recent trials. Nephrol Dial Transplant. 2002;17(9):1558–63 [Review].
39. Pauli-Magnus C, Klumpp S, Alscher DM, Kuhlmann U, Mettang T. Short-term efficacy of tacrolimus ointment in severe uremic pruritus. Perit Dial Int. 2000;20(6):802–3 [Letter].
40. Kuypers DR, Claes K, Evenepoel P, Maes B, Vanrenterghem Y. A prospective proof of concept study of the efficacy of tacrolimus ointment on uraemic pruritus (UP) in patients on chronic dialysis therapy. Nephrol Dial Transplant. 2004;19(7):1895–901 [Clinical Trial Research Support, Non-U.S. Gov't].
41. Silva SR, Viana PC, Lugon NV, Hoette M, Ruzany F, Lugon JR. Thalidomide for the treatment of uremic pruritus: a crossover

randomized double-blind trial. Nephron. 1994;67(3):270–3 [Clinical Trial Randomized Controlled Trial].
42. Gilchrest BA, Rowe JW, Brown RS, Steinman TI, Arndt KA. Ultraviolet phototherapy of uremic pruritus Long-term results and possible mechanism of action. Ann Intern Med. 1979;91(1):17–21 [Clinical Trial Controlled Clinical Trial].
43. Zakrzewska-Pniewska B, Jedras M. Is pruritus in chronic uremic patients related to peripheral somatic and autonomic neuropathy? Study by R-R interval variation test (RRIV) and by sympathetic skin response (SSR). Clin Neurophysiol. 2001;31(3):181–93 [Clinical Trial].
44. Bigliardi-Qi M, Bigliardi PL, Buchner S, Rufli T. Characterization of mu-opiate receptor in human epidermis and keratinocytes. Ann N Y Acad Sci. 1999;885:368–71 [Research Support, Non-U.S. Gov't].
45. Reich A, Szepietowski JC. Non-analgesic effects of opioids: peripheral opioid receptors as promising targets for future antipruritic therapies. Curr Pharm Des. 2012;18(37):6021–4 [Review].
46. Bernstein JE, Swift R. Relief of intractable pruritus with naloxone. Arch Dermatol. 1979;115(11):1366–7 [Case Reports Clinical Trial Controlled Clinical Trial].
47. Andersen LW, Friedberg M, Lokkegaard N. Naloxone in the treatment of uremic pruritus: a case history. Clin Nephrol. 1984;21(6):355–6 [Case Reports Letter].
48. Peer G, Kivity S, Agami O, Fireman E, Silverberg D, Blum M, et al. Randomised crossover trial of naltrexone in uraemic pruritus. Lancet. 1996;348(9041):1552–4 [Clinical Trial Randomized Controlled Trial Research Support, Non-U.S. Gov't].
49. Pauli-Magnus C, Mikus G, Alscher DM, Kirschner T, Nagel W, Gugeler N, et al. Naltrexone does not relieve uremic pruritus: results of a randomized, double-blind, placebo-controlled crossover study. J Am Soc Nephrol. 2000;11(3):514–9 [Clinical Trial Randomized Controlled Trial Research Support, Non-U.S. Gov't].
50. Kumagai H, Ebata T, Takamori K, Muramatsu T, Nakamoto H, Suzuki H. Effect of a novel kappa-receptor agonist, nalfurafine hydrochloride, on severe itch in 337 haemodialysis patients: a phase III, randomized, double-blind, placebo-controlled study. Nephrol Dial Transplant. 2010;25(4):1251–7 [Clinical Trial, Phase III Comparative Study Multicenter Study Randomized Controlled Trial].
51. Zucker I, Yosipovitch G, David M, Gafter U, Boner G. Prevalence and characterization of uremic pruritus in patients undergoing hemodialysis: uremic pruritus is still a major problem for patients with end-stage renal disease. J Am Acad Dermatol. 2003;49(5):842–6 [Multicenter Study].
52. Cohen JB, Janniger CK, Piela Z, Szepietowski JC, Samady JA, Schwartz RA. Dermatologic correlates of selected metabolic events. J Med. 1999;30(3–4):149–56 [Review].
53. Deshmukh SP, Sharma YK, Dash K, Chaudhari NC, Deo KS. Clinicoepidemiological study of skin manifestations in patients of chronic renal failure on hemodialysis. Indian Dermatol Online J. 2013;4(1):18–21.
54. Morton CA, Lafferty M, Hau C, Henderson I, Jones M, Lowe JG. Pruritus and skin hydration during dialysis. Nephrol Dial Transplant. 1996;11(10):2031–6 [Comparative Study].
55. Okada K, Matsumoto K. Effect of skin care with an emollient containing a high water content on mild uremic pruritus. Ther Apher Dial. 2004;8(5):419–22 [Clinical Trial].
56. Hood AF, Hardegen GL, Zarate AR, Nigra TP, Gelfand MC. Kyrle's disease in patients with chronic renal failure. Arch Dermatol. 1982;118(2):85–8.
57. Lynde CB, Pratt MD. Clinical images: acquired perforating dermatosis: association with diabetes and renal failure. Can Med Assoc J. 2009;181(9):615 [Case Reports].
58. Hari Kumar KV, Prajapati J, Pavan G, Parthasarathy A, Jha R, Modi KD. Acquired perforating dermatoses in patients with diabetic kidney disease on hemodialysis. Hemodial Int. 2010;14(1):73–7.
59. Pico MR, Lugo-Somolinos A, Sanchez JL, Burgos-Calderon R. Cutaneous alterations in patients with chronic renal failure. Int J Dermatol. 1992;31(12):860–3 [Review].
60. Deabate MC, Calitri V, Licata C, Fidelio T, Rocchietti M, Pieri F, et al. Scabies in a dialysis unit mystery and prejudice. Minerva Urol Nefrol. 2001;53(2):69–73.
61. Liakopoulos V, Krishnan M, Stefanidis I, Savaj S, Ghareeb S, Musso C, et al. Improvement in uremic symptoms after increasing daily dialysate volume in patients on chronic peritoneal dialysis with declining renal function. Int Urol Nephrol. 2004;36(3):437–43.
62. Ko MJ, Wu HY, Chen HY, Chiu YL, Hsu SP, Pai MF, et al. Uremic pruritus, dialysis adequacy, and metabolic profiles in hemodialysis patients: a prospective 5-year cohort study. PLoS One. 2013;8(8):e71404.
63. Szepietowski JC, Szepietowski T, Reich A. Efficacy and tolerance of the cream containing structured physiological lipids with endocannabinoids in the treatment of uremic pruritus: a preliminary study. Acta Dermatovenerol Croat. 2005;13(2):97–103 [Clinical Trial].
64. Aramwit P, Keongamaroon O, Siritientong T, Bang N, Supasyndh O. Sericin cream reduces pruritus in hemodialysis patients: a randomized, double-blind, placebo-controlled experimental study. BMC Nephrol. 2012;13:119 [Randomized Controlled Trial Research Support, Non-U.S. Gov't].
65. Zhang YQ. Applications of natural silk protein sericin in biomaterials. Biotechnol Adv. 2002;20(2):91–100.
66. Aramwit P, Kanokpanont S, De-Eknamkul W, Srichana T. Monitoring of inflammatory mediators induced by silk sericin. J Biosci Bioeng. 2009;107(5):556–61 [Research Support, Non-U.S. Gov't].
67. Young TA, Patel TS, Camacho F, Clark A, Freedman BI, Kaur M, et al. A pramoxine-based anti-itch lotion is more effective than a control lotion for the treatment of uremic pruritus in adult hemodialysis patients. J Dermatolog Treat. 2009;20(2):76–81 [Comparative Study Randomized Controlled Trial Research Support, Non-U.S. Gov't].
68. Cho YL, Liu HN, Huang TP, Tarng DC. Uremic pruritus: roles of parathyroid hormone and substance P. J Am Acad Dermatol. 1997;36(4):538–43 [Clinical Trial Controlled Clinical Trial Randomized Controlled Trial].
69. Breneman DL, Cardone JS, Blumsack RF, Lather RM, Searle EA, Pollack VE. Topical capsaicin for treatment of hemodialysis-related pruritus. J Am Acad Dermatol. 1992;26(1):91–4 [Clinical Trial Randomized Controlled Trial].
70. Tarng DC, Cho YL, Liu HN, Huang TP. Hemodialysis-related pruritus: a double-blind, placebo-controlled, crossover study of capsaicin 0025% cream. Nephron. 1996;72(4):617–22 [Clinical Trial Randomized Controlled Trial].
71. Kuypers DR. Skin problems in chronic kidney disease. Nature clinical practice. Nephrology. 2009;5(3):157–70 [Review].
72. Gooding SM, Canter PH, Coelho HF, Boddy K, Ernst E. Systematic review of topical capsaicin in the treatment of pruritus. Int J Dermatol. 2010;49(8):858–65 [Research Support, Non-U.S. Gov't Review].
73. Vessal G, Sagheb MM, Shilian S, Jafari P, Samani SM. Effect of oral cromolyn sodium on CKD-associated pruritus and serum tryptase level: a double-blind placebo-controlled study. Nephrol Dial Transplant. 2010;25(5):1541–7 [Randomized Controlled Trial Research Support, Non-U.S. Gov't].
74. Feily A, Dormanesh B, Ghorbani AR, Moosavi Z, Kouchak M, Cheraghian B, et al. Efficacy of topical cromolyn sodium 4% on pruritus in uremic nephrogenic patients: a randomized double-blind study in 60 patients. Int J Clin Pharmacol Ther. 2012;50(7):510–3 [Randomized Controlled Trial].

75. Yosipovitch G, Carstens E, McGlone F. Chronic itch and chronic pain: analogous mechanisms. Pain. 2007;131(1–2):4–7 [Review].
76. Gunal AI, Ozalp G, Yoldas TK, Gunal SY, Kirciman E, Celiker H. Gabapentin therapy for pruritus in haemodialysis patients: a randomized, placebo-controlled, double-blind trial. Nephrol Dial Transplant. 2004;19(12):3137–9 [Clinical Trial Randomized Controlled Trial].
77. Naini AE, Harandi AA, Khanbabapour S, Shahidi S, Seirafiyan S, Mohseni M. Gabapentin: a promising drug for the treatment of uremic pruritus. Saudi J Kidney Dis Transpl. 2007;18(3):378–81 [Randomized Controlled Trial].
78. Hundley JL, Yosipovitch G. Mirtazapine for reducing nocturnal itch in patients with chronic pruritus: a pilot study. J Am Acad Dermatol. 2004;50(6):889–91 [Case Reports].
79. Davis MP, Frandsen JL, Walsh D, Andresen S, Taylor S. Mirtazapine for pruritus. J Pain Symptom Manage. 2003;25(3):288–91 [Case Reports].
80. Dawn AG, Yosipovitch G. Butorphanol for treatment of intractable pruritus. J Am Acad Dermatol. 2006;54(3):527–31.
81. Wanke I, Skabytska Y, Kraft B, Peschel A, Biedermann T, Schittek B. Staphylococcus aureus skin colonization is promoted by barrier disruption and leads to local inflammation. Exp Dermatol. 2013;22(2):153–5 [Letter Research Support, Non-U.S. Gov't].
82. Nickoloff BJ. Cracking the cytokine code in psoriasis. Nat Med. 2007;13(3):242–4 [News].
83. Ada S, Seckin D, Budakoglu I, Ozdemir FN. Treatment of uremic pruritus with narrowband ultraviolet B phototherapy: an open pilot study. J Am Acad Dermatol. 2005;53(1):149–51.

Dyschromias in Renal Disease

8

Mwatsveruka N. Munhutu and Rebat M. Halder

Introduction

Dermatologic signs and diseases associated with dyschromia are evident over the entire spectrum of kidney disease, particularly among patients with chronic kidney disease (CKD). Dyschromias are defined as disorders with *any* alteration of pigmentation in the skin, hair or nails and are either a primary process or due to secondarily induced changes [1]. Normal skin color results from an admixture of several colored pigments or chromophores present within the skin, namely, hemoglobin, carotenoids, and melanins [2]. Dyschromias may either represent the darkening (hyperpigmentation), lightening (hypopigmentation), or loss of pigment (depigmentation) of the skin. An even broader definition includes the various shades of red, pink, and yellow that are evident in lesions with associated erythema or sallow pallor. This chapter will focus on the description and pathophysiologic processes and treatment of the dermatologic diseases associated with dyschromias in the setting of kidney disease. Skin disease in the setting of renal disease has a significant impact on a patient's quality of life with increased morbidity and even mortality. Recognition of pigmentary alterations and their relationship to various skin conditions in the setting of kidney disease is imperative for early diagnosis by astute clinicians for appropriate management of the underlying etiology of the pigmentary alteration.

M.N. Munhutu, M.D., M.P.H. • R.M. Halder, M.D. (✉)
Department of Dermatology, Howard University College of Medicine, 2041 Georgia Avenue NW, Washington, DC 20060, USA
e-mail: mwatsveruka.munhutu@howard.edu; rhalder@howard.edu

General Pigmentary Alterations in Kidney Disease

One of the most common manifestations of dermatologic disease in patients with kidney disorders is a change in skin coloration. Dyspigmentation is typically noted as a darkening of skin color from baseline, especially in patients with CKD who are on dialysis. The hyperpigmentation is photodistributed [3]. The etiology of this darkening is thought to be due to increased melanin in the basal layer and superficial dermis stimulated by increased plasma levels of beta-melanocyte-stimulating hormone [4].

Another commonly noted pigmentary alteration in CKD is the characteristic yellow-hued pallor. This unnatural hue is, in part, due to the underlying anemia of chronic disease from inadequate production of erythropoietin in CKD [5]. However, there is also a complex interplay of chromophores and dermal and subcutaneous carotenoid deposition which may also influence the intensity of this discoloration (Table 8.1).

Xerosis and acquired ichthyosis are common problems that can be associated with hyperpigmentation in the setting of kidney disease. In darker skinned patients there may be a greyish or "ashy" appearance to the dry skin. Many patients experience pruritus secondary to the xerosis and uremia which ultimately leads to mechanical manipulation of skin and associated secondary hyperpigmentation and sometimes lichenification. Symptomatic treatment includes liberal use of emollients to moisturize the skin. Topical antipruritics such as menthol containing lotions provide temporary relief due to a cooling effect when applied to the skin. If pruritus is associated with an underlying severe hyperparathyroidism, parathyroidectomy may be indicated [5]. Narrowband ultraviolet B (NB-UVB) phototherapy may be effective in relieving uremic pruritus but does not alter the associated dyspigmentation and may, in fact, induce further hyperpigmentation due to the tanning response.

J.R. Nunley and E.V. Lerma (eds.), *Dermatological Manifestations of Kidney Disease*,
DOI 10.1007/978-1-4939-2395-3_8, © Springer Science+Business Media New York 2015

Table 8.1 Dyspigmentation associated with renal disease

Discoloration	Dermatologic findings	Etiology	Distribution	Treatment
White	Uremic frosting (rare)	Deposition of urea crystals from sweat on skin	Head and neck	Dialysis
Yellow	Pallor	Anemia, deposition of carotenoids, urochrome	Generalized	Treatment of underlying anemia of chronic disease
Evolving red/purple/green	Ecchymoses	Abnormal hemostasis	Sites of traumatic injury	Normalizing hemostasis
Brown	Hyperpigmentation	Increased circulating β-melanocyte stimulating hormone	Photo-distributed	None, resolves with renal transplantation

Diseases That Affect the Kidney and Skin with Associated Dyschromia

Connective tissue diseases (e.g., systemic lupus erythematosus (SLE), systemic sclerosis) are systemic diseases with significant dermatologic and nephrologic effects. Specific dermatologic findings of these conditions are found in other chapters of this book. They are included here for a complete discussion of dyschromias.

SLE is a systemic connective tissue disease with a wide array of symptoms and signs. Cutaneous involvement is significant and 4 of the 11 diagnostic criteria of SLE are mucocutaneous findings (Table 8.2). Several eruptions of SLE have archetypal descriptions in which dyspigmentation is a prominent finding. The malar rash, classically described as the "butterfly rash," consists of facial erythema across malar cheeks and bridge of the nose. In comparison, discoid lupus typically demonstrates areas of hyperpigmentation and depigmentation especially in darker skinned patients. Other cutaneous manifestations of SLE include periungual telangiectasia, oral mucosal hemorrhages, and a livedoid reaction pattern, most commonly found on the lower legs.

Multidisciplinary treatment approaches are best. From a dermatologic standpoint photoprotection is of utmost importance. Sun avoidance is optimal; however, daily use of a high sun protection factor sunblock should be recommended to those who cannot completely avoid the sun [2]. Skin directed therapy includes the use of potent topical steroids, with topical calcineurin inhibitors being second line topical therapy. First line systemic treatment involves the use of antimalarial drugs; hydroxychloroquine is most commonly used. Ocular toxicity is rare but baseline and follow-up retinal examinations are required to monitor for retinal toxicity; the risk of retinal toxicity may increase with cumulative dose. A more common side effect of hydroxychloroquine is an idiosyncratic development of hyperpigmentation. Other more aggressive treatment options for cutaneous lupus are beyond the scope of this chapter.

Systemic sclerosis, an autoimmune connective tissue disease characterized by anti-Scl-70, anticentromere and antinuclear antibodies, can ultimately lead to progressive sclerosis of the skin and internal organs with significant involvement of the kidney. Established cutaneous disease demonstrates a classic "salt and pepper" mottled dyspigmentation on the trunk and scalp. Raynaud phenomenon is common in systemic sclerosis causing prominent dyspigmentation including pallor, cyanosis, and reactive hyperemia.

Table 8.2 American College of Rheumatology: SLE diagnostic criteria

Malar rash
Discoid rash
Photosensitivity
Oral ulceration
Arthritis
Proteinuria >0.5 g/day or casts
Neurologic disorders
Serositis
Hematologic abnormalities
Immunologic disorders
ANA positivity

SLE systemic lupus erythematosus, *ANA* antinuclear antibody

Treatment with angiotensin inhibitors and angiotensin II receptor antagonists has improved renal morbidity significantly [6]. Skin directed therapies remain unsatisfactory with limited efficacy (Fig. 8.1).

Genodermatoses are inherited disorders that have characteristic skin findings; a subset of these conditions affects the kidney and is associated with pigmentary alteration.

Fabry disease, an X-linked lysosomal storage disorder leads to accumulation of neutral glycosphingolipids in multiple organ systems including the kidney. It is caused by mutations in the α-galactosidase A gene. Patients present with characteristic skin findings of multiple reddish-brown papules in a classic bathing suit distribution. Macular angiomas may also be seen on the proximal extremities, palmar and plantar surfaces, periungually and on the vermillion border of the lips. Cutaneous vascular lesions can be treated with intense pulse light (IPL) and other vascular lasers to improve cosmesis [7].

Familial Mediterranean fever is an inherited disorder due to mutations in the MEFV gene which encodes a pyrin protein important in the inflammatory pathway. The hallmark findings of the disorder are recurrent episodes of serositis, involving the lungs, heart, peritoneum, and joints, with an associated periodic fever. In a subset of patients recurrent

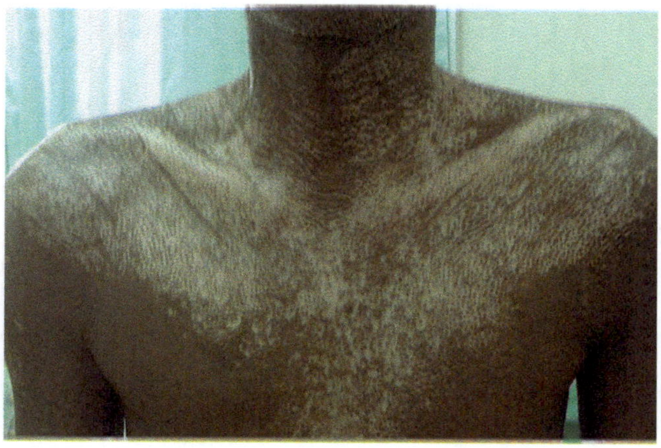

Fig. 8.1 Salt and pepper dyspigmentation in scleroderma. Image reprinted with permission from Jeffrey P. Callen, M.D. University of Louisville School of Medicine, published by *Medscape Reference* (http://emedicine.medscape.com/), 2014, available at: http://emedicine.medscape.com/article/1049648-overview

inflammation results in excess production of amyloid A protein with aberrant deposition in the kidneys leading to eventual renal insufficiency. Patients often present with a "hot ankle rash," consisting of erythematous, erysipelas-like patches on bilateral lower legs. Treatment with colchicine may suppresses attacks and prevent associated amyloid deposition in tissues; anti-interleukin (IL)-1 biologics may be successful in colchicine-resistent cases.

Primary systemic amyloidosis is the most common type of systemic amyloidosis and is usually associated with a plasma cell dyscrasia. There is deposition of light chain amyloid in internal organs including the kidneys which can lead to chronic renal failure; Bence Jones proteins are usually detected in the urine. Cutaneous lesions due to amyloid deposits are rarely seen in primary systemic amyloidosis; however, when present, the most characteristic, and likely pathognomonic, color change is the development of bilateral purpura of the eyelids called "pinch purpura". Similar purpuric lesions and may also be present on the upper trunk, face, and neck. Other less frequent findings are translucent flesh-colored papules on the face, neck, and scalp. Smooth, waxy, infiltrated papules, and plaques may be evident on the palms and fingertips. Skin biopsy may be necessary to make a diagnosis.

Nephrogenic systemic fibrosis is a rare and relatively recently described skin disorder [8]. While the exact etiology is yet to be elucidated, it is associated with exposure to gadolinium based contrast agents used in magnetic resonance imaging in patients with renal insufficiency [8]. Initial cutaneous changes are symmetrical red or deeper colored papules and plaques on the lower extremities with progressive swelling and tightening of the skin. Later stage disease has an indurated peau d'orange appearance of the extremities often with associated hyperpigmentation. Fibrosis may also involve extracutaneous sites including the heart, lungs, and the skeletal muscle and the sclera which can have yellowish plaques. There is no known effective treatment. Therapy is usually directed at optimizing renal function. Other therapies, with limited success include phototherapy, extracorporeal photophoresis, sodium thiosulfate, and rapamycin. Physical therapy is an adjunctive modality highly recommended to maintain functional mobility in affected patients [2, 8, 9].

Vasculitides

This group of disorders is traditionally classified according to the size of the affected vessels. Vasculitides are well known to have associated underlying kidney diseases and prominent characteristic cutaneous findings. There are several major vasculitides that are commonly associated with renal disease and which can have dyspigmentation as a prominent dermatologic sign. The following are discussed in this section.

1. Leukocytoclastic vasculitis
2. Henoch–Schönlein purpura
3. Polyarteritis nodosa
4. Wegener granulomatosis

Leukocytoclastic vasculitis (LCV) is a small vessel vasculitis whose hallmark cutaneous finding is described as "palpable purpura". Affected individuals develop non-blanchable, erythematous, and violaceous papules, most commonly on the distal lower extremities. Lesions evolve with time, turning to a more reddish brown discoloration in older lesions and typically heal with residual hyperpigmentation. Treatment is often directed at the inciting cause; however, skin directed treatment includes mild topical steroids for pruritus or systemic steroids for more severe disease.

Henoch–Schölein purpura (HSP) is a systemic vasculitis caused by the deposition of IgA immune complexes in small blood vessels; a subset of patients develops kidney involvement and may progress to CKD. HSP is usually triggered by a preceding viral or bacterial infection such streptococcal pharyngitis or *Helicobacter pylori* infection. As a subcategory of LCV, findings are similar with palpable purpura distributed classically below the waist on the lower extremities and buttocks. Treatment is generally supportive though systemic corticosteroids and intravenous immunoglobulin (IVIG) may be used for severe systemic disease.

Polyarteritis nodosa is a necrotizing vasculitis of small and medium arteries which often affects the kidneys. There are two major forms of this disease, a benign cutaneous variant, and a more aggressive systemic disease. The exact etiology is unknown but it is thought to be due to deposition of immune complexes in the affected vessels. It has been associated with hepatitis B or C viral infections. Skin findings commonly include 5–10 mm subcutaneous nodules along the blood vessels with dusky overlying erythema and purpura. There may also be ecchymoses and peripheral gangrene with ulcers and characteristic black eschars. Livedo reticularis, a vascular reaction pattern described by a reticular or net-like discoloration is sometimes evident. Lesions occur primarily on the legs and are usually markedly painful. Therapy includes immune suppression and antiviral therapy.

Granulomatosis with polyangiitis (formerly Wegener granulomatosis) is a necrotizing, granulomatous vasculitis with inflammation of the small and medium sized vessels due to antibodies against antineutrophil cytoplasmic proteinase 3 (C-ANCA) with an aggressive clinical course unless diagnosed and treated early with immunosuppressive medications. Although this disease has a prominent pulmonary component, renal manifestations can portend a poor prognosis. Strawberry gingivitis is almost a pathognomonic oral finding for the disorder. Cutaneous findings are infrequent and include targetoid purpuric plaques often with ulceration and necrosis. Treatment is immune suppression. Oral tacrolimus has been reported to be beneficial in the treatment of the ulcerations. Reduction of *Staphylococcus aureus* with oral antibiotics has also been shown to be beneficial in controlling relapse rates in a subset of patients [9].

Cryoglobulinemia is a group of disorders caused by globulins that undergo reversible precipitation from plasma or serum upon cold exposure. Cryoglobulinemia is classified into three types according immunoglobulin subtype. Type I is most commonly encountered in patients with a plasma cell dyscrasias such as multiple myeloma. Types II and III are strongly associated with infection by the hepatitis C virus. Type III is also associated with autoimmune diseases such as SLE and rheumatoid arthritis. Skin involvement is infrequent in type I. The skin findings in type II and III are typically palpable purpura with purpuric papules and plaques and focal areas of skin necrosis. Lesions are usually acrally distributed however; any part of the extremities can be affected. Other findings include a livedo reticularis pattern of dyspigmentation with focal areas of ulcerations and necrosis along the retiform purpura. There is usually a dusky reddish brown background discoloration associated with these findings. The ultimate treatment for cryoglobulinemic vasculitis is to treat the underlying disease (Fig. 8.2).

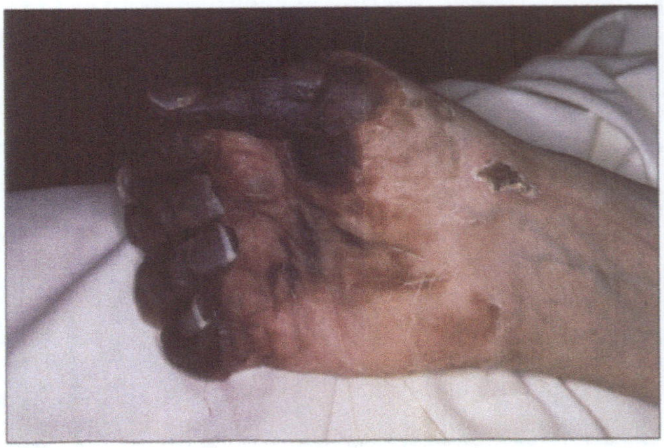

Fig. 8.2 Digital gangrene in type I cryoglobulinemia. Digital gangrene occurring in type I cryoglobulinemia. This complication is observed more rarely in type II and III cryoglobulinemias. Springer, Atlas of Rheumatology, Vol EU, 2002, Chapter 4. Guillevin, L; with kind permission from Springer Science_Business Media B.V.

Skin Diseases with Associated Dyschromia Common or Unique to Uremia

Uremic frost is a pale frostlike deposition of white crystals on the skin caused by high levels of blood urea, related to profound kidney failure. This condition is included in the discussion mainly for historical reference as this is now rarely seen due to the advent of widely accessible hemodialysis. Uremic frost was a morbid prognostic sign prior to the wide availability of dialysis. Treatment is dialysis or immediate renal transplantation.

Uremic pruritus (renal pruritus) is incredibly common in patients with CKD and its often intractable making management challenging. Patients on hemodialysis are disproportionately affected; other risk factors include male gender and elevated serum blood urea nitrogen (BUN) levels [10, 11]. The etiology is unknown but is thought to be multifactorial. Patient often have an underlying hyperparathyroidism, anemia of chronic disease, xerosis and increased blood levels of substance P, magnesium, or aluminum [10]. Additionally, patients often have underlying comorbidities such diabetes mellitus, hypothyroidism, hepatitis, and drug hypersensitivities which all contribute to the pruritus. Skin findings include excoriations which can result in hyperpigmentation, depigmentation, erythema, and lichenification. Treatment involves various topical and systemic medications. NB-UVB light may be effective for uremic pruritus.

Prurigo nodularis is also commonly found in the setting of CKD and pruritus. Patients present with multiple itchy nodules usually on the extremities although the trunk may also be involved. Chronic and repetitive mechanical trauma to the skin from rubbing and scratching eventually leads to lichenification, hyperkeratosis, and pigmentary alterations, including hyperpigmentation and hypopigmentation of the individual lesions. Treatment involves reducing symptoms of itch with topical and systemic medications.

Perforating disorders of renal disease (reactive perforating collagenosis, perforating folliculitis, Kyrle disease) are thought to be separate disorders by some and a spectrum of the same disease process by others [11, 12]. The diagnostic criteria not well defined for the perforating disorders and these entities share clinical similarities. Perforating disorders classically present with umbilicated papules with a central hyperkeratotic crust with peripheral hyperpigmentation. Most lesions are found on the extremities. These disorders are characterized by transepidermal elimination of altered keratin or dermal connective tissue material. Phototherapy with NB-UVB radiation has been reported to be an effective treatment [13].

Calciphylaxis (calcific uremic arteriolopathy) is a vasculopathic process characterized by vascular calcification, thrombosis and cutaneous necrosis. It is seen almost exclusively in patients with end-stage renal disease. The pathogenesis of calciphylaxis is unknown, however; it is likely due to a complex interaction of comorbid factors including hypercalcemia, hyperphosphatemia, an elevated calcium-phosphate product, secondary hyperparathyroidism, in conjunction with a hypercoagulable state [14]. Patients can present with the sudden development of painful black necrotic plaques that progress rapidly. Lesions are excruciatingly tender, extremely firm, and are usually located on the lower extremities although can also be on the trunk and upper extremities. This disorder is associated with a high mortality. Treatment is directed at normalizing the metabolic milieu, as well as identifying and treating hypercoagulable disorders when present. Aggressive wound care management is required for the painful ulcerations. Patients with significantly elevated parathyroid hormone (PTH) may sometimes benefit from parathyroidectomy [14].

Pseudoporphyria is clinically characterized by increased skin fragility, erythema, bullae and erosions on sun exposed skin, mimicking porphyria cutanea tarda (PCT). However, the classic features of hypertrichosis, hyperpigmentation, and sclerodermoid features found in PCT are typically absent in pseudoporphyria. Although urine and serum porphyrins are typically normal in pseudoporphyria, they may be elevated in the patient with CKD due to altered metabolism and reduced clearance [15]. Photoprotection and elimination of any exacerbating factors (usually a medication) are the basis of treatment (Fig. 8.3).

Atheroembolic renal disease (AERD) occurs when small cholesterol plaques are dislodged form vessel walls and are embolized to the small blood vessels of the kidneys. Characteristic skin findings include petechiae, violaceous purpura, and a livedo reticularis vascular pattern with associated ecchymotic dyspigmentation in the form of cyanosis and gangrene in severe cases. Treatment of underlying cardiovascular disease is necessary and avoidance of invasive vascular procedures would be prudent to decrease the risk of embolization of unstable cholesterol plaques.

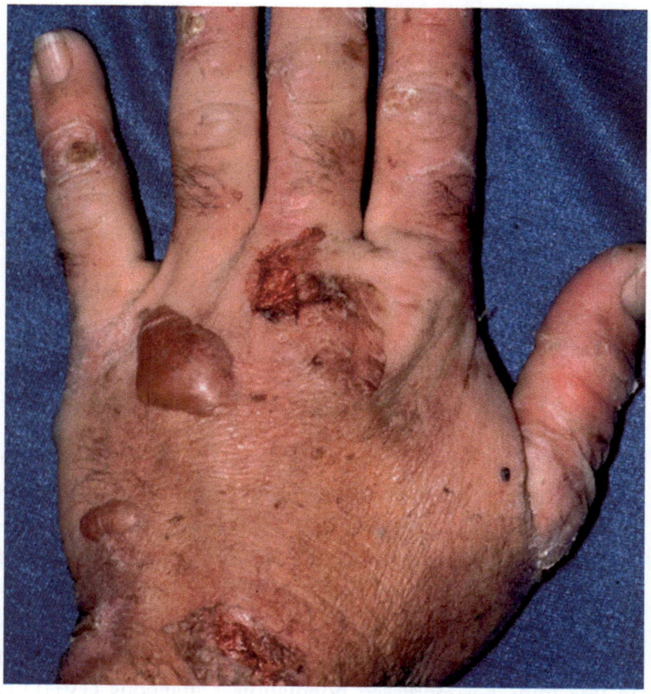

Fig. 8.3 Skin fragility and cutaneous blisters in pseudoporphyria. Image reprinted with permission from Medscape Reference (http://emedicine.medscape.com/), 2013, available at: http://emedicine.medscape.com/article/1049648-overview

Complications with Associated Dyschromia due to Treatment of Renal Carcinoma

Drug-induced pigmentary alterations are sometimes noted in patients with underlying renal disease in the setting of chemotherapeutic treatment for renal carcinoma. The phenomenon of palmar–plantar erythrodysesthesia or "hand–foot syndrome" presents with acral erythema involving the palms and soles with symmetric, well-demarcated erythematous plaques [16]. Often painful, these lesions can be associated with numbness and tingling. Symptoms typically resolve after the discontinuation of the inciting chemotherapeutic agent. Treatment is geared towards symptom control particularly if patient cannot be discontinued from the offending medication. Recent reports have described skin discoloration with the use of the multikinase inhibitors sunitinib and sorafinib which are used in the treatment of renal cancer. Hypopigmentation of the hair or skin has been associated with sunitinib and other blockers of the tyrosine kinase c-Kit [16]. The dyspigmentation is thought to be due to a drug-induced alteration of melanocyte function within the hair follicles. Sunitinib is also known to cause an intense yellow discoloration of the skin due to the deposition of a sunitinib metabolite; there is no available treatment for this adverse effect [16] (Table 8.3).

Graft-versus-host disease (GVHD) is infrequently encountered in patients following solid organ transplantation, especially renal transplantation. However, clinicians need to

Table 8.3 Drugs that can cause palmar–plantar erythrodysesthesia

Capecitabine
Cytarabine
Doxorubicin
Floxuridine
Fluorouracil
Idarubicin
Liposomal doxorubicin
Pazopanib
Sunitinib
Sorafenib
Vemurafenib

maintain a high index of suspicion given the potentially devastating consequences of missing this diagnosis. Cutaneous involvement usually precedes involvement of the gastrointestinal system and recognition of these skin findings is important for early diagnosis. Early acute GVHD may be subtle; the differential diagnosis for cutaneous GVHD includes viral exanthema or drug eruptions, which unfortunately are also common in this immunosuppressed population. Cutaneous GVHD is subdivided into acute and chronic forms, now more by clinical findings, previously by a random 100 day cutoff. Acute GVHD usually presents with prominent cutaneous and gastrointestinal symptoms and consists of four consecutive stages of severity based upon BSA involvement and extent of cutaneous erythroderma. In the initial states of acute GVHD patients present with erythematous macules and patches on the head, face, ears and hands which can evolve into a generalized morbiliform eruption. Palms and soles are frequently affected. Later stages present as generalized erythroderma (Stage 3) and erythroderma with bulla formation mimicking toxic epidermal necrolysis in (Stage 4). Poikilodermatous dyspigmentation, lichenoid dermatitis, scleroderma-like change, and alopecia are more characteristic findings in patients with chronic GVHD. Treatment focuses on preventing graft rejection and optimizing the patient's immunosuppressive regimen. Skin directed therapy is based on the extent of cutaneous involvement; topical steroids, topical calcineurin inhibitors, antihistamines, ultraviolet B phototherapy, and photopheresis may all be considered depending on disease severity.

Nail Discoloration in Kidney Disease [17]

Half and half nails (or Terry half and half nails), occur when the proximal portion of the nail is white secondary to edema and anemia. The distal portion appears dark. These nail changes imply the presence of either renal or liver disease. In the setting of renal disease there is a brown band at the junction of the erythema and the free edge.

Muehrcke lines (or leukonychia striata), are white lines (leukonychia) that extend all the way across the nail, parallel to the lunula. The lines are in the vascular nail bed underneath the nail plate and do not move with nail growth. Muehrcke lines disappear when pressure is placed over the nail, blanching the underlying nail bed.

Splinter hemorrhages are caused by hemorrhage of the distal capillary loop and may be seen in the setting of renal disease.

References

1. Stedman TL. Stedman's medical dictionary for the health professions and nursing. Illustrated 5th ed. Baltimore, MD: Wolters Kluwer; 2005. p. 442.
2. Bolognia JB, Jorizzo JL, Schaffer JV, et al. Dermatology. 3rd ed. Philadelphia, PA: Elsevier Saunders; 2012.
3. Picó MR, Lugo-Somolinos A, Sánchez JL, Burgos-Calderón R. Cutaneous alterations in patients with chronic renal failure. Int J Dermatol. 1992;31(12):860–3.
4. Smith AG, Shuster S, Comaish JS, Plummer NA, Thody AJ, Alvarez-ude F. Plasma immunoreactive β-melanocyte stimulating hormone and skin pigmentation in chronic renal failure. Br Med J. 1975;1:658–9.
5. Cordova KB, Oberg TJ, Malik M, Robinson-Bostom L. Dermatologic conditions seen in end-stage renal disease. Semin Dial. 2009;22:45–55.
6. Shanmugam VK, Steen VD. Renal disease in scleroderma: an update on evaluation, risk stratification, pathogenesis and management. Curr Opin Rheumatol. 2012;24(6):669–76.
7. Morias P, Santos AL, Baudrier T, Mota AV, Oliveira JP, Azevedo F. Angiokeratomas of Fabry successfully treated with intense pulsed light. J Cosmet Laser Ther. 2008;10:218.
8. Kribben A, Witzke O, Hillen U, Barkhausen J, Daul AE, Erbel R. Nephrogenic systemic fibrosis: pathogenesis, diagnosis, and therapy. J Am Coll Cardiol. 2009;53:1621–8.
9. Almouhawis HA, Leao JC, Fedele S, Porter SR. Wegener's granulomatosis: a review of clinical features and an update in diagnosis and treatment. J Oral Pathol Med. 2013;42(7):507–16.
10. Keithi-Reddy SR, Patel TV, Armstrong AW, Singh AK. Uremic pruritus. Kidney Int. 2007;72(3):373–7.
11. Robinson-Bostom L, DiGiovanna JJ. Cutaneous manifestations of end stage renal disease. J Am Acad Dermatol. 2000;43:975–89.
12. Goldsmith DJA, Black MM. Skin disorders in the setting of renal failure: invited editorial. J Eur Acad Dermatol Venereol. 2001; 15:392–8.
13. Rivard J, Lim HW. Ultraviolet phototherapy for pruritus. Dermatol Ther. 2005;18(4):344–54.
14. Weenig RH, Sewell LD, Davis MD, et al. Calciphylaxis: natural history, risk factor analysis, and outcome. J Am Acad Dermatol. 2007;56:569–79.
15. Glynne P, Deacon A, Goldsmith D, Pusey C, Clutterbuck E. Bullous dermatoses in end-stage renal failure: Porphyria or pseudoporphyria? Am J Kidney Dis. 1999;34:155–60.
16. Gutzmer R, Wollenberg A, Ugurel S, Homey B, Ganser A, Kapp A. Cutaneous side effects of new antitumor drugs: clinical features and management. BioDrugs. 2009;23(6):377–89.
17. Mendiratta V, Jain A. Nail dyschromias. Indian J Dermatol Venereol Leprol. 2011;77(6):652–8. doi:10.4103/0378-6323.86473.

Calcinosis Cutis

9

Mitalee P. Christman and Daniela Kroshinsky

Introduction

Calcium is essential in many tissues, including the skin, where it regulates epidermal proliferation, differentiation, and adhesion. When local or systemic insults perturb the factors regulating calcium, they may result in insoluble calcium salt deposition in the skin and subcutaneous tissue, known as calcinosis cutis. The condition is classified into four subtypes based on the presumed mechanism of calcium deposition: dystrophic, metastatic, iatrogenic, and idiopathic. This chapter expands on metastatic calcification, the subtype of calcification most commonly seen in renal disease and includes only limited discussions of subtypes usually seen independent of renal disease or discussed elsewhere in this textbook.

Pathogenesis

Metastatic Calcification

Metastatic calcification is characterized by precipitation of calcium salts in normal skin and soft tissue owing to abnormalities in calcium and/or phosphate metabolism. Decreased phosphate clearance and impaired synthesis of 1,25-OH vitamin D both contribute to derangements in calcium and phosphate levels [1]. Renal failure impairs 1-alpha-hydroxylation of vitamin D, thereby limiting calcium absorption from the intestine. Low serum calcium levels stimulate compensatory secondary hyperparathyroidism, normalizing calcium levels and further increasing phosphate levels. When the solubility product of calcium and phosphate (55 mg^2/dl^2) is exceeded, cutaneous and subcutaneous calcification might result. In patients with chronic renal failure calcinosis cutis might manifest as calciphylaxis or benign nodular calcification.

Calciphylaxis is the most severe form of metastatic calcification, occurring in as many as 4.1 % of patients undergoing hemodialysis, according to one retrospective review of 242 hemodialysis patients [2]. The pathogenesis remains poorly understood but is likely multifactorial—time-averaged elevation of the calcium/phosphate product, a hypercoagulable state due to reduced protein C and S, hyperparathyroidism and skin trauma are all thought to be contributing factors. Multiple risk factors have been identified including female sex, obesity, diabetes, and the use of calcium-based phosphate binders.

Less common causes of metastatic calcification independent of renal disease include milk-alkali syndrome (excessive intake of calcium-containing foods) and hypervitaminosis D (prolonged intake of supratherapeutic doses of vitamin D).

Other Forms of Calcification

Dystrophic calcification is the most common type of calcinosis cutis. It is thought to be secondary to local insults in the absence of derangements in systemic calcium metabolism. The pathogenesis is unclear; however, one proposed mechanism implicates necrotic cell debris that is thought to serve as a nidus for ectopic calcification; further, alterations in collagen, elastin, and the subcutis are thought to promote calcification.

Iatrogenic calcification refers to deposition of calcium salts as a result of medical intervention, usually intravenous calcium chloride or calcium gluconate [3–5]. The etiology is thought to be both locally elevated tissue concentration of calcium, and tissue injury at the site of extravasated calcium.

Idiopathic calcification is the category reserved for cutaneous calcification seen in the absence of an underlying tissue damage or metabolic disorder. It comprises acne-induced, milia-like, tumoral, subepidermal calcified nodules, scrotal calcinosis.

M.P. Christman, A.B., M.D.
Department of Dermatology, Massachusetts General Hospital, 345 Franklin St., Apt. 404, Cambridge, MA 02139, USA
e-mail: mitaleepatil@gmail.com

D. Kroshinsky, M.D., M.P.H. (✉)
Massachusetts General Hospital, Harvard Medical School, 50 Staniford Street, Boston, MA 02114, USA
e-mail: dkroshinsky@partners.org

J.R. Nunley and E.V. Lerma (eds.), *Dermatological Manifestations of Kidney Disease*,
DOI 10.1007/978-1-4939-2395-3_9, © Springer Science+Business Media New York 2015

Clinical Presentation

Soft tissue calcification commonly complicates chronic renal failure: estimates regarding its prevalence range from approximately 40 %, to as high as 80 % in one autopsy study of hemodialysis patients [6]. Please see Chap. 10 for details on clinical presentation and treatment of calciphylaxis.

The most common type of cutaneous calcification seen in CKD is metastatic calcification. Benign nodular calcification, the most common subtype, is defined as cutaneous and subcutaneous tissue calcification in the absence of tissue necrosis. Lesions are typically painless, firm, papules, plaques or nodules that occur most commonly around joints and on the fingertips [7, 8]. Long-standing secondary hyperparathyroidism predisposes to this condition; the number and size of the calcium deposits are directly proportional to the degree of hyperphosphatemia. Similar findings are seen in tumoral calcinosis, an inherited or acquired abnormality of phosphate homeostasis independent of renal function [9]. Although it is often seen in otherwise healthy individuals, it might also be triggered by the uremic mileu.

Dystrophic calcification in CKD is more commonly observed in patients with connective tissue diseases, especially CREST syndrome (calcinosis cutis, Raynaud phenomenon, esophageal dysfunction, sclerodactyly, and telangiectasia) and lupus panniculitis. However, it can also be seen in patients with comorbidities including pancreatic panniculitis, various inherited disorders such as Ehlers-Danlos, cutaneous neoplasms (pilomatricomas, pilar cysts), and infections (onchocerciasis, cysticercosis). Calcified lesions are usually localized to the area affected by the underlying condition.

Iatrogenic calcification occurs as a complication of a procedure, such as extravasation during intravenous administration of solutions containing calcium or phosphate or prolonged contact with calcium chloride electrode paste during electroencephalography [9]. Lesions develop at the site of the inciting event.

Though uncommon, idiopathic calcinosis can also be seen in patients with CKD. Subepidermal calcified nodules present as isolated hard 3–11 mm white-to-yellow papules over the head and extremities, usually in children. These might represent calcified adnexal structures according to one study [10]. Scrotal calcinosis, characterized by marble-like subcutaneous nodules varying in size and number, are thought to arise from epidermal or eccrine cysts. They are usually asymptomatic although minimal pruritus or a white chalky discharge may be noted. Milia-like calcinosis consists of tiny white pearly papules ("milia-like" lesions) on the dorsal surface of the hands and face; they are most commonly seen in patients with Down syndrome. Although there are usually no preexisting lesions, some appear to due to calcification of pre-existing syringomas.

Milia-like calcinosis characterized by tiny white pearly papules ("milia-like" lesions) on the dorsal surface of the hands and face, most commonly seen in the setting of Down syndrome. There are usually no preexisting lesions, although in some patients they appear to arise from calcification of precursor syringomas.

Laboratory Abnormalities

In metastatic calcification, theoretically, precipitation occurs when levels of calcium and phosphate exceed their solubility product, although one study found clinically elevated calcium or phosphate levels in only a fraction of patients with metastatic calcification [11].

Serum calcium and phosphate levels are within normal limits in dystrophic calcification and in idiopathic calcification (except for tumoral calcinosis).

Treatment

Drugs

Aluminum Hydroxide

Dosage: 1.8–2.4 g daily.

Mechanism of action: Aluminum hydroxide taken orally complexes with phosphate to form an insoluble precipitate that limits intestinal absorption of phosphate. The resulting decrease in phosphate levels is thought to hinder or even reverse the development of ectopic calcifications [6].

Effectiveness: There are three case reports of patients with calcinosis cutis related to dermatomyositis and systemic lupus erythematosus (SLE) who responded favorably to oral aluminum hydroxide with size reduction and/or softening of lesions [1, 2, 6]. Therapy ranged between 4 and 9 months.

Adverse Drug Events (ADE): Adverse reactions to aluminum hydroxide might include gastrointestinal (constipation, nausea, cramping, vomiting, discoloration of feces) and metabolic disturbances (hypomagnesemia, hypophosphatemia). Caution must be exercised in patients with compromised renal function, as chronic use might lead to the accumulation of aluminum and resultant toxicity. Alternate therapy should be considered in patients with chronic kidney disease (CKD).

Monitoring: Calcium and phosphate serum levels, as well as aluminum levels, should be monitored when aluminum hydroxide is administered to a patient with CKD.

Bisphosphonates

Dosage: Alendronate 10 mg/day for 1 year [12]; disodium etidronate 10 mg/kg/day for 1 year [13].

Mechanism of action: Bisphosphonates are thought to stop and partially reverse calcification through their inhibitory actions on macrophages and calcium turnover.

Effectiveness: Two case reports show evidence of softening of calcification with bisphosphonates in calcinosis cutis related to dermatomyositis and systemic sclerosis [12, 13].

ADE: Bisphosphonates are usually well tolerated; however, high doses might be accompanied by flu-like symptoms, hypocalcemia, hypophosphatemia, impaired renal function, and nephrotic syndrome. Patients with renal disease at baseline should receive plenty of hydration, slow infusion (if given intravenously), and a lower dose of bisphosphonates to limit further nephrotoxicity.

Monitoring: We recommend monitoring calcium, phosphate, blood urea nitrogen, and creatinine levels.

Diltiazem

Dosage: 2-4 mg/kg daily for 1–2.5 years.

Mechanism of action: Diltiazem is a calcium channel blocker and blocks the entry of calcium into cells.

Effectiveness: Two case reports show resolution of calcification in patients with dermatomyositis [14, 15]. However, a case series describing calcinosis in patients with systemic sclerosis who were prescribed diltiazem for Raynaud phenomenon showed a largely mixed response; calcification resolved in some, worsened in some, yet remained unchanged in others [16]. Dosing variablity may have played a role.

ADE: The most common adverse reactions are cardiovascular (peripheral edema, first degree atrioventricular block) and of the central nervous system (headache and dizziness). Elevations of liver transaminases have also been noted.

Monitoring: We recommend monitoring liver function tests, heart rate, blood pressure, and electrocardiograms.

Extracorporeal Shock Wave Lithotripsy (ESWL)

Dosage: N/A.

Mechanism of action: Shock wave lithotripsy uses high-energy electrical shock waves which when transmitted to calcifications releases energy, causing fragmentation.

Effectiveness: Two patients with calcinosis cutis related to dermatomyositis and CREST (calcinosis cutis, Raynaud, esophageal dysmotililty, sclerodactyly, and telangiectasia) syndrome achieved pain control with shock wave lithotripsy [7, 17].

ADE: Data are limited. However, extrapolating from data on patients receiving ESWL for urinary calculi, collateral tissue damage may be a result of energy release from ESWL [9].

Monitoring: N/A.

Minocycline

Dosage: 50–100 mg/day.

Mechanism of action: Minocycline is a tetracycline antibiotic, which in addition to its antimicrobial effects, binds calcium and inhibits matrix metalloproteinases (MMP) which are involved in connective tissue remodeling, inflammation, and ulceration.

Effectiveness: Nine patients with calcinosis cutis secondary to limited systemic sclerosis received minocycline; eight patients responded favorably with a reduction in lesional size and decreased incidence in ulceration [9].

ADE: Adverse events can be dermatological (hyperpigmentation, anal/vaginal pruritus, tongue and dental discoloration) and systemic (dizzines, tinnitus, lupus-like illness).

Monitoring: We recommend monitoring liver function tests, blood urea nitrogen, and serum creatinine.

Warfarin

Dosage: 1 mg daily for 1 year.

Mechanism of action: The mechanism of action is unclear, as warfarin suppresses vitamin K-dependent carboxylation of matrix G1a protein which inhibits calcification in its carboxylated form.

Effectiveness: Warfarin has shown to be effective for patients with small lesions—two of three patients with calcinosis related to systemic sclerosis responded well to warfarin therapy [3]—but ineffective in larger lesions; no improvement was noted in six patients with long-standing diffuse calcifications secondary to dermatomyositis and systemic sclerosis [4].

ADE: The main adverse reaction due to warfarin is hemorrhage.

Monitoring: We recommend periodically monitoring prothrombin time, international normalized ratio, and hematocrit.

Surgical

Surgical Excision or Curettage

Effectiveness: This is the preferred treatment for idiopathic calcification [5], especially scrotal calcinosis. Subtotal excision of the scrotal wall provides excellent cosmetic results; however, there is conflicting data on the risk of relapse [10]. Surgical excision might also be considered in patients with symptomatic disease refractory to medical treatment, or in cases where the lesions compromise the function of surrounding structures. Single case reports exist of successful surgical excision of calcified deposits in patients with juvenile dermatomyositis [18], systemic lupus erythematosus [19], and CREST syndrome [20].

Adverse effects: Some argue that surgical trauma might induce further calcification. For this reason it might be best to excise a small site prior to attempting a larger excision.

Carbon Dioxide Laser

Effectiveness: The carbon dioxide laser is primarily a cutting instrument owing to its properties of minimal scattering, excellent absorption in water, rapid soft tissue vaporization, and minimal damage of surrounding tissue. Small calcifications on the digits have been successfully treated with carbon dioxide laser. A study using carbon dioxide laser vaporization for 21 sites of digital calcinosis in six patients with limited systemic sclerosis showed complete resolution in 12 sites, partial resolution in 5 sites, a minimal response in 2 sites, and recurrence in 2 sites [21].

Adverse effects: Postoperative hyperpigmentation might be observed in some patients.

Prognosis

Due to the lack of randomized controlled trials to treat this heterogenous condition, no standard therapy has been established for cutaneous calcification. Most therapies are guided by expert opinion, single case reports, or small case series (Reiter [22]). In this environment, treatment of calcinosis cutis must be individualized to each patient at hand.

References

1. Nassim JR, Connolly CK. Treatment of calcinosis universalis with aluminum hydroxide. Arch Dis Child. 1970;45:118–21.
2. Park YM, Lee SJ, Kang H, Cho SH. Large subcutaneous calcification in systemic lupus erythematosus: treatment with oral aluminum hydroxide administration followed by surgical excision. J Korean Med Sci. 1999;14:589–92.
3. Cukierman T, Elinav E, Korem M, Chajek-Shaul T. Low dose warfarin treatment for calcinosis in patients with systemic sclerosis. Ann Rheum Dis. 2004;63:1341–3.
4. Lassoued K, Saiag P, Anglade MC, Roujeau JC, Touraine RL. Failure of warfarin in treatment of calcinosis universalis. Am J Med. 1988;84:795–6.
5. Valdatta L, Buoro M, Thione A, et al. Idiopathic circumscripta calcinosis cutis of the knee. Dermatol Surg. 2003;29:1222–4.
6. Wang WJ, Lo WL, Wong CK. Calcinosis cutis in juvenile dermatomyositis: remarkable response to aluminum hydroxide therapy. Arch Dermatol. 1988;124:1721–2.
7. Sparsa A, Lesaux N, Kessler E, Bonnetblanc JM, Blaise S, Lebrun-Ly V, et al. Treatment of cutaneous calcinosis in CREST syndrome by extracorporeal shock wave lithotripsy. J Am Acad Dermatol. 2005;53:263–5.
8. Smith LH, Drach G, Hall P, Lingeman J, Preminger G, Resnick MI, Segura JW. National High Blood Pressure Education Program (NHBPEP) review paper on complications of shock wave lithotripsy for urinary calculi. Am J Med. 1991;91(6):635.
9. Robertson LP, Marshall RW, Hickling P. Treatment of cutaneous calcinosis in limited systemic sclerosis with minocycline. Ann Rheum Dis. 2003;62:267–9.
10. Ruiz-Genao DP, Rios-Buceta L, Herrero L, Fraga J, Aragues M, Garcia-Diez A. Massive scrotal calcinosis. Dermatol Surg. 2002;28:745–7.
11. Block GA. Prevalence and clinical consequences of elevated Ca x P product in hemodialysis patients. Clin Nephrol. 2000;54: 318–24.
12. Mukamel M, Horev G, Mimouni M. New insight into calcinosis of juvenile dermatomyositis: a study of composition and treatment. J Pediatr. 2001;138:763–6.
13. Rabens SF, Bethune JE. Disodium etidronate therapy for dystrophic cutaneous calcification. Arch Dermatol. 1975;111:357–61.
14. Abdallah-Lotf M, Grasland A, Vinceneux P, Sigal-Grinberg M. Regression of cutis calcinosis with diltiazem in adult dermatomyositis. Eur J Dermatol. 2005;15:102–4.
15. Ichiki Y, Akiyama T, Shimozawa N, Suzuki Y, Kondo N, Kitajima Y. An extremely severe case of cutaneous calcinosis with juvenile dermatomyositis, and successful treatment with diltiazem. Br J Dermatol. 2001;144:894–7.
16. Vayssairat M, Hidouche D, Abdoucheli-Baudot N, Gaitz JP. Clinical significance of subcutaneous calcinosis in patients with systemic sclerosis. Does diltiazem induce its regression? Ann Rheum Dis. 1998;57:252–4.
17. Chan AYK, Li E. Electric shock wave lithotripsy (ESWL) as a pain control measure in dermatomyositis with calcinosis cutis—old method, new discovery. Clin Rheumatol. 2005;24:172–3.
18. Wu JJ, Metz BJ. Calcinosis cutis of juvenile dermatomyositis treated with incision and drainage. Dermatol Surg. 2008;34:575–7.
19. Cousins MA, Jones DB, Whyte MP, Monafo WW. Surgical management of calcinosis cutis universalis in systemic lupus erythematosus. Arthritis Rheum. 1997;40:570–2.
20. Saddic N, Mille JJ, Miller F, Clarke JT. Surgical debridement of painful fingertip calcinosis cutis in CREST syndrome. Arch Dermatol. 2009;145:212–3.
21. Bottomley WW, Goodfield MJD, Sheehan-Dare RA. Digital calcification in systemic sclerosis: effective treatment with good tissue preservation using the carbon dioxide laser. Br J Dermatol. 1996;135:302–4.
22. Reiter N, El-Shabrawi L, Leinweber B, Berghold A, Aberer E. Calcinosis cutis: part II. Treatment options. J Am Acad Dermatol. 2011;65:15–22. quiz 23–4.

Calciphylaxis

10

Julio C. Sartori-Valinotti and Mark Davis

Introduction

Calciphylaxis is currently considered to represent a vasculopathy characterized by calcification, intimal fibrosis and thrombosis of small-sized arterial vessels of the skin and panniculus, leading to painful, necrotic ulcerations, plaques, and subcutaneous nodules. Despite joint efforts from nephrologists, endocrinologists, dermatologists, and basic science research, the specific underlying mechanisms are yet to be fully deciphered, adequate treatment is elusive, and morbidity and mortality remain extremely high.

Hans Selye first introduced the term calciphylaxis in 1962. He described it as "a condition of induced systemic hypersensitivity" whereby connective tissue and stromal elements respond to "challenging agents" with progressive calcification. In his initial experiments in rodents, Selye distinguished the so-called topical calciphylaxis (tissue response to a locally applied challenger) from systemic calciphylaxis, which results from a tissue-specific adaptive response to a systemically circulating factor [1, 2].

Epidemiology

Calciphylaxis was once thought to be a rare condition most frequently encountered in end-stage renal disease (ESRD) patients. Patients with histologically proven calciphylaxis with no evidence of renal impairment are being increasingly recognized. A population-based study from the Rochester Epidemiology Project in Olmsted, MN showed an age-adjusted overall incidence of 4.1 and 5.0 per million for females and males, respectively [3]. Calciphylaxis has an estimated incidence of about 1 % per year in patients with renal failure [4, 5]. A retrospective review of 242 hemodialysis patients indicated a prevalence of 4.1. Interestingly, the same investigators found that calciphylaxis patients were younger and had received hemodialysis longer (on average for 60 additional months) [4]. Due to its occurrence primarily in patients with ESRD, calciphylaxis is also referred to as uremic gangrene syndrome [6], calcific uremic arteriolopathy [7], and calcifying panniculitis which greatly confuses the literature on this condition. Currently the unifying term used for this entity is most commonly calciphylaxis.

Pathogenesis

The pathogenesis of calciphylaxis is complex and multiple pathways in consort with inflammatory cells and cytokines, impaired ability to clear calcium and phosphate as well as defective local inhibitors of calcification are responsible for insidious and progressive calcifying arteriolopathy. Although almost all literature to date focuses on the calcifying arteriolopathy, researchers at Mayo Clinic [8, 9] have emphasized the importance of a critical "tipping point": thrombosis of these calcified vessels, leading to distal ischemia and painful infarctive skin ulcers. It is the ulcerations that leads to the observed mortality and morbidity. Weenig et al. have described this as analogous to a "myocardial infarct of the skin" [10].

The Role of Chronic Inflammation

Systemic inflammation has been blamed for the development of calcification within blood vessels [11]. Elevated levels of c-reactive protein (CRP) are seen in patients with chronic kidney disease (CKD) and rise upon development of skin lesions of calciphylaxis [12]. Increased subclinical coronary artery calcification is associated with higher CRP levels [13]. In non-uremic patients with calciphylaxis, connective tissue diseases are one of the most common reported etiologies [14]. In patients afflicted by rheumatoid arthritis and systemic lupus

J.C. Sartori-Valinotti, M.D. • M. Davis, M.D. (✉)
Department of Dermatology, Mayo Clinic College of Medicine, 200 First Street SW, Rochester, MN 55905, USA
e-mail: SartoriValinotti.Julio@mayo.edu; Davis.mark2@mayo.edu

J.R. Nunley and E.V. Lerma (eds.), *Dermatological Manifestations of Kidney Disease*,
DOI 10.1007/978-1-4939-2395-3_10, © Springer Science+Business Media New York 2015

erythematosus, vascular calcification is more prevalent and may contribute to the overall mortality [15, 16].

Tumor necrosis factor alpha (TNF-α) is implicated in stimulation of osteoclast progenitors and resorption of mineralized matrix [17]. It may also enhance the hypercalcemic effects of parathyroid hormone-related protein (PTHrP) [18]. In addition, TNF-α stimulates osteogenesis in human mesenchymal cells via Wnt5a signaling [19] and upregulates expression of osteoprotegerin (OPG) and tissue-non-specific alkaline phosphatase (TNAP) in vascular smooth muscle cells (VSMC) [20, 21]. Other cytokines may also contribute to vascular calcification. In hemodialysis patients, interleukin (IL)-6 levels are higher [22] and correlate with coronary artery calcification scores [23, 24]. Activated macrophages secrete TNF-α, IL-8, and IL-1B [25]. IL-1B in turn increases TNAP activity and mineralization [26].

The Role of Nuclear Transcription Factors

The nuclear factor kappa-light-chain-enhancer of activated B cells (NF-κB) and the runt-related transcription factor 2 (RUNX2) also known as core-binding factor subunit alpha-1 (CBF-alpha-1) are important players in bone homeostasis.

The membrane-bound receptor activator of NF-κB (RANK) and its ligand (RANKL) form the RANK-RANKL complex. RANKL is the key signal for normal osteoclast development and survival. Its actions are antagonized by the soluble decoy receptor OPG [27], which decreases signaling transduction through RANK [28]. OPG is of pivotal importance in inhibiting bone resorption and is implicated in vascular calcification [29]. In ESRD as well as in other persistent inflammatory states, NF-κB signaling is increased [30]. Hyperphosphatemia in chronic renal patients may promote oxidative stress and NF-κB activation, leading to vascular calcification [31].

OPG levels are increased in subjects with diabetic nephropathy, patients with abdominal aortic aneurysms, and postmenopausal women and may serve as a predictor of vascular events [32–35]. Studies suggest that not only its absolute value but also the ratio of OPG to fetuin-A, a major anti-mineralization protein, is associated with intima–media thickening in patients undergoing hemodialysis [36, 37]. In the presence of prior history of cardiovascular events, high levels of OPG in hemodialysis individuals, is thought to be an independent risk marker of mortality [38]. Notoriously, the association between OPG and vascular calcification persists following renal transplant [39]. Senescence is accompanied by rising levels of OPG, which may contribute to the progression of coronary artery calcification in normotensive, otherwise healthy individuals [40].

Runx2 is crucial in bone metabolism; it is required for osteoblast development and differentiation. Expression of Runx2 is upregulated in arteries of patients with ESRD and calciphylaxis [41]. In vitro, induction of an osteochondrogenic phenotype in smooth muscle cells by high phosphate levels is concomitant with induction of Runx2 [42], suggesting another potential mechanism for development of calciphylaxis in renal patients in whom, almost invariably, phosphate levels are elevated. Conversely, in normophosphatemic murine model of early CKD, Runx2 expression was increased in the aorta media [43]. Similarly, administration of doxercalciferol to uremic rodents results in increased Runx2 messenger RNA (mRNA) and protein expression in the aorta [44]. Taking together, these data underscore the importance of altered calcium–phosphate metabolism at a transcriptional level. More importantly, transition to an osteoblastic phenotype in the vasculature may precede the onset of overt electrolyte derangements. The latter observation provides insight into why new skin lesions arise and old lesions progress despite aggressive control of phosphate–calcium homeostasis.

Altered Calcium–Phosphate Metabolism

It is widely accepted that CKD is the most common cause of metastatic calcification leading to soft tissue calcification (STC). In his hallmark paper, Parfitt described five clinical types of STC in uremic patients: arterial; ocular; periarticular; cutaneous and subcutaneous; and visceral [45]. These forms of STC have been extensively studied, have historically been linked to disturbances in calcium–phosphate homeostasis, and are, indeed, most common than calciphylaxis in ESRD patients. Parfitt himself acknowledged that the mechanisms responsible for these two phenomena may be different and that systemic and local factors operating in concert are likely involved. In agreement with this, ulterior studies have challenged the belief that serum calcium–phosphate product (CPP) is invariably elevated in patients with calciphylaxis.

- *Serum calcium-phosphate product* (*CPP*): Data regarding serum CPP (albumin-corrected calcium x phosphorus levels) in calciphylaxis is controversial with some studies showing that a high product, usually above 70 mg^2/dL^2 [4, 46, 47], is a risk factor for the development of this disease. On the other hand, the majority of hemodialysis patients with equal or higher serum CPP do not suffer from calciphylaxis. A case–control study involving 249 Japanese ESRD patients demonstrated no association with CCP and calciphylaxis at the time of diagnosis [48]. In keeping with this evidence, another case–control study of nine patients with proximal lower extremities and trunk calciphylaxis found that CPP was not significantly different from control hemodialysis subjects [49]. Likewise, in a study of eight female calciphylactic patients undergoing peritoneal dialysis CPP levels were not different relative to controls [50]. Based on these conflicting reports, serum CPP levels may contribute differently to the development of calciphylaxis depending on the race, gender, and/or anatomic location (proximal vs. distal).

- *Parathyroid hormone* (*PTH*): The term renal osteodystrophy encompasses the group of bone mineral abnormalities in patients with CKD/ESRD. Classically, calciphylaxis has been reported in prolonged secondary hyperparathyroidism (high bone turnover state) owing to ESRD. Nonetheless, calciphylaxis is also encountered in patients with adynamic bone disease (low bone turnover state) with suppressed PTH levels and low CPP [51]. PTH levels vary among patients with calciphylaxis, and are not consistently elevated compared to controls [47, 52].
- *Vitamin D*: In ESRD, alterations in vitamin D metabolism stems from impaired renal 1-alpha hydroxylation, leading to decreased 1,25-dihydroxycholecalciferol, the active vitamin D metabolite. Under physiologic conditions, vitamin D promotes intestinal absorption of calcium. Therefore, if active vitamin D is absent or low, hypocalcemia ensues which stimulates PTH secretion (secondary hyperparathyroidism), leading to mobilization of both calcium and phosphate from bone. Consequently, hypovitaminosis D, via changes in calcium–phosphate metabolism, can be linked to the pathogenesis of calciphylaxis. This is not restricted to patients with ESRD since calciphylaxis has been reported in patients with low vitamin D state and normal renal function [53–55]. On the other hand, high-dose vitamin D administration is capable of inducing STC and calciphylaxis in murine models [56, 57]. In an attempt to reestablish normal calcium–phosphate homeostasis, ESRD patients receive vitamin D analogs that could theoretically increase their risk for calciphylaxis if hyperphosphatemia and hypercalcemia ensued. However, newer agents can minimize that risk [58, 59]

Table 10.1 summarizes different disorders of calcium and phosphate metabolism as well as the associated changes in PTH secretion patterns that can be identified in patients with calciphylaxis.

The Role of Anti-mineralization Proteins

Fetuin-A (α2-Heremans-Schmid glycoprotein) is a member of the superfamily of cysteine protease inhibitors. Unlike local inhibitors of calcification, fetuin-A is a ubiquitous serum protein that inhibits calcification at a systemic level by sequestrating circulating calcium and phosphate into colloidal spheres [60]. Mice lacking fetuin-A, although phenotypically normal, developed diffuse STC when fed a vitamin D-rich diet (12897203). In CKD patients, chronic inflammation may promote the development of calciphylaxis via reduction of fetuin-A levels [12]. Clearance of serum fetuin–mineral complex resulting in low serum fetuin-A levels may underlie vitamin D-induced vascular calcification [61]. In an cross-sectional study of 312 stable hemodialysis patients, low levels of fetuin-A were associated with increased cardiovascular mortality [62]. Low fetuin-A levels may also mediate STC in the absence of renal impairment [63].

Another strong inhibitor of vascular calcification is the vitamin K-dependent matrix Gla protein (MGP). This protein is synthesized by chondrocytes, VSMCs, endothelial cells, and fibroblasts [64]. Gamma-carboxylation is necessary for its activation [65]. The mechanisms whereby MGP inhibits vascular mineralization are multifarious including inhibition of calcium–phosphate precipitation and neutralization of bone morphogenic protein (BMP)-2-mediated calcification [66]. BMP-2 is implicated in transition of VSMCs to osteoclast-like cells, a crucial step in the development of vascular calcification. Recently, it has been shown that hyperphosphatemia-induced vascular calcification may be abolished by the calcimimetic calindol via upregulation of MGP synthesis [67].

Thrombosis

An under-recognized aspect of the observed entity of calciphylaxis is thrombosis of the calcified vessels—Mayo Clinic researchers feel this is fundamental to the observed mortality and morbidity. After all, calcification of blood vessel walls alone occurs in many disease processes such as diabetes, but often does not lead to morbidity. In calciphylaxis, it is thrombosis of the blood vessels that is the "tipping point"—leading to skin ulceration, which becomes infected, patients become septic and die. Weenig et al. reported in the Mayo Clinic series that 80 % of skin biopsies in calciphylaxis demonstrate thrombosis. He theorized that the only reason the figure was not 100 % was sampling on skin biopsy.

Why thrombosis? The answer is unknown, but several factors can be considered. First, the calcification of the blood vessels can act as a nidus for thrombosis (analogous to atherosclerosis in the coronary arteries). Second, patients with renal failure and other underlying conditions may be in a pro-thrombotic state-indeed preliminary studies, though few, have demonstrated low protein C and S, or antiphospholipid syndrome.

Clinical Features

Calciphylaxis presents with a spectrum of skin lesions ranging from livedo reticularis- or racemosa-like pattern to deep ulcerations. Very early changes may be clinically imperceptible or manifest as patchy areas with a net-like

Table 10.1 Disorders affecting serum calcium and phosphate levels and parathyroid hormone secretion in patients with calciphylaxis

Disorders affecting serum calcium and phosphate levels and parathyroid hormone secretion				
Disorder or medication	Effect of disorder or medication	Serum calcium	Serum phosphate	PTH production
Hyperparathyroidism				
Primary	PTH-secreting tumors (adenoma, multiple endocrine neoplasia syndrome)	↑	↓	↑
Secondary	Excessive PTH secretion caused by hypocalcemia	↑	↑	↑
Tertiary	Secondary hyperparathyroidism and PTH-secreting tumor	↑	↑	↑
Hypoparathyroidism	After parathyroidectomy, residual glands are suppressed from prior hyperparathyroidism	↓	↑	↓
	Gland destruction caused by heavy metal (copper, iron) toxicity, granuloma, autoimmune disorder	↓	↑	↓
	Magnesium deficiency (PTH secretion depends on normal magnesium levels)	↓	↑	↓
Renal failure	Decreased renal phosphate excretion results in hypocalcemia and secondary hyperparathyroidism	↓	↑	↑
Tumors	PTH is produced by parathyroid adenoma, other tumors	↑	↓	↑
	PTHrP is produced by breast cancer, squamous cell carcinoma, lymphoma, myeloma	↑	↓	nl or ↓
	Caused by tumor secretion of cytokines and PTHrP	↑	↓	nl or ↓
	Vitamin D is produced by lymphomas	↑	↑	nl or ↓
Hypovitaminosis D	Decreased calcium and phosphate absorption from the GI tract and decreased resorption from bone and kidney results in hyperparathyroidism	↓	↓	↑
Aluminum toxicity	Decreased bone responsiveness to vitamin D and PTH	↑	↑	↓
Granulomatous disease	Synthesis of vitamin D2 by granuloma (sarcoidosis, tuberculosis, lymphoma-related granuloma)	↑	↑	↓

Adapted from the JAAD, 58(3), Weenig RH, Pathogenesis of calciphylaxis: Hans Selye to nuclear factor kappa-B, 458–71, Copyright 2008, with permission from Elsevier
GI gastrointestinal, *PTH* parathyroid hormone, *PTHrP* parathyroid hormone-related protein

vascular pattern (livedo reticularis exquisitely tender, indurated) or a broken and branching morphology (livedo racemosa). At this stage, the histopathological correlate is the presence of cutaneous arteriolar stenosis due to intimal fibrosis and media calcification, leading to narrowing of the vessel lumen and reduced blood. When true vascular thrombosis with complete luminal obliteration ensues, purpuric-like lesions and deep and excruciatingly painful ulcerations and subcutaneous nodules appear. They usually retain their retiform configuration, a clue towards the correct diagnosis for the trained eye. Moreover, the same net-like blood vessel calcification configuration can be appreciated in soft-tissue radiographs and may serve as an additional diagnostic tool with a specificity approaching 90 % [68]. Not infrequently, however, they may adopt bizarre shapes with overlying necrotic eschars and dry gangrene.

In terms of distribution, lesions favor areas of high adiposity such as the abdomen, thighs, and buttocks [8, 69, 70] (Fig. 10.1). The head and neck are usually spared. Proximal necrotic lesions (trunk, buttocks, and thighs) are associated with higher mortality as compared to distal (below the knee) and acral disease [71].

Prognosis

The prognosis of calciphylaxis is ominous with mortality rates approaching 46 % at 1 year and 80 % at 2 years from diagnosis [47]. The presence of ulceration portends a bad prognosis with a twofold increase in mortality [72]. Another study documented that 1-year survival rate is about 45 versus 35 % at 5 years [73]. For patients undergoing surgical debridement the 1-year survival rate is nearly 62 % [47].

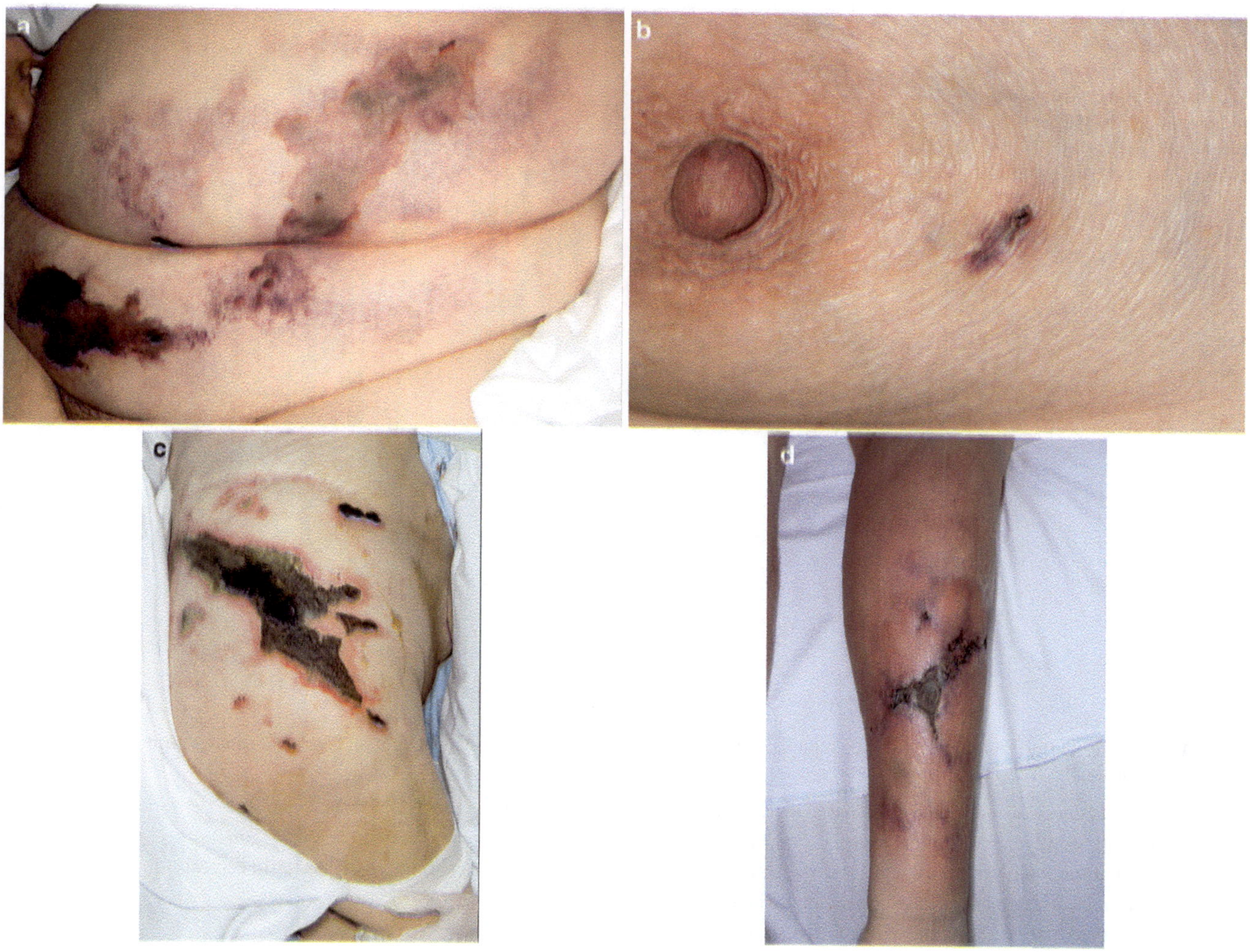

Fig. 10.1 (**a**) Characteristic retiform purpura on the abdomen. (**b**) Small purpuric lesion on the left lateral breast. Note incipient ulceration on the superior aspect. (**c**) Extensive involvement of the left flank and upper thigh with deep ulceration and eschar formation with smaller satellite lesions. (**d**) Involvement of the leg. Note edema and erythema extending beyond the central stellate ulcer

Postmortem Findings

Few studies have been published. Intriguingly however, a study of three patients with calciphylaxis who had postmortem evaluation at Mayo Clinic demonstrated that calciphylaxis only involved the skin: there was no evidence of a similar process internally. The reason for these findings is unclear [74].

Histopathology

Multiple entities can mimic calciphylaxis. Therefore, for definitive diagnosis a deep skin biopsy, including sampling of the subcutaneous tissue, is needed. Histopathologic findings vary depending on the age of the lesion. Early lesions may show only subtle changes. Late lesions are characterized by dermal necrosis and intramural calcium deposition of dermal and pannicular vessels [75] as well as vascular thrombosis and endovascular fibroblastic proliferation [47, 75] (Fig. 10.2). The most common finding overall is the presence of calcifying septal panniculitis [75]. More recently, it has been suggested that when typical features of vascular and extravascular calcification are not evident, the presence of perieccrine calcification may point towards the correct diagnosis [76]. Fragmented and calcified elastic fibers as seen in pseudoxanthoma elasticum may also be a histopathologic finding [77]. A von Kossa stain highlights calcium deposits in the vascular walls and in collagenous septa of subcutaneous tissue [78].

Differential Diagnosis

Fully developed lesions of calciphylaxis have a distinct clinical appearance referred to as retiform purpura. A number of cutaneous disorders share a similar morphology and should be considered in the differential diagnosis (Table 10.2). A thorough history, careful examination of the skin lesions,

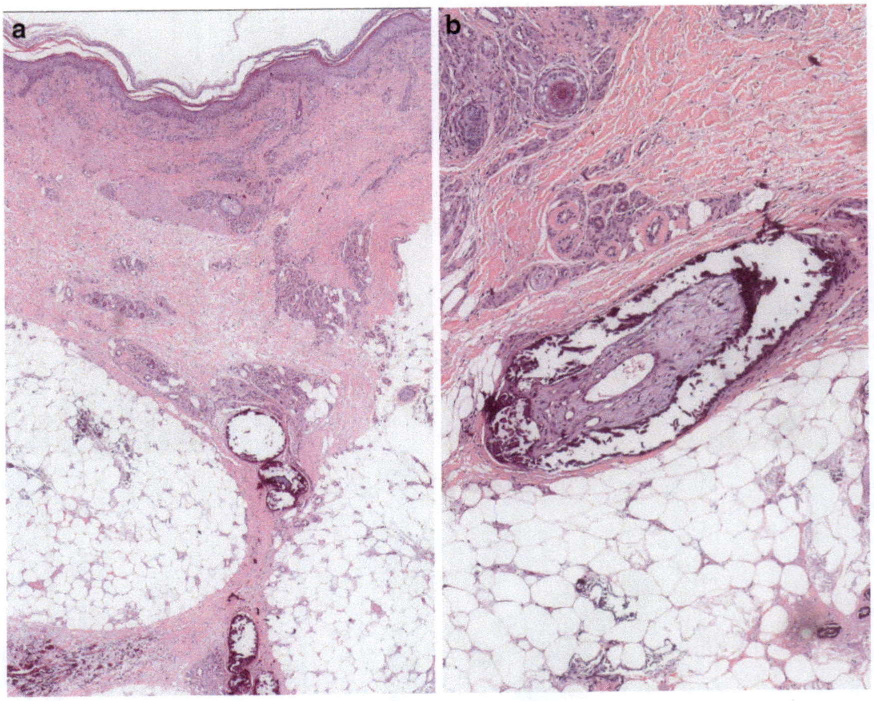

Fig. 10.2 (**a**) Lobular pannicular necrosis with calcified and thrombosed pannicular vessels and mixed lobular pannicular inflammation. (**b**) Higher magnification showing pannicular vessel calcification and thrombosis

Table 10.2 Differential diagnosis of calciphylaxis based on clinical morphology. Most common conditions that present with "retiform purpura"

Differential diagnosis of calciphylaxis based on clinical morphology. Most common conditions that present with "retiform purpura"
– Vasculitis (Wegener granulomatosis, polyarteritis nodosa, Churg–Strauss syndrome, microscopic polyangiitis)
– Antiphospholipid syndrome, lupus anticoagulant, protein C and S dysfunction, heparin necrosis, warfarin necrosis
– Cold-related vascular occlusion (cryoglobulinemia, cryofibrinogenemia)
– Cutaneous anthrax, ecthyma gangrenosum, disseminated strongyloidiasis, mucormycosis
– Panniculitis
– Purpura fulminans
– Pyoderma gangrenosum
– Livedoid vasculopathy
– Thromboangiitis obliterans

risk factor analysis, and histopathologic evaluation will render the correct diagnosis. In the right clinical setting, visual recognition alone will be highly suggestive but incisional biopsy (to include subcutaneous fat) is necessary for confirmatory purposes.

Associated Conditions and Risk Factors

ESRD is the most important and widely recognized condition associated with calciphylaxis [47, 79]. Within this patient population several risk factors have been linked to an increased risk for development of calciphylaxis including: white race [49], liver disease, systemic steroid use, CPP greater than 70 mg^2/dL^2, serum aluminum more than 25 ng/mL, obesity [47], female gender, peritoneal dialysis, diabetes mellitus, concurrent therapy with calcium salts and vitamin D [50, 80], increased serum phosphate levels, elevated alkaline phosphatase [73], warfarin therapy, poor nutritional status [48], and increased sedimentation rate [81].

Non-uremic calciphylaxis cases have also been reported in patients with normal renal and parathyroid function and in association with connective tissue disorders (systemic lupus erythematosus, rheumatoid arthritis, giant cell arteritis), hematologic malignancies (multiple myeloma, chronic myelocytic leukemia), diabetes (without concomitant renal failure), primary hyperparathyroidism, vitamin D deficiency, protein C and S deficiency, warfarin therapy, factor V Leiden deficiency, Crohn disease, primary autoimmune myelofibrosis, and liver disease [14, 46, 49, 53, 82–88]. It is expected that this list will continue to expand with increased recognition of this condition.

Table 10.3 Suggested evaluation for patients with suspected calciphylaxis

Suggested evaluation for patients with suspected cutaneous calciphylaxis
– Detailed history including past and current medications (warfarin, calcium and vitamin D supplements, phosphate binders, systemic steroids)
– Liver enzymes, alkaline phosphatase, and bilirubin
– Erythrocyte Sedimentation rate
– Serum glucose
– Serum creatinine and BUN
– Serum calcium, phosphorus and PTH
– Coagulation studies: prothrombin time, protein C and S levels, lupus anticoagulant, anticardiolipin, anti β2-glycoprotein; consider more comprehensive hypercoagulable state testing
– Nutritional status assessment: body mass index, serum albumin, vitamin D levels
– Skin biopsy: Deep, to include subcutaneous tissue
– Plain soft-tissue radiographs to look for netlike pattern of calcification
– In non-uremic patients and based on clinical suspicion: Consider serum protein electrophoresis, special coagulation studies (factor V Leiden, homocysteine, etc.), antinuclear antibodies, and rheumatoid factor

BUN blood urea nitrogen, *PTH* parathyroid hormone

Evaluation

Table 10.3 lists a recommended initial workup for patients in whom calciphylaxis is suspected. In the authors' opinion a deep skin, preferentially excisional, biopsy to include subcutaneous tissue is of utmost importance in establishing the diagnosis.

Treatment

Management of calciphylaxis is challenging; multiple authors now suggest that multidisciplinary collaboration is essential. The main goals of treatment are identification and correction of underlying metabolic derangements, addressing vessel thrombosis that is leading to the ulcerations, arresting disease progression, wound care, pain control, and prevention of gangrene formation and fatal sepsis. To this end, aggressive wound care are of utmost importance.

In practice, efforts must be focused additionally on pain control, symptomatic management, and palliative care.

Renal Replacement Therapy and Normalization of Metabolic Disturbances

Traditionally, the standard of care for calciphylaxis has focused on restoration of the calcium–phosphate homeostasis by intensified hemodialysis [53, 89], restriction of calcium intake [90], low-calcium dialysates [91, 92], use of non-calcium-containing phosphate binders and correction of secondary hyperparathyroidism via calcimimetics or surgical parathyroidectomy when indicated.

Cinacalcet enhances the sensitivity of the calcium sensing receptor to extracellular calcium, thereby reducing serum calcium and PTH levels and normalizing secondary hyperparathyroidism. Paracalcitriol is a synthetic analog of calcitriol capable of selectively activating vitamin D receptors and, therefore, vitamin D responsive pathways, which in turn results in inhibition of PTH secretion. These calcimimetics have been reported to be valuable when use as part of a multimodal approach [93–96].

Parathyroidectomy has the potential advantage of eliminating excess PTH, thus normalizing calcium–phosphate levels. Unfortunately, the results are rather conflicting with some studies documenting improvement in wound healing and survival [97, 98], whereas others reporting no statistical difference [47, 99]. Importantly, it is not an innocuous procedure and complications may arise including poor wound healing, infection and metabolic alterations, to name a few [100]. Notably, complete resolution of severe calciphylaxis has been reported following kidney transplantation, but only in some case reports [101].

Bisphosphonates increase OPG production, thereby decreasing extraosseous mineralization [111]. In a case series of eight patients with calciphylaxis, administration of bisphosphonates resulted in rapid pain control and arrest of disease progression as soon as 2 weeks into treatment with no recurrence documented up to 9 years upon cessation of treatment [112]. Contrary to this observation, a patient with parathyroid adenoma developed calciphylaxis 9 months into treatment with bisphosphonates [113].

Sodium Thiosulfate

Since its first successful use for the treatment of calciphylaxis in 2004 (15168392), a beneficial role for sodium thiosulfate (STS) intravenously or by intraperitoneal infusion [102] has been increasingly documented in case reports and some case series. STS is a potent antioxidant and may improve the endothelial dysfunction associated with calciphylaxis [103]. It is also a chelator that binds calcium to form highly soluble calcium thiosulfate salts that are easily excreted by the kidneys or extracted by hemodialysis thereby improving wall vessel calcification. There are reports on its use in both uremic [104, 105] and non-uremic forms of calciphylaxis [106, 107]. It is generally well tolerated but its administration can be complicated with the development of non-anion gap metabolic acidosis [108]. However, other studies have failed to demonstrate improve survival.

Management of Thrombosis

Thrombosis is the final common pathway which results in tissue necrosis, infarctive skin ulcerations and consequent pain, morbidity and mortality. Therefore, thrombolysis and prevention of future thrombosis are essential management goals.

Hypercoagulability may contribute to the development of the disease [109, 110]; thus, it is conceivable to hypothesize that restoration of blood flow via thrombolysis would halt disease progression. A case report from Mayo Clinic researchers showed marked improvement in cutaneous ulcers and pain with administration of tissue plasminogen activator (tPA) [9]. This observation was further supported by a retrospective study of 15 patients that demonstrated that daily low-dose of tPA may be useful when used in conjunction with other therapies [8]. However, a mortality benefit has not been documented to date.

Wound Care

As with other treatment modalities, conflicting data and opinions exist regarding wound debridement in the management of calciphylactic ulcers. Experience at the Mayo Clinic documented that surgical debridement was associated with 1-year survival of approximately 62 % compared with only 27 % in patients who did not receive such intervention [47]. In a different study of 26 patients, surgical debridement was also associated with improved survival [97]. Aggressive wound debridement followed by split-skin transplantation has also been advocated [114]. Hyperbaric oxygen therapy has emerged as an adjunct in the management of calciphylactic ulcers. It enhances wound healing when delivered in combination with other therapies [115].

Pain Control and Palliative Care

Given the poor prognosis and severe pain associated with calciphylaxis, pain control and palliative care should actively be involved in the care of these patients to ensure mitigation of their discomfort and improvement of their quality of life [116].

Other Treatment Modalities

There are single case reports or small case series on the use of low-density lipoprotein-apheresis [117], sterile maggot therapy [118], and corticosteroids [80].

Conclusion

Calciphylaxis is a life-threatening condition characterized by cutaneous arteriolar calcification complicated by arteriolar thrombosis, leading to skin infarction, ulceration, and consequent mortality. Calciphylaxis has a complex biopathogenesis stemming from increased CPPs to interaction between several inflammatory molecules. The final pathway is the formation of painful ulcers that are prone to harbor microorganisms, leading to local infection and fatal sepsis. In order to provide the best possible outcome in patient care, a multidisciplinary approach is needed.

References

1. Selye H. The dermatologic implications of stress and calciphylaxis. J Invest Dermatol. 1962;39:259–75.
2. Selye H, Gabbiani G, Strebel R. Sensitization to calciphylaxis by endogenous parathyroid hormone. Endocrinology. 1962;71:554–8.
3. Reed KB, Davis MD. The incidence of physician-diagnosed calciphylaxis: a population-based study. J Am Acad Dermatol. 2007; 57(2):365–6.
4. Angelis M, Wong LL, Myers SA, Wong LM. Calciphylaxis in patients on hemodialysis: a prevalence study. Surgery. 1997; 122(6):1083–9. discussion 9-90.
5. Levin A, Mehta RL, Goldstein MB. Mathematical formulation to help identify the patient at risk of ischemic tissue necrosis–a potentially lethal complication of chronic renal failure. Am J Nephrol. 1993;13(6):448–53.
6. Torok L, Kozepessy L, Suhajda K. [Secondary hyperparathyroidism manifesting as cutaneous gangrene in a patient on hemodialysis (uremic gangrene syndrome)]. Hautarzt. 1990;41(12):689–91.
7. Esteve V, Almirall J, Luelmo J, Saez A, Andreu X, Garcia M. [Calcific uraemic arteriolopathy (calciphylaxis): incidence, clinical features and long term outcomes]. Nefrologia. 2007;27(5): 599–604.
8. el-Azhary RA, Arthur AK, Davis MD, McEvoy MT, Gibson LE, Weaver AL, et al. Retrospective analysis of tissue plasminogen activator as an adjuvant treatment for calciphylaxis. JAMA Dermatol. 2013;149(1):63–7.
9. Sewell LD, Weenig RH, Davis MD, McEvoy MT, Pittelkow MR. Low-dose tissue plasminogen activator for calciphylaxis. Arch Dermatol. 2004;140(9):1045–8.
10. Weenig RH. Pathogenesis of calciphylaxis: Hans Selye to nuclear factor kappa-B. J Am Acad Dermatol. 2008;58(3):458–71.
11. Shantsila E, Lip GY. Systemic inflammation as a driver of vascular calcification: a proof of concept. J Intern Med. 2009;266(5): 453–6.
12. Slough S, Servilla KS, Harford AM, Konstantinov KN, Harris A, Tzamaloukas AH. Association between calciphylaxis and inflammation in two patients on chronic dialysis. Adv Perit Dial. 2006;22:171–4.

13. Wang TJ, Larson MG, Levy D, Benjamin EJ, Kupka MJ, Manning WJ, et al. C-reactive protein is associated with subclinical epicardial coronary calcification in men and women: the Framingham Heart Study. Circulation. 2002;106(10):1189–91.
14. Nigwekar SU, Wolf M, Sterns RH, Hix JK. Calciphylaxis from nonuremic causes: a systematic review. Clin J Am Soc Nephrol. 2008;3(4):1139–43.
15. Paccou J, Brazier M, Mentaverri R, Kamel S, Fardellone P, Massy ZA. Vascular calcification in rheumatoid arthritis: prevalence, pathophysiological aspects and potential targets. Atherosclerosis. 2012;224(2):283–90.
16. Yiu KH, Wang S, Mok MY, Ooi GC, Khong PL, Lau CS, et al. Relationship between cardiac valvular and arterial calcification in patients with rheumatoid arthritis and systemic lupus erythematosus. J Rheumatol. 2011;38(4):621–7.
17. van der Pluijm G, Most W, van der Wee-Pals L, de Groot H, Papapoulos S, Lowik C. Two distinct effects of recombinant human tumor necrosis factor-alpha on osteoclast development and subsequent resorption of mineralized matrix. Endocrinology. 1991;129(3):1596–604.
18. Uy HL, Mundy GR, Boyce BF, Story BM, Dunstan CR, Yin JJ, et al. Tumor necrosis factor enhances parathyroid hormone-related protein-induced hypercalcemia and bone resorption without inhibiting bone formation in vivo. Cancer Res. 1997;57(15): 3194–9.
19. Briolay A, Lencel P, Bessueille L, Caverzasio J, Buchet R, Magne D. Autocrine stimulation of osteoblast activity by Wnt5a in response to TNF-alpha in human mesenchymal stem cells. Biochem Biophys Res Commun. 2013;430(3):1072–7.
20. Lencel P, Hardouin P, Magne D. Do cytokines induce vascular calcification by the mere stimulation of TNAP activity? Med Hypotheses. 2010;75(6):517–21.
21. Zhang J, Fu M, Myles D, Zhu X, Du J, Cao X, et al. PDGF induces osteoprotegerin expression in vascular smooth muscle cells by multiple signal pathways. FEBS Lett. 2002;521(1–3):180–4.
22. Lee CT, Chua S, Hsu CY, Tsai YC, Ng HY, Kuo CC, et al. Biomarkers associated with vascular and valvular calcification in chronic hemodialysis patients. Dis Markers. 2013;34(4): 229–35.
23. Krasniak A, Drozdz M, Pasowicz M, Chmiel G, Michalek M, Szumilak D, et al. Factors involved in vascular calcification and atherosclerosis in maintenance haemodialysis patients. Nephrol Dial Transplant. 2007;22(2):515–21.
24. Stompor T, Pasowicz M, Sullowicz W, Dembinska-Kiec A, Janda K, Wojcik K, et al. An association between coronary artery calcification score, lipid profile, and selected markers of chronic inflammation in ESRD patients treated with peritoneal dialysis. Am J Kidney Dis. 2003;41(1):203–11.
25. Nadra I, Mason JC, Philippidis P, Florey O, Smythe CD, McCarthy GM, et al. Proinflammatory activation of macrophages by basic calcium phosphate crystals via protein kinase C and MAP kinase pathways: a vicious cycle of inflammation and arterial calcification? Circ Res. 2005;96(12):1248–56.
26. Ding J, Ghali O, Lencel P, Broux O, Chauveau C, Devedjian JC, et al. TNF-alpha and IL-1beta inhibit RUNX2 and collagen expression but increase alkaline phosphatase activity and mineralization in human mesenchymal stem cells. Life Sci. 2009; 84(15–16):499–504.
27. Collin-Osdoby P, Rothe L, Anderson F, Nelson M, Maloney W, Osdoby P. Receptor activator of NF-kappa B and osteoprotegerin expression by human microvascular endothelial cells, regulation by inflammatory cytokines, and role in human osteoclastogenesis. J Biol Chem. 2001;276(23):20659–72.
28. Liu C, Walter TS, Huang P, Zhang S, Zhu X, Wu Y, et al. Structural and functional insights of RANKL-RANK interaction and signaling. J Immunol. 2010;184(12):6910–9.
29. Wu M, Rementer C, Giachelli CM. Vascular calcification: an update on mechanisms and challenges in treatment. Calcif Tissue Int. 2013;93(4):365–73.
30. Sowers KM, Hayden MR. Calcific uremic arteriolopathy: pathophysiology, reactive oxygen species and therapeutic approaches. Oxid Med Cell Longev. 2010;3(2):109–21.
31. Zhao MM, Xu MJ, Cai Y, Zhao G, Guan Y, Kong W, et al. Mitochondrial reactive oxygen species promote p65 nuclear translocation mediating high-phosphate-induced vascular calcification in vitro and in vivo. Kidney Int. 2011;79(10):1071–9.
32. Gordin D, Soro-Paavonen A, Thomas MC, Harjutsalo V, Saraheimo M, Bjerre M, et al. Osteoprotegerin is an independent predictor of vascular events in Finnish adults with type 1 diabetes. Diabetes Care. 2013;36(7):1827–33.
33. Kadoglou NP, Papadakis I, Moulakakis KG, Ikonomidis I, Alepaki M, Moustardas P, et al. Arterial stiffness and novel biomarkers in patients with abdominal aortic aneurysms. Regul Pept. 2012;179(1–3):50–4.
34. Albu A, Fodor D, Bondor C, Craciun AM. Bone metabolism regulators and arterial stiffness in postmenopausal women. Maturitas. 2013;76(2):146–50.
35. Tousoulis D, Siasos G, Maniatis K, Oikonomou E, Kioufis S, Zaromitidou M, et al. Serum osteoprotegerin and osteopontin levels are associated with arterial stiffness and the presence and severity of coronary artery disease. Int J Cardiol. 2013;167(5): 1924–8.
36. Kim HR, Kim SH, Han MJ, Yoon YS, Oh DJ. The ratio of osteoprotegerin to Fetuin-A is independently associated with vascular stiffness in hemodialysis patients. Nephron Clin Pract. 2013;123(3–4):165–72.
37. Pateinakis P, Papagianni A, Douma S, Efstratiadis G, Memmos D. Associations of fetuin-A and osteoprotegerin with arterial stiffness and early atherosclerosis in chronic hemodialysis patients. BMC Nephrol. 2013;14:122.
38. Winther S, Christensen JH, Flyvbjerg A, Schmidt EB, Jorgensen KA, Skou-Jorgensen H, et al. Osteoprotegerin and mortality in hemodialysis patients with cardiovascular disease. Clin Nephrol. 2013;80(9):161–7.
39. Meneghini M, Regalia A, Alfieri C, Barretta F, Croci D, Gandolfo MT, et al. Calcium and osteoprotegerin levels predict the progression of the abdominal aortic calcifications after kidney transplantation. Transplantation. 2013;96(1):42–8.
40. Stepien E, Fedak D, Klimeczek P, Wilkosz T, Banys RP, Starzyk K, et al. Osteoprotegerin, but not osteopontin, as a potential predictor of vascular calcification in normotensive subjects. Hypertens Res. 2012;35(5):531–8.
41. Chen NX, Moe SM. Uremic vascular calcification. J Investig Med. 2006;54(7):380–4.
42. Li X, Giachelli CM. Sodium-dependent phosphate cotransporters and vascular calcification. Curr Opin Nephrol Hypertens. 2007;16(4):325–8.
43. Fang Y, Ginsberg C, Sugatani T, Monier-Faugere MC, Malluche H, Hruska KA. Early chronic kidney disease-mineral bone disorder stimulates vascular calcification. Kidney Int. 2013;85(1):142–50.
44. Mizobuchi M, Finch JL, Martin DR, Slatopolsky E. Differential effects of vitamin D receptor activators on vascular calcification in uremic rats. Kidney Int. 2007;72(6):709–15.
45. Parfitt AM. Soft-tissue calcification in uremia. Arch Intern Med. 1969;124(5):544–56.
46. Ahmed S, O'Neill KD, Hood AF, Evan AP, Moe SM. Calciphylaxis is associated with hyperphosphatemia and increased osteopontin expression by vascular smooth muscle cells. Am J Kidney Dis. 2001;37(6):1267–76.
47. Weenig RH, Sewell LD, Davis MD, McCarthy JT, Pittelkow MR. Calciphylaxis: natural history, risk factor analysis, and outcome. J Am Acad Dermatol. 2007;56(4):569–79.

48. Hayashi M, Takamatsu I, Kanno Y, Yoshida T, Abe T, Sato Y. A case-control study of calciphylaxis in Japanese end-stage renal disease patients. Nephrol Dial Transplant. 2012;27(4):1580–4.
49. Bleyer AJ, Choi M, Igwemezie B, de la Torre E, White WL. A case control study of proximal calciphylaxis. Am J Kidney Dis. 1998;32(3):376–83.
50. Zacharias JM, Fontaine B, Fine A. Calcium use increases risk of calciphylaxis: a case-control study. Perit Dial Int. 1999;19(3): 248–52.
51. Mawad HW, Sawaya BP, Sarin R, Malluche HH. Calcific uremic arteriolopathy in association with low turnover uremic bone disease. Clin Nephrol. 1999;52(3):160–6.
52. Byrne H, Lloyd S. Calciphylaxis: calcific uraemic arteriolopathy–a case study. J Ren Care. 2007;33(2):74–7.
53. Malabu UH, Roberts LJ, Sangla KS. Calciphylaxis in a morbidly obese woman with rheumatoid arthritis presenting with severe weight loss and vitamin D deficiency. Endocr Pract. 2011; 17(4):e104–8.
54. Zechlinski JJ, Angel JR. Calciphylaxis in the absence of renal disease: secondary hyperparathyroidism and systemic lupus erythematosus. J Rheumatol. 2009;36(10):2370–1.
55. Shah DS, Williamson DJ. A rare cause of ulceration with a promising new treatment. Calciphylaxis due to secondary hyperparathyroidism caused by vitamin D deficiency. Clin Exp Dermatol. 2010;35(3):e90–3.
56. Price PA, Buckley JR, Williamson MK. The amino bisphosphonate ibandronate prevents vitamin D toxicity and inhibits vitamin D-induced calcification of arteries, cartilage, lungs and kidneys in rats. J Nutr. 2001;131(11):2910–5.
57. Price PA, Faus SA, Williamson MK. Bisphosphonates alendronate and ibandronate inhibit artery calcification at doses comparable to those that inhibit bone resorption. Arterioscler Thromb Vasc Biol. 2001;21(5):817–24.
58. Block GA, Martin KJ, de Francisco AL, Turner SA, Avram MM, Suranyi MG, et al. Cinacalcet for secondary hyperparathyroidism in patients receiving hemodialysis. N Engl J Med. 2004; 350(15):1516–25.
59. Lindberg JS, Culleton B, Wong G, Borah MF, Clark RV, Shapiro WB, et al. Cinacalcet HCl, an oral calcimimetic agent for the treatment of secondary hyperparathyroidism in hemodialysis and peritoneal dialysis: a randomized, double-blind, multicenter study. J Am Soc Nephrol. 2005;16(3):800–7.
60. Heiss A, DuChesne A, Denecke B, Grotzinger J, Yamamoto K, Renne T, et al. Structural basis of calcification inhibition by alpha 2-HS glycoprotein/fetuin-A. Formation of colloidal calciprotein particles. J Biol Chem. 2003;278(15):13333–41.
61. Price PA, Williamson MK, Nguyen TM, Than TN. Serum levels of the fetuin-mineral complex correlate with artery calcification in the rat. J Biol Chem. 2004;279(3):1594–600.
62. Ketteler M, Bongartz P, Westenfeld R, Wildberger JE, Mahnken AH, Bohm R, et al. Association of low fetuin-A (AHSG) concentrations in serum with cardiovascular mortality in patients on dialysis: a cross-sectional study. Lancet. 2003;361(9360):827–33.
63. Brandenburg V, Al-Fakhri N, Nemeth K, Goettsch C, Schurgers LJ, Vermeer C, et al. Calcification inhibitors in vascular calciphylaxis associated with normal renal function. Thromb Haemost. 2012;108(6):1241–3.
64. Schurgers LJ, Uitto J, Reutelingsperger CP. Vitamin K-dependent carboxylation of matrix Gla-protein: a crucial switch to control ectopic mineralization. Trends Mol Med. 2013;19(4):217–26.
65. Chatrou ML, Winckers K, Hackeng TM, Reutelingsperger CP, Schurgers LJ. Vascular calcification: the price to pay for anticoagulation therapy with vitamin K-antagonists. Blood Rev. 2012;26(4):155–66.
66. Zebboudj AF, Imura M, Bostrom K. Matrix GLA protein, a regulatory protein for bone morphogenetic protein-2. J Biol Chem. 2002;277(6):4388–94.
67. Ciceri P, Elli F, Brenna I, Volpi E, Brancaccio D, Cozzolino M. The calcimimetic calindol prevents high phosphate-induced vascular calcification by upregulating matrix GLA protein. Nephron Exp Nephrol. 2012;122(3–4):75–82.
68. Shmidt E, Murthy NS, Knudsen JM, Weenig RH, Jacobs MA, Starnes AM, et al. Net-like pattern of calcification on plain soft-tissue radiographs in patients with calciphylaxis. J Am Acad Dermatol. 2012;67(6):1296–301.
69. Janigan DT, Hirsch DJ, Klassen GA, MacDonald AS. Calcified subcutaneous arterioles with infarcts of the subcutis and skin ("calciphylaxis") in chronic renal failure. Am J Kidney Dis. 2000;35(4):588–97.
70. Budisavljevic MN, Cheek D, Ploth DW. Calciphylaxis in chronic renal failure. J Am Soc Nephrol. 1996;7(7):978–82.
71. Hafner J, Keusch G, Wahl C, Burg G. Calciphylaxis: a syndrome of skin necrosis and acral gangrene in chronic renal failure. Vasa. 1998;27(3):137–43.
72. Guldbakke KK, Khachemoune A. Calciphylaxis. Int J Dermatol. 2007;46(3):231–8.
73. Mazhar AR, Johnson RJ, Gillen D, Stivelman JC, Ryan MJ, Davis CL, et al. Risk factors and mortality associated with calciphylaxis in end-stage renal disease. Kidney Int. 2001;60(1):324–32.
74. Andersen LK, Lehman JS, Davis MD. Calciphylaxis is a cutaneous process without involvement of internal organs in a retrospective study of postmortem findings in three patients. Acta Derm Venereol. 2013;94(3):298–302.
75. Au S, Crawford RI. Three-dimensional analysis of a calciphylaxis plaque: clues to pathogenesis. J Am Acad Dermatol. 2002; 47(1):53–7.
76. Mochel MC, Arakaki RY, Wang G, Kroshinsky D, Hoang MP. Cutaneous calciphylaxis: a retrospective histopathologic evaluation. Am J Dermatopathol. 2013;35(5):582–6.
77. Fernandez KH, Liu V, Swick BL. Nonuremic calciphylaxis associated with histologic changes of pseudoxanthoma elasticum. Am J Dermatopathol. 2013;35(1):106–8.
78. Boccara O, Prost-Squarcioni C, Battistella M, Brousse N, Rongioletti F, Fraitag S. Calcinosis cutis: a rare reaction to subcutaneous injections of calcium-containing heparin in patients with renal failure. Am J Dermatopathol. 2010;32(1):52–5.
79. Adrogue HJ, Frazier MR, Zeluff B, Suki WN. Systemic calciphylaxis revisited. Am J Nephrol. 1981;1(3–4):177–83.
80. Fine A, Zacharias J. Calciphylaxis is usually non-ulcerating: risk factors, outcome and therapy. Kidney Int. 2002;61(6):2210–7.
81. Kalajian AH, Malhotra PS, Callen JP, Parker LP. Calciphylaxis with normal renal and parathyroid function: not as rare as previously believed. Arch Dermatol. 2009;145(4):451–8.
82. Mallett A, John GT, Ranganathan D, Kark A, Berquier I, Casey J, et al. Sustained remission of systemic lupus erythematosus related calciphylaxis. Lupus. 2012;21(4):441–4.
83. Aliaga LG, Barreira JC. Calciphylaxis in a patient with systemic lupus erythematosus without renal insufficiency or hyperparathyroidism. Lupus. 2012;21(3):329–31.
84. Brouns K, Verbeken E, Degreef H, Bobbaers H, Blockmans D. Fatal calciphylaxis in two patients with giant cell arteritis. Clin Rheumatol. 2007;26(5):836–40.
85. Nichols B, Saadat P, Vadmal MS. Fatal systemic nonuremic calciphylaxis in a patient with primary autoimmune myelofibrosis. Int J Dermatol. 2011;50(7):870–4.
86. Smith VM, Oliphant T, Shareef M, Merchant W, Wilkinson SM. Calciphylaxis with normal renal function: treated with intravenous sodium thiosulfate. Clin Exp Dermatol. 2012;37(8):874–8.
87. Hafiji J, Deegan P, Brais R, Norris P. Warfarin-induced calciphylaxis successfully treated with sodium thiosulphate. Australas J Dermatol. 2013;54(2):133–5.
88. Wollina U. [Cutaneous calciphylaxis]. Hautarzt. 2010;61(12): 1063–71. quiz 72.

89. Baldwin C, Farah M, Leung M, Taylor P, Werb R, Kiaii M, et al. Multi-intervention management of calciphylaxis: a report of 7 cases. Am J Kidney Dis. 2011;58(6):988–91.
90. Acher-Chenebaux A, Maillard H, Potier A, Nzeyimana H, Cazals F, Celerier P. [Cutaneous calciphylaxis treated by autologous keratinocytes graft and subtotal parathyroidectomy]. Ann Dermatol Venereol. 2006;133(3):260–3.
91. Yeh SM, Hwang SJ, Chen HC. Treatment of severe metastatic calcification in hemodialysis patients. Hemodial Int. 2009;13(2): 163–7.
92. Wang HY, Yu CC, Huang CC. Successful treatment of severe calciphylaxis in a hemodialysis patient using low-calcium dialysate and medical parathyroidectomy: case report and literature review. Ren Fail. 2004;26(1):77–82.
93. Kakagia D, Kriki P, Thodis E, Roumeliotis A, Vargemezis V. Calcific uremic arteriolopathy treated with cinacalcet, paricalcitol, and autologous growth factors. J Cutan Med Surg. 2011;15(2):121–4.
94. Savoia F, Gaddoni G, Patrizi A, Misciali C, Odorici G, Tampieri G, et al. Calciphylaxis in dialysis patients, a severe disease poorly responding to therapies: report of 4 cases. G Ital Dermatol Venereol. 2013;148(5):531–6.
95. Zitt E, Konig M, Vychytil A, Auinger M, Wallner M, Lingenhel G, et al. Use of sodium thiosulphate in a multi-interventional setting for the treatment of calciphylaxis in dialysis patients. Nephrol Dial Transplant. 2013;28(5):1232–40.
96. Vargemezis V, Liakopoulos V, Kriki P, Panagoutsos S, Leontsini M, Passadakis P, et al. Pivotal role of paricalcitol in the treatment of calcific uremic arteriolopathy in the presence of a parathyroid adenoma. Am J Kidney Dis. 2010;55(1):144–7.
97. Lal G, Nowell AG, Liao J, Sugg SL, Weigel RJ, Howe JR. Determinants of survival in patients with calciphylaxis: a multivariate analysis. Surgery. 2009;146(6):1028–34.
98. Girotto JA, Harmon JW, Ratner LE, Nicol TL, Wong L, Chen H. Parathyroidectomy promotes wound healing and prolongs survival in patients with calciphylaxis from secondary hyperparathyroidism. Surgery. 2001;130(4):645–50. discussion 50-1.
99. Kang AS, McCarthy JT, Rowland C, Farley DR, van Heerden JA. Is calciphylaxis best treated surgically or medically? Surgery. 2000;128(6):967–71. discussion 71-2.
100. Vedvyas C, Winterfield LS, Vleugels RA. Calciphylaxis: a systematic review of existing and emerging therapies. J Am Acad Dermatol. 2012;67(6):e253–60.
101. Bhat S, Hegde S, Bellovich K, El-Ghoroury M. Complete resolution of calciphylaxis after kidney transplantation. Am J Kidney Dis. 2013;62(1):132–4.
102. Dethloff SB. Calcific uremic arteriolopathy: treatment with intraperitoneal sodium thiosulfate in a patient on peritoneal dialysis. Nephrol Nurs J. 2012;39(4):323–5. 347.
103. Hayden MR, Goldsmith DJ. Sodium thiosulfate: new hope for the treatment of calciphylaxis. Semin Dial. 2010;23(3):258–62.
104. Scola N, Gackler D, Stucker M, Kreuter A. Complete clearance of calciphylaxis following combined treatment with cinacalcet and sodium thiosulfate. J Dtsch Dermatol Ges. 2011;9(12): 1030–1.
105. Burnie R, Smail S, Javaid MM. Calciphylaxis and sodium thiosulphate: a glimmer of hope in desperate situation. J Ren Care. 2013;39(2):71–6.
106. Hackett BC, McAleer MA, Sheehan G, Powell FC, O'Donnell BF. Calciphylaxis in a patient with normal renal function: response to treatment with sodium thiosulfate. Clin Exp Dermatol. 2009; 34(1):39–42.
107. Stanciu M, Gagne-Henley A, Therien G. Unusual case of proximal calciphylaxis without renal failure. J Cutan Med Surg. 2011;15(5):290–2.
108. Rogers NM, Coates PT. Calcific uraemic arteriolopathy: an update. Curr Opin Nephrol Hypertens. 2008;17(6):629–34.
109. Harris RJ, Cropley TG. Possible role of hypercoagulability in calciphylaxis: review of the literature. J Am Acad Dermatol. 2011;64(2):405–12.
110. Goli AK, Goli SA, Shah LS, Byrd Jr RP, Roy TM. Calciphylaxis: a rare association with alcoholic cirrhosis. Are deficiencies in protein C and S the cause? South Med J. 2005;98(7):736–9.
111. Viereck V, Emons G, Lauck V, Frosch KH, Blaschke S, Grundker C, et al. Bisphosphonates pamidronate and zoledronic acid stimulate osteoprotegerin production by primary human osteoblasts. Biochem Biophys Res Commun. 2002;291(3):680–6.
112. Torregrosa JV, Duran CE, Barros X, Blasco M, Arias M, Cases A, et al. Successful treatment of calcific uraemic arteriolopathy with bisphosphonates. Nefrologia. 2012;32(3):329–34.
113. Muscat M, Brincat M, Degaetano J, Vassallo J, Calleja-Agius J. An unusual site for calciphylaxis: a case report. Gynecol Endocrinol. 2013;29(2):91–2.
114. Wollina U, Helm C, Hansel G, Koch A, Schonlebe J, Haroske G, et al. Deep ulcer shaving combined with split-skin transplantation in distal calciphylaxis. Int J Low Extrem Wounds. 2008;7(2): 102–7.
115. Arenas MD, Gil MT, Gutierrez MD, Malek T, Moledous A, Salinas A, et al. Management of calcific uremic arteriolopathy (calciphylaxis) with a combination of treatments, including hyperbaric oxygen therapy. Clin Nephrol. 2008;70(3):261–4.
116. Polizzotto MN, Bryan T, Ashby MA, Martin P. Symptomatic management of calciphylaxis: a case series and review of the literature. J Pain Symptom Manage. 2006;32(2):186–90.
117. Iwagami M, Mochida Y, Ishioka K, Oka M, Moriya H, Ohtake T, et al. LDL-apheresis dramatically improves generalized calciphylaxis in a patient undergoing hemodialysis. Clin Nephrol. 2012;81(3):198–202.
118. Picazo M, Bover J, de la Fuente J, Sans R, Cuxart M, Matas M. Sterile maggots as adjuvant procedure for local treatment in a patient with proximal calciphylaxis. Nefrologia. 2005;25(5): 559–62.

11 Acquired Perforating Disorders

Mieke L.F. Flour and Dirk R.J. Kuypers

Definition

Acquired perforating dermatosis (APD) of chronic kidney disease (CKD) is characterized by transepidermal elimination of degenerative or foreign material from the dermis; some authors use the term Kyrle disease synomously. APD typically occurs in adults unlike the hereditary reactive dermatoses such as elastosis perforans serpiginosa (EPS) and RPC which occur in children and adolescence [1].

The classification of these dermatoses is based on the nature of the eliminated material and the type of epidermal disruption. They are called "primary" perforating dermatosis because the main disease process consists of perforation of the dermo-epidermal junction and transepidermal elimination of collagen and/or elastic fibers or other material. In the "secondary" perforating dermatosis with a different pathogenesis this elimination process is an occasional phenomenon, as in perforating granuloma, pseudoxanthoma elasticum, some infectious diseases or following laser treatment.

Epidemiology, Incidence, Prevalence

Although the exact prevalence and incidence of APD is unknown, it is reportedly uncommon. APD occurs in 5–10 % of patients maintained on hemodialysis [2, 3]; age of onset ranges from 29–96 years, with a peak frequency in the sixth decade of life.

Sex distribution is considered equal. There seems to be no racial variations in the incidence.

M.L.F. Flour, M.D. (✉)
Department of Dermatology, University Hospitals Leuven, Schoonzichtlaan 43, 3020 Winksele, Leuven, Belgium
e-mail: mie.flour@skynet.be

D.R.J. Kuypers, M.D., Ph.D.
Department of Nephrology and Renal Transplantation, University Hospitals Leuven, Leuven, Belgium

Clinical Presentation

Clinical presentations of APD are not uniform; it may resemble any of the four perforating disorders: Kyrle disease (KD), RPC, perforating folliculitis (PF), or EPS. In one individual patient the lesions seem to be of the same type, although it might be possible to find several histological types if more biopsies were performed [4] (Fig. 11.1).

Characteristic clinical findings, proposed by Faver et al. to be seen as diagnostic criteria are: hyperkeratotic or cup-shaped centrally depressed papules, transepidermal elimination of basophilic collagen bundles, manifestation in adults over 18 years of age [5, 6].

APD typically starts as small papules of 1 mm which develop in a few weeks into umbilicated papules and plaques with firmly adherent "crusts" measuring up to 0.5–2.0 cm in diameter; lesions may occasionally coalesce to form plaques of several centimeters. The border is erythematous and slightly elevated, as a ridge. The color of the crust varies from light to black to brown-green, sometimes with an oyster-shell appearance. The number of lesions ranges from just a few to many. Lesions typically are grouped, solitary disseminated papules are less common; some lesions form as a manifestation of the Köbner phenomenon. Forceful removal of the plug will result in a bleeding crater. Elevated, plateau-like, or depressed lesions occur. After detachment of the crust, a crater-like lesion remains, healing by 2 months leaving an atrophic, depressed, hypopigmented or hyperpigmented scar. Although each individual lesion has a limited evolution time, the eruption in one individual may last many years (Fig. 11.2).

J.R. Nunley and E.V. Lerma (eds.), *Dermatological Manifestations of Kidney Disease*,
DOI 10.1007/978-1-4939-2395-3_11, © Springer Science+Business Media New York 2015

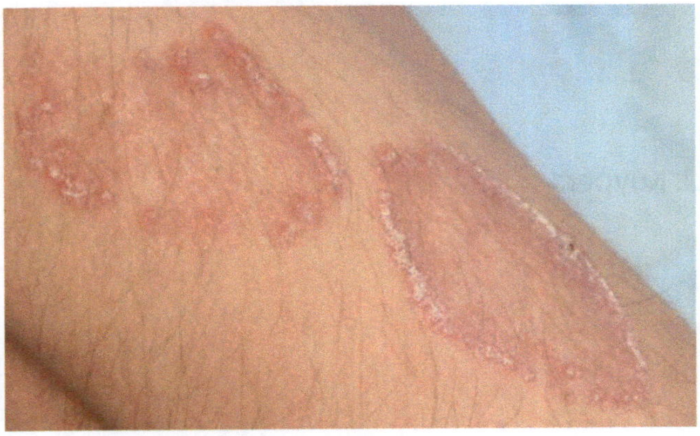

Fig. 11.1 Elastosis perforans serpiginosa. Conditions such as elastosis perforans serpiginosa (EPS) may be confused with acquired perforating dermatosis (APD). However, the annular distribution seen here is common in EPS, yet rare in APD. Courtesy of Julia R. Nunley, M.D.

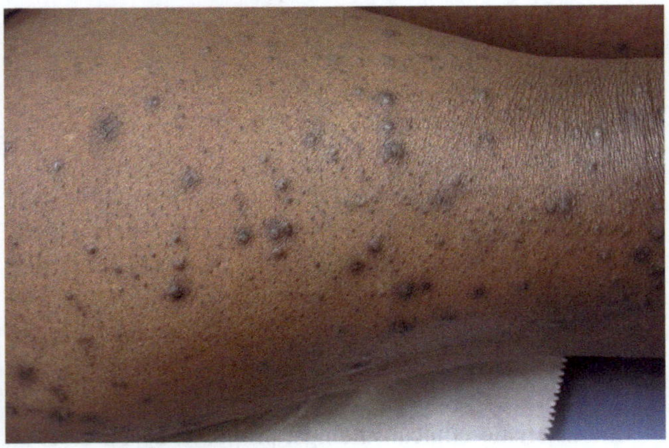

Fig. 11.2 Seen here are typical cone-shaped hyperpigmented, hyperkeratotic papules of acquired perforating dermatosis in a diabetic on hemodialysis. Courtesy of Julia R. Nunley, M.D.

Sites commonly affected include the extensor aspects of the extremities, the trunk, shoulder girdle, the gluteal region, and sometimes the head. Mucous membranes, folds or intertriginous areas, and palmoplantar regions are spared.

Pruritus is the presenting symptom in about three-fourths of patients, although pruritus is not universal; a minority of patients are asymptomatic and others report pain. Some with pruritus report sporadic bouts of severe, unrelenting itch.

Pathogenesis, Etiology

The pathogenesis is unclear but several hypotheses have been developed to explain the phenomenon.

Suggested causes include: a genetic predisposition (to be distinguished from the inherited forms), associated diseases, and occasionally certain medications [7].

The main abnormality in the primary reactive perforating disorders is a focal damage to or alteration of the extracellular matrix collagen fibers, or deposition of material foreign to normal dermis, and a subsequent elimination of this altered material through the epidermis.

There is indirect evidence that mild superficial trauma plays a role: the frequent association with pruritus and scratching; development of lesions on reachable sites and superficial trauma-prone areas; the observed Köbner phenomenon; and the lack of lesion development following deeper wounds such as surgical incisions.

Alterations of extracellular matrix-components may be secondary to inflammation, metabolic alteration, neoplastic cells, or deposition of aberrant external substances. These papillary dermal changes induce an active epidermal response consisting of downward proliferation to engulf and isolate the material, thereby creating perforating transepithelial channels to extrude the altered components. The proliferative epidermis is sometimes seen as pseudoepitheliomatous hyperplasia surrounding the central plug.

Mehregan identifies this as an active process, distiguishable from the more "passive" transmigration and desquamation through epidermal turnover experienced by small particles such as hemosiderin, or the active migration and epidermal elimination of motile cells such as neutrophils or infectious such as *Treponema pallidum* [6]. Following the elimination of material in these cases, the epidermis will return to normal, although sometimes leaving a scar.

Through which signal transepidermal elimination is induced is a matter of debate. Exogenous foreign material, deposition of urate crystals or calcium hydroxyapatite, both infectious and non-infectious granulomas, altered dermal components all are stimuli for the epidermis to respond with downward proliferation, engulfing and elimination of these altered substances. Close proximity to the dermal–epidermal interaction zone seems to be a condition sine qua non: according to experimental studies the critical level would be that of the hair papillae; deep granulomas, deeper trauma, or foreign material will not induce the response [8].

In APD associated with CKD, deposition of substances that cannot be removed with dialysis is a proposed theory. Matrix and epidermal changes related to metabolic diseases have been suggested to play a role. Hyaline degeneration of collagen fibers in advanced diabetes may be due to glycation and lipoxidation of proteins and other compounds, resulting in advanced glycation end products (AGEs). The resulting Mailliard adducts remain in proteins with a long half-life and change their physical/biochemical properties. The induced molecular cross-linking impairs the solubility, susceptibility, and reaction ability of these altered structural biological proteins and fibers. In patients with chronic renal insufficiency, the elimination of these Maillard products is impaired. One hypothesis is that microtrauma to the skin may trigger the elimination of such altered collagen fibers.

Diabetic microangiopathy is considered to be a predisposing factor facilitating necrosis or necrobiosis of metabolically altered subepidermal components by minor trauma.

Histopathology

Characteristic feature of the perforating dermatoses is the transepidermal elimination of various substances such as keratin, collagen, and elastic fibers. Histological features of APD are not uniform; they may resemble any of the four perforating disorders mentioned above. Histopathological examination will vary according to evolution and clinical subtype, resembling specific perforating disorders (PF, APD, KD, EPS).

Histologic findings are relative to the evolutionary stage of the lesion.

Early lesions show complete disappearance of the basal lamina and although desmosomes are intact, bundles of collagen fibers appear in widened intercellular spaces. In excoriated lesions (due to scratching) eosinophilic necrotic material may be seen containing pycnotic nuclei of inflammatory cells and degenerated collagen bundles lying in continuity with those in the dermis. The epidermis in these excoriated lesions may show any stage of regenerative healing.

The fully develop umbilicated papule shows a typical cup-shaped interruption in the epidermis containing cellular debris and basophilic collagen bundles in its center. Content includes cellular debris, neutrophilic granulocytes, and sometimes bacteria. The degenerated collagen fibers are oriented vertically, perpendicular to the skin surface which is parakeratotic in the central zone of this plug, in what appears to be narrow tunnels of elimination.

The lateral borders are sharply delineated with epithelial hyperplasia, sometimes with hypergranulosis and hyperkeratosis. There is often a mild superficial inflammatory infiltrate of mixed cells, with lymphocytes, neutrophils, and histiocytes.

In resolving lesions the crater is shallow, containing remnants of degenerated collagen and parakeratotic keratin, while the base of the plug consists of almost regenerated epidermis, with a partially organized basement membrane. A repair phenomenon will reconstitute the epidermis and close the eliminating channels. Along with epidermal turnover the hyperkeratotic plug gradually will slough off.

The clinical and histopathological subtype of APD is determined by the content of the eliminated material.

The lesions resembling KD show epidermal invagination filled with a keratotic plug containing cellular debris and neutrophils, but no collagen nor elastin. In those presenting like RPC, the cup-shaped invagination of the epidermis is filled with a plug containing keratin, cellular debris and neutrophils; vertically oriented collagen bundles can be seen at the base of the cup, which are eliminated in a transepidermal way. The refractile hyalinized collagen fiber bundles in the base of the plug stain basophilic with hematoxylin–eosin and red with Van Gieson staining.

Lesions resembling PF show a dilated infundibulum filled with necrotic debris, orthokeratotic and parakeratotic keratin, and inflammatory cell debris. This follicular content is exposed to the dermis, and the resulting inflammatory reaction is a perifollicular mononuclear of mixed type of inflammatory infiltration believed to lead to transepidermal elimination.

In APD associated with CKD, only rarely will elimination of degenerated elastic fibers and cellular debris be seen as a cup-shaped epidermal invagination; this is more characteristic of EPS. However, when present, histochemical staining reveals an increase in coarse and degenerative dermal elastic fibers.

There are inconsistencies in reported vascular changes, inflammatory reactions and restorative features. Reported vascular changes include vessel wall thickening and positive periodic acid-Schiff (PAS) staining. Inflammatory reactions may consist of a mixed infiltrate of mononuclear cells, neutrophils, and occasionally eosinophils. Collagen bundle degradation has been reported at the base of some elimination channels and reactive granulation tissue, as seen in wound healing has also been described. This fact may explain the recently reported findings of fibronectin and transforming growth factor beta 3 in lesions of APD.

Associated Disorders

In a published case series [9] most of the patients (86 %) suffering from APD had at least one systemic disease, of which chronic renal failure and diabetes mellitus (DM) were the most commonly associated morbidities; of those with chronic renal failure, all were on dialysis.

Diseases and disorders which are commonly associated with APD include (1) primary pruritic dermatoses such as atopic dermatiitis and scabies; (2) metabolic disorders such as DM, uremia per se, thyroid and hepatic diseases; (3) infections such as human immunodeficiency virus (HIV) and tuberculosis; (4) malignancies including solid tumors and both lymphoproliferative and myeloproliferative disorders; (5) localized trauma from laser treatment or lesional currettage; (6) medications including clopirogrel, indinavir, sirolimus and calcium-channel blockers, most commonly amlodipine. Special consideration is necessary for medications metabolized by the cytochrome P450 system when liver enzymes are elevated [10, 11].

It has been estimated that APD occurs in 5–10 % of dialysis patients. Most patients develop APD after the initiation of dialysis, although rare cases have been reported to predate dialysis. The most common cause of renal failure in patients with APD is DM; however APD has developed in patients with renal failure due to hypertension, glomerulonephritis or polycystic kidney disease. Diabetic dialysis patients who develop APD uniformly have had a long-standing DM-related complication such as nephropathy, retinopathy, neuropathy, and/or peripheral vascular disease before the development of APD.

Associated pruritus is regarded as a precipitating factor due to repetitive trauma from scratching, although not all patients have severe itch. The pruritus is most likely associated with the underlying disease, like diabetes, renal failure, Hodgkin disease, and other reported itching disorders. The scratching has been reported to be responsible for repeated microtrauma, inducing focal degeneration of collagen fibers. Experimental microtrauma can trigger the clinical onset of APD [12–14]. The localization of the lesion at "reachable sites," the manifest Köbner phenomenon, and improvement of lesions after successful antipruritic treatment are all arguments supporting this hypothesis.

Trauma to superficial dermis and subsequent repair mechanism are consistent with immunohistochemical studies showing growth factors and enzymes characteristic for wound healing in the extracellular matrix, like increased intralesional transforming growth factor (TNF)-β3 expression, or markers of increased intralesional fibroblast activity [15, 16].

Differential Diagnosis

The characteristic clinical appearance and morphology of the lesions, their localization and distribution are very suggestive for a clinical diagnosis of APD.

Lesions must also be distinguished from secondary perforating disorders, tumors, or inflammatory dermatoses, as mentioned previously.

Treatment

Treatment is challenging, not to say disappointing, and multimodal; guidlines are non-existent due to the lack of clinical data supporting any treatment option.

Treating the underlying internal or oncological disease, if at all possible, would be the primary focus.

Management of the pruritus by topical and systemic treatment will for some patients stop the trauma inducing scratching. Uremic pruritus has a complex pathophysiology [17] discussed at depth in Chap. 7, 16. Results of antipruritic treatment have been controversial or anecdotal. Preparations containing urea, capsaicin, and polidocanol have been advocated. Systemic treatment using sedating antihistamines may help in some cases. More recent reports have claimed—but also denied—efficacy of tacrolimus ointment for uremic pruritus in patients on chronic dialysis therapy. Phototherapy with ultraviolet B (UVB) [18–21] in varying treatment schedules, e.g., starting with five times daily for 2 weeks then three times weekly for 4 weeks has been used for its anti-inflammatory and antipruritic effects.

Keratolytic preparations have been used to ease removal of the plug, if necessary under occlusion: salicylic acid (5–7 % in vaseline), urea (10–15 %), topical tretinoin 0.01–0.1 % cream. Curettage is not easy and will leave some bleeding area since the plug is adherent to underlying dermis in fully developed lesions.

Anti-inflammatory therapy may include topical corticosteroids class 2–3, or even intralesional injections of triamcinolone suspension. Some have applied topical corticosteroids like betamethasone valerate cream 0.1 % twice daily for 4 weeks (in combination with UVB phototherapy).

UVB phototherapy has been advocated in diabetic patients on dialysis [22]: presumably acting on the pruritus, adding anti-inflammatory and antiproliferative effects.

Others have reported the use of systemic oral steroids, like prednisone 20–50 mg daily [21].

Retinoids may be applied as topical preparation to ease removal of the crust and for their antiproliferative effect. Systemic treatment with retinoids have been tried [23, 24] with varying results.

Oral allopurinol (100 mg daily) has had conflicting results: although some cases healed with treatment, allopurinol treatment for hyperuricemia did not prevent the development of APD in others.

Anecdotal evidence, via isolated cases, suggests that other treatment options may be effective for APD including oral antibiotics such as erythromycin, tetracycline, and doxycycline and miscellaneous options including hydroxychloroquine, diphenylsulfone, or methotrexate [11, 13, 25, 26].

References

1. Rapini RP, Herbert AA, Drucker CR. Acquired perforating dermatosis: evidence for combined transepidermal elimination of both collagen and elastic fibers. Arch Dermatol. 1989;125:1074–8.
2. Morton CA, Henderson IS, Jones MC, Lowe JG. Acquired perforating dermatosis in a British dialysis population. Br J Dermatol. 1996;135(5):671–7.
3. Poliak SC, Lebwohl MG, Parris A, Prioleau PG. Reactive perforating collagenosis associated with diabetes mellitus. N Engl J Med. 1982;306(2):81–4.
4. Patterson JW. Progress in the perforating dermatoses. Arch Dermatol. 1989;125:1121–3.
5. Faver IR, Daoud MS, Su WDP. Acquired reactive perforating collagenosis. Report of six cases and review of the literature. J Am Acad Dermatol. 1994;30:575–80.

6. Mehregan AH, Schwartz OD, Livingood CS. Reactive perforating collagenosis. Arch Dermatol. 1967;96:277–82.
7. Woo TY, Rasmussen JE. Disorders of transepidermal elimination. Part 1. Int J Dermatol. 1985;24(5):267–79.
8. Marks R, Schellander F. The epidermal response in subepidermal inflammation. Br J Dermatol. 1973;83:363–76.
9. Saray Y, Seçkin D, Bilezikçi B. Acquired perforating dermatosis: clinicopathological features in twenty-two cases. J Eur Acad Dermatol Venereol. 2006;20:679–88.
10. Calista D, Morri M. Acquired reactive perforating collagenosis induced by indinavir in 2 patients with HIV disease. Eur J Dermatol. 2008;18:84–5.
11. Lübbe J, Sorg O, Male PJ, et al. Sirolimus-induced inflammatory papules with acquired reactive perforating collagenosis. Dermatology. 2008;216:239–42.
12. Krüger K, Tebbe B, Krengel S, et al. Erworbene reaktive perforierende dermatose. Erfolgreiche behandlung mit allopurinol in 2 fällen. Hautarzt. 1999;50:115–20.
13. Bovenmyer DA. Reactive perforating collagenosis: experimental production of the lesion. Arch Dermatol. 1970;102:313–7.
14. Yuzuk S, Trau H, Stempler D, et al. Reactive perforating collagenosis. Int J Dermatol. 1985;24:584–6.
15. Gambichler T, Birkner L, Stücker M, et al. Up-regulation of transforming growth factor-β3 and extracellular matrix proteins in acquired reactive perforating collagenosis. J Am Acad Dermatol. 2009;60:463–9.
16. Kawakami T, Soma Y, Mizoguchi M, Saito R. Immunohistochemical analysis of transforming growth factor-beta 3 expression in acquired reactive perforating collagenosis. Br J Dermatol. 2001;144:197–9.
17. Kuypers D. Skin problems in chronic kidney disease. Nat Clin Pract Nephrol. 2009;5(3):157–70. doi:10.1038/ncpneph1040. Epub 2009 Feb 3.
18. Scola N, Gambichler T, Altmeyer P, et al. Erworbene reaktive perforierende Kollagenose nach Herpes zoster als isotopische Antwort ? Hautarzt. 2011;62:683–7.
19. Schlotmann K, Megahed M, Goerz G. Ungewöhnlicher Fall einer erworbenen reaktiven perforierenden Kollagenose. HuG. 1996;71: 786–8.
20. Gambichler T, Altmeyer P, Kreuter A. Treatment of acquired perforating dermatosis with narrowband ultraviolet B. J Am Acad Dermatol. 2005;52:363–4.
21. Cullen SI. Successful treatment of reactive perforating collagenosis with tretinoin. Cutis. 1979;23:187–93.
22. Cochran RJ, Rucker SB, Wilkin JK. Reactive perforating collagenosis of diabetes and renal failure. Cutis. 1983;31:55–8.
23. Büchau AS, Lewerenz V, Kruse R, et al. Reaktive perforierende Kollagenose. Hautarzt. 2005;56:963–5.
24. Nebel R, Fiedler E, Danz B, et al. Erworbene reaktive perforierende Kollagenose bei Diabetes mellitus und dialysepflichtige Niereninsuffizienz. Dtsch Med Wochenschr. 2007;132: 2624–6.
25. Brinkmeier T, Schaller J, Herbst RA, Frosch PJ. Successful treatment of acquired reactive perforating collagenosis with doxycycline. Acta Derm Venereol. 2002;82:393–5.
26. Armano H, Nagai Y, Kishi C, Ishikawa O. Acquired reactive perforating collagenosis in dermatomyositis. J Dermatol. 2011;38(12): 1199–201.

Nephrogenic Systemic Fibrosis

12

Avery LaChance, Ali K. Abu-Alfa, and Shawn E. Cowper

Abbreviations

AKI	Acute kidney injury
ANA	Antinuclear antibody
CDC	Centers for disease control
CF	Circulating fibrocyte
CKD	Chronic kidney disease
eGFR	estimated glomerular filtration rate
EMEA	European Medicines Agency
EMG	Electromyelogram
ESRD	End-stage renal disease
FDA	Food and Drug Administration
GBCA	Gadolinium based contrast agent
Gd	Gadolinium
GFR	Glomerular filtration rate
H&E	Hematoxylin and eosin
IEP	Immunoelectrophoresis
IF	Immunofixation
LDS	Lipodermatosclerosis
MR	Magnetic resonance
MRA	Magnetic resonance angiography
MRI	Magnetic resonance imaging
NFD	Nephrogenic fibrosing dermopathy
NSF	Nephrogenic systemic fibrosis
PHA	Public health advisory
POC	Point of care
SCX	Scleromyxedema
SPEP	Serum protein electrophoresis
SS	Systemic sclerosis
TGFβ1	Transforming growth factor beta-1
TIMP-1	Tissue inhibitor of metalloproteinases-1

A. LaChance, M.D., M.P.H.
Harvard Combined Dermatology Residency, Harvard Medical School, Massachusetts General Hospital, 55 Fruit Street, Boston, MA 02114, USA
e-mail: avery.lachance@gmail.com

A.K. Abu-Alfa, M.D.
Division of Nephrology and Hypertension, Department of Internal Medicine, American University of Beirut, Cairo Street, PO Box 11-0236, Beirut, Riad El-Solh, 1107 2020, Lebanon

Section of Nephrology, Yale University School of Medicine, 330 Cedar Street, BB 114, PO Box 208029, New Haven, CT 06520-8029, USA
e-mail: abualfa@aub.edu.lb; ali.abu-alfa@yale.edu

S.E. Cowper, M.D. (✉)
Department of Dermatology, Yale University School of Medicine, Yale Dermatopathology Service, 15 York Street, LMP 5031, PO Box 208059, New Haven, CT 06520-8059, USA

Department of Pathology, Yale University School of Medicine, Yale Dermatopathology Service, 15 York Street, LMP 5031, PO Box 208059, New Haven, CT 06520-8059, USA
e-mail: shawn.cowper@yale.edu

Introduction

Nephrogenic systemic fibrosis (NSF) emerged and virtually disappeared within a span of approximately 15 years. The quick extinction of this perplexing clinical entity is attributed to clinical recognition, epidemiologic surveillance, association studies on causation, and the passage of professional and regulatory guidelines informed by the work of numerous physicians, scientists, and regulatory officials.

The lessons learned from the appearance of NSF, especially regarding the potential for iatrogenic disease or toxicity secondary to the use of renally cleared medications, remain relevant. Physicians, pharmaceutical manufacturers and regulators were confounded by a series of circumstances and trends that laid the groundwork for the emergence of NSF: (1) gadolinium based contrast agents (GBCAs) were administered without caution for use or dose adjustment in the renal population despite the fact that they had not been specifically tested in this setting; (2) ever-increasing doses of GBCAs were employed in the off-label use of GBCAs for magnetic resonance angiography (MRA); (3) the unusual nature of the clinical manifestations of NSF did not suggest a medication toxicity; and (4) the link between the administration of GBCAs and their subsequent toxic effects was

J.R. Nunley and E.V. Lerma (eds.), *Dermatological Manifestations of Kidney Disease*,
DOI 10.1007/978-1-4939-2395-3_12, © Springer Science+Business Media New York 2015

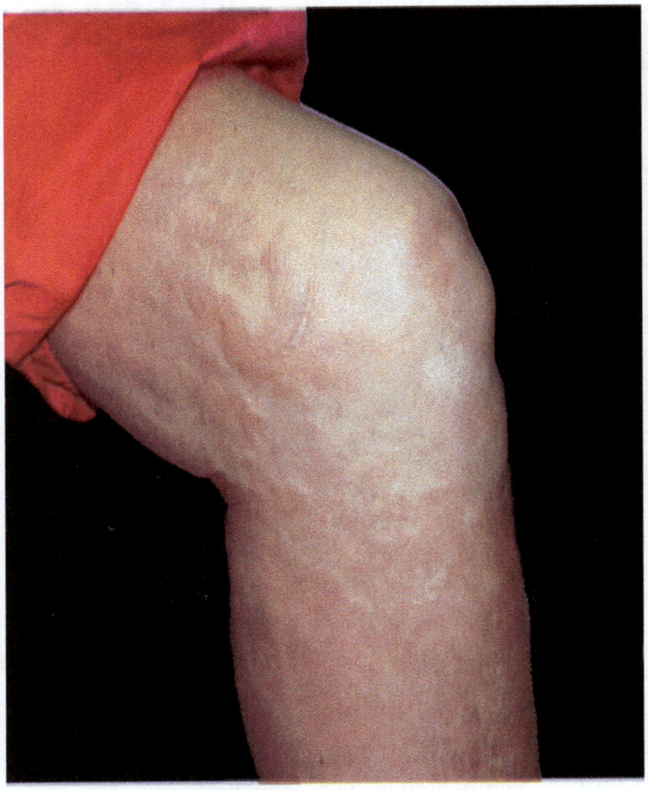

Fig. 12.1 NSF patients exhibited cutaneous thickening and hardening, chiefly on the extremities. (Reprinted from the Lancet, Vol 356(9234), Cowper SE, Robin HS, Steinberg SM, Su LD, Gupta S, LeBoit PE. Scleromyxoedema-like cutaneous diseases in renal-dialysis patients, Pages 1000-1, 2000, with permission from Elsevier)

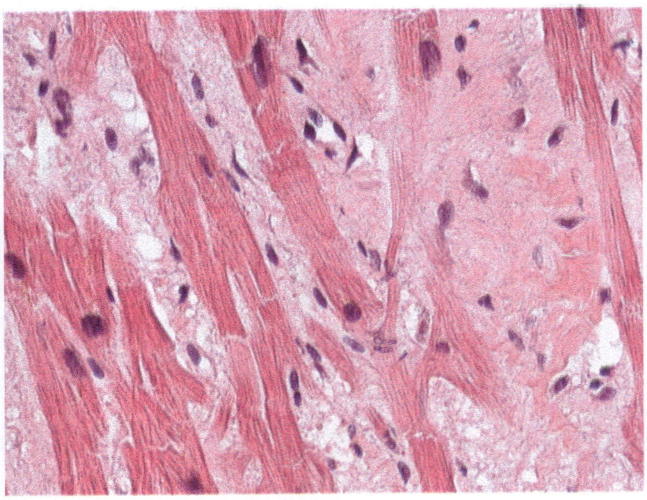

Fig. 12.2 Fibrosis involving the heart of a deceased NSF patient. (With permission of the International Center for Nephrogenic Systemic Fibrosis Research (ICNSFR.org))

slow to be recognized because of the several weeks to months time delay of NSF onset, the complexity of medical care in this challenging population, and the administration of GBCAs in radiology departments, outside of the purview of the patients' usual care providers.

While we may celebrate the departure of NSF, its future reemergence can be anticipated if certain currently available GBCAs are accidentally administered in the setting of renal disease, or if future GBCA formulations are not evaluated for toxicity in this setting. In addition, the long-term effects of gadolinium retention are still unknown, and the possibility of renal or non-renal patients accumulating this rare metal and developing as-yet-unsuspected conditions should be considered. For these reasons, physicians should remain alert for the reemergence of this rare condition and for the appearance of potential new toxicities that may develop in the complex medical and treatment scenarios of the future.

History

NSF, initially observed in 1997, was described by Cowper, et al. as a "scleromyxedema-like" cutaneous disease in a letter to the Lancet in 2000 [1] (Fig. 12.1). The initial paper described 14 patients with hemodialysis-dependent end-stage renal disease (ESRD). These patients, in four different American medical centers, displayed a similar pattern of cutaneous thickening and hardening localized to the extremities [1]. Cutaneous biopsies demonstrated a common histopathological pattern that included increased numbers of dermal fibroblast-like cells, collagen remodeling, and mucin deposition [1]. Despite its clinical and histopathological resemblance to scleromyxedema (SCX), an absence of the typical monoclonal gammopathy of SCX, and differences in lesional distribution prompted researchers to declare a new and distinct clinical entity [1].

Following this initial report, the investigators partnered with the Centers for Disease Control (CDC) to create a case definition, ultimately resulting in the recognition of eight additional cases with a similar constellation of symptoms [2]. Although all of the patients identified in the original cohort were receiving hemodialysis at the time of disease onset, this expanded group included some patients receiving hemodialysis, some receiving peritoneal dialysis, and a few patients with chronic kidney disease (CKD) who had never before been dialyzed [2].

In 2001, the disease was named nephrogenic fibrosing dermopathy (NFD) accounting for (1) the characteristic non-inflammatory cutaneous fibrosis and its exclusive occurrence (2) in the setting of severe kidney disease [2]. Although the cause of NSF would not be determined until 2006, this defining paper hypothesized a possible infectious and/or toxic etiology in light of its rapid, recent emergence and clustering around dialysis centers [2].

In 2003, the first NFD autopsy was performed [3]. In addition to cutaneous fibrosis, the findings of significant fibrosis of the diaphragm, psoas muscle, renal tubules and testes underscored the systemic nature of the process [3]. The disease was renamed "nephrogenic systemic fibrosis" to better reflect the extent of the disease process (Fig. 12.2).

That same year, a chart review of cases present in the International NSF Registry (icnsfr.org) demonstrated a preponderance of certain comorbidities in patients with NSF. Patients had a greater likelihood of hypercoagulability, and increased rates of thrombosis and vascular surgery were noted in the days to weeks preceding NSF onset. They also seemed to display a disproportionately high brain tumor incidence than would be expected among patients with ESRD or CKD [4]. This, in addition to continued geographic clustering, strengthened the hypothesis that a toxic exposure could be fueling NSF [4–6].

In the fall of 2005, a lecture was presented at the New England Dermatologic Society meeting at Yale University, during which a strong correlation between imaging studies just prior to the onset of NSF was described—publicly implicating GBCAs as the suspected etiopathogenic trigger of NSF [7].

In January 2006, Grobner et al. published the first medical report implicating GBCAs as the potential cause of NSF [8]. This study included a case series of nine ESRD patients who developed NSF within 3 months following GBCA administration for MRA studies [8]. This observation was further substantiated in a paper from Denmark published in November 2006 describing a similar temporal association between exposure to GBCAs in patients with ESRD and the development of NSF [9].

These publications were of particular interest given the history of GBCA sales in the United States. In 1996, shortly before the identification of NSF, a paper declaring high-dose GBCAs to be significantly less nephrotoxic than iodinated contrast agents had been published [10, 11]. This observation implied that GBCAs were safe for use in renally compromised individuals, prompting the nearly reflexive use of these agents in patients with any degree of renal insufficiency in the years to follow [10, 11]. Thus, just as GBCAs were being preferentially employed for imaging studies in patients with kidney disease, the initial publications linking GBCAs and NSF began to appear. Ironically, GBCAs remained the agent of choice in many centers even in anuric ESRD patients who had no residual renal function to protect.

In June 2006, the U.S. Food and Drug Administration (FDA) issued its first advisory on the use of GBCAs in patients with kidney failure [12]. The public health advisory suggested that GBCAs should only be used if absolutely necessary in patients with advanced kidney failure, as defined by dialysis dependence or patients with a glomerular filtration rate (GFR) of 15 cc/min or less [12]. Additionally, the warning suggested that physicians should consider prompt initiation of dialysis following gadolinium contrast MRAs in patients with kidney dysfunction [12].

In 2007, two articles linking gadolinium to the onset of NSF strengthened the epidemiological data [13, 14]. The first article used a field emission scanning electron microscope equipped with energy dispersive spectroscopy to determine that the element, gadolinium (Gd) was detectable within the tissue of patients (Fig. 12.3) with NSF up to 11 months following exposure to GBCAs [13]. The second study used inductively coupled plasma mass spectrometry to illustrate that Gd levels were quantifiable within the tissue of patients with NSF [14]. Importantly, Gd levels were found to be highest in the tissue regions most affected by fibrosis [14]. Up until that time, pharmaceutical companies had assumed that no residual Gd would be retained in the body so long after the exposure.

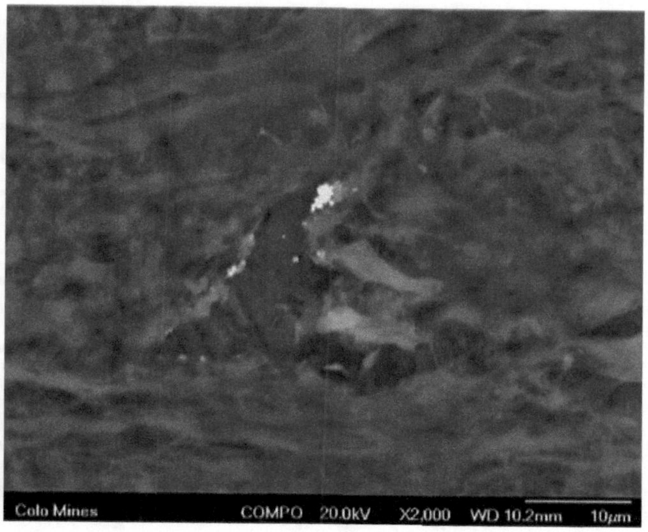

Fig. 12.3 Field emission scanning photomicrograph showing aggregated particles of gadolinium associated with a cell body of a probable macrophage located within dermal fibrosis (Original magnification: ×32,000). (Reprinted from Journal of the American Academy of Dermatology, Vol 56(1), High WA, Ayers RA, Chandler J, Zito G, Cowper SE. Gadolinium is detectable within the tissue of patients with nephrogenic systemic fibrosis, Pages 21-6, 2007, with permission from Elsevier and the American Academy of Dermatology)

That same year, the European Medicines Agency (EMEA) reviewed the safety profile for GBCAs in patients with kidney dysfunction, ultimately contraindicating the use of gadodiamide, gadopentetate dimeglumine, and gadoversetamide in patients with an estimated glomerular filtration rate (eGFR) < 30 mL/min/1.73 m^2 in February, June, and July of 2007, respectively [10]. In 2010, the FDA followed suit, requiring all GBCAs to be labeled with warnings surrounding the risk of developing NSF for patients with acute kidney injury (AKI) or CKD stages 4–5 exposed to gadolinium, taking the additional step of specifically contraindicating gadodiamide, gadopentetate dimeglumine, and gadoversetamide use in patients with kidney disease [15]. The FDA also advised health-care professionals to evaluate kidney function in patients at risk of having kidney disease prior to the administration of GBCAs; to avoid using GBCAs in patients at risk for kidney failure; to monitor patients for signs and symptoms of NSF following GBCA administration; and to limit the dose of GBCAs used for imaging purposes [15].

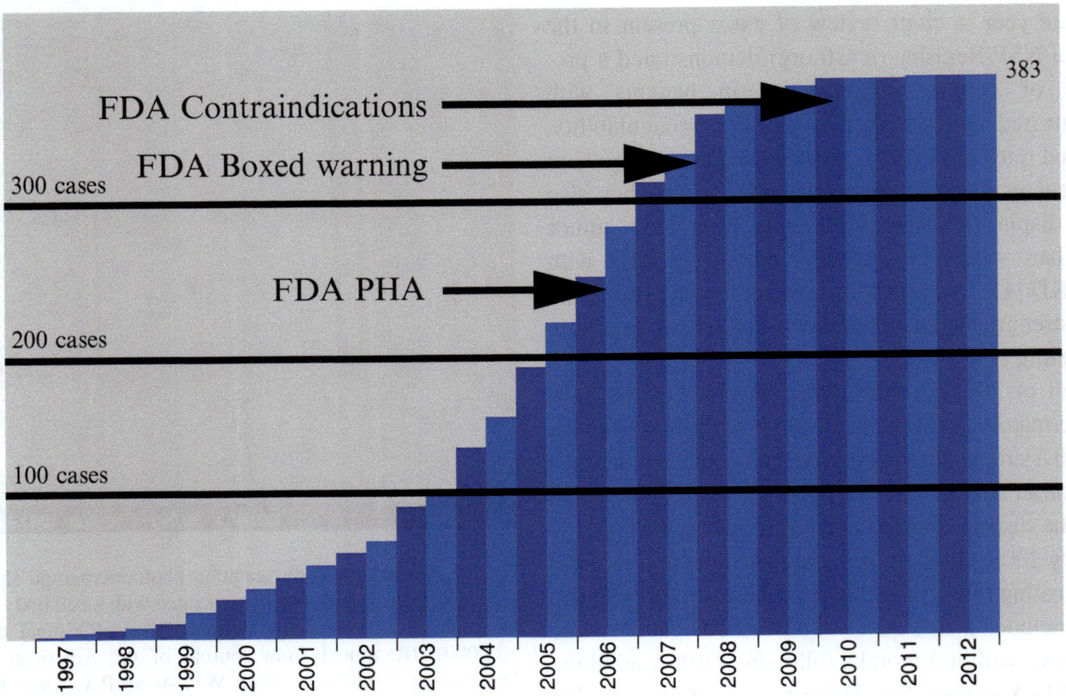

Fig. 12.4 Chart showing cumulative NSF cases reported to the NSF Registry by date of onset through 2012. Important FDA announcements are marked on the timeline. (With permission of the International Center for Nephrogenic Systemic Fibrosis Research (ICNSFR.org)). *FDA* Food and Drug Administration, *PHA* Public Health Advisory

Prior to 2007, sales figures for gadodiamide, the most commonly used GBCA, were on the rise [16]. However, following the publication of these regulatory guidelines, a reduction in overall sales of gadodiamide occurred [16]. In addition, as use patterns and protocols for GBCA administration changed following the publication of international guidelines, NSF incidence rates decreased significantly (Fig. 12.4), with a virtual disappearance of new cases reported to the registry by 2010 [16–20].

Physiology/Pathogenesis

Gadolinium Based Contrast Agents

The development of NSF requires: (1) GBCA exposure in the setting of (2) reduced renal function. In its ionic form, Gd^{3+} is a known toxin due to its ability to block voltage-gated calcium channels [21]. The high number of unpaired electrons in Gd^{3+} has the advantage of modifying proton relaxation time, a parameter that made it an ideal magnetic resonance imaging (MRI) contrast agent, providing the toxicity could be avoided [21]. Binding the Gd^{3+} to an organic ligand (chelate) seemed to enable the safe use of Gd in this context [9, 22]. Chelated gadolinium was initially believed to be safe for use in all patients, even those with kidney disease, and provided an alternative to nephrotoxic iodine-based contrast agents [11]. The tight bond between Gd and its ligand, and the relatively short half-life of GBCAs in healthy individuals, made these agents safe for use in imaging studies [9]. As a result, the FDA approved GBCAs for use as a contrast agent in MRI studies. However, because GBCAs were considered to have such a high safety profile, these agents were also routinely employed in MRA, an off-label use that required dosing at 2–3 times the FDA approved dosage for routine MRI examinations [23].

Nine GBCAs are currently available (Fig. 12.5), all of which are approved for use in the United States (Table 12.1) [24]. Following the initial publications linking gadolinium exposure to NSF and subsequent observations that suggested breakdown of the gadolinium-chelate complex (dechelation) might be partly to blame, additional studies began to focus on prolonged GBCA stability [9, 10, 24–26]. The risk for developing NSF is highest among patients who had received one of the three high-risk linear GBCAs, with essentially no or extremely rare verified cases of NSF following the use of the more stable macrocyclic agents, implicating a key role for stability of GBCAs in the pathogenesis of NSF [24].

Currently available GBCAs enclose a single Gd atom within a proprietary organic ligand in either a linear or macrocyclic arrangement. Macrocyclic chelates enclose the Gd atom within a carbon ring. This arrangement confers stability, as multiple bonds must be broken simultaneously in order to release ionic gadolinium. Conversely, linear chelates wrap around the gadolinium atom, and can be sequentially unzipped from Gd by breaking single bonds. Both linear and

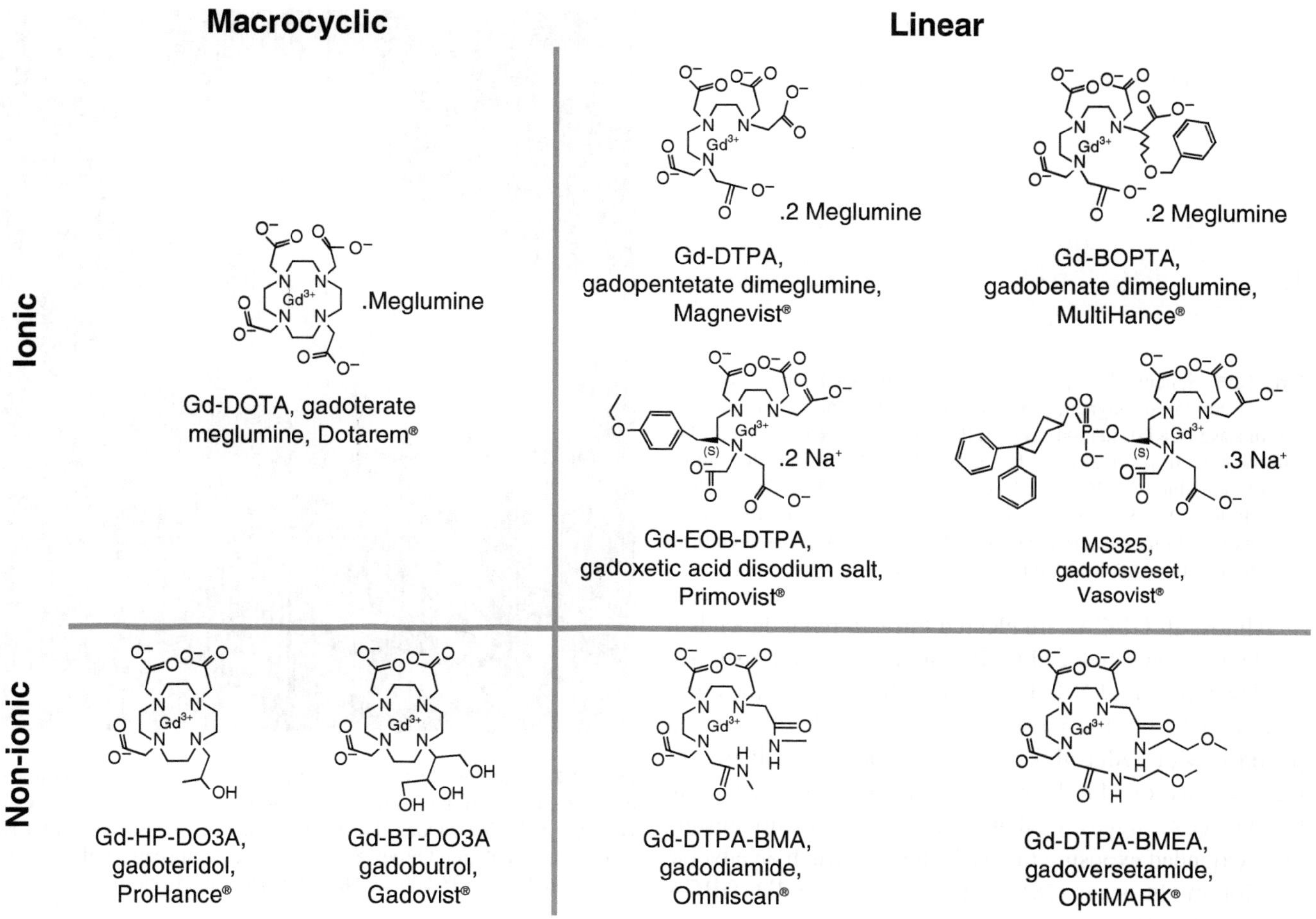

Fig. 12.5 Chemical structures of available GBCAs. (Reprinted from Radiologic clinics of North America, Vol 47(5), Idée JM, Port M, Dencausse A, Lancelot E, Corot C. Involvement of gadolinium chelates in the mechanism of nephrogenic systemic fibrosis: an update, Pages 855-69, 2009, with permission from Elsevier)

Table 12.1 Classification of GBCAs by structure and charge

Generic name	Trade name	Structure/charge
Gadodiamide	Omniscan™	Linear nonionic
Gadoversetamide	OptiMARK™	Linear nonionic
Gadofosveset trisodium	Ablavar®/Vasovist®	Linear ionic
Gadoxetic acid disodium	Eovist®/Primovist®	Linear ionic
Gadopentetate dimeglumine	Magnevist®	Linear ionic
Gadobenate dimeglumine	MultiHance®	Linear ionic
Gadobutrol	Gadovist®/Gadavist®	Macrocyclic nonionic
Gadoteridol	ProHance®	Macrocyclic nonionic
Gadoterate meglumine	Dotarem®	Macrocyclic ionic

(Adapted from Advances in Chronic Kidney Disease, Vol 18(3), Abu-Alfa AK. Nephrogenic systemic fibrosis and gadolinium-based contrast agents, Pages 188-98, 2011, with permission from Elsevier)

macrocyclic chelates can also be either "ionic" or "non-ionic," the latter generally regarded as being less stable [24].

Three GBCAs in particular have been implicated in the development of NSF: Gadodiamide (Omniscan™—GE Healthcare Inc., Princeton, NJ), gadopentetate dimeglumine (Magnevist®—Bayer Healthcare, Wayne, NJ), and gadoversetamide (OptiMARK™—Mallinckrodt, St. Louis, MO) [10, 24]. Of these three agents, two (gadodiamide and gadoversetamide) utilize a linear non-ionic chelate, and one (gadopentetate dimeglumine) utilizes a linear ionic chelate [10].

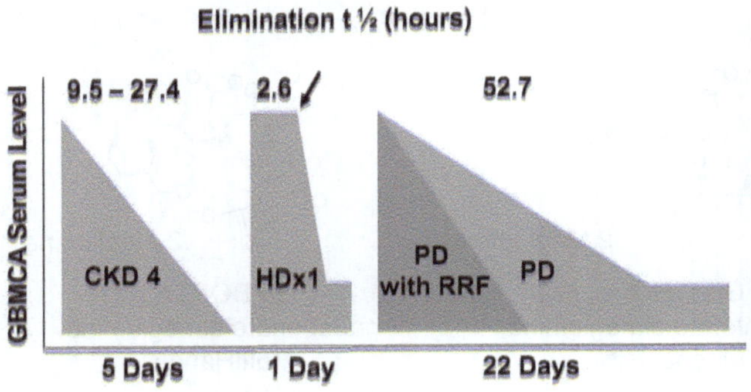

Fig. 12.6 Schematic representation of prolonged elimination of gadolinium-based magnetic resonance contrast agents in chronic kidney disease (CKD), hemodialysis (HD), and peritoneal dialysis (PD), with or without residual renal function (RRF). *Arrow* indicates initiation of hemodialysis. (Reprinted from Journal of the American College of Radiology, Vol 5(1), Abu-Alfa A. The impact of NSF on the care of patients with kidney disease, Pages 45-52, 2008, with permission from Elsevier and the American College of Radiology)

Almost all GBCAs are cleared through renal dependent mechanisms and reduced GFR is a known prerequisite for the development of NSF [27]. In healthy subjects, the elimination half-life for most GBCAs is 1.3 h ± 0.25 h. In patients with reduced kidney function, the half-life of GBCAs was found to be prolonged up to 34.3 h ± 22.9 h in CKD stage 4, suggesting that reduced renal function results in an extended exposure to GBCA during which an adverse reaction might occur [28]. In patients with ESRD, GBCA will only be cleared when dialysis is performed, and it can take up to four hemodialysis sessions for removal of one GBCA dose [28].

Although a majority of patients have developed NSF in the setting of ESRD, approximately 20 % of patients experience disease onset in the setting of AKI or CKD stages 4 or 5 [24]. A model for calculating risk in patients (Fig. 12.6) with varying levels of CKD has been developed, based upon an estimated risk of 2.4 % for developing NSF in ESRD patients exposed to a high risk GBCA. Utilizing estimated prevalence for CKD in the US and distribution of NSF among patients with various levels of kidney function based on reports in the literature, the model predicts that patients with CKD 4 have a 1 in 2,492 risk of developing NSF after exposure to GBCA. The risk for patients with CKD stage 3 drops to between 1 in 100,000 and 1 in 700,000, suggesting that a patient with CKD stage 3 who is exposed to a single dose of a stable GBCA is not at an increased risk for developing NSF [18, 24]. For patients with ESRD, peritoneal dialysis-dependent patients were found to be at a 7.5 % increased risk of developing NSF as compared to hemodialysis-dependent patients [6]. Finally, only 2–18 % of patients with reduced renal function who are exposed to GBCAs ultimately develop NSF, suggesting that additional factors contribute to the pathogenesis of this disease [24, 26, 29–33].

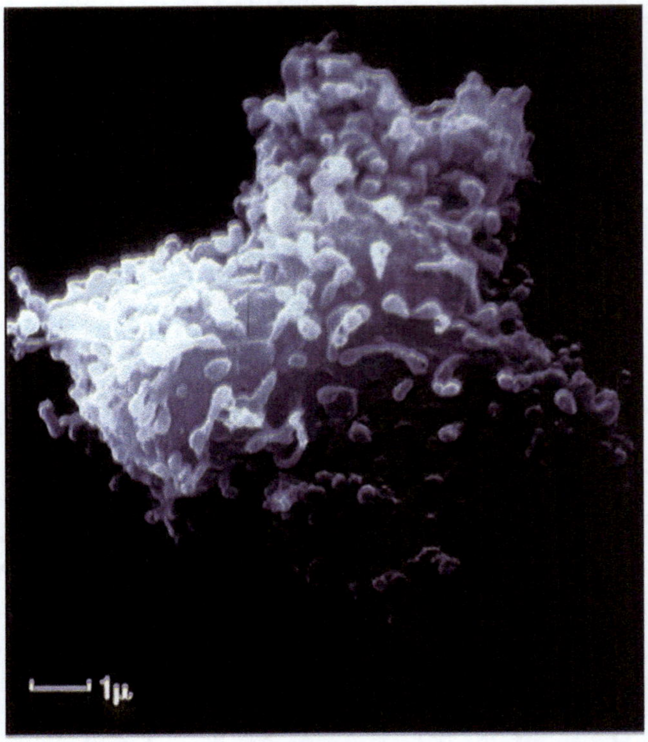

Fig. 12.7 Scanning electron micrograph of a human circulating fibrocyte. (Reprinted from the International Journal of Biochemistry & Cell Biology, Vol 36(4), Quan TE, Cowper S, Wu SP, Bockenstedt LK, Bucala R. Circulating fibrocytes: collagen-secreting cells of the peripheral blood, Pages 598-606, 2004, with permission from Elsevier)

Circulating Fibrocytes

In 2003, circulating fibrocytes (CF) were identified as the likely effector cells in NSF [34]. CFs were first described in 1994 as a subpopulation of circulating leukocytes (Fig. 12.7) with the ability to differentiate into fibroblast-like cells to facilitate wound repair at the local level [35]. However, in addition to normal wound repair, CFs have also been implicated in the propagation of several fibrosing conditions [36]. In 2003, the observation that the spindle-shaped cells seen in biopsies from patients with NSF stained for both CD34 and procollagen I (Fig. 12.8) led to the hypothesis that aberrant CF activity was to blame [34, 36]. Why this population of cells was emerging from the circulation and homing to the particular sites of fibrosis in NSF was unclear [34].

Shortly after the epidemiologic link between GBCAs and NSF was identified, a cell culture study by Edward et al. explored some of the key differences between NSF and control fibroblasts as well as the effects of gadolinium on fibroblast function [37]. The study showed that fibroblasts from patients with NSF demonstrated higher levels of hyaluronan and collagen production than those from controls. Additionally, control fibroblasts demonstrated increased production of these matrix materials after exposure to the serum of patients with NSF. Finally, when control fibroblasts were exposed to gadodiamide itself, they were shown to have increased growth, matrix production, and an enhanced ability to differentiate into myofibroblasts [37]. Additional studies confirmed the stimulatory role of gadolinium on the proliferation of fibroblasts [38] and the in vitro pro-fibrotic activity of the gadolinium-chelate complex [39].

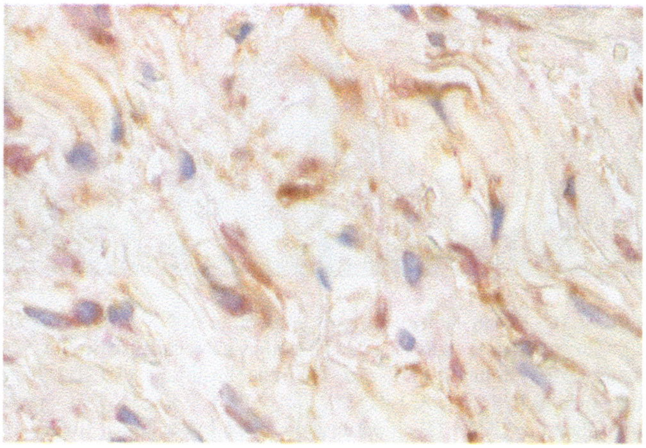

Fig. 12.8 Double immunoperoxidase staining for CD34 (*brown*) and procollagen (*red*) shows staining for CD34 is most marked along the dendritic processes while that for procollagen is localized to the cytoplasm. (From Cowper SE, Bucala R. Nephrogenic fibrosing dermopathy: suspect identified, motive unclear. American Journal of Dermatopathology 25(4), Page 358, 2003. Reprinted with permission)

Animal Studies

To date, most of the animal studies of NSF were planned and executed by contrast manufacturers. Until recently, these depended on a sub-totally nephrectomized rat model [22, 40–43]. However, this model did not fully capture the clinical picture present in NSF. A subtotal nephrectomy leaves the animal with a diminished GFR (as compared to an absent GFR in ESRD patients) and is not accompanied by the same degree of hyperphosphatemia typically observed in ESRD patients [22]. Nevertheless, these models were collectively able to demonstrate that the GBCA gadodiamide was capable of producing histopathological changes in the 5/6 nephrectomized animals similar to those found in human patients with NSF (Fig. 12.9) [44]. Additionally, deposition of gadolinium in the skin of these animals was measured and found to be highest for animals dosed with gadodiamide and other linear agents, when compared to levels found in animals exposed to macrocyclic agents [22].

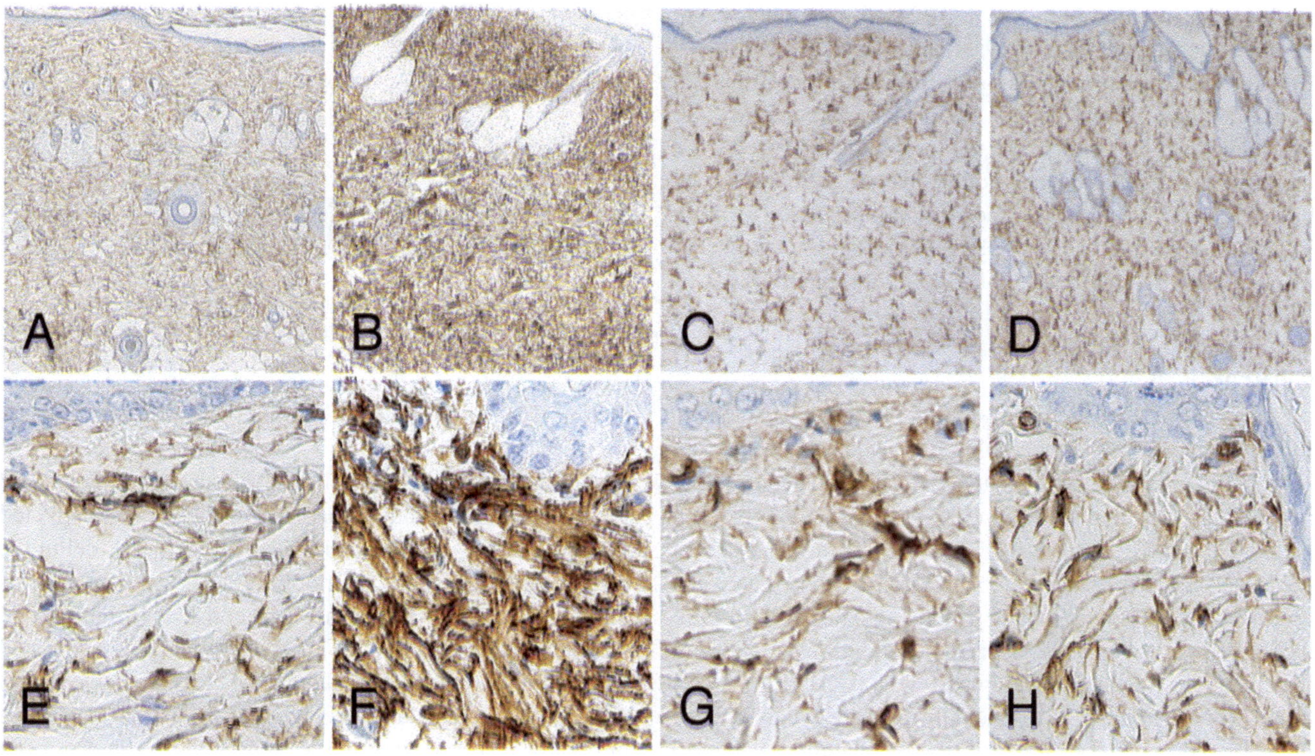

Fig. 12.9 Microscopic skin findings in rats after final administration of each agent. High-magnification images show strong diffuse CD34-positivity among spindle cells of the dermis in the gadodiamide group (**b, f**). Column 1: control, Column 2: gadodiamide, Column 3: gadoxetate sodium, Column 4: Gadoteridol. (Images **a–d** ×50 magnification, Images **e–h** ×400 magnification). (Reprinted from Magnetic Resonance Imaging, Vol 31(8), Sato T, Ito K, Tamada T, Kanki A, Watanabe S, Nishimura H, Tanimoto D, Higashi H, Yamamoto A. Tissue gadolinium deposition in renally impaired rats exposed to different gadolinium-based MRI contrast agents: evaluation with inductively coupled plasma mass spectrometry (ICP-MS), Pages 1412-7, 2013, with permission from Elsevier)

More recently, Fretellier et al. have been able to achieve a more accurate rat model replication of NSF pathology [22]. This group's model utilized rats on an adenine-enriched diet for 8, 14, or 16 days to produce differing degrees of renal failure within the context of hyperphosphatemia. Rats with differing degrees of renal failure were then exposed to either gadodiamide or saline. Serial biopsies were obtained to allow for histologic examination and quantification of gadolinium within the tissue using inductively coupled plasma mass spectrometry. This trial demonstrated that rats with more severe kidney dysfunction had more severe profibrotic skin lesions and systemic toxicity. Additionally, rats that developed the most severe pathology were also found to have higher gadolinium levels by mass spectrometry than rats without cutaneous changes. Akin to humans, affected rats demonstrated overexpression of profibrotic cytokines including transforming growth factor beta-1 (TGF-β1) and tissue inhibitor of metalloproteinases-1 (TIMP-1) [22].

Another trial by this group examined the effects of exposing the rats with the greatest degree of kidney dysfunction to each of the available GBCAs. As opposed to the gadodiamide trial with differing degrees of renal compromise, these rats did not produce cutaneous changes, likely due to the high degree of toxicity and early mortality in this trial [22]. However, the authors were able to perform relaxometry studies that revealed that both linear GBCAs (gadodiamide and gadopentetate) underwent slow, gradual dechelation (defined by a release of the gadolinium ion from its organic chelate) in the adenine-induced renal failure rats. Conversely, all macrocyclic agents remained stable and did not produce a measurable degree of dechelation in vivo. To date, this model has most closely mimicked the pathologic process of NSF in vivo and provided additional insight into possible mechanisms at play behind the role of gadolinium in NSF [22].

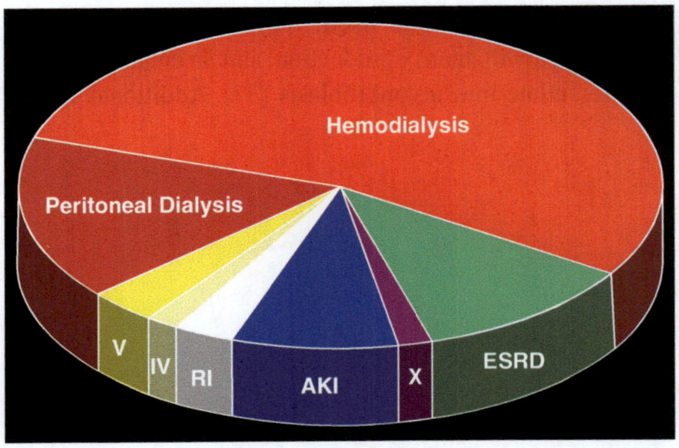

Fig. 12.10 Renal status of patients upon onset of NSF. Hemodialysis (52 %); peritoneal dialysis (16 %); end-stage renal disease (11 %); acute kidney injury (AKI) (10 %); renal insufficiency/CKD stage unknown (RI) (8 %); CKD stage IV (1.5 %); CKD stage V (3 %); post-transplant (X) (3 %). (With permission of the International Center for Nephrogenic Systemic Fibrosis Research (ICNSFR.org)). *ESRD* end-stage renal disease, *AKI* acute kidney injury

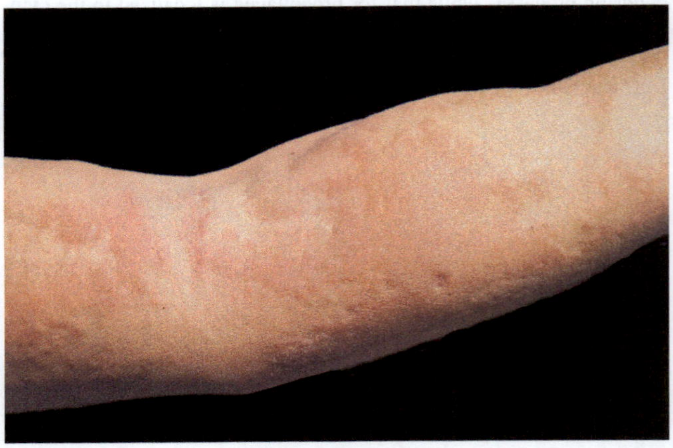

Fig. 12.11 The forearm of a patient manifesting the thickened, *brawny* plaques of NSF. The surface can appear "cobblestoned" or have a "peau d' orange" texture. (From Cowper SE, Su LD, Bhawan J, Robin HS, LeBoit PE. Nephrogenic fibrosing dermopathy. American Journal of Dermatopathology 23(5), Page 383-93, 2001. Reprinted with permission)

Clinical

In 2003, 6 years of demographic data were analyzed from Yale's International NSF registry to develop an epidemiologic profile for this disease [4]. The age range of NSF patients at disease onset is 8–87 years, with a mean age of 46.4 years [4]. No gender or racial predilections have been observed [4]. The majority of patients diagnosed with NSF have ESRD at the time of diagnosis [24]. However, approximately 20 % of patients develop NSF with CKD stages 4 or 5 or AKI (Fig. 12.10) [24]. Additionally, patients with NSF have an increased likelihood of: (1) hypercoagulability leading to clotting complications; (2) vascular surgical procedures in the weeks to months prior to NSF diagnosis; (3) and brain tumors. The currently accepted interpretation of these observations is that each is associated with magnetic resonance (MR) imaging or angiography that eventually leads to a GBCA exposure.

The earliest observable clinical effects of NSF include erythema, edema, and palpable warmth of the affected extremity, often leading clinicians to suspect cellulitis. Patients with NSF also commonly describe pain or pruritus in affected areas, and over time, joint complaints that include pain and stiffening. Almost all patients develop indurated plaques with a woody consistency (Fig. 12.11). These have a predilection for the distal extremities, with the legs more commonly involved than the arms. Induration and fibrosis adjacent to joints can become severe enough to produce irreversible contractures (Fig. 12.12). Many patients have deteriorated from being fully ambulatory to wheelchair-restricted within a few weeks to months. Other common findings include "cobblestoning," where the skin develops

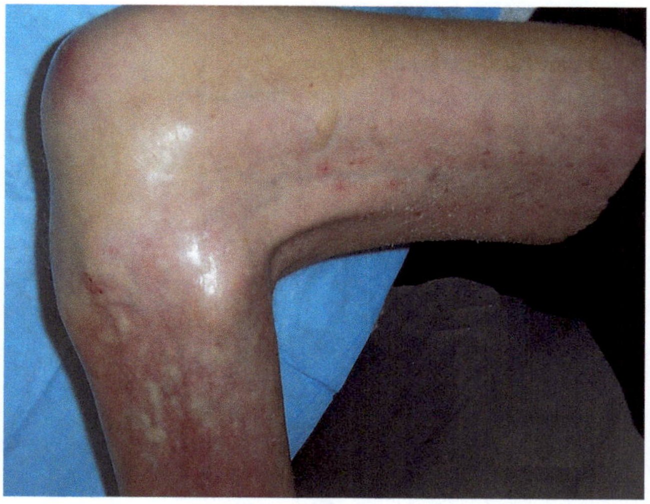

Fig. 12.12 In "end-stage NSF," the skin becomes fibrotic, and subcutaneous tissue is diminished. Contracture of the knee is illustrated. (Reprinted from Journal of the American College of Radiology, Vol 5(1), Girardi M. Nephrogenic systemic fibrosis: a dermatologist's perspective, Pages 40-4, 2008, with permission from Elsevier and the American College of Radiology)

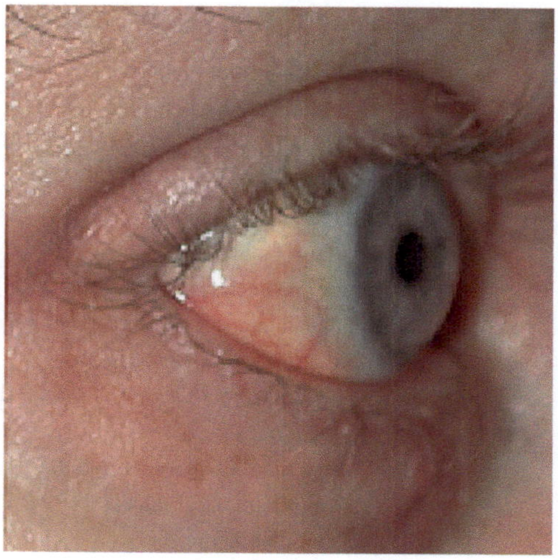

Fig. 12.13 Scleral plaques (minor criterion). There are new onset *white-yellow* scleral plaques with dilated capillary loops in a patient age <45 years. Over this age, the sign becomes less specific due to overlapping features with actinically induced pingueculae. (Reprinted from Journal of the American Academy of Dermatology, Vol 65(6), Girardi M, Kay J, Elston DM, Leboit PE, Abu-Alfa A, Cowper SE. Nephrogenic systemic fibrosis: clinicopathological definition and workup recommendations, Pages 1095-1106, 2011, with permission from Elsevier and the American Academy of Dermatology)

raised papules over an area of induration visually resembling a cobblestoned sidewalk, and "peau d'orange," wherein surface changes overlying deep cutaneous tethering come to resemble the texture of an orange peel [4, 27].

Cutaneous manifestations can also include puckering or linear banding, superficial plaques and/or patches, and dermal papules. Cutaneous manifestations only rarely involve the trunk or face [1, 4, 27]. Scleral plaques have been described in a number of patients with NSF (Fig. 12.13) [45]. Because patients with NSF can present with a constellation of symptoms, a diagnostic system combining major and minor clinical criteria has been established [27]. Clinical evaluation, however, is not sufficient to fully exclude competing clinical differentials (Table 12.2). All patients who present with clinical findings suggestive of NSF should undergo an incisional or deep punch biopsy of involved skin to obtain a specific diagnosis. A combination of clinical (Tables 12.3 and 12.4) and histopathological features (Table 12.5) informed by concurrent historical and laboratory evaluation (Table 12.6), should accurately identify most putative cases of NSF.

Clinical Differential Diagnoses

A number of entities that have been identified as clinical mimics of NSF should be excluded (Table 12.2) prior to making a definitive diagnosis of NSF [27]. These include, but are not limited to:

1. *Lipodermatosclerosis (LDS) or chronic venous stasis*: In LDS, skin findings typically localize in a symmetric fashion to the lower extremities below the knees and classically consist of ruddy brown-red hyperpigmentation and indurated plaques. The lower legs may come to resemble the shape of inverted champagne bottles. Of note, joint contractures are absent in LDS and patients may present with varicosities in the lower extremities proximal to areas of induration [27].
2. *Scleromyxedema (SCX) (lichen myxedematosus)*: SCX patients present with multiple, small (2–3 mm), firm, grouped papules, often with a linear distribution on the hands, arms, upper trunk, neck, and/or face. Patients with SCX may also demonstrate glabellar furrowing. Of note, the distribution of cutaneous involvement can be a useful feature in distinguishing between SCX and NSF as the latter typically spares the face, neck, and trunk [27].
3. *Scleroderma (systemic sclerosis-SS)*: SS can manifest in either its limited form, with cutaneous involvement exclusive to the face and hands, or its diffuse form, with additional involvement of the trunk and proximal extremities. Clinically, patients present with multiple findings including (1) diffuse hyperpigmentation or salt/pepper dyspigmentation (characterized by areas of hypopigmentation with retention of pigment surrounding hair follicles) of the forehead or in a shawl distribution on the upper back; (2) sclerodactyly; (3) induration of the trunk and/or face with a decreased oral aperture; (4) dilated capillary loops in a periungual distribution; and (5) Raynaud phenomenon (characterized by color changes

Table 12.2 NSF: clinical and histopathological differential diagnoses

Clinical differential diagnoses	Histopathological differential diagnoses
Lipodermatosclerosis/chronic venous stasis	Lipodermatosclerosis/chronic venous stasis
Scleromyxedema	Scleromyxedema
Eosinophilic fasciitis	Eosinophilic fasciitis
Scleroderma (systemic sclerosis)	Morphea/scleroderma
Scleredema diabeticorum	Scleredema diabeticorum
Porphyria cutanea tarda (sclerodermoid)	Eosinophilia-myalgia syndrome
Morphea/Lichen sclerosus et atrophicus	Lipodermatosclerosis
Chronic graft-versus-host disease	Chronic graft-versus-host disease
Stiff skin syndrome/congenital fascial dystrophy	Stiff skin syndrome/congenital fascial dystrophy
Diabetic digital sclerosis	Septal panniculitis
Pruritus of renal disease/neuropathy	Pseudoxanthoma elasticum
β_2-microglobulin amyloidosis	Calciphylaxis
Dupuytren contracture	Dermatofibrosarcoma protuberans

Adapted from Journal of the American Academy of Dermatology, Vol 65(6), Girardi M, Kay J, Elston DM, Leboit PE, Abu-Alfa A, Cowper SE. Nephrogenic systemic fibrosis: clinicopathological definition and workup recommendations, Pages 1095-1106, 2011, with permission from Elsevier and the American Academy of Dermatology

Table 12.3 Clinical criteria, scoring summary

Major criteria	Minor criteria
Patterned plaques	Puckering/linear banding
Joint contractures	Superficial plaque/patch
"Cobblestoning"	Dermal papules
Marked induration/"Peau d'orange"	Scleral plaques (only if $<$ age 45 years)

Adapted from Journal of the American Academy of Dermatology, Vol 65(6), Girardi M, Kay J, Elston DM, Leboit PE, Abu-Alfa A, Cowper SE. Nephrogenic systemic fibrosis: clinicopathological definition and workup recommendations, Pages 1095-1106, 2011, with permission from Elsevier and the American Academy of Dermatology

Table 12.4 Determining the clinical score (refer to Table 12.3)

Score	Scenario	Clinical interpretation
4	More than one major criterion	Highly consistent with NSF
3	One major criterion	Consistent with NSF
2	More than one minor criterion	Suggestive of NSF
1	One or no minor criteria	Inconsistent with NSF
0	Diagnostic of another entity	NSF excluded

Adapted from Journal of the American Academy of Dermatology, Vol 65(6), Girardi M, Kay J, Elston DM, Leboit PE, Abu-Alfa A, Cowper SE. Nephrogenic systemic fibrosis: clinicopathological definition and workup recommendations, Pages 1095-1106, 2011, with permission from Elsevier and the American Academy of Dermatology

NSF nephrogenic systemic fibrosis

of the distal fingers triggered by vasospasm). Of note, as with SCX, lesions of SS have a distribution that is distinct from NSF. Clinicians should use caution when distinguishing sclerodactyly from the joint contractures typical of NSF [27].

4. *Scleredema diabeticorum*: Patients with scleredema diabeticorum have a history of diabetes mellitus and present with thickened plaques and areas of induration over their upper back and neck. Again, this would be an unusual distribution for NSF [27].

5. *Morphea/lichen sclerosus et atrophicus*: Patients present with paucilesional, asymmetrically distributed, dyspigmented, indurated plaques. Generally plaques are arranged in a linear fashion. The distribution of morphea or lichen sclerosus et atrophicus is generally more limited and asymmetric than that of NSF [27].
6. *Chronic graft-versus-host disease*: Patients present with lichenoid papules and erosive-indurated plaques with truncal predominance. This disorder can only occur in those who have received a prior allogeneic bone marrow or stem cell transplant [27].
7. *Dupuytren contracture*: Patients present with subcutaneous bands of fibrosis on the palms resulting in contractures of the fingers and hands. Lesions are confined to the hands and tend to develop over a course of years [27].
8. *Pruritus of renal disease/neuropathy*: Patients present with generalized erosions/ulcers secondary to chronic scratching [27].
9. *β2-microglobulin amyloidosis*: Patients present with subcutaneous masses around the shoulders, palms, and wrists without cutaneous involvement [27].

Table 12.5 Determining the histopathological score

Score	Histological interpretation
4 or 5	Highly consistent with NSF
3	Consistent with NSF
2	Suggestive of NSF
1	Inconsistent with NSF
0	NSF excluded (Diagnostic of another entity)

Adapted from Journal of the American Academy of Dermatology, Vol 65(6), Girardi M, Kay J, Elston DM, Leboit PE, Abu-Alfa A, Cowper SE. Nephrogenic systemic fibrosis: clinicopathological definition and workup recommendations, Pages 1095-1106, 2011, with permission from Elsevier and the American Academy of Dermatology

Increased dermal cellularity, thick and thin collagen fibers, septal involvement, and CD34 positivity in a tram-track pattern receive a score of +1 for each feature present. Osseous metaplasia (lollipop bodies) receives a score of +3 if present. This *weighted* score reflects the more specific nature of this finding. Preserved elastic tissue results in no net change in score. If elastic tissue is absent or reduced, the score is *reduced* by 1

NSF nephrogenic systemic fibrosis

Histology

Because NSF can only be confidently diagnosed by clinicopathological correlation, biopsies must be obtained from all suspected cases. The cutaneous pathology of NSF extends from the dermis into the subcutaneous fat. Thus, an incisional or deep punch biopsy is essential. In addition, because samples collected from below the knee may be challenging to fully differentiate from LDS, the greatest diagnostic certainty will be obtained in specimens collected above this level. Lastly, biopsy material should be evaluated by a dermatopathologist utilizing published clinicopathological criteria.

Histopathologically, NSF is characterized by a proliferation of bland dermal spindle cells associated with variable numbers of epithelioid cells (Fig. 12.14). The increased cellularity is seen in combination with thickened collagen bundles surrounded by clefts, often with an increased number of thin collagen fibers (Fig. 12.15) [1]. These findings often extend into the subcutaneous fat along septa and can sometimes be limited to this area (Fig. 12.16). Encroachment on fat lobules is common. Elastic fibers are preserved and can be readily identified with stains specific for elastic tissue [2]. The epithelioid cells, which are usually the less dominant cell type, are CD68+ and show histological features commonly seen in histiocytes. Typically, biopsies show a paucity of other inflammatory cells [27].

Table 12.6 NSF clinical assessment: laboratory investigation

All cases: eGFR at time of symptom onset	Use MDRD formula unless clinically inappropriate or patient already on dialysis (see text)
Differential diagnosis under consideration	*Consider performing these tests if suggested by physical exam and/or history*
Lipodermatosclerosis/chronic venous stasis	Venous duplex ultrasound with reflux testing
Scleromyxedema (lichen myxedematosus)	SPEP and serum IF or immunoelectrophoresis (IF/IEP) for monoclonal gammopathy
Eosinophilic fasciitis	CBC and WBC differential count, absolute eosinophil count
Scleroderma/morphea	ANA titer and pattern, including anti-centromere antibodies; anti-topoisomerase 1 (SCL-70) antibodies
Pruritus of renal disease/neuropathy	EMG
Sclerodermoid porphyria cutanea tarda	Quantitation of uroporphyrinogen I in the urine; in anuric patients, stool isocoproporphyrin III and plasma uroporphyrin levels

Adapted from Journal of the American Academy of Dermatology, Vol 65(6), Girardi M, Kay J, Elston DM, Leboit PE, Abu-Alfa A, Cowper SE. Nephrogenic systemic fibrosis: clinicopathological definition and workup recommendations, Pages 1095-1106, 2011, with permission from Elsevier and the American Academy of Dermatology

Legend: Several disorders enter into the clinical differential diagnosis of NSF. As noted on line 1, all cases of potential NSF should have an eGFR calculated at the time of symptom onset. The remaining listed clinical differentials have specific laboratory studies that may be helpful in verifying or excluding the diagnosis of NSF

ANA antinuclear antibody, *CBC* complete blood count, *eGFR* estimated glomerular filtration rate, *EMG* electromyogram, *IEP* immunoelectrophoresis, *IF* immunofixation, *MDRD* modification of diet in renal disease, *SPEP* serum protein electrophoresis, *WBC* white blood count

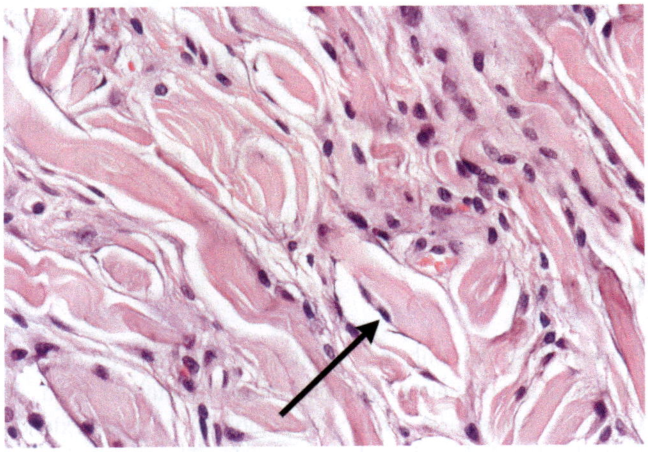

Fig. 12.14 H&E-stained section showing increased dermal cellularity with thickened collagen bundles with surrounding clefts. Spindled cells with hyperchromatic nuclei can be seen closely apposed to collagen bundles (*arrow*). Larger epithelioid cells with oval nuclei are arrayed between the collagen bundles. (From Cowper SE, Su LD, Bhawan J, Robin HS, LeBoit PE. Nephrogenic fibrosing dermopathy. American Journal of Dermatopathology 23(5), Page 383-93, 2001. Reprinted with permission)

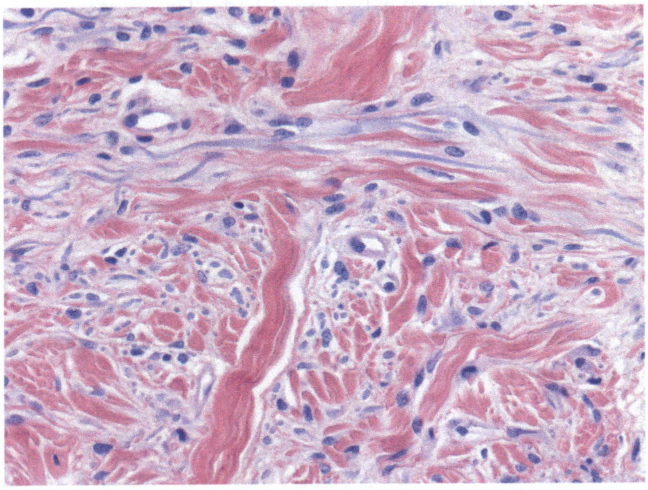

Fig. 12.15 Thick and thin collagen bundles and elastic fibers. The presence of normal elastic, seen here as *gray blue* fibers parallel to *pink* collagen fibers, does not affect the overall histological score. Elastic fibers only affect histological scoring when absent (score −1 if absent). (H&E stain; original magnification: ×100) (Reprinted from Journal of the American Academy of Dermatology, Vol 65(6), Girardi M, Kay J, Elston DM, Leboit PE, Abu-Alfa A, Cowper SE. Nephrogenic systemic fibrosis: clinicopathological definition and workup recommendations, Pages 1095-1106, 2011, with permission from Elsevier and the American Academy of Dermatology)

The spindle cells observed in NSF show dual immunohistochemical expression for procollagen I and CD34 (Fig. 12.8), a pattern identical to that seen in bone marrow derived "circulating fibrocytes" (CFs) [34]. The procollagen I expression localizes to the cytoplasm, whereas the CD34 expression is membranous, most prominently identified along extremely thin dendritic processes [34]. Dermal CFs are typically arranged parallel to the epidermis, with CD34+ dendritic processes extending along elastic fibers. This pattern of parallel dendritic staining is known as "tram-tracking." (Fig. 12.17) [27].

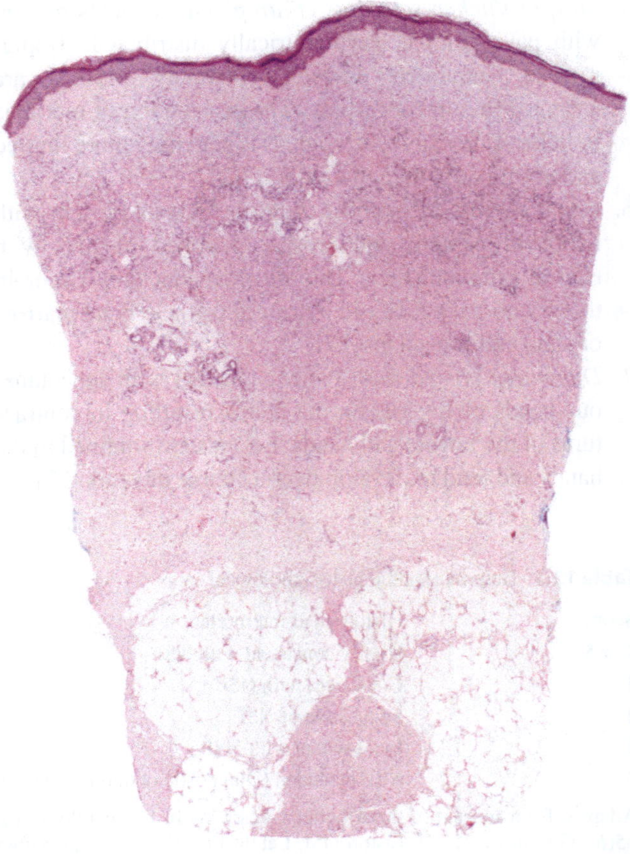

Fig. 12.16 At scanning magnification, a marked increase in dermal spindle cells is associated with thickened collagen bundles in the reticular dermis. The process extends through the subcutis along thickened septa. There is no inflammatory infiltrate. (From Cowper SE, Su LD, Bhawan J, Robin HS, LeBoit PE. Nephrogenic fibrosing dermopathy. American Journal of Dermatopathology 23(5), Page 383-93, 2001. Reprinted with permission)

The persistent pattern of CD34 expression, together with an absence of inflammatory cells and preservation of elastic and collagen clefts, distinguishes NSF from morphea and SS. CD34 expression in a pattern identical to NSF can be seen in SCX, although in that condition findings are confined to the dermis (illustrating why a deep subcutaneous biopsy is crucial in these cases). Lesional distribution and protein electrophoresis are helpful in reaching a definitive diagnosis in this challenging histological differential.

In 2009, "sclerotic bodies" were first described as a histologic finding in NSF [46]. A presentation in 2011 proposed the term "lollipop bodies" to illustrate their characteristic appearance [47]. These round to ovoid eosinophilic bodies are bordered by a single layer of bland matrix producing cells and pierced by

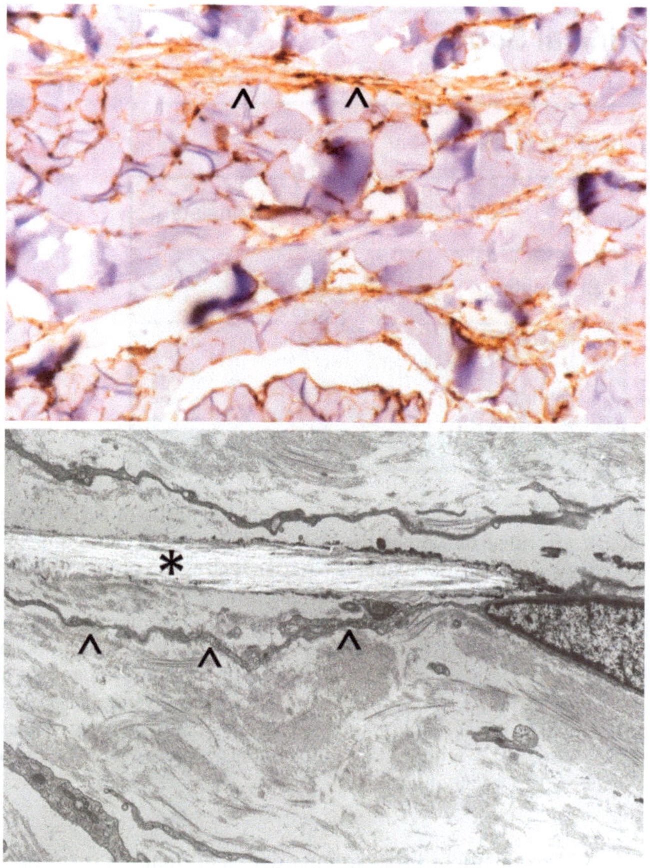

Fig. 12.17 (*Top*) CD-34 positive dendritic processes (*arrowheads*) closely apposed to elastic fibers. The dendritic processes also encircle bundles of collagen. (*Bottom*) An electron micrograph illustrates an elastic fiber (*asterisk*) with dendritic processes (*arrowheads*) running above and below in a parallel arrangement. (From Cowper SE, Su LD, Bhawan J, Robin HS, LeBoit PE. Nephrogenic fibrosing dermopathy. American Journal of Dermatopathology 23(5), Page 383-93, 2001. Reprinted with permission)

one or more elastic fibers—giving lollipop bodies their pathognomonic appearance (Fig. 12.18) [47, 48]. The eosinophilic, hyalinized matrix comprising the solid part of the structure stains identically to collagen by trichrome methods, and the enveloping flattened cells resemble osteoblasts, leading to the hypothesis that lollipop bodies represent non-mineralized osteoid forming around an elastic nidus. Lollipop bodies can be found in both the reticular dermis and subcutaneous tissue in patients with NSF, however, most of these lesions cluster within the reticular dermis [47]. These bodies, until recently thought to be specific for NSF, have been described in a single patient with renal failure and GBCA exposure that did not have clinical NSF [49]. A review of slides from 309 NSF patients found lollipop bodies in 16 cases, yielding a 5 % sensitivity [47].

A histopathological scoring system has been devised to facilitate accurate diagnosis. This system assigns one point for the presence of each of the findings characteristic of NSF described above, and a more highly weighted three points for the more specific finding of lollipop bodies (Table 12.5).

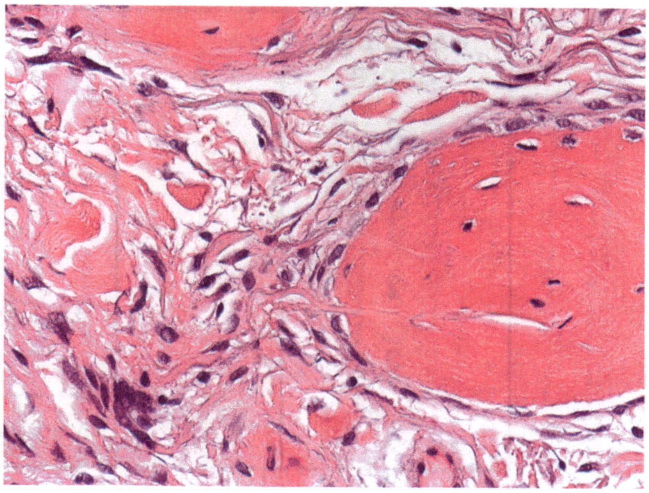

Fig. 12.18 Osseous metaplasia (Lollipop bodies). Non-mineralized osseous tissue forms around elastic fibers, some of which protrude beyond the zone of ossification. If this highly specific feature is noted, the histological score should be increased by 3. (H&E stain; original magnification: ×400.) (Reprinted from Journal of the American Academy of Dermatology, Vol 65(6), Girardi M, Kay J, Elston DM, Leboit PE, Abu-Alfa A, Cowper SE. Nephrogenic systemic fibrosis: clinicopathological definition and workup recommendations, Pages 1095-1106, 2011, with permission from Elsevier and the American Academy of Dermatology)

Neither the histopathologic nor clinical findings alone are sufficiently characteristic to diagnose NSF and exclude competing differentials [27]. An NSF clinicopathological definition (Fig. 12.19) which combines histopathologic and clinical criteria has been developed and should inform the work up and diagnosis of patients with suspected NSF [27].

Laboratory Abnormalities

Laboratory evaluation in NSF is mostly limited to excluding competing differentials. It can also be helpful in determining a patient's renal status at the time of NSF onset. Renal evaluation would include the blood urea nitrogen (BUN) and creatinine levels—the latter is also used to calculate the eGFR. If a GBCA exposure can be documented in the 2–6 weeks prior to NSF onset, the brand of contrast used, the dose administered, and the eGFR at the time of exposure are especially helpful. If the patient is known to be in ESRD, focus should be placed on documenting the patient's disease state at the time of exposure or diagnosis, including the mode of dialysis, and the dialysis schedule and duration. Because occasional patients with AKI have developed NSF after exposure to GBCAs, normal renal function at the time of NSF workup does not rule out a diagnosis of NSF. Patients without CKD/ESRD or AKI who present with findings suggestive of NSF are extremely rare, and should be carefully evaluated by physicians with expertise in diagnosing NSF.

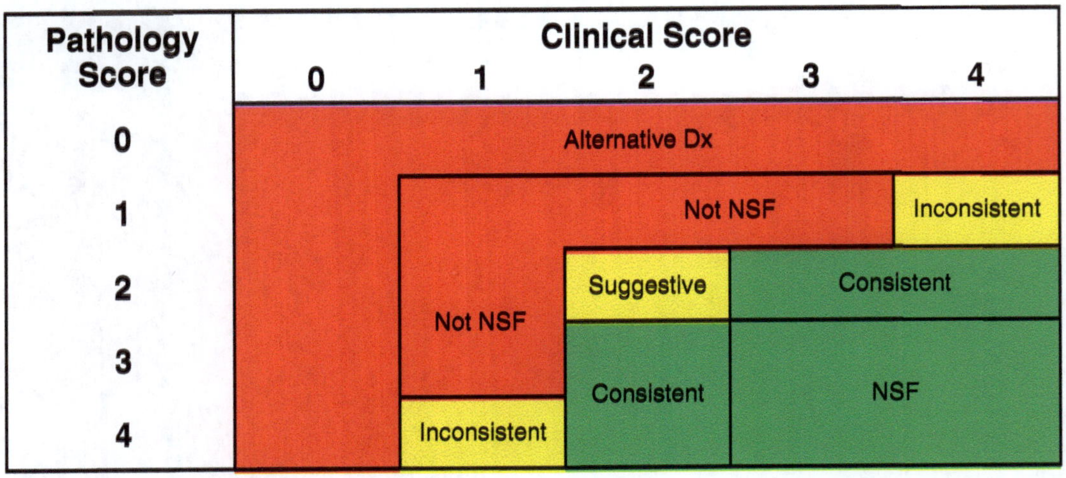

Fig. 12.19 Diagnosis and reporting grid. Clinical and histologic scoring: the clinical score (0–4) is derived from major and minor clinical criteria listed in Table 12.3. The histologic score (0–4) is derived from criteria listed in Table 12.4. Using the grid: clinical score is located across *top row of grid*, whereas histologic score is located along left vertical column. Intersection of these two values within the chart results in one of six diagnostic possibilities. For epidemiologic purposes, those in *green* should be scored as confirmed nephrogenic systemic fibrosis (NSF) cases. Those in *yellow* should be closely re-examined and perhaps re-biopsied. Until more compelling evidence is obtained, these will not have satisfied criteria for NSF and should be considered non-diagnostic of NSF. Those in *red* are ruled out either for lack of criteria or because another diagnosis can be made. Examples of case scoring are provided in the source article, including two important clinical scenarios: NSF with an absence of documentable renal disease and postmortem evaluation of suspected NSF. (Reprinted from Journal of the American Academy of Dermatology, Vol 65(6), Girardi M, Kay J, Elston DM, Leboit PE, Abu-Alfa A, Cowper SE. Nephrogenic systemic fibrosis: clinicopathological definition and workup recommendations, Pages 1095-1106, 2011, with permission from Elsevier and the American Academy of Dermatology)

Important laboratory information that may assist in excluding competing differentials is listed in Table 12.6. For patients with symptoms confined to the lower extremities, particularly below the knees, a venous duplex ultrasound with reflux testing can be considered to help differentiate NSF from LDS or chronic venous stasis [50].

Serum protein electrophoresis (SPEP) and immunofixation or immunoelectrophoresis (IF/IEP) and free light chain measurements are useful parameters to detect a monoclonal gammopathy. Approximately 80 % of patients with SCX will present with a monoclonal gammopathy, often of the IgG-lambda subtype [51]. Conversely, serum from patients with NSF has not been shown to demonstrate abnormal paraproteins.

A white blood cell count with differential can be useful if eosinophilic fasciitis is being considered. Patients with eosinophilic fasciitis will often demonstrate peripheral eosinophilia—a finding not typically observed in NSF [52]. Serological autoantibody abnormalities may accompany scleroderma, morphea, and mixed connective tissue disease, including antinuclear antibody (ANA), anti-histone antibodies, anti-double stranded deoxyribonucleic acid (DNA) antibodies, anti-centromere antibodies, and anti-topoisomerase 1 (Scl-70) antibodies [53, 54]. To date, no autoantibodies have been described in patients with NSF with the exception of those who have another documented illness, such as lupus erythematosus.

Scleredema diabeticorum occurs in the setting of diabetes mellitus. Thus, fasting glucose and/or hemoglobin A1c should be considered for patients with a clinical picture characteristic for this and not known to be diabetic [55]. Finally, patients with peripheral neuropathy as the etiology for peripheral pain or pruritus can present with abnormalities on electromyogram (EMG) studies [56].

Prevention

The key to preventing NSF is to avoid the use of a high risk GBCA in a patient at risk. While patients with ESRD are readily identifiable because of their dialysis-dependence, identifying patients with CKD or AKI can present a particular challenge, especially in the outpatient and emergency settings. As screening questionnaires to identify asymptomatic renal disease may miss a significant number of at risk patients [57, 58], specific point of care (POC) tests for creatinine and eGFR have been adopted at some centers [57, 58]. Currently the FDA mandates screening for renal disease prior to exposing patients to GBCAs. For those deemed to be at risk for kidney disease because of age or other comorbidities, laboratory testing is required.

In general, GBCAs should be avoided in patients with AKI, ESRD, and stages 4 or 5 CKD. In cases where GBCA-enhanced imaging is desired in an at-risk patient, physicians must conduct a risk–benefit analysis that considers the following questions: (1) Are alternative imaging options available? (2) Is there morbidity associated with not pursuing contrast enhanced MRI study, including missing important diagnostic information? (3) What is the risk of contrast induced nephropathy if conventional radiology with iodinated contrast is pursued as an alternative? Ideally, this decision should involve the patient, the primary physician, the nephrologist, and the radiologist. If a GBCA-enhanced MR study is judged to be the best diagnostic imaging test, the radiologist should avoid administering contraindicated high-risk GBCAs (Omniscan™, Magnevist®, OptiMARK™). In such cases, macrocyclic GBCAs may be a safer alternative. Additionally, dosing of GBCAs for patients with a reduced GFR should not exceed 0.1 mmol/kg. Finally, repeat dosing within a short period of time should be avoided whenever possible.

Although there are no supporting studies, hemodialysis within 2 h of exposure would be judicious in at risk ESRD and possibly AKI patients following the administration of GBCAs [24]. Additionally, all patients with renal disease should be monitored for the development of signs and symptoms of NSF following exposure to GBCAs. Although no GBCA has been deemed "safe" for use in patients with AKI, CKD 4 or 5, or ESRD, the above guidelines can help to minimize the overall risk of NSF in patients with a reduced GFR. As NSF becomes a remote memory, it will be important for physicians to periodically reinforce the need for these guidelines to prevent the re-emergence of NSF in years to come.

Treatment and Prognosis

To date there is no "cure" once a patient has developed NSF. Virtually every published treatment study is small, uncontrolled, and retrospective. The most promising treatment strategies surround improving renal function. One group described the course of two different patients with NSF upon improvement in their kidney function [59, 60]. In this case series, one hemodialysis patient developed NSF that improved clinically following a recovery of renal function, despite persistent histopathologic features of NSF in her clinically normal-appearing skin [59]. Another patient improved clinically following a successful living-related kidney transplant [59]. These cases, as well as the unpublished experiences of many investigators, directly link improved renal function to NSF resolution despite the mixed and incomplete results described in the published literature [25, 61]. For patients with ESRD, transplantation early in the course of NSF may be the best option for delaying disease progression by circumventing the irreversible deposition of collagen.

In light of current theories about NSF onset, limiting the exposure time to administered gadolinium would seem to be a prudent strategy for avoiding NSF. Although no supporting data have been developed to date, dialysis within 2 hours of GBCA administration is still recommended for patients with reduced renal function who cannot avoid exposure [15, 24]. The practical application of this strategy varies depending on the severity of renal dysfunction, the stability of the contrast agent used, and the dialysis status of the patient [24]. The decision regarding whether or not to initiate dialysis following GBCA exposure should be individualized [24].

Because of the high degree of morbidity [62] caused by the immobility associated with NSF, a critical first line treatment is physical therapy. One study described two patients, who, with the assistance of 4–12 weeks of physical therapy (in addition to ongoing treatment with imitanib) showed improvements in range of motion and strength that translated into diminished functional impairments. Specific interventions were tailored to the individual, but included aggressive range-of-motion exercises, ultrasound, dynamic splinting, strength training, occupational therapy, and functional training [63]. The attractiveness of physical therapy as an intervention is that it is readily available, can be used in concert with other interventions, has proven benefit, and has no significant side effects. Unfortunately, very little is currently published on the optimal use of this promising intervention.

With the successful avoidance of new cases of NSF, the likelihood of future prospective clinical trials in this mysterious disease is rapidly shrinking. There have been numerous single case studies, as well as several small trials, but virtually all therapeutic studies suffer from having small case numbers, or being retrospective, non-blinded or confounded (in some cases all four)! Because an in-depth discussion of these numerous empirical interventions is beyond the scope of this chapter, the interested reader is referred to the medical literature for further information. Some of the interventions to be found there are listed in Table 12.7. One note of caution, however, is that, as noted above, improving renal function, by itself, can lead to clinical improvement in NSF. When evaluating any therapeutic claims, the reader should carefully consider the patient's concurrent underlying renal function to critically assess whether any clinical improvement is truly attributable to the agent under study.

To date, NSF has proven to be a progressive disease with a lack of effective treatment options. Progressive fibrosis leading to joint contractures produces a significant degree of morbidity. A case series following ten patients noted that eight patients were wheelchair-bound within 1 year of diagnosis secondary to limited joint mobility produced by joint contractures [62].

Conclusion

Although there has been a dramatic reduction in NSF incidence in recent years, a theoretical risk of resurgence exists should regulatory and/or preventative efforts wane as the memory of this disease grows distant. Physicians and public health professionals should maintain a heightened awareness for iatrogenic disease in patients with reduced kidney

Table 12.7 Therapeutic modalities that have been reported in the treatment of NSF

Renal transplantation	
Physical therapy	
Extracorporeal photopheresis	
Plasmapheresis (therapeutic plasma exchange)	
Imatinib mesylate	
Photodynamic therapy with methyl aminolevulinate	
Pentoxifylline	Sodium thiosulfate
UVA-1	PUVA
PUVA with retinoids	IVIG
Corticosteroids (topical, intralesional, and systemic)	
Methotrexate (systemic)	
Azathioprine	
Calcipotriene	
Alefacept	
Rapamycin	
Acetazolamide	

NSF nephrogenic systemic fibrosis, *UVA-1* ultraviolet A1, *PUVA* psoralen in conjunction with ultraviolet A, *IVIG* intravenous immunoglobulin

function who are given medications or agents that are primarily renally cleared. As technologically sophisticated treatment regimens expand into the developing world, this preventative strategy of avoidance and surveillance, as well as regulatory oversight, will need to keep pace.

References

1. Cowper SE, Robin HS, Steinberg SM, Su LD, Gupta S, LeBoit PE. Scleromyxoedema-like cutaneous diseases in renal-dialysis patients. Lancet. 2000;356(9234):1000–1. PubMed PMID: 11041404. Epub 2000/10/21. eng.
2. Cowper SE, Su LD, Bhawan J, Robin HS, LeBoit PE. Nephrogenic fibrosing dermopathy. Am J Dermatopathol. 2001;23(5):383–93. PubMed PMID: 11801769. Epub 2002/01/22. eng.
3. Ting WW, Stone MS, Madison KC, Kurtz K. Nephrogenic fibrosing dermopathy with systemic involvement. Arch Dermatol. 2003;139(7):903–6. PubMed PMID: 12873886.
4. Cowper SE. Nephrogenic fibrosing dermopathy: the first 6 years. Curr Opin Rheumatol. 2003;15(6):785–90. PubMed PMID: 14569211. Epub 2003/10/22. eng.
5. LeBoit PE. What nephrogenic fibrosing dermopathy might be. Arch Dermatol. 2003;139(7):928–30. PubMed PMID: 12873893.
6. Centers for Disease Control and Prevention. Nephrogenic fibrosing dermopathy associated with exposure to gadolinium-containing contrast agents—St. Louis, Missouri, 2002–2006. MMWR Morb Mortal Wkly Rep. 2007;56:137–41.
7. Cowper S. Nephrogenic fibrosing dermopathy: latest developments. New England Dermatological Society; October 1, 2005. New Haven, CT: Yale University; 2005.
8. Grobner T. Gadolinium—a specific trigger for the development of nephrogenic fibrosing dermopathy and nephrogenic systemic fibrosis? Nephrol Dial Transplant. 2006;21(4):1104–8. PubMed PMID: 16431890. Epub 2006/01/25. eng.
9. Marckmann P, Skov L, Rossen K, Dupont A, Damholt MB, Heaf JG, et al. Nephrogenic systemic fibrosis: suspected causative role of gadodiamide used for contrast-enhanced magnetic resonance imaging. J Am Soc Nephrol. 2006;17(9):2359–62. PubMed PMID: 16885403.
10. Thomsen HS, Morcos SK, Almen T, Bellin MF, Bertolotto M, Bongartz G, et al. Nephrogenic systemic fibrosis and gadolinium-based contrast media: updated ESUR Contrast Medium Safety Committee guidelines. Eur Radiol. 2013;23(2):307–18. PubMed PMID: 22865271.
11. Prince MR, Arnoldus C, Frisoli JK. Nephrotoxicity of high-dose gadolinium compared with iodinated contrast. J Magn Reson Imaging. 1996;6(1):162–6. PubMed PMID: 8851422.
12. Administration UFaD. Public Health Advisory—Gadolinium-containing Contrast Agents for Magnetic Resonance Imaging (MRI). 6/8/2006.
13. High WA, Ayers RA, Chandler J, Zito G, Cowper SE. Gadolinium is detectable within the tissue of patients with nephrogenic systemic fibrosis. J Am Acad Dermatol. 2007;56(1):21–6. PubMed PMID: 17097388.
14. High WA, Ayers RA, Cowper SE. Gadolinium is quantifiable within the tissue of patients with nephrogenic systemic fibrosis. J Am Acad Dermatol. 2007;56(4):710–2. PubMed PMID: 17289213. Epub 2007/02/10. eng.
15. Administration USFaD. FDA Drug Safety Communication: New warnings for using gadolinium-based contrast agents in patients with kidney dysfunction [Guidance update]. US FDA [updated 12/2010 December 26, 2010]. http://www.fda.gov/Drugs/DrugSafety/ucm223966.htm.
16. Weller A, Barber JL, Olsen OE. Gadolinium and nephrogenic systemic fibrosis: an update. Pediatr Nephrol. 2013;29:1927–37. PubMed PMID: 24146299.
17. Martin DR, Krishnamoorthy SK, Kalb B, Salman KN, Sharma P, Carew JD, et al. Decreased incidence of NSF in patients on dialysis after changing gadolinium contrast-enhanced MRI protocols. J Magn Reson Imaging. 2010;31(2):440–6. PubMed PMID: 20099361. Pubmed Central PMCID: 3698801.
18. Altun E, Martin DR, Wertman R, Lugo-Somolinos A, Fuller 3rd ER, Semelka RC. Nephrogenic systemic fibrosis: change in incidence following a switch in gadolinium agents and adoption of a gadolinium policy—report from two U.S. universities. Radiology. 2009;253(3):689–96. PubMed PMID: 19789233.
19. Abujudeh HH, Rolls H, Kaewlai R, Agarwal S, Gebreananya ZA, Saini S, et al. Retrospective assessment of prevalence of nephrogenic systemic fibrosis (NSF) after implementation of a new guideline for the use of gadobenate dimeglumine as a sole contrast agent

for magnetic resonance examination in renally impaired patients. J Magn Reson Imaging. 2009;30(6):1335–40. PubMed PMID: 19937927.
20. Becker S, Walter S, Witzke O, Kreuter A, Kribben A, Mitchell A. Application of gadolinium-based contrast agents and prevalence of nephrogenic systemic fibrosis in a cohort of end-stage renal disease patients on hemodialysis. Nephron Clin Pract. 2012;121(1–2): c91–4. PubMed PMID: 23182840.
21. Idee JM, Port M, Medina C, Lancelot E, Fayoux E, Ballet S, et al. Possible involvement of gadolinium chelates in the pathophysiology of nephrogenic systemic fibrosis: a critical review. Toxicology. 2008;248(2–3):77–88. PubMed PMID: 18440117.
22. Fretellier N, Bouzian N, Parmentier N, Bruneval P, Jestin G, Factor C, et al. Nephrogenic systemic fibrosis-like effects of magnetic resonance imaging contrast agents in rats with adenine-induced renal failure. Toxicol Sci. 2013;131(1):259–70. PubMed PMID: 22977165.
23. Weinreb JC, Abu-Alfa AK. Gadolinium-based contrast agents and nephrogenic systemic fibrosis: why did it happen and what have we learned? J Magn Reson Imaging. 2009;30(6):1236–9. PubMed PMID: 19938035.
24. Abu-Alfa AK. Nephrogenic systemic fibrosis and gadolinium-based contrast agents. Adv Chronic Kidney Dis. 2011;18(3):188–98. PubMed PMID: 21531325. Epub 2011/05/03. eng.
25. Collidge TA, Thomson PC, Mark PB, Traynor JP, Jardine AG, Morris ST, et al. Gadolinium-enhanced MR imaging and nephrogenic systemic fibrosis: retrospective study of a renal replacement therapy cohort. Radiology. 2007;245(1):168–75. PubMed PMID: 17704357.
26. Deo A, Fogel M, Cowper SE. Nephrogenic systemic fibrosis: a population study examining the relationship of disease development to gadolinium exposure. Clin J Am Soc Nephrol. 2007;2(2):264–7. PubMed PMID: 17699423. Epub 2007/08/21. eng.
27. Girardi M, Kay J, Elston DM, Leboit PE, Abu-Alfa A, Cowper SE. Nephrogenic systemic fibrosis: clinicopathological definition and workup recommendations. J Am Acad Dermatol. 2011;65(6): 1095.e7–1106.
28. Joffe P, Thomsen HS, Meusel M. Pharmacokinetics of gadodiamide injection in patients with severe renal insufficiency and patients undergoing hemodialysis or continuous ambulatory peritoneal dialysis. Acad Radiol. 1998;5(7):491–502. PubMed PMID: 9653466.
29. Marckmann P, Skov L, Rossen K, Heaf JG, Thomsen HS. Case-control study of gadodiamide-related nephrogenic systemic fibrosis. Nephrol Dial Transplant. 2007;22(11):3174–8. PubMed PMID: 17483196. Epub 2007/05/08. eng.
30. Swaminathan S, Ahmed I, McCarthy JT, Albright RC, Pittelkow MR, Caplice NM, et al. Nephrogenic fibrosing dermopathy and high-dose erythropoietin therapy. Ann Intern Med. 2006;145(3): 234–5. PubMed PMID: 16880475. Epub 2006/08/02. eng.
31. Rydahl C, Thomsen HS, Marckmann P. High prevalence of nephrogenic systemic fibrosis in chronic renal failure patients exposed to gadodiamide, a gadolinium-containing magnetic resonance contrast agent. Invest Radiol. 2008;43(2):141–4. PubMed PMID: 18197066.
32. Todd DJ, Kagan A, Chibnik LB, Kay J. Cutaneous changes of nephrogenic systemic fibrosis: predictor of early mortality and association with gadolinium exposure. Arthritis Rheum. 2007;56(10):3433–41. PubMed PMID: 17907148.
33. Vakil V, Sung JJ, Piecychna M, Crawford JR, Kuo P, Abu-Alfa AK, et al. Gadolinium-containing magnetic resonance image contrast agent promotes fibrocyte differentiation. J Magn Reson Imaging. 2009;30(6):1284–8. PubMed PMID: 19937928. Pubmed Central PMCID: 2787835.
34. Cowper SE, Bucala R. Nephrogenic fibrosing dermopathy: suspect identified, motive unclear. Am J Dermatopathol. 2003;25(4):358. PubMed PMID: 12876500. Epub 2003/07/24. eng.
35. Bucala R, Spiegel LA, Chesney J, Hogan M, Cerami A. Circulating fibrocytes define a new leukocyte subpopulation that mediates tissue repair. Mol Med. 1994;1(1):71–81. PubMed PMID: 8790603. Pubmed Central PMCID: 2229929.
36. Quan TE, Cowper S, Wu SP, Bockenstedt LK, Bucala R. Circulating fibrocytes: collagen-secreting cells of the peripheral blood. Int J Biochem Cell Biol. 2004;36(4):598–606. PubMed PMID: 15010326. Epub 2004/03/11. eng.
37. Edward M, Quinn JA, Mukherjee S, Jensen MB, Jardine AG, Mark PB, et al. Gadodiamide contrast agent 'activates' fibroblasts: a possible cause of nephrogenic systemic fibrosis. J Pathol. 2008;214(5):584–93. PubMed PMID: 18220317. Epub 2008/01/29. eng.
38. Li JX, Liu JC, Wang K, Yang XG. Gadolinium-containing bioparticles as an active entity to promote cell cycle progression in mouse embryo fibroblast NIH3T3 cells. J Biol Inorg Chem. 2010;15(4):547–57. PubMed PMID: 20076980.
39. Newton BB, Jimenez SA. Mechanism of NSF: new evidence challenging the prevailing theory. J Magn Reson Imaging. 2009;30(6):1277–83. PubMed PMID: 19937925.
40. Fretellier N, Idee JM, Guerret S, Hollenbeck C, Hartmann D, Gonzalez W, et al. Clinical, biological, and skin histopathologic effects of ionic macrocyclic and nonionic linear gadolinium chelates in a rat model of nephrogenic systemic fibrosis. Invest Radiol. 2011;46(2):85–93. PubMed PMID: 20938344.
41. Pietsch H, Lengsfeld P, Steger-Hartmann T, Lowe A, Frenzel T, Hutter J, et al. Impact of renal impairment on long-term retention of gadolinium in the rodent skin following the administration of gadolinium-based contrast agents. Invest Radiol. 2009;44(4):226–33. PubMed PMID: 19252439.
42. Grant D, Johnsen H, Juelsrud A, Lovhaug D. Effects of gadolinium contrast agents in naive and nephrectomized rats: relevance to nephrogenic systemic fibrosis. Acta Radiol. 2009;50(2):156–69. PubMed PMID: 19160079.
43. Haylor J, Dencausse A, Vickers M, Nutter F, Jestin G, Slater D, et al. Nephrogenic gadolinium biodistribution and skin cellularity following a single injection of Omniscan in the rat. Invest Radiol. 2010;45(9):507–12. PubMed PMID: 20697223.
44. Sato T, Ito K, Tamada T, Kanki A, Watanabe S, Nishimura H, et al. Tissue gadolinium deposition in renally impaired rats exposed to different gadolinium-based MRI contrast agents: evaluation with inductively coupled plasma mass spectrometry (ICP-MS). Magn Reson Imaging. 2013;31(8):1412–7. PubMed PMID: 23643157.
45. Streams BN, Liu V, Liegeois N, Moschella SM. Clinical and pathologic features of nephrogenic fibrosing dermopathy: a report of two cases. J Am Acad Dermatol. 2003;48(1):42–7. PubMed PMID: 12522369.
46. Bhawan J, Swick BL, Koff AB, Stone MS. Sclerotic bodies in nephrogenic systemic fibrosis: a new histopathologic finding. J Cutan Pathol. 2009;36(5):548–52. PubMed PMID: 19476523.
47. Milless T, LaChance A, Moeckel G, Cowper SE. The lollipop lesion: its prevalence and potential diagnostic significance in nephrogenic systemic fibrosis. American Society of Dermatopathology Annual Meeting; Seattle, WA; 2011.
48. Kartono F, Basile A, Roshdieh B, Schwimer C, Shitabata PK. Findings of osseous sclerotic bodies: a unique sequence of cutaneous bone formation in nephrogenic systemic fibrosis. J Cutan Pathol. 2011;38(3):286–9. PubMed PMID: 20726931.
49. Bhawan J, Perez-Chua TA, Goldberg L. Sclerotic bodies beyond nephrogenic systemic fibrosis. J Cutan Pathol. 2013;40(9):812–7. PubMed PMID: 23808625.
50. Duncan AA. Commentary on "Reflux testing and imaging for endovenous ablation". Perspect Vasc Surg Endovasc Ther. 2007;19(1):71–2. PubMed PMID: 17437985.
51. Pomann JJ, Rudner EJ. Scleromyxedema revisited. Int J Dermatol. 2003;42(1):31–5. PubMed PMID: 12581140.

52. Paudyal BP, Gyawalee M, Sigdel K. Eosinophilic fasciitis: a rare fibrosing disorder. Kathmandu Univ Med J. 2012;10(39):73–5. PubMed PMID: 23434968.
53. Dharamsi JW, Victor S, Aguwa N, Ahn C, Arnett F, Mayes MD, et al. Morphea in adults and children cohort III: nested case-control study—the clinical significance of autoantibodies in morphea. JAMA Dermatol. 2013;149(10):1159–65. PubMed PMID: 23925398.
54. Savas N, Dagli U, Ertugrul E, Kuran S, Sahin B. Autoantibody profile in systemic sclerosis as a marker for esophageal and other organ involvement in Turkish populations. Dig Dis Sci. 2007;52(11): 3081–6. PubMed PMID: 17393310.
55. Murphy-Chutorian B, Han G, Cohen SR. Dermatologic manifestations of diabetes mellitus: a review. Endocrinol Metab Clin North Am. 2013;42(4):869–98. PubMed PMID: 24286954.
56. Crone C, Krarup C. Neurophysiological approach to disorders of peripheral nerve. Handb Clin Neurol. 2013;115:81–114. PubMed PMID: 23931776.
57. Kalisz KR, Davarpanah AH, Usman AA, Collins JD, Carroll TJ, Carr JC. Detection of renal dysfunction by point-of-care creatinine testing in patients undergoing peripheral MR angiography. AJR Am J Roentgenol. 2011;197(2):430–5. PubMed PMID: 21785090.
58. Chang P, Saddleton E, Laumann AE, Schmitz B, West DP, Belknap SM, et al. Comparison of the sensitivity of a pre-MRI questionnaire and point of care eGFR testing for detection of impaired renal function. Acad Radiol. 2012;19(10):1181–5. PubMed PMID: 22831822.
59. Othersen JB, Maize JC, Woolson RF, Budisavljevic MN. Nephrogenic systemic fibrosis after exposure to gadolinium in patients with renal failure. Nephrol Dial Transplant. 2007;22(11): 3179–85. PubMed PMID: 17890246.
60. Knopp EA, Cowper SE. Nephrogenic systemic fibrosis: early recognition and treatment. Semin Dial. 2008;21(2):123–8. PubMed PMID: 18226008.
61. Richmond H, Zwerner J, Kim Y, Fiorentino D. Nephrogenic systemic fibrosis: relationship to gadolinium and response to photopheresis. Arch Dermatol. 2007;143(8):1025–30. PubMed PMID: 17709661.
62. Schieren G, Wirtz N, Altmeyer P, Rump LC, Weiner SM, Kreuter A. Nephrogenic systemic fibrosis—a rapidly progressive disabling disease with limited therapeutic options. J Am Acad Dermatol. 2009;61(5):868–74. PubMed PMID: 19836645.
63. Ramaizel L, Sliwa JA. Rehabilitation in nephrogenic systemic fibrosis. PM R. 2009;1(7):684–6. PubMed PMID: 19627963.

Blistering Disorders (Porphyria Cutanea Tarda and Pseudoporphyria)

13

Christine A. DeWitt, Kara M. Trapp, and Melissa A. Muszynski

Abbreviations

ESRD	End-stage renal disease
HBV	Hepatitis B virus
HCV	Hepatitis C virus
HIV	Human immunodeficiency virus
PAS	Periodic acid-Schiff
PCT	Porphyria cutanea tarda
UROD	Uroporphyrinogen III decarboxylase
UVA	Ultraviolet A
UVB	Ultraviolet B

Introduction

Porphyria cutanea tarda (PCT), first described and characterized by Waldenstrom in 1937, presents as a disorder with a multitude of cutaneous manifestations, including characteristic pruritic vesicles occurring on sun-exposed skin [1]. In addition to skin involvement, PCT is characterized by hepatic pathologies. PCT represents the most common variant of the porphyrias, a collection of disorders related to deficiencies in one of eight enzymes involved in heme biosynthetic pathway (Fig. 13.1). Individuals with PCT exhibit reduced levels of uroporphyrinogen III decarboxylase (UROD), the enzyme that converts uroporphyrinogen to coproporphyrinogen, leading to a buildup of porphyrin by-products.

Several PCT variants exist, including an acquired form denoted as "sporadic" or "Type 1 PCT" and an inherited autosomal dominant form denoted as "familial" or "Type 2 PCT." A much less common familial variant, "Type 3 PCT," is hypothesized to occur from the inheritance of an unidentified gene [2]. Irrespective of subtype, clinical manifestations typically occur when hepatic UROD activity decreases to 20 % of normal or less [3]. A variety of factors are known to precipitate PCT in all subtypes including environmental exposures, infections, nutritional influences, and other medical comorbidities.

The relationship between PCT and hemodialysis is well established in the scientific literature [4–28]. Though less common, there is also a reported association with peritoneal dialysis [29–32]. Furthermore, patients with impaired renal function, irrespective of dialysis treatment, may develop PCT due to inefficient excretion of porphyrin by-products [33].

Zelickson first described pseudoporphyria in 1964 after a patient taking nalidixic acid was observed to have the clinical findings of PCT, yet no porphyrin abnormalities were identified. Pseudoporphyria has indistinguishable clinical and histologic findings from PCT, but laboratory analysis does not demonstrate the abnormalities in porphyrin metabolism that defines PCT [34]. Pseudoporphyria has been classically reported in association with excessive exposure to ultraviolet A (UVA) from tanning beds, medication use, and in patients with chronic kidney disease.

In those patients with chronic renal disease, pseudoporphyria has also been termed "bullous dermatosis of end-stage renal disease" and is associated primarily with hemodialysis. Gilchrest first demonstrated the association between pseudoporphyria and hemodialysis in 1975, in a report of five patients presenting with PCT but exhibiting normal porphyrin levels [35]. Pseudoporphyria has also been observed in patients undergoing peritoneal dialysis as well as in patients with impaired renal function without exposure to dialysis [36–39]. Although it is a disorder characterized by normal porphyrin metabolism, dialysis patients

C.A. DeWitt, M.D. (✉)
Department of Dermatology, Georgetown University/Washington Hospital Center, 5530 Wisconsin Ave, Suite 660, Chevy Chase, MD 20815, USA
e-mail: christine.a.dewitt@gunet.georgetown.edu

K.M. Trapp, B.A.
Georgetown University School of Medicine, 3900 Reservoir Road NW, Washington, DC 20057, USA

M.A. Muszynski, M.D.
Department of Dermatology, Georgetown University Hospital/Washington Hospital Center, 110 Irving St. NW, 2B-44, Washington, DC 20010, USA

J.R. Nunley and E.V. Lerma (eds.), *Dermatological Manifestations of Kidney Disease*,
DOI 10.1007/978-1-4939-2395-3_13, © Springer Science+Business Media New York 2015

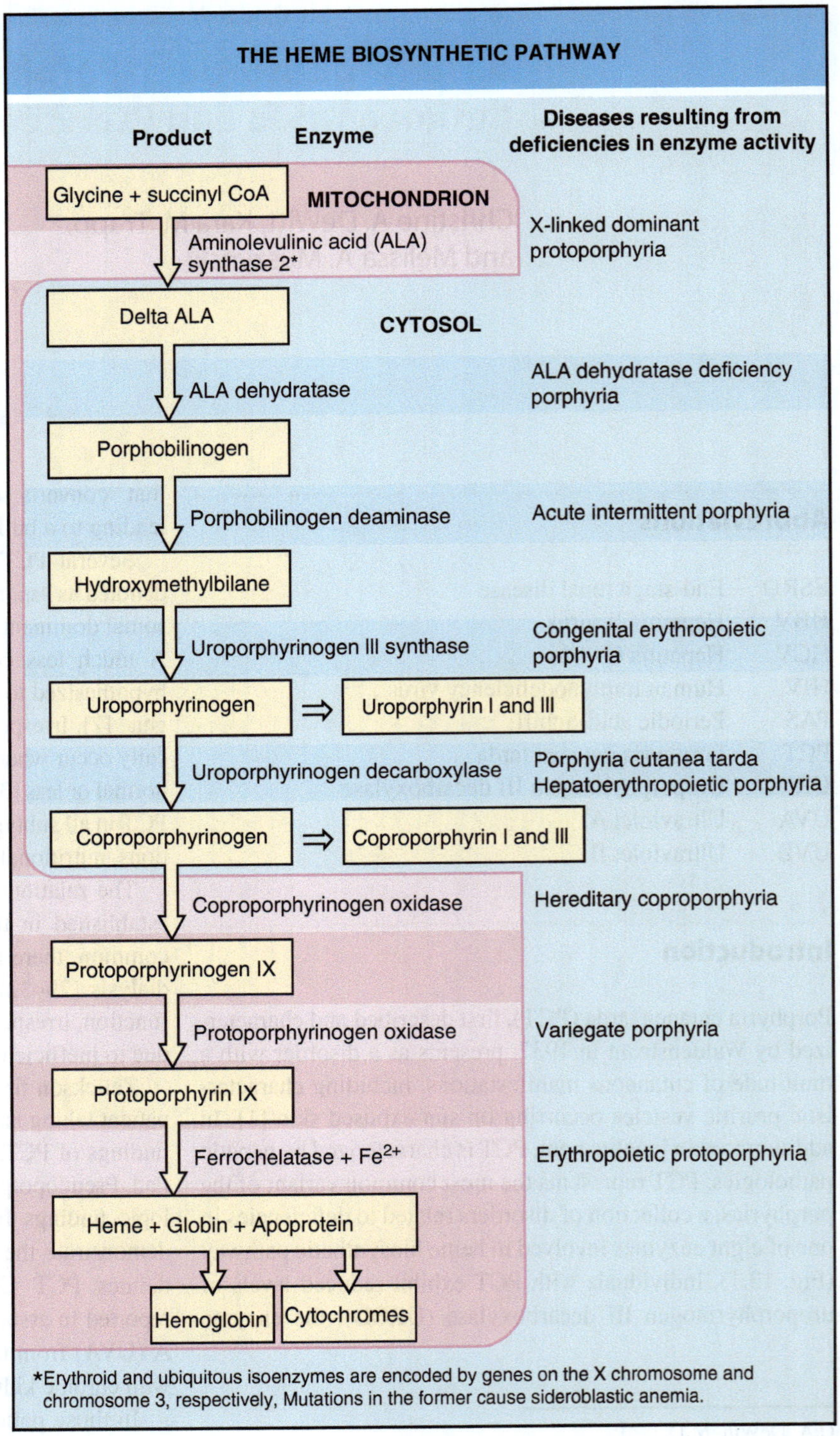

Fig. 13.1 Heme biosynthetic pathway (published in Dermatology, 3rd ed., Bolognia J and Gutierrez PAP, Porphyria, 718, Copyright Elsevier (2012))

with pseudoporphyria may exhibit mildly elevated serum porphyrin levels due to the poor porphyrin clearance associated with dialysis [19].

Epidemiology

While PCT is the most common of the porphyrias, it is considered to be an uncommon condition. The estimated prevalence of PCT is approximately 1 in 10,000 individuals [40]. Approximately 80 % of PCT patients have the sporadic (Type I) form, and the remaining 20 % are predominantly the familial (Type II) type. In both types, PCT most often presents during the third to fourth decade of life [41]. In the past, PCT demonstrated a greater frequency in men. However, current rates of PCT are approximately equal across both genders [41]. The increasing frequency among woman is hypothesized to reflect the greater use of oral contraceptives [41].

The incidence of PCT in patients undergoing hemodialysis has been reported to range from 1.2 to 18 % [18].

In the pre-erythropoietin era, the prevalence of PCT in dialysis patients may have been a more common occurrence due to the frequency of transfusion-related iron overload and perhaps transfusion-related hepatitis C infection [42].

A retrospective review of 20 patients with pseudoporphyria demonstrated a mean age of diagnosis to be 50 years, with a range of 33–71 years [43]. Though more common in adults, pseudoporphyria has been described in children. In a subset of children taking naproxen for joint pain associated with juvenile idiopathic arthritis, 11 % of naproxen users developed pseudoporphyria. The overall incidence and prevalence of pseudoporphyria is variable depending on the proposed inciting agent, such as medication use or ultraviolet A (UVA) exposure, but in all causes, fair skin appears to be an independent risk factor [45–48]. In patients with end-stage renal disease (ESRD) on hemodialysis, pseudoporphyria has been reported to occur at a rate from 1.2 % to as high as 18 %; pseudoporphyria occurs less frequently in those on peritoneal dialysis [49]. This discrepancy may be related to the lower levels of plasma uroporphyrin seen in patients receiving peritoneal dialysis [37].

Pathogenesis

Porphyria Cutanea Tarda

PCT is characterized as a multifactorial disorder related to either an inherited or acquired deficiency of UROD caused by both genetic and nongenetic factors. The abnormal physiology of PCT is related to the accumulation of porphyrins in the liver, plasma, and skin due to reduced activity of UROD. Approximately one-fifth of individuals with PCT have an inherited UROD mutation and exhibit UROD activity at 50 % of normal in all tissues from birth. The remaining majority of individuals with PCT have the sporadic form and exhibit reduced UROD activity only in hepatocytes. Porphyrin molecules have very intense absorption bands in the visible and ultraviolet A (UVA) electromagnetic spectrum especially in the Soret band, between 400 and 410 nm. Pathogenic porphyrin accumulation in the skin absorbs both visible and ultraviolet light, causing the main cutaneous signs and symptoms of PCT.

In both the sporadic and familial forms, the clinical expression of PCT requires additional susceptibility factors, genetic and/or environmental, to reduce UROD activity to 20 % of normal. In a study of 143 patients with PCT, the most frequent inciting agents included ethanol use, smoking, chronic hepatitis C virus (HCV) infection, and hemochromatosis HFE mutations; three or more susceptibility factors were recognized in 70 % of patients [50]. These proposed etiologic agents promote the accumulation of excess iron or oxidative stress in hepatocytes.

Hepatic iron overload is present in almost all cases of PCT, often with stores nearly twice that of normals. Iron has many proposed roles in the pathogenesis of PCT. Perhaps most importantly, iron directly inhibits UROD enzymatic activity and acts as a catalyst for the formation of reactive oxygen species that damages hepatic tissue [51]. Additional genetic associations with PCT that affect iron accumulation include hemochromatosis HFE gene mutations. Many patients with PCT, either genetic or acquired, are frequently found to have concurrent HFE gene mutations.

Alcohol has often been observed to precipitate PCT. Along with diminishing UROD activity after acute ingestion or in chronic alcoholics, ethanol may induce the enzyme aminolevulinic acid (ALA)-synthetase. This leads to porphyrin accumulation without the ability to complete the heme synthesis cascade due to inhibited UROD. Chronic alcoholism has also been associated with increased iron absorption and suppressed erythropoiesis.

Additional triggers reported to precipitate PCT include exposure to estrogens, environmental pollutants, human immunodeficiency virus (HIV) infection, and concurrent medical conditions including diabetes mellitus, systemic lupus erythematosus, hepatic steatosis, bone marrow disorders, and myeloproliferative disorders.

In patients with impaired renal function, PCT has several interconnected pathogenic mechanisms but in part results from impaired porphyrin clearance. Furthermore, patients with ESRD requiring renal replacement therapy may have even higher porphyrin levels since current dialytic techniques (hemodialysis or peritoneal dialysis) are substandard in clearing porphyrins from circulation [33]. Indeed, porphyrin clearance across the dialysis membrane in a hemodialysis patient with PCT was demonstrated to be 100 times less than the renal clearance of porphyrin molecules in PCT patients with normal renal function [20]. Furthermore, individuals undergoing chronic hemodialysis are at an increased risk of developing acquired forms of UROD deficiency due to hepatotoxicity from various exposures, such as alcohol, statins, estrogens, viruses, or iron overload [19]. Other mechanisms proposed to induce abnormal porphyrin metabolism in dialysis patients include the reduction of UROD from azotemia [52], exposure to phototoxic medications, and aluminum load [53].

Pseudoporphyria

Although the mechanism is not fully understood, pseudoporphyria has been associated independently with various medications, excessive sun exposure, ultraviolet A (UVA) radiation, chronic kidney disease, and dialysis [49]. Additional reported associations include phototherapy with ultraviolet B (UVB), hormone replacement, human immunodeficiency virus (HIV) and HCV infections, and other coexisting medical conditions including systemic lupus erythematosus, vitiligo, sarcoidosis, Sjögren syndrome, and hepatoma.

The pathogenesis of pseudoporphyria in individuals with chronic kidney disease is not fully established. However, several mechanisms have been proposed and may not be mutually exclusive. These theories have included a primary drug-induced pathogenesis, as this population is often concurrently managed with many drugs known to be associated with pseudoporphyria, such as nifedipine, furosemide, and erythropoietin; an increase in oxidative stress due to dialysis-associated glutathione depletion; and in those patients undergoing dialysis, a potential role of aluminum hydroxide that is found in the dialysate and that has demonstrated phototoxicity in animal models [49]. It is important to note that the association between erythropoietin and pseudoporphyria may be of minor significance as pseudoporphyria appeared in the literature prior to the introduction of erythropoietin [49]. Both peritoneal dialysis and hemodialysis reduce glutathione levels in the blood and erythrocytes; the resultant glutathione deficiency creates an increased susceptibility to oxidative stress in these patients and may facilitate photo-oxidative cutaneous injury [54, 55]. The development of pseudoporphyria in nondialyzed individuals with chronic kidney disease has been reported in the scientific literature, suggesting that renal dysfunction may play a more significant role in the induction of pseudoporphyria than previously hypothesized; however, there may have also been a drug-induced component lending evidence to the multifactorial mechanisms in this patient population [37].

Clinical

The predominant clinical characteristics of all forms of PCT usually involve photocutaneous and liver manifestations. There are several characteristic skin findings, but the most commonly observed features include skin fragility and blistering on the hands, present in the vast majority of cases (Fig. 13.2a, b) [56]. Along with the observable skin changes, a notable symptom reported frequently by patients is increased pruritus of the affected skin. Though many uremic patients have chronic pruritus, the development of PCT may heighten symptoms. Other classic features of PCT include facial hypertrichosis, most notably on the temples (Fig. 13.3a, b); photodistributed hyperpigmentation; premature aging; and milial cysts and comedones (Fig. 13.4). Less common, but still characteristic, findings include sclerodermoid changes, facial blisters, scarring alopecia, and photo-onycholysis (Fig. 13.5) [56, 57]. Because of the underlying porphyrin accumulation, patients may report the darkening of their urine. This finding may not be as specific in oliguric or anuric patients. In PCT, the liver is the other predominant organ system affected. The range of hepatic findings is diverse and may include steatosis, fibrosis, siderosis, and as a late manifestation, cirrhosis [58]. Complete hepatic evaluation must be performed as these patients may be at risk for an underlying hepatocellular carcinoma [59]. These liver findings often relate to the underlying inciting PCT trigger, such as HCV, alcohol abuse, iron overload, or hemochromatosis. There may be additional clinical findings more specific to these conditions as opposed to being directly related to PCT [60].

The clinical characteristics of pseudoporphyria greatly resemble PCT. In pseudoporphyria, the most frequent clinical characteristic is photodistributed blistering that occurs in nearly every patient. Also characteristically observed are scarring, photosensitivity, and skin fragility. Though not as common, milia may develop and are often directly related to the presence of scarring [43]. In contrast to PCT, noticeably absent clinical features include hypertrichosis, hyperpigmentation, and sclerodermoid changes [42].

Differential Diagnosis

The differential diagnosis for PCT includes other forms of the porphyrias (including variegate porphyria, congenital erythropoietic porphyria, hepatoerythropoietic porphyria, and hereditary coproporphyria), pseudoporphyria, other bullous skin disorders (including bullous pemphigoid, bullous drug eruption, epidermolysis bullosa, epidermolysis bullosa

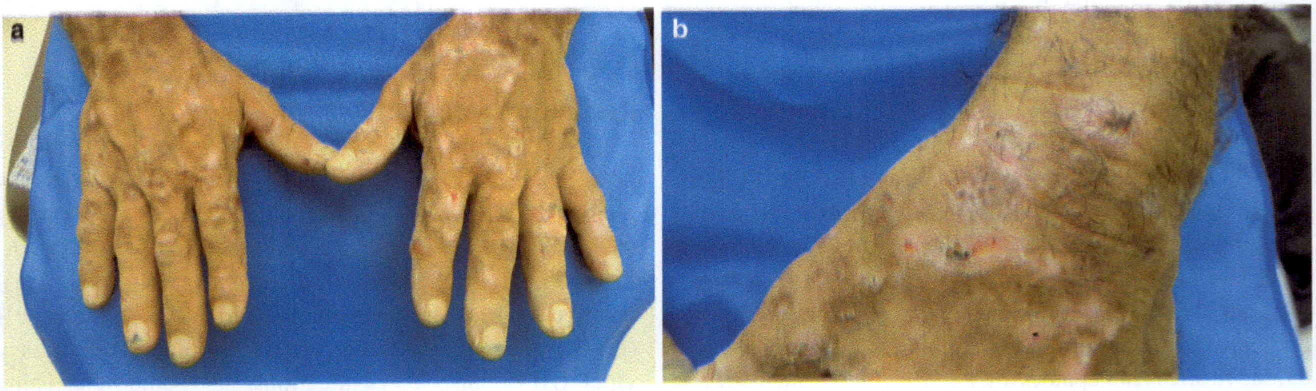

Fig. 13.2 PCT classically presents with skin fragility and vesicles on the dorsal surface of hands

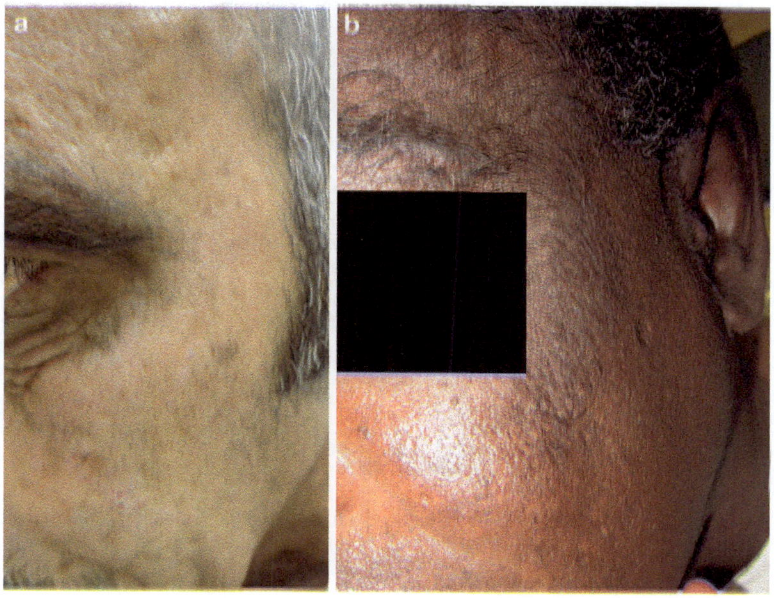

Fig. 13.3 Hypertrichosis is another characteristic feature of PCT and can involve the forehead, temples, and upper cheeks

acquisita, and bullous lupus erythematosus), and hydroa vacciniforme, a rare chronic photodermatosis.

Laboratory analysis of urinary and fecal porphyrin levels allows for differentiation of PCT and pseudoporphyria from other subtypes of porphyrias [41]. To distinguish PCT and pseudoporphyria from other vesiculobullous disorders, a skin biopsy for histology and direct immunofluorescence is recommended [42]. Immunohistochemical analysis of tissue submitted for direct immunofluorescence would differentiate autoimmune immunobullous disorders from PCT. Genetic immunobullous diseases can generally be differentiated based on time of onset, as most are present at or near birth. Hydroa vacciniforme is considered a disease of childhood, is associated with Epstein–Barr virus, and rarely has hepatic involvement.

Workup

The workup for PCT and pseudoporphyria includes clinical data, laboratory analysis, imaging studies, and histopathologic data. PCT and pseudoporphyria frequently simulate various subepidermal bullous disorders; thus, complete integration of clinical, histopathologic, and biochemical information is necessary for accurate diagnosis. Of note, results from 24 h urinary collections in the setting of significantly low renal clearance, especially in those who are oliguric or anuric, are not reliable.

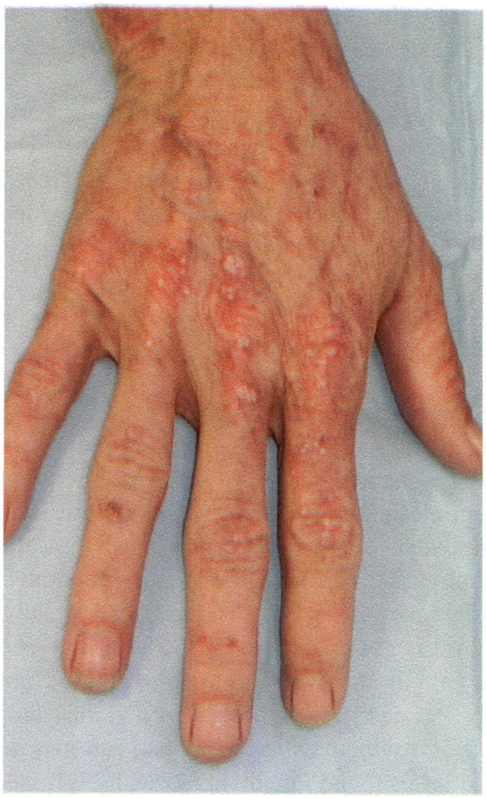

Fig. 13.4 Milia formation is a common occurrence following extensive blistering in PCT. Courtesy of Julia R. Nunley, M.D.

Histology

PCT has various clinical findings, but a punch biopsy of the edge of photodistributed vesicles often demonstrates the pathognomonic features that aid in diagnosis. Histology of these vesicobullae demonstrates a cell-poor subepidermal bullae with festooning of dermal papillae, minimal inflammatory infiltration, and periodic acid-Schiff (PAS)-positive thickening of the papillary vessel wall [61] (Fig. 13.6). Intraepidermal eosinophilic collections of basement membrane type IV collagen, denoted as "caterpillar bodies," are frequently observed [62].

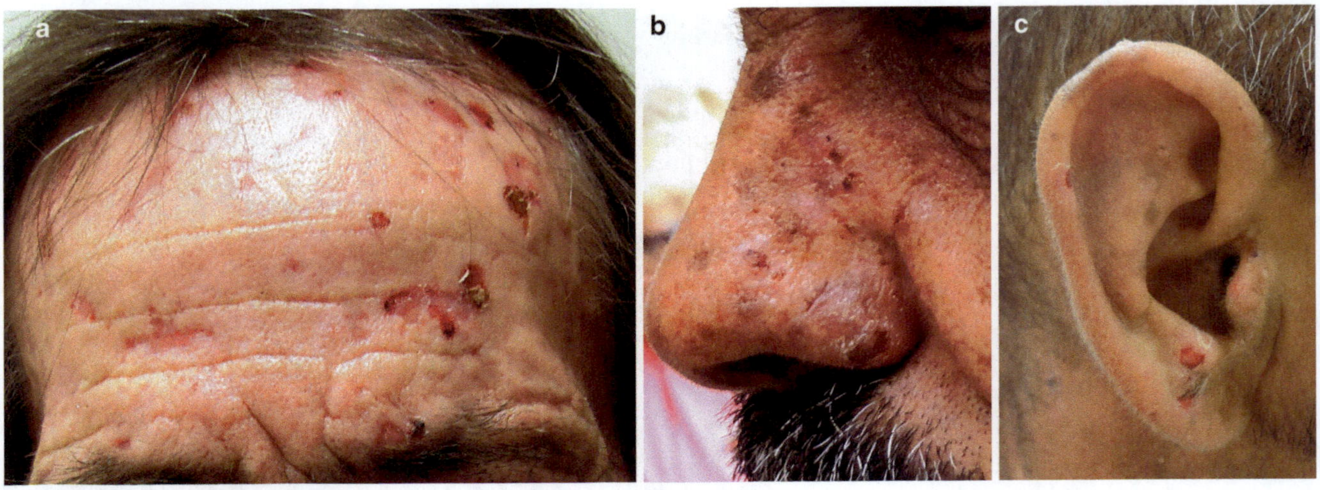

Fig. 13.5 Photo-onycholysis, a sun-induced nail dystrophy, is seen along with erosions and milial cysts on the bilateral dorsal hands

Direct immunofluorescence frequently demonstrates linear IgG, C3, and fibrinogen along the dermal perivascular area and dermoepidermal junction [42], with less frequent observations of IgA and IgM deposition [63].

The histologic profile of pseudoporphyria is nearly identical to PCT and cannot be reliably used to differentiate the two disorders. One minor difference reported is less blood vessel wall thickening with PAS staining in pseudoporphyria as compared to cases of PCT [61].

Laboratory Abnormalities

PCT is a disorder characterized by abnormalities in biochemical porphyrin levels. The urinary porphyrin profile demonstrates marked elevations in uroporphyrin I with less significant elevations in uroporphyrin III, 8-carboxyl uroporphyrin, and 7-carboxyl porphyrin [61]. Additionally, plasma uroporphyrin and fecal isocoproporphyrin IIII demonstrate elevations [42]. The urinary porphobilinogen (PBG) level is normal and the ALA level may be slightly elevated [3]. Erythrocyte porphyrin levels are normal or modestly elevated. It is important to note that uroporphyrin levels in asymptomatic ESRD patients may resemble or exceed levels found in individuals with PCT and normal renal function, as uroporphyrins are not sufficiently excreted via hemodialysis [65].

In anuric patients, fecal analysis for elevated levels of isocoproporphyrin III and plasma analysis for uroporphyrin are important diagnostic measures [32]. Fecal analysis remains the most accurate diagnostic marker of PCT in patients with chronic kidney disease as plasma uroporphyrin levels normally exhibit marked elevations due to impaired renal and dialytic clearance [64].

Additionally, workup for hemochromatosis may demonstrate positive results, given the strong association between hereditary hemochromatosis HFE gene mutations and PCT [66]. For the diagnosis of familial PCT, genetic sequencing of the UROD gene is necessary and is typically present as a heterozygous mutation.

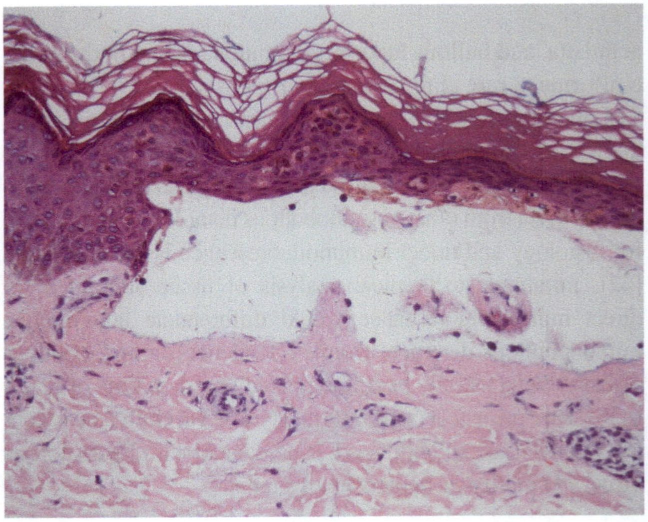

Fig. 13.6 Cell-poor subepidermal bullae with festooning of dermal papillae

Because liver involvement frequently accompanies PCT, investigation of hepatic activity is recommended. Laboratory tests include complete blood count, serum ferritin, serum iron, liver function profile, and screening for HCV, HBV (hepatitis B virus), and HIV infections. Most patients with PCT exhibit iron overload, which can be observed by high normal or moderate elevations in serum iron and ferritin levels. An analysis of serum alpha-fetoprotein is beneficial in screening for hepatocellular carcinoma [67].

Another diagnostic measure for PCT includes examination of urine under Wood lamp illumination in the dark, but after exposure to natural light (Fig. 13.7). If adequately con-

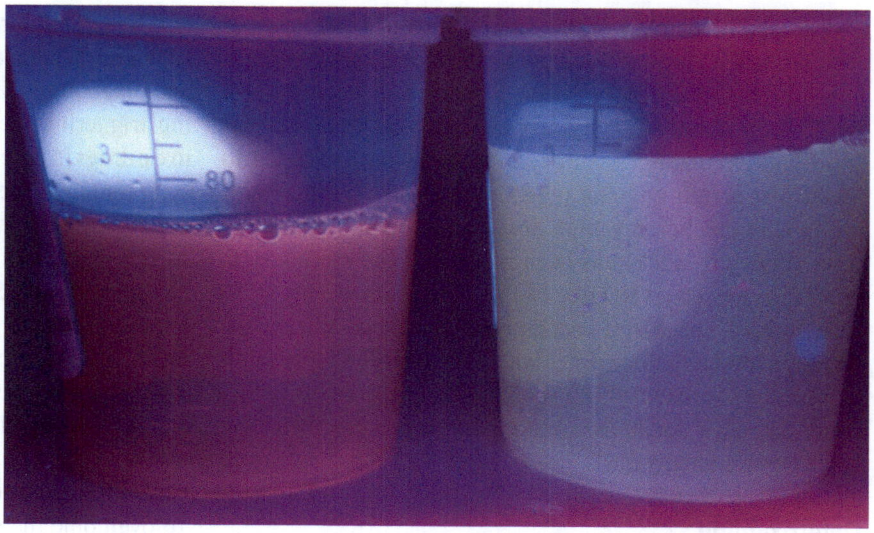

Fig. 13.7 Pink fluorescence of patient urine (*left*) compared to normal urine (*right*) under a Wood lamp illumination

centrated, the urine of PCT patients will exhibit a pink to red fluorescence under a ultraviolet A (UVA) source and will turn red to brown after exposure to natural light for several hours [41]. However, it is important to note that these tests are neither sensitive nor specific.

Pseudoporphyria is a disorder characterized by normal biochemical porphyrin levels in the serum, urine, and stool. The diagnosis of pseudoporphyria in ESRD patients on dialysis is challenging because many of these individuals exhibit elevated plasma porphyrins despite having normal porphyrin metabolism [68]. Additionally, when comparing uroporphyrin levels in dialysis patients, hemodialysis patients frequently exhibit greater plasma uroporphyrin levels than patients undergoing peritoneal dialysis [37]. Thus, mildly elevated serum porphyrin levels should be anticipated in dialysis patients with bullous lesions who are diagnosed with pseudoporphyria [19]. Plasma porphyrin and fecal porphyrin levels should be assayed in ESRD patients, as urinary levels may be inaccurate. Liver enzyme analysis for individuals with pseudoporphyria is most often normal; however, abnormalities have been observed [49].

Imaging Studies

Imaging of the liver may be recommended in certain cases of PCT to evaluate hepatic iron content, size, and hepatic carcinoma.

Treatment

Porphyria Cutanea Tarda

Primary management of PCT in renal disease involves a combination of eliminating or reducing triggers, reducing iron load, and removing excess porphyrin accumulation. In some refractory cases, kidney transplantation may be a consideration.

Trigger Avoidance

If a known trigger of PCT has been identified, every effort should be made to minimize or eliminate the causative agent. Estrogen use should be discontinued, at least until complete remission is achieved, and attempts should be made to avoid hepatotoxic drugs. Active viral disease, such as with HIV and HCV, should be identified and appropriate therapy for these infections should be a part of the management plan. Sun protection is often of paramount importance. Beyond sun avoidance and protective clothing, ultraviolet A (UVA)-absorbing sunscreens, such as those containing avobenzone or zinc oxide, may be the best option when patients do plan to be exposed. Other lifestyle changes that should be encouraged include smoking cessation and strict alcohol avoidance.

Reducing Iron Load

Phlebotomy

After exogenous exacerbating factors are removed or discontinued, medical therapies employed to reduce iron load are the treatment of choice [69]. Even in patients with ESRD on either hemodialysis or peritoneal dialysis, the first line of treatment is therapeutic phlebotomy, as long at the hemoglobin is adequate. By using phlebotomy to reduce iron stores, the heme synthetic pathway normalizes both by augmenting UROD activity, an enzyme that is inhibited by iron, and through regeneration of new hepatic UROD [70]. Caution must be exercised with repeated phlebotomies in patients with renal disease due to the challenge of concurrent chronic anemia that is frequently observed. Most patients with renal failure are unable to tolerate the standard protocol of once or twice weekly removal of 500 mL of blood. Instead, small-volume phlebotomy, ranging from 100 to 350 mL, every 2–3 weeks is employed while aiming for target serum hemoglobin between 10 and 11 g/dL. Nevertheless, both standard volume and small-volume phlebotomy have induced clinical remission in PCT patients associated with chronic kidney disease [21, 22, 30].

For those patients with severe anemia, the use of recombinant human erythropoietin in conjunction with small-volume phlebotomies has been a successful strategy [14, 69–72]. By stimulating erythropoiesis, tissue iron is mobilized and circulating erythrocyte numbers are increased to levels that permit ongoing phlebotomy. When used concurrently with phlebotomy, high dose erythropoietin (150 U/kg three times per week) has been reported to be more efficacious than low dose (50 U/kg two to three times weekly) [70] Interestingly, successful anecdotes of erythropoietin monotherapy (150 U/kg three times weekly) have been reported in hemodialysis-related PCT [10–12, 73]. Phlebotomy is discontinued once serum iron and ferritin levels reach slightly low to low-normal values.

Deferoxamine

In patients with severe anemia or who are unable to undergo phlebotomy, use of deferoxamine, a ferrous iron chelator, may be an alternative. Deferoxamine has demonstrated measurable success in the scientific literature as a treatment method for dialysis-related PCT [6, 15, 23, 24, 31]. Remission of hemodialysis-related PCT has been reported following treatment with 40 mg/kg intravenous deferoxamine every week for 6 weeks [24]. There is one report of low dose hydroxychloroquine (400 mg weekly) used in conjunction with 40 mg/kg deferoxamine intravenously every week for 6 weeks in a patient with chronic dialysis-related PCT. Resolution of symptoms occurred within six cycles of treatment [6].

Reducing Porphyrins

Antimalarials

In patients unable to tolerate or that are refractory to phlebotomy, the antimalarial drugs, chloroquine or hydroxychloroquine, may be cautiously considered. These agents form water-soluble complexes with hepatic porphyrins, thereby promoting their renal excretion and have been successfully used in the treatment of PCT. However, in patients with chronic kidney disease on dialysis, the chloroquine-porphyrin complexes may not be effectively eliminated from the body, potentially rendering treatment unsuccessful [6, 26, 27, 70]. Furthermore, chloroquine may cause paradoxical harm to patients with PCT through direct liver toxicity and hepatic porphyrin release [7].

When antimalarials are used, appropriate dosage is key to ensuring patient safety. For use in PCT, the dose is significantly less (e.g., hydroxychloroquine 200–400 mg weekly in single or divided doses) as compared to the traditional regimen used for connective tissue diseases (e.g., hydroxychloroquine 200–400 mg daily). When used in combination with other treatment modalities, hydroxychloroquine has been shown to improve clinical characteristics of PCT. In one report, there was resolution of blisters and a decrease in serum porphyrin levels in a case of hemodialysis-associated PCT after 2 months of twice weekly phlebotomy, low dose oral hydroxychloroquine, high-flux hemodialysis, and erythropoietin [7]. In addition to low dose hydroxychloroquine and phlebotomy, improvement can also be seen when reducing triggering factors such as photo exposure and hepatotoxic drugs [5]. Because the skin is often the most troublesome symptom, treatment with hydroxychloroquine 400 mg once a week in combination with a topical calcineurin inhibitor, such as pimecrolimus 1 % cream, significantly improved blistering in an ESRD patient with PCT and anemia [63]. It has even been suggested that treatment with topical pimecrolimus and low dose oral hydroxychloroquine may represent a suitable alternative to conventional phlebotomy in patients with PCT associated with renal dysfunction and anemia [63].

High-Flux Hemodialysis

To overcome the problem of porphyrin accumulation due to ineffective clearance, therapies designed to facilitate large molecular weight "middle" molecule clearance have also been employed for the treatment of hemodialysis-related PCT. High-flux hemodialysis has been shown to be more effective at removing plasma porphyrins than conventional hemodialysis [74]. One report demonstrated a 37 % decrease in plasma porphyrins from predialysis levels after the replacement of conventional hemodialysis with a standard cellulose acetate dialyzer to high-flux hemodialysis with a polysulfone dialyzer for 4 weeks. Furthermore, a return to conventional hemodialysis resulted in a rise in plasma porphyrins to prestudy levels [74].

Plasma Exchange

Plasma exchange has also been successfully used in hemodialysis-associated PCT [8, 17, 25]. Interestingly after just two treatments, 48 h apart, one patient demonstrated a rapid decrease in plasma porphyrin levels and dramatic clinical improvement. The patient was able to achieve remission for several months without additional therapy [25].

In circumstances in which the aforementioned treatments are unsuccessful, renal transplantation may be required in exceptional cases [28]. Cholestyramine, often used for binding bile salts and lowering cholesterol, may have a beneficial role in PCT by blocking enterohepatic circulation of porphyrins. Use of 12 g daily in divided doses produced rapid resolution of clinical findings in PCT patients with normal renal function. Unfortunately results in patients with ESRD have been disappointing [70]. Although charcoal hemoperfusion successfully removed uroporphyrin from plasma in vitro, an isolated report of use in a patient with hemodialysis-related PCT was not effective.

Pseudoporphyria

N-acetylcysteine

The administration of oral *N*-acetylcysteine, a metabolic precursor of glutathione, has been demonstrated to induce clinical remission of hemodialysis-associated pseudoporphyria, peritoneal dialysis-associated pseudoporphyria, and pseudoporphyria associated with nonhemodialyzed renal insufficiency [36, 37, 75–79]. In these studies, dosages ranged from 600 to 1,200 mg daily, 400 to 600 mg twice daily, and 200 mg four times a day. Resolution of lesions occurred over a time span of 20 days to 2 months, and treatments were continued over a period of 4 weeks to 1 year with most studies reporting no adverse side effects. It is important to note that in a case of peritoneal dialysis-associated pseudoporphyria, lesions initially resolved with oral *N*-acetylcysteine treatment; however, after 1 month of treatment, the patient contracted bacterial peritonitis and was switched from peritoneal dialysis to hemodialysis [36]. Following the onset of the infection, the lesions recurred despite the continuation of treatment; the authors hypothesize this result to reflect new oxidative stress and a change in dialysis treatment [36].

High-Flux Hemodialysis

N-acetylcysteine has also been used in conjunction with additional therapies for the treatment of hemodialysis-associated pseudoporphyria [76]. One such combination included 200 mg oral *N*-acetylcysteine four times a day, topical steroids for 1 week, and a replacement of low-flux (less than 250 mL/min) conventional hemodialysis three times per week with high-flux (300 mL/min) hemodialysis three times per week using a polysulfone membrane. This led to complete resolution of skin lesions after 3 weeks of treatment and sustained remission over a 24 month of follow-up [76].

Antimalarials

While *N*-acetylcysteine has induced remission of pseudoporphyria in many cases, other alternatives may need to be considered. There has been a report of hemodialysis-associated pseudoporphyria treated with twice daily 400 mg oral *N*-acetylcysteine for 3 months without resolution of symptoms that ultimately required a change of therapy to low dose chloroquine (200 mg weekly). Resolution of the blisters occurred after 1 month of this therapy [80].

Glutathione

The literature also demonstrates the use of glutathione as a treatment for hemodialysis-associated pseudoporphyria. The administration of oral glutathione 300 mg daily and avoidance of sun exposure has been reported to resolve the blisters and ulcers in hemodialysis-associated pseudoporphyria. Glutathione may cause nausea and vomiting; however, no adverse side effects were demonstrated in this study [81].

Additional recommendations and preventative measures for the treatment of pseudoporphyria include particular avoidance of ultraviolet A (UVA), general sun protective measures including the use of a broad-spectrum sunscreen, and possibly a switch to high-flux dialysis in cases of hemodialysis-associated pseudoporphyria.

Prognosis

For PCT associated with hemodialysis, peritoneal dialysis, and/or ESRD, clinical remission has been reported in many cases following treatment with small-volume phlebotomies in conjunction with erythropoietin therapy [14, 69–72]. Additionally, treatments involving solely small-volume phlebotomies [21, 30] and solely erythropoietin [10–12, 73] have induced remission. Urine and plasma porphyrins gradually decline, and continue to decline even after phlebotomy is stopped. Cutaneous improvement often lags behind porphyrin normalization and can take several months or even years before the skin returns to normal.

Deferoxamine treatment has also demonstrated remission [6, 15, 23, 24, 31]; however, four groups have reported no improvement with lower doses (0.5–1.5 g intravenously with each dialysis) of deferoxamine [10–12, 14]. The antimalarial drugs, chloroquine and hydroxychloroquine, have not demonstrated success when used independently [6, 26, 27, 70]; however the use of hydroxychloroquine in conjunction with additional treatment modalities and reducing ongoing exposure to known triggers has demonstrated success in the medical literature [5, 7, 63].

In cases of drug-induced pseudoporphyria, discontinuation of the inciting medication typically results in clinical remission over a time period of weeks to months, with an average of 8 weeks [37]. For pseudoporphyria associated with hemodialysis or peritoneal dialysis, clinical remission has been reported in many cases following treatment with *N*-acetylcysteine at various dosages and at varying lengths of administration [76–79]. Discontinuation of this therapy has resulted in recurrence of lesions in several cases [36, 75, 79]; however, one study proposes the investigation and evaluation of the influence of a possible bias, such as sun exposure or alcohol intake, needed to confirm their results [79]. Clinical remission following 2 weeks of treatment with 300 mg daily oral glutathione has also been demonstrated in the scientific literature [81]. The authors propose oral glutathione as a suitable alternative to *N*-acetylcysteine for the treatment of pseudoporphyria [81].

References

1. Waldenström J. Studien über Porphyrie, Dissertation. Acta Medica Scandinavica. 1937;82:1–254.
2. Ryan Caballes F, Sendi H, Bonkovsky HL. Hepatitis C, porphyria cutanea tarda and liver iron: an update. Liver Int. 2012;32(6):880–93.

3. Balwani M, Desnick RJ. The porphyrias: advances in diagnosis and treatment. Hematology Am Soc Hematol Educ Program. 2012;2012:19–27.
4. Huang YC, Wang CC, Sue YM. Porphyria cutanea tarda in a hemodialysis patient. QJM. 2013;106(6):591–2.
5. Talmaci L, Davenport A, Burns A. The case | A blistering problem in a hemodialysis patient. The diagnosis | Porphyria cutanea tarda. Kidney Int. 2010;78(11):1195–6.
6. Labidi J. Porphyria cutanea tarda in a chronic hemodialysis patient. Saudi J Kidney Dis Transpl. 2010;21(5):919–22.
7. Tarwater K, Misra S, Misra M. Type I (sporadic) porphyria cutanea tarda in a hemodialysis patient: a case report. Hemodial Int. 2008;12 Suppl 2:S38–42.
8. Suga C, Ikezawa Z. Porphyria cutanea tarda in hemodialyzed patients. Nihon Rinsho. 1995;53(6):1484–90.
9. Koszo F, Foldes M, Morvay M, Judak R, Vakis G, Dobozy A. Chronic hemodialysis-related porphyria/pseudoporphyria. Orv Hetil. 1994;135(39):2131–6.
10. Peces R, Enriquez de Salamanca R, Fontanellas A, Sanchez A, de la Torre M, Caparros G, et al. Successful treatment of haemodialysis-related porphyria cutanea tarda with erythropoietin. Nephrol Dial Transplant. 1994;9(4):433–5.
11. Yaqoob M, Smyth J, Ahmad R, McClelland P, Fahal I, Kumar KA, et al. Haemodialysis-related porphyria cutanea tarda and treatment by recombinant human erythropoietin. Nephron. 1992;60(4):428–31.
12. Piazza V, Villa G, Galli F, Segagni S, Bovio G, Poggio F, et al. Erythropoietin as treatment of haemodialysis-related porphyria cutanea tarda. Nephrol Dial Transplant. 1992;7(5):438–42.
13. Kawabe M, Matsumoto Y, Yasue T, Toriyama T, Kondo M. Porphyria cutanea tarda in a chronic hemodialysis patient. Nihon Hifuka Gakkai Zasshi. 1990;100(5):589–96.
14. Anderson KE, Goeger DE, Carson RW, Lee SM, Stead RB. Erythropoietin for the treatment of porphyria cutanea tarda in a patient on long-term hemodialysis. N Engl J Med. 1990;322(5):315–7.
15. Stockenhuber F, Kurz R, Grimm G, Moser G, Balcke P. Successful treatment of hemodialysis-related porphyria cutanea tarda with deferoxamine. Nephron. 1990;55(3):321–4.
16. Kano T, Yamane Y, Suzuki M, Yaoita H. Porphyria cutanea tarda in a chronic hemodialysis patient. Nihon Hifuka Gakkai Zasshi. 1989;99(7):819–26.
17. Toriyama F, Nonaka S, Murayama F, Irifune H, Ohgami T, Kakimoto S, et al. A case of porphyria cutanea tarda associated with hemodialysis in chronic renal failure. Nihon Hifuka Gakkai Zasshi. 1987;97(11):1189–92.
18. Poh-Fitzpatrick MB, Masullo AS, Grossman ME. Porphyria cutanea tarda associated with chronic renal disease and hemodialysis. Arch Dermatol. 1980;116(2):191–5.
19. Ryali ME, Whittier WL. Bullous skin lesions in a patient undergoing chronic hemodialysis. Semin Dial. 2010;23(1):83–7.
20. Topi GC, Alessandro GL, Cancarini GC, De Costanza F, Griso D, Ravelli M. Porphyria cutanea tarda in a haemodialysed patient. Br J Dermatol. 1981;104(5):579–80.
21. Riccioni N, Donati G, Soldani S, Scatena P, Arcabasso GD. Treatment of hemodialysis-related porphyria cutanea tarda with small repeated phlebotomies. Nephron. 1987;46(2):125–7.
22. Lichtenstein JR, Babb EJ, Felsher BF. Porphyria cutanea tarda (PCT) in a patient with chronic renal failure on haemodialysis. Br J Dermatol. 1981;104(5):575–8.
23. Praga M, Enriquez de Salamanca R, Andres A, Nieto J, Oliet A, Perpina J, et al. Treatment of hemodialysis-related porphyria cutanea tarda with deferoxamine. N Engl J Med. 1987;316(9):547–8.
24. Pitche P, Corrin E, Wolkenstein P, Revuz J, Bagot M. Successful treatment of haemodialysis-related porphyria cutanea tarda with deferoxamine. Ann Dermatol Venereol. 2003;130(1 Pt 1):37–9.
25. Disler P, Day R, Burman N, Blekkenhorst G, Eales L. Treatment of hemodialysis-related porphyria cutanea tarda with plasma exchange. Am J Med. 1982;72(6):989–93.
26. Garcia Parrilla J, Ortega R, Pena ML, Rodicio JL, de Salamanca RE, Olmos A, et al. Porphyria cutanea tarda during maintenance haemodialysis. Br Med J. 1980;280(6228):1358.
27. King J, Day RS, Milne FJ, Bezwoda WR, Viljoen JD, Kramer S. Delayed onset of overt porphyria cutanea tarda in a patient on long-term haemodialysis. A case report. S Afr Med J. 1983;63(19):743–6.
28. Stevens BR, Fleischer Jr AB, Piering F, Crosby DL. Porphyria cutanea tarda in the setting of renal failure. Response to renal transplantation. Arch Dermatol. 1993;129(3):337–9.
29. Kelly MA, O'Rourke KD. Treatment of porphyria cutanea tarda with phlebotomy in a patient on peritoneal dialysis. J Am Acad Dermatol. 2001;44(2 Suppl):336–8.
30. Ruggian JC, Fishbane S, Demento FJ, Maesaka JK, Frei GL. Porphyria cutanea tarda in a patient on chronic ambulatory peritoneal dialysis. J Am Soc Nephrol. 1996;7(3):397–402.
31. Andreoli SP, Cohen M. Intraperitoneal deferoxamine therapy for iron overload in children undergoing CAPD. Kidney Int. 1989;35(6):1330–5.
32. Glynne P, Deacon A, Goldsmith D, Pusey C, Clutterbuck E. Bullous dermatoses in end-stage renal failure: porphyria or pseudoporphyria? Am J Kidney Dis. 1999;34(1):155–60.
33. Markova A, Lester J, Wang J, Robinson-Bostom L. Diagnosis of common dermopathies in dialysis patients: a review and update. Semin Dial. 2012;25(4):408–18.
34. Zelickson AS. Phototoxic reaction with nalidixic acid. JAMA. 1964;190:556–7.
35. Gilchrest B, Rowe JW, Mihm Jr MC. Bullous dermatosis of hemodialysis. Ann Intern Med. 1975;83(4):480–3.
36. Guiotoku MM, Pereira Fde P, Miot HA, Marques ME. Pseudoporphyria induced by dialysis treated with oral *N*-acetylcysteine. An Bras Dermatol. 2011;86(2):383–5.
37. Katoulis AC, Ferra D, Toumbis E, Papadavid E, Kanelleas A, Panayiotides I, et al. Pseudoporphyria associated with nonhemodialyzed renal insufficiency, successfully treated with oral *N*-acetylcysteine. Case Rep Dermatol Med. 2013;2013:271873.
38. Harvey E, Bell CH, Paller AS, LaVoo EJ, Hanna W, Balfe JW, et al. Pseudoporphyria cutanea tarda: two case reports on children receiving peritoneal dialysis and erythropoietin therapy. J Pediatr. 1992;121(5 Pt 1):749–52.
39. Keczkes K, Farr M. Bullous dermatosis of chronic renal failure. Br J Dermatol. 1976;95(5):541–6.
40. Elder GH. The cutaneous porphyrias. Semin Dermatol. 1990;9(1):63–9.
41. Frank J, Poblete-Gutiérrez P. Porphyria cutanea tarda—when skin meets liver. Best Pract Res Clin Gastroenterol. 2010;24(5):735–45.
42. Cordova KB, Oberg TJ, Malik M, Robinson-Bostom L. Dermatologic conditions seen in end-stage renal disease. Semin Dial. 2009;22(1):45–55.
43. Schanbacher CF, Vanness ER, Daoud MS, Tefferi A, Su WP. Pseudoporphyria: a clinical and biochemical study of 20 patients. Mayo Clin Proc. 2001;76(5):488–92.
44. Schad SG, Kraus A, Haubitz I, Trcka J, Hamm H, Girschick HJ. Early onset pauciarticular arthritis is the major risk factor for naproxen-induced pseudoporphyria in juvenile idiopathic arthritis. Arthritis Res Ther. 2007;9(1):R10.
45. Poh-Fitzpatrick MB, Ellis DL. Porphyrialike bullous dermatosis after chronic intense tanning bed and/or sunlight exposure. Arch Dermatol. 1989;125(9):1236–8.
46. Murphy GM, Wright J, Nicholls DS, McKee PH, Messenger AG, Hawk JL, et al. Sunbed-induced pseudoporphyria. Br J Dermatol. 1989;120(4):555–62.

47. Girschick HJ, Hamm H, Ganser G, Huppertz HI. Naproxen-induced pseudoporphyria: appearance of new skin lesions after discontinuation of treatment. Scand J Rheumatol. 1995;24(2):108–11.
48. Levy ML, Barron KS, Eichenfield A, Honig PJ. Naproxen-induced pseudoporphyria: a distinctive photodermatitis. J Pediatr. 1990;117(4):660–4.
49. Green JJ, Manders SM. Pseudoporphyria. J Am Acad Dermatol. 2001;44(1):100–8.
50. Jalil S, Grady JJ, Lee C, Anderson KE. Associations among behavior-related susceptibility factors in porphyria cutanea tarda. Clin Gastroenterol Hepatol. 2010;8(3):297–302. 302.e1.
51. Sassa S. Modern diagnosis and management of the porphyrias. Br J Haematol. 2006;135(3):281–92.
52. Day RS, Eales L. Porphyrins in chronic renal failure. Nephron. 1980;26(2):90–5.
53. Rosenlof K, Fyhrquist F, Tenhunen R. Erythropoietin, aluminium, and anaemia in patients on haemodialysis. Lancet. 1990; 335(8684):247–9.
54. Ceballos-Picot I, Witko-Sarsat V, Merad-Boudia M, Nguyen AT, Thevenin M, Jaudon MC, et al. Glutathione antioxidant system as a marker of oxidative stress in chronic renal failure. Free Radic Biol Med. 1996;21(6):845–53.
55. Clermont G, Lecour S, Lahet J, Siohan P, Vergely C, Chevet D, et al. Alteration in plasma antioxidant capacities in chronic renal failure and hemodialysis patients: a possible explanation for the increased cardiovascular risk in these patients. Cardiovasc Res. 2000;47(3):618–23.
56. Munoz-Santos C, Guilabert A, Moreno N, To-Figueras J, Badenas C, Darwich E, et al. Familial and sporadic porphyria cutanea tarda: clinical and biochemical features and risk factors in 152 patients. Medicine (Baltimore). 2010;89(2):69–74.
57. Bygum A, Christiansen L, Petersen NE, Hørder M, Thomsen K, Brandrup F. Familial and sporadic porphyria cutanea tarda: clinical, biochemical and genetic features with emphasis on iron status. Acta Derm Venereol. 2003;83(2):115–20.
58. Lee KG, Hyun JJ, Seo YS, Keum B, Yim HJ, Jeen YT, et al. Liver cirrhosis induced by porphyria cutanea tarda: a case report and review. Gut Liver. 2010;4(4):551–5.
59. Murphy GM. The cutaneous porphyrias: a review. The British Photodermatology Group. Br J Dermatol. 1999;140(4):573–81.
60. Cassiman D, Vannoote J, Roelandts R, Libbrecht L, Roskams T, Van den Oord J, et al. Porphyria cutanea tarda and liver disease. A retrospective analysis of 17 cases from a single centre and review of the literature. Acta Gastroenterol Belg. 2008;71(2):237–42.
61. Robinson-Bostom L, DiGiovanna JJ. Cutaneous manifestations of end-stage renal disease. J Am Acad Dermatol. 2000;43(6):975–86. quiz 987–90.
62. Fung MA, Murphy MJ, Hoss DM, Berke A, Grant-Kels JM. The sensitivity and specificity of "caterpillar bodies" in the differential diagnosis of subepidermal blistering disorders. Am J Dermatopathol. 2003;25(4):287–90.
63. Chou TC, Su YS, Wu SM, Wang CC, Lee CH. Successful treatment of refractory blisters in porphyria cutanea tarda with topical pimecrolimus combined with oral hydroxychloroquine: an alternative to phlebotomy in patients with renal insufficiency and anemia. Eur J Dermatol. 2012;22(4):567–8.
64. Elder GH. Porphyria cutanea tarda. Semin Liver Dis. 1998; 18(1):67–75.
65. Gafter U, Mamet R, Korzets A, Malachi T, Schoenfeld N. Bullous dermatosis of end-stage renal disease: a possible association between abnormal porphyrin metabolism and aluminium. Nephrol Dial Transplant. 1996;11(9):1787–91.
66. Mehrany K, Drage LA, Brandhagen DJ, Pittelkow MR. Association of porphyria cutanea tarda with hereditary hemochromatosis. J Am Acad Dermatol. 2004;51(2):205–11.
67. Gisbert JP, Garcia-Buey L, Alonso A, Rubio S, Hernandez A, Pajares JM, et al. Hepatocellular carcinoma risk in patients with porphyria cutanea tarda. Eur J Gastroenterol Hepatol. 2004; 16(7):689–92.
68. Harber LC, Bickers DR. Porphyria and pseudoporphyria. J Invest Dermatol. 1984;82(3):207–9.
69. Hamzi MA, Alayoud A, Asseraji M, Akhmouch I, Oualim Z. Porphyria cutanea tarda in a hemodialysis patient with hepatitis C virus: efficacy of treatment with multiple phlebotomies and erythropoietin. Saudi J Kidney Dis Transpl. 2013; 24(1):121–3.
70. Shieh S, Cohen JL, Lim HW. Management of porphyria cutanea tarda in the setting of chronic renal failure: a case report and review. J Am Acad Dermatol. 2000;42(4):645–52.
71. Poux JM, Demontis R, Cadranel JF, Ghazali A, Fievet P, Nordmann Y. Porphyria cutanea tarda in a dialyzed patient with hepatitis C virus infection: dramatic efficacy of small repeated phlebotomies. Am J Med. 1997;103(2):163–4.
72. Lee PK, Abrahams I, Bickers DR. Porphyria cutanea tarda occurring in a patient with renal failure, systemic lupus erythematosus and chronic hepatitis C infection treated with hemodialysis. Cutis. 1999;64(4):237–9.
73. Sarkell B, Patterson JW. Treatment of porphyria cutanea tarda of end-stage renal disease with erythropoietin. J Am Acad Dermatol. 1993;29(3):499–500.
74. Carson RW, Dunnigan EJ, DuBose Jr TD, Goeger DE, Anderson KE. Removal of plasma porphyrins with high-flux hemodialysis in porphyria cutanea tarda associated with end-stage renal disease. J Am Soc Nephrol. 1992;2(9):1445–50.
75. Tremblay JF, Veilleux B. Pseudoporphyria associated with hemodialysis treated with *N*-acetylcysteine. J Am Acad Dermatol. 2003;49(6):1189–90.
76. Massone C, Ambros-Rudolph CM, Di Stefani A, Mullegger RR. Successful outcome of haemodialysis-induced pseudoporphyria after short-term oral *N*-acetylcysteine and switch to high-flux technique dialysis. Acta Derm Venereol. 2006;86(6): 538–40.
77. Cooke NS, McKenna K. A case of haemodialysis-associated pseudoporphyria successfully treated with oral *N*-acetylcysteine. Clin Exp Dermatol. 2007;32(1):64–6.
78. Felix RH, Silva Jr MF, Almeida JB, Neto PB. Pseudoporphyria associated with hemodialysis. Kidney Int. 2011;79(1):140.
79. Vadoud-Seyedi J, de Dobbeleer G, Simonart T. Treatment of haemodialysis-associated pseudoporphyria with *N*-acetylcysteine: report of two cases. Br J Dermatol. 2000;142(3):580–1.
80. El Kabbaj D, Laalou A, Alouane Z, Bahadi A, Oualim Z. Hemodialysis-associated pseudoporphyria resistant to *N*-acetylcysteine. Saudi J Kidney Dis Transpl. 2011;22(2):311–4.
81. Kasuya A, Hashizume H, Hirakawa S, Tokura Y. Haemodialysis-induced pseudoporphyria successfully treated with glutathione. Eur J Dermatol. 2012;22(1):137–8.

Nail Diseases Among Renal Patients

14

Avner Shemer, Nicole Sakka, and C. Ralph Daniel III

Henoch-Schönlein Purpura

Henoch-Schönlein purpura (HSP) is a vasculitic disease commonly seen in childhood which can affect the skin, gastrointestinal tract, the kidneys, and multiple joints. Among the hallmark findings in HSP is the non-thrombocytopenic purpuric eruption involving the buttocks and lower extremities, polyarthralgias, abdominal pain, and renal involvement with glomeronephritis. The exact pathogenesis of HSP remains poorly understood but is believed to be secondary to an unknown antigenic stimulus which causes elevation of circulating immunoglobulin A (IgA) and complement resulting in deposition within the vasculature [1]. Skin biopsies often reveal leukocytoclastic vasculitis with perivascular infiltrate while indirect immunofluorescence demonstrates deposition of IgA and complement (C3) within the blood vessel wall. In most cases, the disease is self-limiting with only one-third of patients having recurrent illnesses. A more protracted course of illness has been associated with renal involvement with about 1–3 % progressing to end stage renal disease [2]. Affected patients can also present with nailfold telangiectasias in up to 50 % of the cases.

A. Shemer, M.D. (✉)
Department of Dermatology, Sheba Medical Center, Sackler School of Medicine, Tel-Aviv University, Tel Hashomer, Ramat-Gan 52621, Israel
e-mail: ashemer1@gmail.com

N. Sakka, M.D., Ph.D.
Department of Dermatology, Sheba Medical Center, Tel-Hashomer, Tel Aviv 52621, Israel
e-mail: nicsakka@hotmail.com

C.R. Daniel III, M.D.
University of Mississippi Medical Center, 971 Lakeland Drive #659, Jackson, MS 39216, USA

University of Alabama at Birmingham, AL, USA
e-mail: crd322@aol.com

Nailfold changes in patients with HSP have been observed with the use of nailfold videocapillaroscope. Morphologic capillary abnormalities characterized by the presence of tortuosity, edema, derangement of capillaries, and blanching of the capillary network have been seen during acute and chronic follow up [1, 3].

Hypoalbuminemia

Muehrcke nail: Muehrcke lines are characterized by the presence of two transverse bands of pallor that run parallel to the lunula separated from each other by normal pink nail. Robert Muehrcke was the first to describe these lines in 1956 in 32 patients with chronic severe hypoalbuminemia [4]. Of those 32 patients, 23 had nephrotic syndrome and 9 had hypoalbuminemia from other causes. He also noted that these lines occurred with serum albumin levels less than 2.2 g/dL. He also observed that when patients were treated with intravenous albumin or corticosteroids, the lines disappeared, especially after serum albumin increased to greater than 2.2 g/dL. Conditions known to be associated with chronic hypoalbuminemia such as nephrotic syndrome, cirrhosis, or severe malnutrition may result to their presentation [5]. Muehrcke lines have also been described in acrodermatitis enteropathica [6]. It is believed that since zinc is 85 % albumin bound, a significant chronic decrease in serum levels of zinc results leads to hypoalbuminemia. Lines tend to disappear when albumin levels increase. However, they have also been reported even in the absence of hypoalbuminemia particularly in patients treated with multiple cytotoxic chemotherapeutic agents [5] and also in Hodgkin disease, liver disease, end-stage renal failure, and heart transplantation [6]. Muehrcke lines are most commonly observed involving the second, third, and fourth fingernails and frequently spare the thumbnail [5]. If pressure is applied to the nail, the surrounding healthy nail blanches, leading to a homogenously-white colored nail. The pathogenesis of Muehrcke lines is not completely understood but is believed to be caused by vascular compression

J.R. Nunley and E.V. Lerma (eds.), *Dermatological Manifestations of Kidney Disease*,
DOI 10.1007/978-1-4939-2395-3_14, © Springer Science+Business Media New York 2015

within the nail bed as a result of local edema [5]. Because the lines result as an abnormality of the vascular bed of the nail rather than the nail matrix, the lines fail to move with nail growth. Histologically, the underlying nail matrix and nail bed are unremarkable. Muehrcke lines should be differentiated from Mees lines which are white, nonblanching, transverse bands running parallel to the lunula across the entire nail bed with no palpable ridges. Another important difference is that whereas involvement of the thumb is common with Mees lines, it is rare with Muehreke lines.

Nephrotic Syndrome

Yellow nail syndrome: It is characterized by the triad of slow-growing dystrophic yellow nails, lymphedema, and pleural effusions. The nails of both upper and lower extremities are most commonly involved [7]. Pleural effusions tend to be associated with pulmonary diseases such as restrictive and obstructive lung diseases, bronchiectasis as well as rhinosinusitis [7]. The pathogenesis of yellow nail syndrome is still unknown. The nails are thickened, overcurved, and the cuticle tends to disappear. Color can vary between yellow to dark-yellow green. Diagnosis is based solely on clinical grounds. Although most cases are idiopathic it has been reported in association with acquired immunodeficiency syndrome [8], rheumatoid arthritis [9], tuberculosis [10], penicillamine [11], Guillain-Barre syndrome [12], and fetal hydrops [13]. It has also been described in patients with nephrotic syndrome [7], hypoplastic kidney [14], xanthogranulomatous pyelonephritis [15], and artificial arteriovenous fistula in a hemodialysis patient [16]. The discolored appearance of the nails tend to resolve with improvement of the renal disease.

Muehrcke nail: Muehrcke lines are white, transverse paired lines on the fingernails that run parallel to the distal lunula. Muehrcke lines are commonly seen in patients with nephrotic syndrome, partivularly in relation to hypoalbuminemia, although it has also been described in those with nephritic disease. Muehrcke lines have also been described in renal transplant recipients [6]. For more detailed reference regarding Muehrcke lines, see the section "Hypoalbuminemia."

Renal Failure

Half-and-half nails, absence of lunula, and splinter hemorrhage are the most frequent associated nail changes in patients with chronic renal failure [17, 18].

Half-and-half nail: Half-and-half nail, also known as brown arcs or Lindsay nails, is one of the most common nail pathologies encountered among patients with chronic renal failure

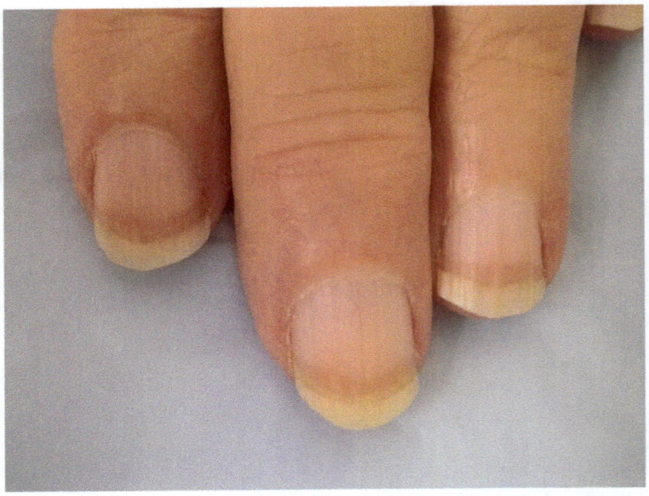

Fig. 14.1 Half-and-half nails. Seen here are the classic changes of half-and-half nails associated with renal failure. Visualization of the lunula is lost; the proximal nail appears white compared to the darker distal area. (Courtesy of Julia R. Nunley, M.D.)

and those on maintenance hemodialysis [19]. Half-and-half nail was first reported by Bean in 1963 in two patients who presented with azotemia. Although it was initially thought to be pathognominic of uremia, it has been demonstrated in patients without any evidence of renal involvement, such as Kawasaki disease, liver cirrhosis, zinc deficiency, Behçet disease, yellow nail syndrome, and Crohn disease [19, 20]. Half and half nails have also been seen in normal individuals, and in some cases, no distinct disease association could be demonstrated [21]. In half-and-half nails, the proximal half of the nail is white, while the distal portion is reddish-brown. The discoloration does not fade with pressure [22]. Generally, 20–40 % of the nail surface is affected [20]. If the distal band occupies less than 20 % of the nail bed, it is then referred to as Terry nail. In Terry nail, the nail abnormality is characterized by a white nail with a distal band of 1–2 mm in length of a normal pink colored nail. Terry nail has been associated with liver cirrhosis, congestive heart failure, diabetes mellitus, and advanced age. A precise clinical differentiation between half-and-half nail and Terry nail can be difficult. The exact cause of half-and-half nail disorder remains unclear, but some authors have postulated that the whiteness may be caused by excessive development of connective tissue between the nail and the bone, resulting in reduced blood supply in the subcapillary plexus [20]. In addition, it has been suggested that increased tissue concentration of β-melanocyte-stimulating hormone may have a contributory role [23]. Histologically, the red color in the distal band was found to be related to increase in capillaries and thickening of their walls [22]. It has also been demonstrated that in the distal part of the nail plate there is melanin believed to be due to increase of melanocyte activity and deposition of excess pigment in the nail plate which has been described in association with renal failure [24] (Fig. 14.1).

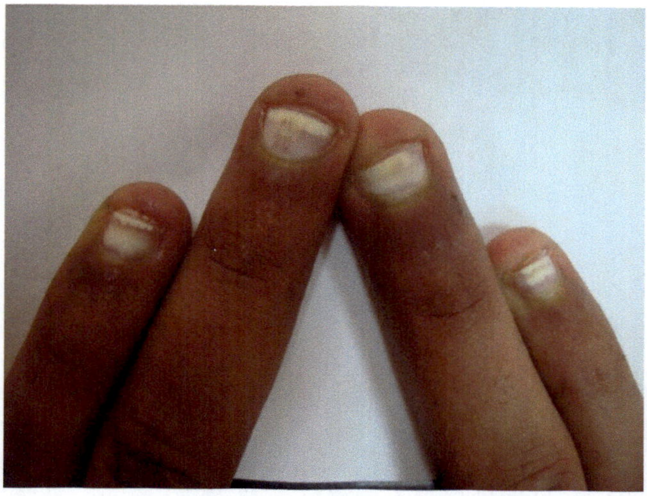

Fig. 14.2 Transverse leukonychia. (Springer Berlin Heidelberg, Color Atlas of Nails, 2010, 45–61, Tosti A, et al.)

Leukonychia, transverse: Leukonychia transverse is a frequently noted nail pathology that can be observed in patients with acute or chronic renal failure as well as renal transplant recipients. It is characterized by the presence of a white single 1–2 mm wide transverse nail plate band. Leukonychia has also been described in patients with acute arsenic toxicity (Mees lines), hepatic cirrhosis, and in association with immunosuppressive medications such as cyclosporine and prednisolone [19]. Other associated conditions include human immunodeficiency virus (HIV) infection, sickle cell anemia, pellagra, nail damage from handling paraquat, and during the course of various chemotherapeutic agents [17, 25–27]. Leukonychia is believed to result from abnormal keratinization of the nail plate [17] (Fig. 14.2).

Nail-patella syndrome (NPS): NPS is a rare autosomal dominant disorder with a reported incidence of 1 in 50,000 live births [28, 29]. Sporadic occurrence accounts for approximately 20 % of the cases and because of the dominant type of inheritance, the children of affected individuals have a 50 % chance of developing the disease [28]. NPS is caused by loss-of-function mutations in the *LMX1B* gene linked to the distal end of the long arm of Chromosome 9 in the region 9q 34. Animal studies have shown that the *LMX1B* gene plays an important role in the dorsal-ventral pattering of limb development, morphogenesis and function of the glomerular basement membrane, as well as the development of the anterior segment of the eye [18]. Classical NPS involves nails, bone abnormalities of patellae, elbow, iliac, and less frequently renal and ocular involvement. Clinical manifestations can be observed during childhood or adolescence. Nail anomalies have been reported in up to 95 % of NPS patients [28]. Nail dysplasia and patellar aplasia or hypoplasia are the most commonly encountered nail abnormalities and are essential features for diagnosis. Nail dystrophy is more pronounced in the fingernails, and patellar abnormalities which may be asymmetrical can be present in up to 90 % of affected individuals [29]. Nail dysplasia is usually present at birth. A pathognomonic sign for NPS is the presence of triangular nail lunulae. The thumbs are more severely affected and the degree of involvement usually decreases progressively from the thumb to the 5th digit. Toenails are rarely affected. Skeletal abnormalities associated with NPS frequently involve the pelvis, elbow, and feet. A pathognomonic sign for NPS is the presence of iliac horns which are triangular bony protuberances of the posterior ilium and is found in 70–80 % of patients [28, 29]. They are located at the side of attachment of the gluteus medius muscle and project posterolaterally. Approximately 70 % of patients with NPS exhibit some degree of elbow involvement which can include limitation of extension, pronation and supination, cubitus valgus, and antecubital pterygia. Other skeletal abnormalities include rib hypoplasia, clubfoot deformities, shoulder girdle dysplasia, scoliosis, clavicular horns, and affected patients are also predisposed to increased incidence of fractures [29]. Ocular involvement includes open angle glaucoma and ocular hypertension. Renal involvement occurs in about 30–60 % of patients and presents with proteinuria and/or microscopic hematuria, edema, and hypertension. Renal involvement is the most serious aspect of NPS, as it can progress to nephrotic syndrome in up to 20 % of patients, and about 10 % of patients will progress to renal failure requiring subsequent renal replacement therapy, e.g., dialysis or renal transplantation [29]. Renal biopsies reveal nonspecific microscopic findings mostly related to the degree of renal failure, including focal and segmental sclerosis, proliferative glomerulonephritis with crescent formation with the only consistent histopathological feature being the focal thickening of glomerular basement membrane [28]. Under the electron microscope, the glomerular basement membrane appears irregularly thickened with electro-lucent areas giving the typical "moth-eaten" appearance [29]. Within the glomerular basement membrane and the mesangium, cross-banded fibrillar collagen-like material has been found in patients with glomerular involvement but not associated with nail or skeletal abnormalities. At the present time, conservative management of proteinuria and hypertension with angiotensin-converting inhibitors and angiotensin receptor blockers is indicated. Renal transplantation is considered a viable therapeutic modality in patients with end-stage renal failure as the disease may not recur in the transplanted kidney [29].

Digital clubbing and Pseudoclubbing: Clubbing is an overcurvature of the nails in the transverse and longitudinal axes with preservation of the angle between the nail palate and the proximal nail fold (Lovibond angle). Such an angle is

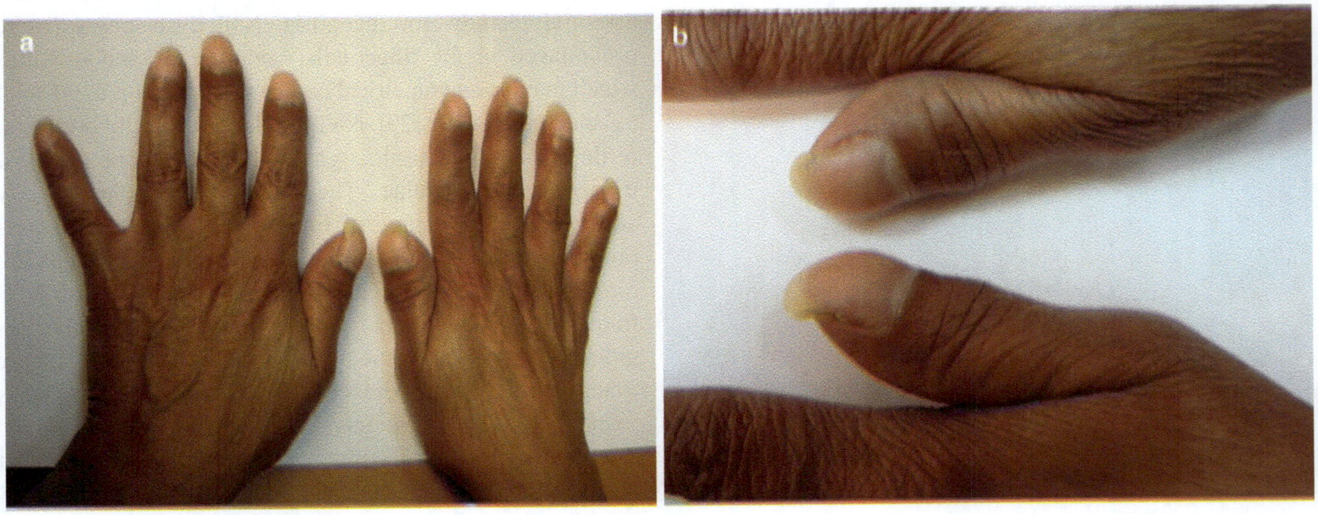

Fig. 14.3 Clubbing

usually less than 160°. In clubbing, this angle exceeds 180°, while in pseudoclubbing, it is less than 180° [30]. Clubbing was first described in the first century BC by Hippocrates and has been commonly described with pulmonary diseases, cyanotic heart disease, liver cirrhosis, but it can also be due to congenital causes and in some instances, it is idiopathic [31]. Both digital clubbing and pseudoclubbing have been described in patients with secondary hyperparathyroidism due to chronic renal failure [30–32]. Pseudoclubbing has been reported to occur in 0.6 % of dialysis patients [32] and can manifest as painful digits tender to palpation. In contrast to clubbing which tends to be symmetrical, pseudoclubbing usually presents as an asymmetric involvement of the fingers. Radiographically, there is resorption of the terminal tufts, i.e., acro-osteolysis. Other known associations include thyroid carcinoma, primary hypothyroidism, sarcoidosis, subungual hemangioma, scleroderma, and certain chromosome anomalies [33–39] (Fig. 14.3).

Hemodialysis

Nail diseases in patients on maintenance hemodialysis are common and may affect from 52 to 71.4 % of patients [17, 40]. The most frequent onychopathy observed in hemodialysis patients include half-and-half nail, absence of lunula, splinter hemorrhage, and onycholysis [17–19].

Half-and-half nail: Half-and-half nail is the most common nail abnormality observed among hemodialysis patients with an estimated frequency that varies between 15 and 50.6 % among different series [41–45]. In half-and-half nails the proximal half of the nail is white, while the distal portion is reddish-brown. Generally, 20–40 % of the nail surface is affected [20]. There has been no demonstrable association between the dose and duration of hemodialysis and frequency of half and half nail [17, 19, 44, 46]. Some studies have shown that half-and-half nails can completely disappear after successful renal transplantation [17, 41]. The exact cause of this nail disorder remains unclear. For more detailed reference regarding half-and-half nail, see the section "Renal Failure" (Fig. 14.1).

Absent lunula: It is characterized by the absence of the visible portion of the nail matrix, and has been associated with metabolic disturbances as well as anemia related to underlying chronic renal failure [17, 47]. Absent lunula can also be found as a normal variant especially among people of Africo-Caribbean and Caucasian decent [6, 19, 40] but hemodialysis patients have a higher rate of occurrence compared to the general population. It has also been demonstrated to occur at any time during the course of chronic renal failure progression to end stage renal disease [17, 19] (Fig. 14.4).

Splinter hemorrhages: These appear as dark red, filiform, longitudinal lines in the distal region of the nail plate. Splinter hemorrhages can be seen in patients on hemodialysis or peritoneal dialysis and have been reported to occur with a prevalence of up to 20 % [17, 19]. Longer duration of dialytic therapy is not associated with the occurrence of splinter hemorrhages [11]. In hemodialysis patients, splinter hemorrhages are believed to result from microtrauma [17, 19]. The exact pathogenesis remains unclear but capillary fragility and thrombocyte dysfunction has been implicated in the development of splinter hemorrhages [17, 19]. They have also been reported in chronic glomerulonephritis, e.g., focal

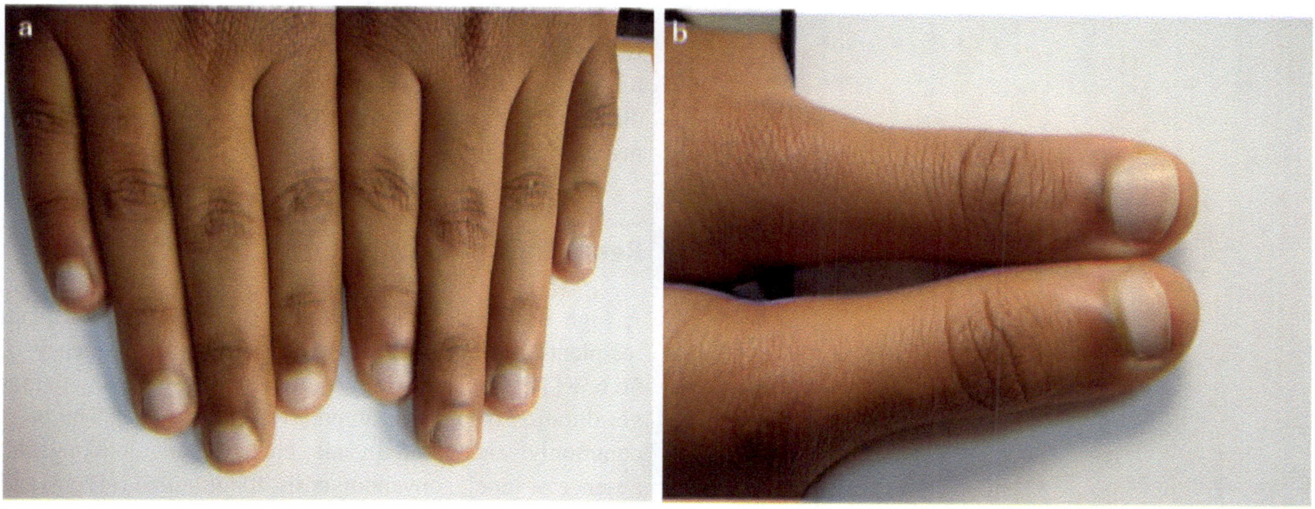

Fig. 14.4 Absence of lunula

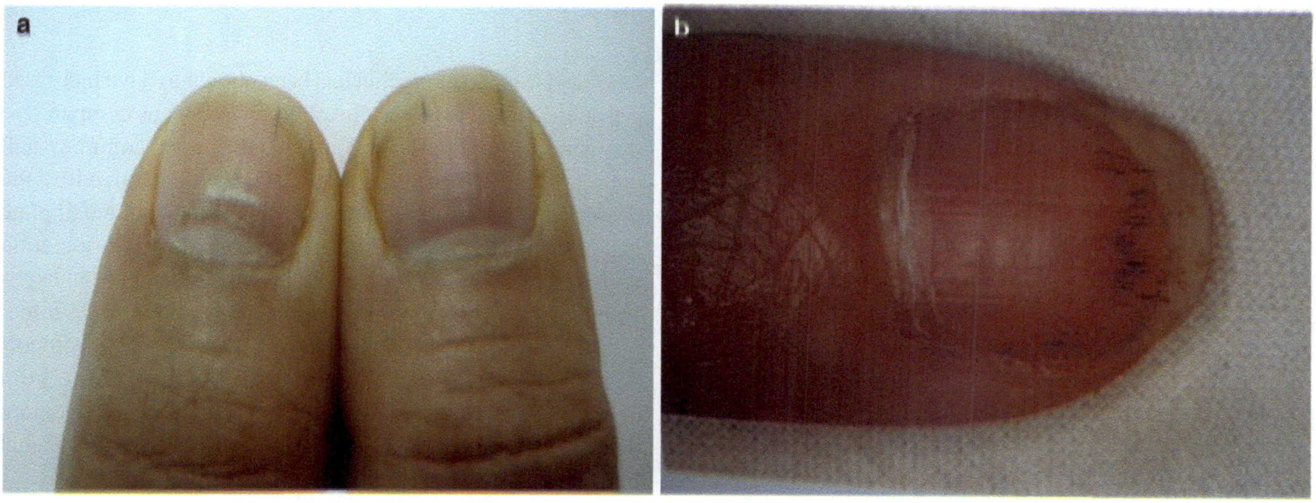

Fig. 14.5 Splinter hemorrhages

segmental glomerulosclerosis. Other associations include bacterial endocarditis, antiphospholipid antibody syndrome, trichinosis, onychomatricoma, and external trauma [46] (Fig. 14.5).

Onycholysis: Normally, the nail plate adheres strictly to the nail bed and this represents as an anatomical barrier. Its disruption results in nail plate detachment with onycholysis. Onycholysis is commonly seen in hemodialysis patients and can result from different local and systemic causes. Captopril has been described to induce reversible onycholysis [48, 49]. Medications causing photosensitivity can induce photo-onycholysis which has been described in hemodialysis patients receiving large doses of cephalordine or cloxacillin [50, 51] (Fig. 14.6).

Brittle nails: Brittle nails are alteration of the nails consistency and have been associated with up to 11.7 % of hemodialysis patients [19, 40]. Etiological factors associated with brittle nails include hypochromic anemia [40], malnutrition, peripheral vascular disease, and low circulating levels of iron and zinc [52] (Fig. 14.7).

Onychomycosis: Onychomycosis has a high prevalence among patients on maintenance hemodialysis. The frequency of onychomycosis in this population can range between 6.2 and 52 % [17, 44, 43, 53]. This may be due to impaired cellular immunity characterized by lymphopenia, decreased B-cell activity, and alteration of T-cell subsets [44]. The most common pathogen isolated in affected patients was *Trichophyton rubrum* followed by *Trichophyton mentagrophytes*, *Scytalidium dimidiatum*, and

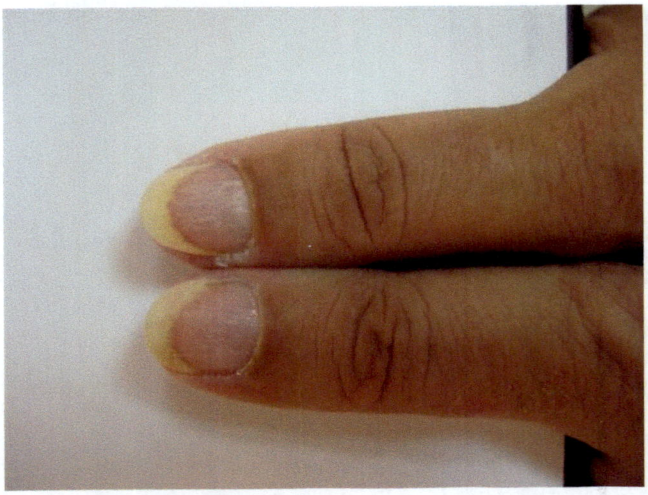

Fig. 14.6 Onycholysis

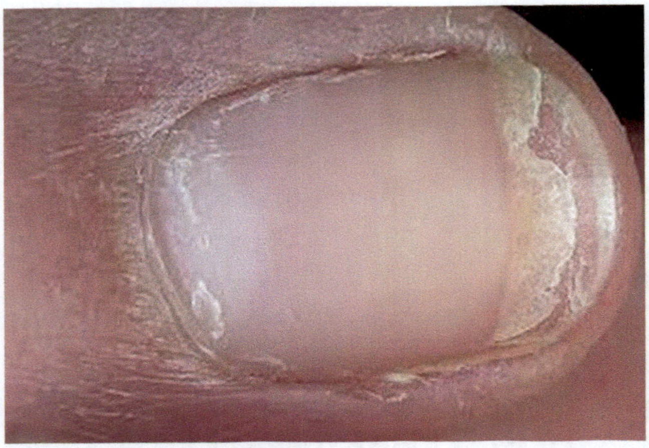

Fig. 14.7 Brittle nail

Candida species [44, 53]. Dermatophytes are more frequently isolated from the toenails whereas *Candida* species from the fingernails. Increase of the dialysis duration and presence of diabetes mellitus are known factors for occurrence of onychomycosis [53] (Fig. 14.8).

Renal Transplantation

A high incidence of nail changes among renal transplant recipients has been reported with an overall frequency of 56.6 % [17]. Nail pathology increases with age and with longer duration of immunosuppressive therapy [17]. The most commonly encountered nail changes are leukonychia, absence of lunula, onychomycosis, longitudinal ridging, and Muehrcke lines [6, 17]. Absence of lunula and longitudinal ridging are also frequent [6]. The occurrence of splinter hemorrhage and half-and-half nails is much less in renal transplant patients as compared to those on maintenance dialysis.

Leukonychia: Leukonychia has been shown to have increased prevalence rates in renal transplant recipients as compared to the general population [6] and is the most common nail pathology in this population [17]. It is characterized by the presence of a single 1–2 mm wide transverse white nail plate band. It has been documented to occur also in association with acute and chronic renal failure, hepatic cirrhosis, exposure to various medications, exposure to toxins, HIV infection, and during the course of various chemotherapy protocols [25–27, 54, 55]. Leukonychia is thought to result from abnormal keratinization of the nail plate [17]. For more detailed reference on leukonychia, see the section "Renal Failure" (Fig. 14.2).

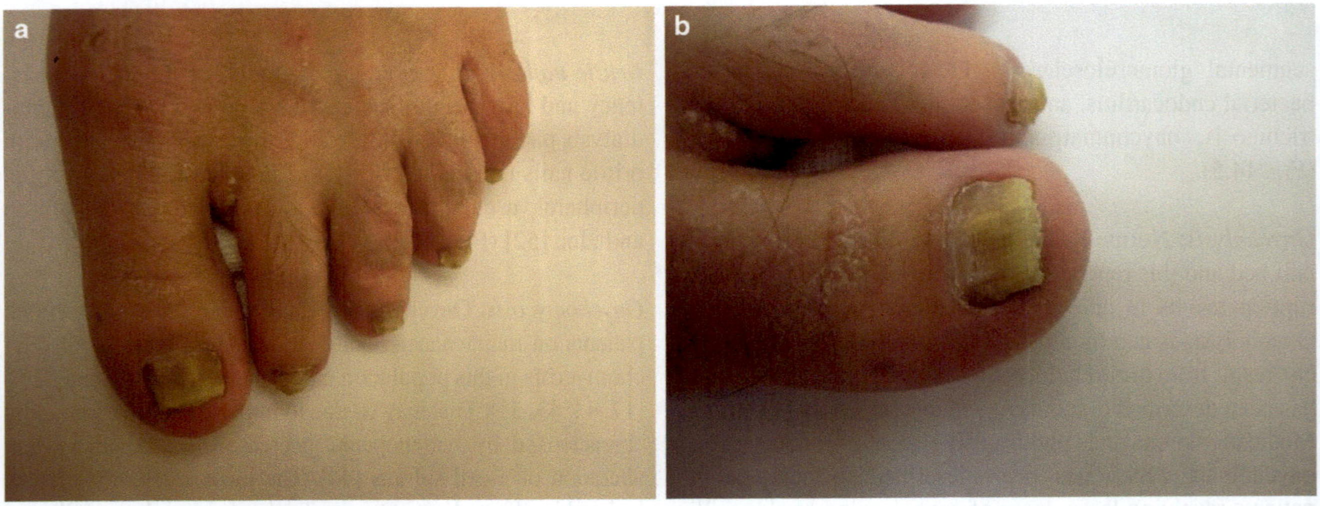

Fig. 14.8 Onychomycotic toenails

Absence of lunula: There is increased frequency of absent lunula among renal transplant patients [6]. It is characterized by the absence of the visible portion of the nail matrix. Several other diseases have been associated with absence of lunula such as atherosclerosis, chronic obstructive pulmonary disease, and rheumatoid arthritis [6]. Absence of lunula was particularly observed with increased frequency in older renal transplant recipients. Interestingly, such increased prevalence was not related to duration of immunosuppression or any treatment protocols [17] (Fig. 14.4).

Superficial fungal infections: A significantly higher incidence of opportunistic infections such as superficial fungal infections, e.g., *Pityrosporum ovale* and *Candida albicans* have also been noted with increased frequency in renal transplant recipients [6, 17]. The increased incidence of mycologically proven *onychomycosis* and superficial fungal infections in renal transplant recipients can be explanted on the basis of decreased cell-mediated immunity brought about by immunosuppressive therapy [6, 17]. Pityriasis versicolor is the most common isolated fungal infection followed by oral candidiasis, onychomycosis, and interdigital toe-web infection [55]. *Trichophyton rubrum* is the most common dermatophyte causing tinea unguium in this population [6, 56–58]. Some studies however, have shown *Trichophyton mentagrophytes* to be quite common [59, 60] (Fig. 14.8).

Muehrcke nail: Muehrcke lines are paired white transverse lines that have been seen in renal transplant recipients, end-stage renal failure, and Hodgkin disease [6]. It is believed to be caused by localized edema involving the nail bed thereby applying pressure to underlying vasculature, resulting in a decreased erythema of the nail bed [61].

Drug-induced onychopathy: Sirolimus is an immunosuppressive drug used commonly in renal transplantation as well as in rheumatoid arthritis. Dermatological side effects associated with sirolimus include edema, acne, aphthous ulceration, and vasculitis [62]. Sirolimus-induced onychopathy has been described in renal transplant recipients, and the most frequent nail abnormalities were matrix alterations (slow growth, onychomalacia, onychorrhexis), nail bed alterations (onycholysis), vascular charges (erythema, splinter hemorrhages), and periungual anomalies (pyogenic granuloma) [62, 63].

Onychoschizia: Onychoschizia is fracture of the distal nail plate into lamellae (splitting into layers of the free edge of the nail). Its occurrence has been reported in association with microtrauma, use of detergents or chemicals, anemia, polycythemia, and poor peripheral blood supply. Onychoschizia was initially described in children who are renal transplant recipients, in whom toenails were primarily affected [64]. There has been no demonstrable association between immunosuppresive regimens and occurence of onychoschizia.

Metastatic Carcinoma

Cutaneous metastases to the nail unit are rare. Subungual metastases (cutaneous metastasis of the nail unit) most frequently occur in patients with primary tumors of the lung (41 %), genitourinary tract 17 %, of which the kidney represented 11 %, followed by breast, head, and neck (parotic gland, hypopharynx, larynx, oral cavity), sarcoma (chondrosarcoma), and melanoma [65]. Primary renal cell carcinoma and squamous cell carcinoma (originating from the lung and the head and neck area) are the most frequent histologic types [65]. Lung cancer is the most common cancer associated with metastatic tumor of the hands while genitourinary was the commonest metastatic tumor of the feet. The presence of cutaneous metastases in patients with established malignancy is indicative of recurrence or progression of the malignancy [66, 67]. It is not uncommon for a to be the initial manifestation of an underlying undiagnosed primary malignancy or to present at a similar time frame as the diagnosis of the primary cancer [68]. Subungual metastases typically present as painful lesions of the distal digit that may involve a single digit or multiple digits of the hand or foot or both. These tumors predominantly involve the digits of the upper extremities. Metastatic tumors involving the nail unit most commonly involve the nail plate and often metastasizes to the adjacent joint space of the bone and can spread to the surrounding soft tissue [65]. Symptoms of subungual metastases result from tumor infiltration of the nail bed or as a result of space occupying lesion or as metastases to the distal bone. The most common appearance of the lesion is either as an erythematous enlargement or swelling of the distal digit or as a red to violaceous nodule that distorts either the nail plate or the soft tissue of the distal digit, or both [65]. Additionally, it can present with discoloration of the nail plate or nail bed and the periungual soft tissue. Frequently the clinical presentation of a subungual metastasis is misleading and can be mistaken for an abscess, paronychia, or osteomyelitis. The clinician should have a high index of clinical suspicion for metastasis to the nail unit and clues to the diagnosis include lack of improvement with antibiotics or surgical drainage and symptoms that are disproportionate to the degree of the appearance of the lesion. When a metastasis of the nail unit is suspected, histological examination should be promptly performed and samples should be taken from either the nail bed or the surrounding soft tissue of the distal digit. Once the diagnosis of subungual metastasis is established, the patient should be aggressively managed as an oncology patient. Combination chemotherapy, radiotherapy to bony metastasis, and surgical intervention has been recommended. Surgical management includes nail avulsion, excision or curettage of the tumor, and amputation of the involved digit. The prognosis of subungual metastasis is poor with an estimated survival of less than 6 months from the time of detection. A case report of acral verrucous malignant melanoma has been described in an immunosuppressed patient after renal transplantation [69].

References

1. Zampetti A, Rigante D, Bersani G, Rendeli C, Feliciani C, Stabile A. Longitudinal study of microvascular involvement by nailfold capillaroscopy in children with Henoch-Schönlein purpura. Clin Rheumatol. 2009;28:1101–5.
2. Trapani S, Micheli A, Grisolia F, Resti M, Chiappini E, Falcini F, De Martino M. Henoch Schonlein purpura in childhood: epidemiological and clinical analysis of 150 cases over a 5-year period and review of literature. Semin Arthritis Rheum. 2005;35:143–53.
3. Martino F, Agolini D, Tsalikova E, Bederti O, Principessa L, Martino E, Carnevali E, Giardini O. Nailfold capillaroscopy in Henoch-Schönlein purpura: a follow-up study of 31 cases. J Pediatr. 2002;141:145.
4. Muehrcke RC. The finger-nails in chronic hypoalbuminaemia; a new physical sign. Br Med J. 1956;1:1327–8.
5. Short N, Shah C. Muehrcke lines. Am J Med. 2010;123:991–2.
6. Gaveau D, Piette F, Cortot A, Dumur V, Bergoend H. Cutaneous manifestations of zinc deficiency in ethylic cirrhosis. Ann Dermatol Venereol. 1987;114:39–53.
7. Yáñez S, Val-Bernal JF, Fernández-Llaca H. Yellow nails and minimal change nephrotic syndrome. Nephron. 1999;82:180–2.
8. Chernosky ME, Finley VK. Yellow nail syndrome and acquired immunodeficiency disease. J Am Acad Dermatol. 1986;14:844–6.
9. Mattingly PC, Bossingham DH. Yellow nail syndrome in rheumatoid arthritis: report of three cases. Ann Rheum Dis. 1979;38:475–8.
10. Pang SM. Yellow nail syndrome resolution following treatment of pulmonary tuberculosis. Int J Dermatol. 1993;32:605–6.
11. Ilchyshyn A, Vickers CF. Yellow nail syndrome associated with penicillamine therapy. Acta Derm Venereol. 1983;63:554–5.
12. Woollons A, Darley CR. Yellow nail syndrome following Guillain-Barrésyndrome. Clin Exp Dermatol. 1997;22:253–4.
13. Govaert P, Leroy JG, Pauwels R, Vanhaesebrouck P, De Praeter C, Van Kets H, Goeteyn M. Perinatal manifestations of maternal yellow nail syndrome. Pediatrics. 1992;89:1016–8.
14. Cockram CS, Richards P. Yellow nails and nephrotic syndrome. Br J Dermatol. 1979;101:707–9.
15. Danenberg HD, Eliashar R, Flusser G, Rosenmann E, Chajek-Shaul T. Yellow nail syndrome and xanthogranulomatous pyelonephritis. Postgrad Med J. 1995;71:110–1.
16. Mehta V, Vasanth V, Balachandran C. Yellow nails following hemodialysis in chronic renal failure: is it yellow nail syndrome or a variant? Dermatol Online J. 2008;14:19.
17. Saray Y, Seçkin D, Güleç AT, Akgün S, Haberal M. Nail disorders in hemodialysis patients and renal transplant recipients: a case-control study. J Am Acad Dermatol. 2004;50:197–202.
18. Lee BH, Cho TJ, Choi HJ, Kang HK, Lim IS, Park YH, Ha IS, Choi Y, Cheong HI. Clinico-genetic study of nail-patella syndrome. J Korean Med Sci. 2009;24(Suppl):82–6.
19. Salem A, Al Mokadem S, Attwa E, Abd El Raoof S, Ebrahim HM, Faheem KT. Nail changes in chronic renal failure patients under haemodialysis. J Eur Acad Dermatol Venereol. 2008;22:1326–31.
20. Pellegrino M, Taddeucci P, Mei S, Peccianti C, Fimiani M. Half-and-half nail in a patient with Crohn disease. J Eur Acad Dermatol Venereol. 2010;24:1366–7.
21. Zágoni T, Sipos F, Tarján Z, Péter Z. The half-and-half nail: a new sign of Crohn disease? Report of four cases. Dis Colon Rectum. 2006;49:1071–3.
22. Markova A, Lester J, Wang J, Robinson-Bostom L. Diagnosis of common dermopathies in dialysis patients: a review and update. Semin Dial. 2012;25:408–18.
23. Kurban MS, Boueiz A, Kibbi AG. Cutaneous manifestations of chronic kidney disease. Clin Dermatol. 2008;26:255–64.
24. Alston H, Burns A. Half and half nails. Nephrol Dial Transplant. 2011;4:361.
25. Benatti C, Gnocchi M, Travaglino E, Invernizzi R, Ascari E. Chemotherapy-induced leukonychia. Haematologica. 2004; 89:16.
26. Mautner GH, Lu I, Ort RJ, Grossman ME. Transverse leukonychia with systemic infection. Cutis. 2000;65:318–20.
27. Cribier B, Mena ML, Rey D, Partisani M, Fabien V, Lang JM, Grosshans E. Nail changes in patients infected with human immunodeficiency virus. A prospective controlled study. Arch Dermatol. 1998;134:1216–20.
28. Bongers EM, Gubler MC, Knoers NV. Nail-patella syndrome. Overview on clinical and molecular findings. Pediatr Nephrol. 2002;17:703–12.
29. Granata A, Nori G, Ravazzolo R, Marini M, Castellino S, Sicurezza E, Fiore CE, Mignani R. Nail-patella syndrome and renal involvement. Description of three cases and literature review. Clin Nephrol. 2008;69:377–82.
30. Santiago MB, Lima I, Feitosa AC, Braz Ade S, Miranda LG. Pseudoclubbing: is it different from clubbing? Semin Arthritis Rheum. 2009;38:452–7.
31. Grekas D, Avdelidou A. Digital clubbing as an unusual complication associated with severe secondary hyperparathyroidism: report of two cases. Hemodial Int. 2007;11:193–7.
32. Chow KM, Szeto CC, Li PK. Pseudoclubbing of fingers. Nephrology. 2007;12:206.
33. Backman U, Butler G, Fletchner P, McMullin J. A case study with delayed renal graft function as a consequence of severe secondary hyperparathyroidism. Artif Organs. 1995;19:72–5.
34. Wong E, Milkes D. Photo quiz. New-onset digital clubbing. Am Fam Physician. 2001;64:141–2.
35. Rault R, Carpenter B. Pseudoclubbing in chronic renal failure. Q J Med. 1989;73:1063–9.
36. Lieberman J, Krauthammer M. Pseudoclubbing in a patient with sarcoidosis of the phalangeal bones. Arch Intern Med. 1983;143:1017–9.
37. Richards AJ. A case of thyroid carcinoma and primary hyperparathyroidism with pseudoclubbing. Br J Clin Pract. 1971;25:34–6.
38. Piraccini BM, Antonucci A, Rech G, Iorizzo M, Neri I, Patrizi A, Tosti A. Congenital pseudoclubbing of a fingernail caused by subungual hemangioma. J Am Acad Dermatol. 2005;53(2 Suppl 1):123–6.
39. Lo Monaco A, Govoni M, Trotta F. Digital clubbing or digital "pseudoclubbing" in systemic sclerosis. J Clin Rheumatol. 2006; 12:97.
40. Tercedor J, López Hernández B, Manuel Ródenas J. Nail diseases in haemodialysis patients: case-control study. Br J Dermatol. 2001;144:445–6.
41. Lubach D, Strübbe J, Schmidt J. The "half and half nail" phenomenon in chronic hemodialysis patients. Dermatologica. 1982;164: 350–3.
42. Stewart WK, Raffle EJ. Brown nail-bed arcs and chronic renal disease. Br Med J. 1972;1:784–6.

43. Bencini PL, Montagnino G, Citterio A, Graziani G, Crosti C, Ponticelli C. Cutaneous abnormalities in uremic patients. Nephron. 1985;40:316–21.
44. Dyachenko P, Monselise A, Shustak A, Ziv M, Rozenman D. Nail disorders in patients with chronic renal failure and undergoing haemodialysis treatment: a case-control study. J Eur Acad Dermatol Venereol. 2007;21:340–4.
45. Thomas EA, Pawar B, Thomas A. A prospective study of cutaneous abnormalities in patients with chronic kidney disease. Indian J Nephrol. 2012;22:116–20.
46. Martinez MA, Gregório CL, Santos VP, Bérgamo RR, Machado Filho CD. Nail disorders in patients with chronic renal failure undergoing hemodialysis. An Bras Dermatol. 2010;85:318–23.
47. Robinson-Bostom L, DiGiovanna JJ. Cutaneous manifestations of end-stage renal disease. J Am Acad Dermatol. 2000;43:975–86.
48. Brueggemeyer CD, Ramirez G. Onycholysis associated with captopril. Lancet. 1984;1:1352–3.
49. Borders JV. Captopril and onycholysis. Ann Intern Med. 1986;105:305–6.
50. Piraccini BM, Iorizzo M, Starace M, Tosti A. Drug-induced nail diseases. Dermatol Clin. 2006;24:387–91.
51. Rutherford T, Sinclair R. Photo-onycholysis due to indapamide. Australas J Dermatol. 2007;48:35–6.
52. Nicolopoulos J, Goodman GJ, Howard A. Diseases of the generative nail apparatus. Part 1. Nail matrix. Australas J Dermatol. 2001; 43:81–90.
53. Picó MR, Lugo-Somolinos A, Sánchez JL, Burgos-Calderón R. Cutaneous alterations in patients with chronic renal failure. Int J Dermatol. 1992;31:860–3.
54. Unamuno P, Fernández-López E, Santos C. Leukonychia due to cytostatic agents. Clin Exp Dermatol. 1992;17:273–4.
55. Chapman S, Cohen PR. Transverse leukonychia in patients receiving cancer chemotherapy. South Med J. 1997;90:395–8.
56. Güleç AT, Demirbilek M, Seçkin D, Can F, Saray Y, Sarifakioglu E, Haberal M. Superficial fungal infections in 102 renal transplant recipients: a case-control study. J Am Acad Dermatol. 2003;49: 187–92.
57. SentamilSelvi G, Kamalam A, Ajithados K, Janaki C, Thambiah AS. Clinical and mycological features of dermatophytosis in renal transplant recipients. Mycoses. 1999;42:75–8.
58. McLelland J, Chu AC. Fungal infection in renal transplant patients. Br J Dermatol. 1988;118:734.
59. Virgili A, Zampino MR, La Malfa V, Strumia R, Bedani PL. Prevalence of superficial dermatomycoses in 73 renal transplant recipients. Dermatology. 1999;199:31–4.
60. Shuttleworth D, Philpot CM, Salaman JR. Cutaneous fungal infection following renal transplantation: a case control study. Br J Dermatol. 1987;117:585–90.
61. Daniel CR, Sams WM, Scher PK. Nail is systemic disease. In: Nails: therapy, diagnosis, surgery. Philadelphia: WB Saunders; 1997. pp. 219–250.
62. Mahé E, Morelon E, Lechaton S, Sang KH, Mansouri R, Ducasse MF, Mamzer-Bruneel MF, de Prost Y, Kreis H, Bodemer C. Cutaneous adverse events in renal transplant recipients receiving sirolimus-based therapy. Transplantation. 2005;79:476–82.
63. Mahé E, Morelon E, Lechaton S, Kreis H, De Prost Y, Bodemer C. Sirolimus-induced onychopathy in renal transplant recipients. Ann Dermatol Venereol. 2006;133:531–5.
64. Menni S, Beretta D, Piccinno R, Ghio L. Cutaneous and oral lesions in 32 children after renal transplantation. Pediatr Dermatol. 1991;8:194–8.
65. Cohen PR. Metastatic tumors to the nail unit: subungual metastases. Dermatol Surg. 2001;27:280–93.
66. Cohen PR. Cutaneous manifestations of internal malignancy. In: Callen JP, Bone RC, editors. Current practice of medicine, vol. 2. Philadelphia: Current Medicine; 1996. p. 19.1–19.13.
67. Cohen PR. Skin clues to primary and metastatic malignancy. Am Fam Physician. 1995;51:1199–204.
68. Cohen PR, Buzdar AU. Metastatic breast carcinoma mimicking an acute paronychia of the great toe: case report and review of subungual metastases. Am J Clin Oncol. 1993;16:86–91.
69. Merkle T, Landthaler M, Eckert F, Braun-Falco O. Acral verrucous malignant melanoma in an immunosuppressed patient after kidney transplantation. J Am Acad Dermatol. 1991;24:505–6.

Alopecias

15

Kimberly Scott Salkey

Introduction

Very little is written about the impact of chronic kidney disease (CKD) on patient's hair. Perhaps this is because such patients often have many other manifestations of their disease that are considered far more serious. In fact, hair is an important component of self-image. For patients with CKD, recognizing types and patterns of hair loss and their likely underlying causes is essential. This chapter addresses alopecias that occur as a consequence of the sequelae of CKD.

In most of the circumstances presented here, hair loss occurs in the form of telogen effluvium. Telogen effluvium occurs when anagen hairs prematurely enter the telogen phase. Patients experience diffuse, heavy hair shedding although they do not reach the point of total baldness.

Malnutrition

Iron Deficiency

Iron deficiency is a frequent occurrence in patients with renal failure who are on hemodialysis (HD) [1]. This occurs as a result of several factors. Patients are deficient in endogenous erythropoietin, necessitating a supplement. Administration of exogenous (recombinant humanized) erythropoietin results in accelerated hematopoiesis and subsequent increased iron demands. In addition, blood loss from dialysis and blood draws, and poor dietary iron intake all contribute to iron deficiency. The latter may also contribute to anemia of chronic disease in patients who are not on HD.

K.S. Salkey, M.D. (✉)
Department of Dermatology, Eastern Virginia Medical School,
721 Fairfax Avenue, Suite 200, Norfolk, VA 23507, USA
e-mail: salkeyks@evms.edu

The role of iron deficiency in hair growth and loss has long been debated. The relation between the two was initially postulated in 1963 by Hard [2]. Iron deficiency has been implicated as a potential contributor to many forms of alopecia including alopecia areata, female pattern hair loss, and telogen effluvium. More recently, a study done by Kantor et al. found that mean ferritin levels in female patients with alopecia areata and those with female pattern hair loss was significantly lower than levels in control patients [3]. Deloche et al. had similar results with a survey of over 5,000 women. Of those with excessive hair loss (specific diagnoses not indicated), 59 % had low ferritin [4]. Conversely, a number of authors have also contested any connection between iron levels and alopecia. In 2010, Olsen and colleagues evaluated 381 patients and found no correlation between iron deficiency and female pattern hair loss or chronic telogen effluvium [5]. Sinclair and colleagues reported similar results in 2002 after evaluation of nearly 200 patients [6].

In the cases where a relationship between iron deficiency and alopecia has been demonstrated, the proposed mechanism relates to the role of iron in normal physiology—oxygen delivery to tissues. Impaired tissue oxygenation can result in deficiency in heme proteins and even impairment in T cell function [7]. Clinical features are variable, including localized shedding, diffuse hair shedding, and patchy hair loss. As one might expect, iron supplementation for cases of alopecia attributable to iron deficiency ought to bring about improvement; however, a comprehensive study to demonstrate this has yet to be done. Most experts agree that a ferritin level between 30 and 70 μg/L is adequate. Higher levels are required in patients with comorbidities such as hepatitis C [8].

Zinc Deficiency

Zinc is a vital micronutrient, of which deficiency can impact nearly every organ system. Results of severe deficiency include mental lethargy, loss of appetite, sexual dysfunction

J.R. Nunley and E.V. Lerma (eds.), *Dermatological Manifestations of Kidney Disease*,
DOI 10.1007/978-1-4939-2395-3_15, © Springer Science+Business Media New York 2015

(delayed sexual maturity, hypogonadism, impotence), and immune dysfunction. Hair loss is also among these sequelae.

Patients with chronic renal disease are subject to zinc deficiency mainly as a result of decreased dietary intake. The recommended diet for patients often restricts intake of food sources high in zinc such as dairy products, legumes, and nuts. Also, patients may have decreased appetite leading to decreased intake of zinc rich foods. In a recent editorial, Steiber reported zinc deficiency in 40–78 % of HD patients [9].

The exact role of zinc in human physiology is multifold. It functions in enzyme catalysis, protein structure, and enzyme regulation [10]. Alopecia due to zinc deficiency is usually gradual in onset, paralleling the development of deficiency. Clinical findings are of diffuse, generalized scalp hair loss. Eyebrows and eyelashes may also be affected. Fortunately, it is rapidly reversed with zinc supplementation. Zinc supplementation increases serum values and subsequently improves hair loss that is attributable to zinc deficiency. Patients demonstrate improvement in symptoms often before zinc levels even reach normal serum levels [11].

Drug Induced

Drugs Used in End-Stage Renal Disease

Erythropoietin

To date, only four patients have been reported who experienced alopecia attributed to erythropoietin-α (Epo). The exact mechanism by which Epo may disrupt hair growth remains to be seen. Its impact on the hypothalamic–pituitary axis is well established. Resultant changes including effects on hormone levels may be the cause. Alternatively, it may have an idiosyncratic effect [12].

One report, a case series of three women of Southeast Asian descent, described two women who developed rapidly progressive, near total alopecia within 1 month of beginning Epo. Iron levels were normal in one case (not mentioned in the other) and thyroid studies were normal in both cases. The third patient in this case series had a more complicated course, receiving numerous red blood cell transfusions in addition to increasing doses of Epo. She had long standing patchy hair loss and then developed sudden, complete scalp hair loss over the course of a few days. This patient also had low ferritin, but there was no change in her hair when this was corrected [12].

A separate case report describes a 60-year-old man with nephrotic syndrome secondary to membranous nephropathy. In the first 3 weeks of erythropoietin therapy, he began to develop hair shedding. Within 4 months, he developed alopecia universalis—loss of all scalp and body hair. Interestingly, laboratory evaluation revealed low zinc; however, supplementation for 2 months did not bring about any improvement. Finally, the patient was changed from erythropoietin α to erythropoietin β and then enjoyed good hair regrowth [13].

More studies are required to establish whether these cases represent a true, but possibly underreported consequence of Epo therapy.

Antihypertensives

According to the National Kidney Foundation, preferred antihypertensive drugs are

- Diabetic kidney disease—Angiotensin converting enzyme inhibitor (ACEI) or angiotensin receptor blocker (ARB).
- Non-diabetic kidney disease—ACEI or ARB.
- Kidney transplant recipient—no preferred agent.

Recommended agents for use in addition to the preferred drug include diuretics, then beta blocker or calcium channel blocker [14].

Of these, ACEI (specifically captopril) and beta blockers have the most frequent reports of associated alopecia.

Angiotensin Converting Enzyme Inhibitors (and Angiotensin Receptor Blockers)

Captopril has been used widely in the management of hypertension since its Food and Drug Administration (FDA) approval in 1981. While it rapidly gained favor for its (at the time) unique mechanism of action, it was not without side effects. As with other ACEI, cough is the most common side effect. It is also frequently associated with dysgeusia (metallic taste, loss of taste). Several cutaneous reactions to captopril have also been reported—mainly rashes in various forms including lichenoid and morbilliform. There are a few reports of alopecia attributed to captopril although the exact mechanism of such loss is not known.

The mechanism of action of ACEI is exerted when the drug binds to a zinc moiety on the angiotensin converting enzyme. As a consequence, zinc deficiency has been reported as a side effect, particularly in patients with renal failure who may already have reduced zinc reserves [15]. As mentioned in a previous section, zinc deficiency alone may be a cause of hair loss.

In 1990, Motel reported the case of a 68-year-old woman who developed a morbilliform eruption in addition to diffuse hair shedding when captopril was added to her antihypertensive regimen of furosemide and potassium [16]. Similarly, Ahmad reported a patient who developed heavy hair shedding within 4 weeks of starting enalapril. In both cases, the loss stopped when the ACEI was discontinued. The patient reported by Ahmad had hair shedding recur upon rechallenge [17]. Interestingly, Leaker and colleague reported a patient who developed hair loss while taking captopril that resolved when she was switched to enalapril. Urine and serum zinc levels in this patient were within normal limits [18]. Zinc levels were not reported in the other cases.

In each case, alopecia presented as diffuse and precipitous and began within 4 weeks of starting the offending medication. This suggests that in patients who are experiencing hair loss and have been on stable doses of ACEI over a long period (several months or more), a cause other than the ACEI should be investigated. It appears that alopecia corrects itself without intervention aside from discontinuation of the medication.

β Adrenergic Receptor Inhibitors

Metoprolol and propranolol have both been associated with telogen effluvium [19, 20]. In most cases, hair loss attributed to beta blockers follows the usual pattern of telogen effluvium with acute onset, rapid loss of up to 50 % of hairs followed by complete regrowth. English and colleague reported a case of more extensive hair loss—90 % in addition to eyebrow and eyelash loss attributed to propranolol [21]. The beta blocker nadolol has been reported to cause extensive hair loss, not in a telogen effluvium pattern, but associated with a biopsy-confirmed scalp dermatitis. Both the alopecia and dermatitis rapidly resolved when nadolol was discontinued [22].

Alopecia in various forms has been associated with multiple beta blocker medications. In all cases, alopecia resolves with cessation of the medication.

Diuretics

Furosemide is one of the most commonly prescribed diuretics. There are no reports of alopecia specifically attributed to furosemide. In the case reported by Motel, the patient developed alopecia when captopril was added to furosemide. The author suggests that an unknown interaction between the two may have been the cause of the alopecia. Interestingly, there is one report in the veterinary literature of furosemide causing rash and alopecia in a dog [23].

In contradistinction to furosemide, there are many reports of the potassium sparing diuretic, spironolactone as having therapeutic efficacy for treatment of hair loss. It is generally understood to be effective in managing some cases of female pattern hair loss. This effect is exerted through its competitive inhibition of the androgen receptor [24].

Calcium Channel Blockers

Calcium channel blockers are frequently associated with peripheral edema. The frequency and severity of the edema depend on the specific agent and dose prescribed [25]. Aside from edema, this class of medications is relatively benign from a cutaneous adverse effect standpoint. Alopecia is reported as a side effect in less than 1 % of patients [26].

Minoxidil

While the use of oral minoxidil is limited to recalcitrant cases of hypertension, its efficacy as a topical therapy for hair loss is well documented. Hypertrichosis reportedly occurs in about 70 % of patients taking oral minoxidil [27].

Lipid-Lowering Agents

HMG-CoA reductase inhibitors, also known as statins, are very commonly used cholesterol-lowering agents. Approximately six different statin medications are commercially available in the USA, all with subtle differences in their efficacy and side effect profile. Alopecia is mentioned in the package insert for all but rosuvastatin. In the lovastatin and pravastatin inserts, alopecia is reported as 0.5–1 % and <2 % incidence, respectively. This was not statistically significant compared to placebo in the case of lovastatin. Both the fluvastatin and simvastatin package inserts mention alopecia in post marketing reports and point out that frequency and causal relationship cannot be reliably estimated from these reports. The atorvastatin insert mentions alopecia as an "additional adverse effect reported" which is separate from the "most frequent adverse effects associated."

Despite these warnings in the prescribing information, reports of alopecia attributed to statins in the literature are rare. A 2002 report reviews the case of a woman with minimal change disease in whom therapy with furosemide, prednisone, benazepril, and atorvastatin was initiated. Within 2 weeks, she developed progressive alopecia that resolved when atorvastatin was discontinued and other medications were not changed. Hair loss occurred again upon rechallenge with atorvastatin. The loss resolved with atorvastatin was permanently discontinued [28].

There is conflicting data specifically for the role of simvastatin in alopecia. While alopecia is documented in post marketing reports, there are several published cases indicating that its use in combination with ezetimibe may be therapeutic for cases of alopecia areata [29, 30]. This is particularly interesting because a conclusion of the Study of Heart and Renal Protection (SHARP) study was that the long-term combination of simvastatin and ezetimibe reduced the risk of cardiac adverse events in people with CKD [31].

Drugs Used in Dialysis

Heparin

Low-molecular-weight heparins dalteparin, tinzaparin, and enoxaparin have all been reported to cause alopecia in the form of telogen effluvium. In one case, a 9-year-old girl who was treated with dalteparin for sinus venous thrombosis developed profuse hair loss within 10 weeks of beginning the drug [32]. Alopecia began to resolve within 2 weeks of dalteparin discontinuation.

A separate report describes five adult women on HD who developed hair loss while on long-term dalteparin therapy. Four of the patients had similar patterns of diffuse and patchy hair loss that began within 6–12 weeks of dalteparin initiation. When dalteparin was discontinued in favor of regional citrate anticoagulation, these patients experienced complete

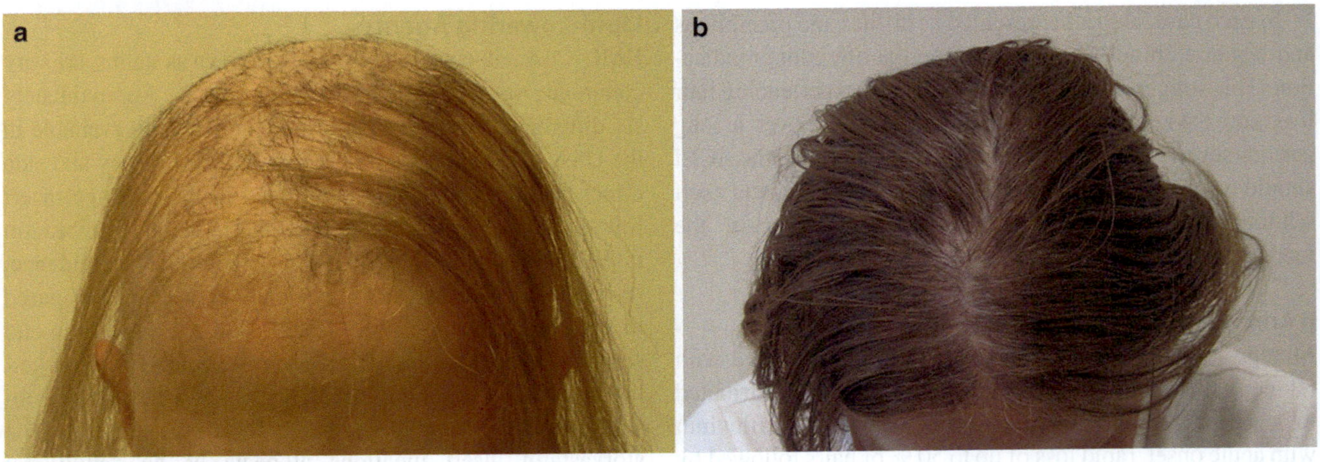

Fig. 15.1 (**a**) Widespread, diffuse hair loss in a renal transplant patient taking tacrolimus. (**b**) Excellent response to minoxidil

hair regrowth within 6–12 weeks. One of these patients again developed precipitous hair loss upon rechallenge with dalteparin. The fifth reported patient in this series had "poor hair growth" along with hair shedding. In her case, shedding ceased when dalteparin was discontinued but she did not experience any hair regrowth [33].

In 2006, Wang and Po reported a series of three patients who developed alopecia as a consequence of enoxaparin. Each patient was treated with enoxaparin for central venous thrombosis and all developed patchy, non-scarring alopecia within 3 weeks of initiation. After 3 weeks of treatment with enoxaparin, therapy was switched to warfarin. In all three cases, hair growth returned to normal within 4 weeks after enoxaparin was discontinued [34]. Interestingly, Sarris and colleagues reported the case of a 66-year-old patient who developed diffuse alopecia attributed to tinzaparin that resolved with enoxaparin was substituted [35].

Alopecia attributed to low-molecular-weight heparins occurs within 1–3 months of initiation of therapy. Hair loss is usually characterized by precipitous and patchy, non-scarring loss and resolves within 1–3 months of drug discontinuation.

Drugs Used After Renal Transplant

Tacrolimus

Tacrolimus is a macrolide antibiotic whose primary mechanism of action is through inhibition of calcineurin phosphatase. Subsequently, calcium dependent events are inhibited [36]. This medication is commonly used as part of the immunosuppression regime after renal transplantation.

There is evidence to suggest tacrolimus can account for hair growth in some cases and loss in others. In cases where tacrolimus is credited for hair growth, the mechanism of such growth is attributed to reversal of autoimmune alopecia. Clinicians have attempted to exploit this mechanism while avoiding the side effects of systemic administration by using topical tacrolimus to treat alopecia areata. Unfortunately, these attempts are generally unsuccessful [37].

The mechanism by which tacrolimus may cause alopecia is less clear. One postulated mechanism is through induction of vasoconstriction. This theory is supported by a case series in which 12 of 13 simultaneous pancreas–kidney transplant patients who experienced alopecia attributed to tacrolimus improved with administration of minoxidil whose proposed mechanism of action is through vasodilation. The final patient in that group recovered only when tacrolimus was discontinued in favor of cyclosporine [38].

The incidence of alopecia in renal transplant patients on tacrolimus varies widely from 1.4 to 22 %. It appears to be more likely in female patients [38]. Specific patterns of alopecia are seldom reported but it seems that patients generally experience widespread, diffuse hair loss (Fig. 15.1a). As stated above, a large cohort of patients responded well to treatment with topical minoxidil (Fig. 15.1b).

Other reports indicate many patients recover from alopecia when tacrolimus doses are minimized. Finally, some cases require complete discontinuation of tacrolimus. When cyclosporine is used as a tacrolimus replacement, patients are able to take advantage of its hypertrichosis side effect.

Infectious

Hepatitis B

Although alopecia is not associated with viral hepatitis B (HBV) per se, it has been reported following HBV vaccination. Wise and colleagues reviewed spontaneous reports submitted to FDA, the Centers for Disease Control and Prevention, and the Vaccine Adverse Event Reporting

System [39]. They identified 46 cases of alopecia attributed to the HBV vaccine. Twenty-five percent of these patients demonstrated repeated hair loss upon rechallenge. The authors propose some type of immunologic target overlap between the vaccine and the hair follicle but the exact pathogenesis is unclear.

The details of each case varied widely from elapsed time between vaccination and hair loss, pattern of hair loss and extent of recovery although most patients had a full recovery. Other authors have reported similar incidences of alopecia following HBV vaccination [40].

Hepatitis C

It is estimated that about 40 % of patients with hepatitis C (HCV) exhibit extra-hepatic manifestations. In the realm of dermatology, the most common associations are mixed cryoglobulinemia presenting as vasculitis, porphyria cutanea tarda, and lichen planus [41]. Alopecia areata is an autoimmune disease in which patients acutely develop sharply demarcated round patches of non-scarring alopecia than can become confluent. Hair anywhere on the body can be affected. There are scant reports of alopecia areata specifically attributed to HCV virus infection. Paoletti and colleagues studies a cohort of 96 patients with HCV and found that two had alopecia areata [42]. Conversely, Jadali found that of 45 patients with alopecia areata, none had anti-HCV antibodies in their serum [43]. Figure 15.2 demonstrates a patient with HCV, alopecia areata and vitiligo.

Callen and colleagues reported one case of scarring alopecia attributed HCV infection. The patient developed porphyria cutanea tarda with sclerodermoid features involving the scalp (Fig. 15.2) [44].

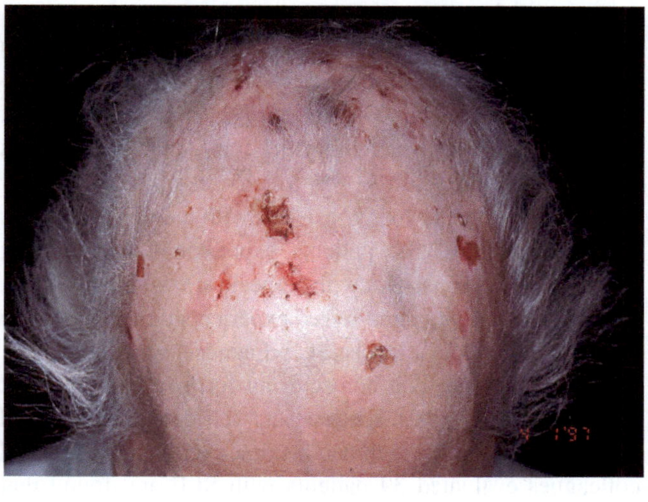

Fig. 15.2 Erosions and scaring alopecia in a patient with hepatitis C infection

Given the association between lichen planus and HCV, one might expect an increased incidence of lichen planopilaris in patients with HCV. This, however, is not the case. Perhaps it is underreported given the well-established association between lichen planus and HCV infection.

More often, alopecia is associated with treatments for hepatitis. There are many cases of alopecia universalis (loss of all scalp and body hair) in association with pegylated interferon and ribivarin treatment [45, 46]. Enhanced cytotoxic T cell activity is among the mechanisms of action for pegylated interferon. This, in addition to causing an immune shift from Th2 to Th1 response, is identified as the mechanism of this form of alopecia.

In reported cases of alopecia universalis attributed to pegylated interferon and ribivarin, patchy hair loss began after 4–6 months of treatment. Within 3 months, loss of scalp and body hair was complete. Spontaneous hair regrowth began 3–9 months after the treatment was completed.

Human Immunodeficiency virus (HIV)

Alopecia is a frequent finding in patients with HIV infection. There are many potential contributing factors including the HIV infection itself, secondary infections, immune and endocrine dysfunction, and medications. Nutritional deficiencies may also contribute. Alopecia may occur in the form of telogen effluvium with dystrophy of the hair shafts, texture changes of the hair, and alopecia areata.

In 1996, Smith and colleagues published their clinical and histologic findings of ten patients with HIV and alopecia [47]. All ten patients were diagnosed with telogen effluvium with telogen hair counts ranging from 24 to 50 %. In all cases, there was some degree of dystrophy of the hair shafts. They used scanning electron microscopy to demonstrate a range of findings from small, local defects to marked dystrophy and transverse fractures (Fig. 15.3). All of the patients reported straightening of their hair which was attributed to the changes in the hair shaft.

Mirmirani et al. evaluated hair changes in 196 HIV infected women and 50 non-infected women in the Women's Interagency HIV Study (WIHS) [48]. Twenty-eight percent of women with HIV reported finer hair compared with only 12 % of the non-infected group. This was significantly associated with higher viral loads. Interestingly, long eyelash was the only other statistically significant finding as it was also associated with higher viral loads. Other changes in hair texture (straighter, curlier, coarser) were reported but did not reach statistical significance.

Straighter, finer hair is a frequent finding in HIV disease, but the same changes have been reported outside of HIV disease and should not be considered pathognomonic [49].

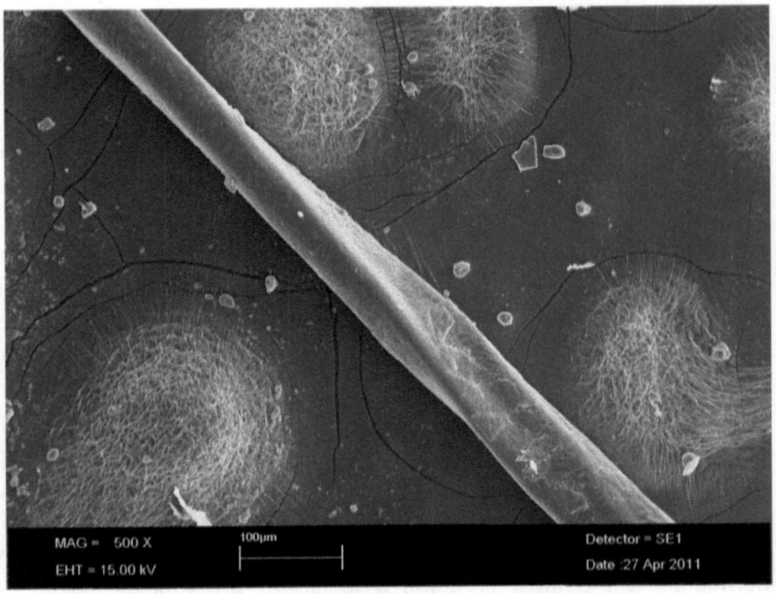

Fig. 15.3 Dystrophic hair showing twisting and a longitudinal ridge in a patient with HIV and alopecia. Scanning electron micrograph. Original magnification 500×

Alopecia areata and alopecia universalis have been reported in association with HIV. An early case of alopecia universalis attributed to HIV infection was reported by Ostlere et al. Two years after the patient tested positive for HIV infection, he developed a typical course of patchy hair loss which rapidly degenerated into loss of all scalp and body hair [50]. Several similar cases have been reported since. There are a few theories regarding the mechanism by which HIV infection induces alopecia areata. Most emphasize a change in the immune cell balance (T helper versus T suppressor cells or CD4/CD8 ratios). In one case, a patient developed trichomegaly (seen in advanced immunosuppression) in addition to alopecia areata which requires immune activation. This case highlights the selective pathogenesis of HIV infection [51].

In patients with HIV infection, alopecia can occur in a number of different forms. There are no set criteria for HIV induced alopecia; therefore, in association with appropriate risk factors, clinicians should always consider HIV as a cause of alopecia.

Autoimmune

Systemic Lupus Erythematosus

Alopecia in the setting of systemic lupus erythematosus (SLE) can take on many forms. It is easiest to consider it in terms of non-scarring versus scarring types. In non-scarring alopecia, hair follicles are retained and the potential for hair regrowth remains. The opposite is true of scarring alopecia in which hair follicles are replaced with scars.

Telogen effluvium is a form of non-scarring alopecia in which patients experience diffuse hair shedding in response to any number of psychological or physiological stressors. It is a frequent occurrence with flares of SLE [52]. Telogen effluvium resolves once lupus is controlled although patients may lose 30 % or more of their hair. Complete regrowth can be expected, assuming the underlying cause is corrected, within 6–12 months. Telogen effluvium overlaps significantly with the phenomenon termed "lupus hair." Lupus hair refers to short, brittle hairs along the frontal hair line that also seem to occur during flares of disease. It is associated with recession of the frontal hair line. Hairs in this region are either broken or replaced with vellus hairs. This hair also regrows in a normal fashion once the SLE is under control.

Yun et al documented hair loss events in 122 patients with SLE before and after their SLE diagnosis [53]. In total, 104 patients experienced some form of hair loss. Eighty-six patients experienced hair loss after the SLE diagnosis was made, the majority (65 %) of which was characterized by diffuse, non-scarring loss consistent with telogen effluvium. Fifteen percent of the patients experienced non-scarring patchy alopecia consistent with alopecia areata. Interestingly, 26 % of the patients interviewed experienced more than two patterns of alopecia after the SLE diagnosis was made.

Alopecia areata is a non-scarring form of hair loss that generally presents with acute onset, well demarcated, round patches of alopecia which can become confluent. Werth and colleagues evaluated 39 patients with SLE and found that alopecia areata developed in 10 % (4/39) [54]. Histopathology demonstrated a granular deposition of IgG which is only rarely seen in alopecia areata. Patients responded to standard alopecia areata treatment (i.e., intralesional corticosteroids). A larger study has not been published.

Seven percent of patients in the Yun study experienced discoid lupus, a form of scarring alopecia. Other sources suggest a similar incidence ranging from 4 to 14 % of patients with SLE having discoid lupus on the scalp [55]. Conversely, discoid lupus *without* SLE is not uncommon, although the exact incidence is difficult to pinpoint. There appears to be some overlap between the immunologic mediators of lupus and lupus nephritis. IL-17, a pro-inflammatory cytokine, has been demonstrated to have an important role in both entities [56].

Discoid lupus on the scalp most commonly affects young adult women with onset between ages 20 and 30 years. Classic lesions show an erythematous plaque that evolves into a centrally depressed, depigmented, alopecic plaque. There is associated follicular plugging. The mnemonic PASTE has been suggested to describe discoid lupus lesions: plugging, atrophy, scale, telangiectasia, erythema [52]. An erythematous or hyperpigmented active edge is retained. Conchal bowl of the ear involvement is also common, occurring in about 50 % of patients with scalp involvement. Symptoms range from none to pruritus and pain.

Biopsy can help distinguish discoid lupus from other forms of scarring alopecia such as central centrifugal cicatricial alopecia and lichen planopilaris. The histology of discoid lupus demonstrates epidermal atrophy, dermal fibrosis, and follicular plugging as might be expected given the clinical appearance. Other key features are basement membrane thickening, basal vacuolization, and mucin deposition in the papillary dermis.

Alopecia in the setting of SLE may present in many different ways. The most frequent presentation is that of telogen effluvium which is incited by a lupus flare and is self-resolving once the flare is controlled. Alopecia areata in SLE responds to treatment in the same way that non-lupus related alopecia areata responds. Discoid lupus results in permanent scarring which cannot be reversed. Early intervention may limit its progression.

Infiltrative

Amyloidosis

Given that any organ system can be affected by systemic amyloidosis, one might expect alopecia to be a common finding. On the contrary, it is not. There are only a few published case reports describing alopecia in the constellation of signs and symptoms of systemic amyloidosis.

The first case of systemic amyloidosis causing alopecia was reported in 1991 by Hunt and colleagues [57]. The patient presented with diffuse, non-scarring alopecia involving the scalp and body. Hair pull test on the scalp was positive.

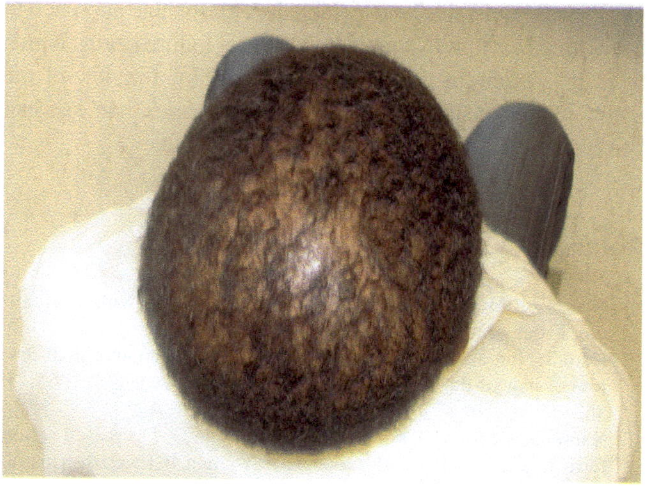

Fig. 15.4 Diffuse alopecia of the scalp in a patient with amyloidosis

The patient also demonstrated pinch purpura and easy bruising, cutaneous features commonly associated with systemic amyloidosis. Two scalp biopsies (taken 7 months apart) both demonstrated perifollicular deposition of amyloid.

Lutz and Pittelkow describe a patient who presented with gradual, progressive alopecia beginning 6 years before any other signs or symptoms of amyloidosis were identified. The alopecia involved scalp and body hair. An initial scalp biopsy was read as nonspecific and the patient failed a trial of 2 % minoxidil. With time, the patient also developed brittle fingernails and erythema and thickening of the palms. A subsequent biopsy from the scalp with special staining (Thioflavine-T and Congo red) confirmed the diagnosis [58]. Figure 15.4 shows a patient with a similar pattern of alopecia.

Barja and colleagues reported a case in which the patient presented with a 1 year history of dyspnea, dysphagia, and weakness [59]. On exam, the patient had diffusely decreased density of scalp hair and fingernail dystrophy which had been present for years. Scalp biopsy was diagnostic in this case, demonstrating amyloid deposition.

As with the patients reported, alopecia in the setting of systemic amyloidosis presents with diffuse, non-scarring alopecia. Often scalp and body hair is affected. Hair pull test is usually positive. Histopathology demonstrates perifollicular amyloid deposition. Minoxidil is not effective. Instead, therapy should be directly targeted to the disease process underlying the amyloidosis.

Summary

In any population, alopecia can have many different causes. For those with renal disease, the most common culprits are medications; however, infectious, autoimmune, and infiltrative etiologies should also be considered. A reasonable approach to evaluating hair loss in a patient with renal failure begins with a thorough review of medications followed by a review of the entire medical history. Fortunately in most cases, hair loss can be reversed by addressing the underlying cause.

References

1. Nissenson AR, Strobos J. Iron deficiency in patients with renal failure. Kidney Int Suppl. 1999;69:S18–21.
2. Hard S. Non-anemic iron deficiency as an etiologic factor in diffuse loss of hair of the scalp in women. Acta Derm Venereol. 1963;43: 562–9.
3. Kantor J, Kessler LJ, Brooks DG, Cotsarelis G. Decreased serum ferritin is associated with alopecia in women. J Invest Dermatol. 2003;121(5):985–8.
4. Deloche C, Bastien P, Chadoutaud S, Galan P, Bertrais S, Hercberg S, et al. Low iron stores: a risk factor for excessive hair loss in non-menopausal women. Eur J Dermatol. 2007;17(6):507–12.
5. Olsen EA, Reed KB, Cacchio PB, Caudill L. Iron deficiency in female pattern hair loss, chronic telogen effluvium, and control groups. J Am Acad Dermatol. 2010;63(6):991–9.
6. Sinclair R. There is no clear association between low serum ferritin and chronic diffuse telogen hair loss. Br J Dermatol. 2002;147(5): 982–4.
7. Dallman PR. Biochemical basis for the manifestations of iron deficiency. Annu Rev Nutr. 1986;6:13–40.
8. Hung KY, Wu DJ, Wu KD, Chen WY, Tsai TJ. Serum ferritin level required for adequate response to recombinant human erythropoietin in haemodialysis patients with hepatitis C virus infection. Nephrol Dial Transplant. 1998;13(10):2709–10.
9. Roozbeh J, Sharifian M, Sagheb MM, Shabani S, Hamidian Jahromi A, Afshariani R, et al. Comment on: does zinc supplementation affect inflammatory markers in hemodialysis patients? Ren Fail. 2011;33(4):466–7.
10. Haase H, Rink L. Zinc signals and immune function. Biofactors. 2013;40(1):27–40.
11. Daniells S, Hardy G. Hair loss in long-term or home parenteral nutrition: are micronutrient deficiencies to blame? Curr Opin Clin Nutr Metab Care. 2010;13(6):690–7.
12. Whitwam W, Lewis M, Rabb H. Alopecia in three women of Southeast Asian descent with chronic renal failure: possible association with erythropoietin use. Am J Kidney Dis. 2001;37(1):E9.
13. Reddy V, Turney JH. Epoietin-alpha-associated total alopecia. Nephrol Dial Transplant. 2001;16(7):1525.
14. NKF K/DOQI Guidelines. [Internet] 2002. http://www.kidney.org/professionals/kdoqi/guidelines_bp/guide_11.htm.
15. Smit AJ, Hoorntje SJ, Donker AJ. Zinc deficiency during captopril treatment. Nephron. 1983;34(3):196–7.
16. Motel PJ. Captopril and alopecia: a case report and review of known cutaneous reactions in captopril use. J Am Acad Dermatol. 1990;23(1):124–5.
17. Ahmad S. Enalapril and reversible alopecia. Arch Intern Med. 1991;151(2):404.
18. Leaker B, Whitworth JA. Alopecia associated with captopril treatment. Aust N Z J Med. 1984;14(6):866.
19. Graeber CW, Lapkin RA. Metoprolol and alopecia. Cutis. 1981;28(6):633–4.
20. Hilder RJ. Propranolol and alopecia. Cutis. 1979;24(1):63–4.
21. England JR, England JD. Alopecia and propranolol therapy. Aust Fam Physician. 1982;11(3):225–6.
22. Shelley ED, Shelley WB. Alopecia and drug eruption of the scalp associated with a new beta-blocker, nadolol. Cutis. 1985;35(2): 148–9.
23. Ochoa PG, Arribas MT, Mena JM, PÈrez MG. Cutaneous adverse reaction to furosemide treatment: new clinical findings. Can Vet J. 2006;47(6):576–8.
24. Sinclair R, Patel M, Dawson TL, Yazdabadi A, Yip L, Perez A, et al. Hair loss in women: medical and cosmetic approaches to increase scalp hair fullness. Br J Dermatol. 2011;165 Suppl 3:12–8.
25. Sica DA. Calcium-channel blocker related peripheral edema: can it be resolved? J Clin Hypertens. 2003;5(4):291–5.
26. Litt JZ. Litt's pocketbook of drug eruptions and interactions. 3rd ed. New York: The Parthenon Publishing Group; 2004.
27. Olsen EA, Delong E, Weiner MS. Reply to A falling out following minoxidil: Telogen effluvium. J Am Acad Dermatol. 1987;16(1): 145–6.
28. Segal AS. Alopecia associated with atorvastatin. Am J Med. 2002;113(2):171.
29. Ali A, Martin JM. Hair growth in patients alopecia areata totalis after treatment with simvastatin and ezetimibe. J Drugs Dermatol. 2010;9(1):62–4.
30. Robins DN. Case reports: alopecia universalis: hair growth following initiation of simvastatin and ezetimibe therapy. J Drugs Dermatol. 2007;6(9):946–7.
31. Baigent C, Landray MJ, Reith C, Emberson J, Wheeler DC, Tomson C, et al. The effects of lowering LDL cholesterol with simvastatin plus ezetimibe in patients with chronic kidney disease (Study of Heart and Renal Protection): a randomised placebo-controlled trial. Lancet. 2011;377(9784):2181–92.
32. Barnes C, Deidun D, Hynes K, Monagle P. Alopecia and dalteparin: a previously unreported association. Blood. 2000;96(4):1618–9.
33. Apsner R, H^rl WH, Sunder-Plassmann G. Dalteparin-induced alopecia in hemodialysis patients: reversal by regional citrate anticoagulation. Blood. 2001;97(9):2914–5.
34. Wang YY, Po HL. Enoxaparin-induced alopecia in patients with cerebral venous thrombosis. J Clin Pharm Ther. 2006;31(5):513–7.
35. Sarris E, Tsele E, Bagiatoudi G, Salpigidis K, Stavrianaki D, Kaklamanis L, et al. Diffuse alopecia in a hemodialysis patient caused by a low-molecular-weight heparin, tinzaparin. Am J Kidney Dis. 2003;41(5):E15.
36. Thomson AW, Bonham CA, Zeevi A. Mode of action of tacrolimus (FK506): molecular and cellular mechanisms. Ther Drug Monit. 1995;17(6):584–91.
37. Price VH, Willey A, Chen BK. Topical tacrolimus in alopecia areata. J Am Acad Dermatol. 2005;52(1):138–9.
38. Tricot L, LebbÈ C, Pillebout E, Martinez F, Legendre C, Thervet E. Tacrolimus-induced alopecia in female kidney-pancreas transplant recipients. Transplantation. 2005;80(11):1546–9.
39. Wise RP, Kiminyo KP, Salive ME. Hair loss after routine immunizations. JAMA. 1997;278(14):1176–8.
40. Geier DA, Geier MR. A case-control study of serious autoimmune adverse events following hepatitis B immunization. Autoimmunity. 2005;38(4):295–301.
41. Palekar NA, Harrison SA. Extrahepatic manifestations of hepatitis C. South Med J. 2005;98(10):1019–23.
42. Paoletti V, Mammarella A, Basili S, Paradiso M, Di Franco M, De Matteis A, et al. Prevalence and clinical features of skin diseases in chronic HCV infection. A prospective study in 96 patients. Panminerva Med. 2002;44(4):349–52.
43. Jadali Z, Mansouri P, Jadali F. There is no relationship between hepatitis C virus and alopecia areata. Eur J Dermatol. 2006;16(1):94–5.
44. Jackson JM, Callen JP. Scarring alopecia and sclerodermatous changes of the scalp in a patient with hepatitis C infection. J Am Acad Dermatol. 1998;39(5 Pt 2):824–6.

45. Kartal ED, Alpat SN, Ozgunes I, Usluer G. Reversible alopecia universalis secondary to PEG-interferon alpha-2b and ribavirin combination therapy in a patient with chronic hepatitis C virus infection. Eur J Gastroenterol Hepatol. 2007;19(9):817–20.
46. Demirturk N, Aykin N, Demirdal T, Cevik F. Alopecia universalis: a rare side effect seen on chronic hepatitis C treatment with peg-IFN and ribavirin. Eur J Dermatol. 2006;16(5):579–80.
47. Smith KJ, Skelton HG, DeRusso D, Sperling L, Yeager J, Wagner KF, et al. Clinical and histopathologic features of hair loss in patients with HIV-1 infection. J Am Acad Dermatol. 1996;34(1):63–8.
48. Mirmirani P, Hessol NA, Maurer TA, Berger TG, Greenblatt RM, Price VH. Hair changes in women from the Women's Interagency HIV Study. Arch Dermatol. 2003;139(1):105–6.
49. Green SL, Nelson DL. Straightening of the hair is not pathognomonic for HIV infection. Clin Infect Dis. 2002;35(10):1276–7.
50. Ostlere LS, Langtry JA, Staughton RC, Samrasinghe PL. Alopecia universalis in a patient seropositive for the human immunodeficiency virus. J Am Acad Dermatol. 1992;27(4):630–1.
51. Grossman MC, Cohen PR, Grossman ME. Acquired eyelash trichomegaly and alopecia areata in a human immunodeficiency virus-infected patient. Dermatology. 1996;193(1):52–3.
52. Moghadam-Kia S, Franks AG. Autoimmune disease and hair loss. Dermatol Clin. 2013;31(1):75–91.
53. Yun SJ, Lee JW, Yoon HJ, Lee SS, Kim SY, Lee JB, et al. Cross-sectional study of hair loss patterns in 122 Korean systemic lupus erythematosus patients: a frequent finding of non-scarring patch alopecia. J Dermatol. 2007;34(7):451–5.
54. Werth VP, White WL, Sanchez MR, Franks AG. Incidence of alopecia areata in lupus erythematosus. Arch Dermatol. 1992;128(3):368–71.
55. Yell JA, Mbuagbaw J, Burge SM. Cutaneous manifestations of systemic lupus erythematosus. Br J Dermatol. 1996;135(3):355–62.
56. Crispìn JC, Oukka M, Bayliss G, Cohen RA, Van Beek CA, Stillman IE, et al. Expanded double negative T cells in patients with systemic lupus erythematosus produce IL-17 and infiltrate the kidneys. J Immunol. 2008;181(12):8761–6.
57. Hunt SJ, Caserio RJ, Abell E. Primary systemic amyloidosis causing diffuse alopecia by telogen arrest. Arch Dermatol. 1991;127(7):1067–8.
58. Lutz ME, Pittelkow MR. Progressive generalized alopecia due to systemic amyloidosis. J Am Acad Dermatol. 2002;46(3):434–6.
59. Barja J, Piñeyro F, Almagro M, Sacristán F, Rodríguez-Lojo R, Fernández-Jorge B, et al. Systemic amyloidosis with an exceptional cutaneous presentation. Dermatol Online J. 2013;19(1):11.

Uremic Frost

16

Kristie Lynn Slivka Delaney, Edgar V. Lerma, and Julia R. Nunley

Introduction and Epidemiology

First described by Hirschsprung in 1865, uremic frost is a now rare dermatologic manifestation of severe azotemia characterized by a friable white crystalline material on the skin [1–4]. In the pre-dialysis era, uremic frost was a commonly manifested dermatologic finding in end-stage renal disease (ESRD) patients [1]. However, it is rarely seen today. This is because uremic frost typically develops when the blood urea nitrogen level is greater than 200 mg/100 mL [1], although it can be seen at lower blood urea nitrogen levels as well [4, 5]. Thus, with the invention of hemodialysis (HD), and the now vast accessibility and early intervention of HD, this condition rarely manifests itself [1–5].

Today uremic frost is most frequently seen in undeveloped countries or in patients noncompliant with dialysis [1, 2]. The exact incidence is unknown [3, 6], but one study from India ($n = 100$) found a 3 % incidence of uremic frost in ESRD patients undergoing HD [1], while a second study from Nigeria ($n = 120$) found a 0.8 % incidence of uremic frost in ESRD patients undergoing HD [7].

K.L.S. Delaney, M.D. (✉)
Internal Medicine, UIC/Advocate Christ Hospital, Advocate Christ Medical Center, 4440 W 95th Street, 131NO, Oak Lawn, IL 60453, USA
e-mail: kslivka@gmail.com

E.V. Lerma, M.D.
Section of Nephrology, Department of Medicine, Advocate Christ Medical Center, University of Illinois at Chicago, Oak Lawn, IL, USA
e-mail: nephron0@gmail.com

J.R. Nunley, M.D.
Department of Dermatology, Virginia Commonwealth University Medical Center, Nelson Clinic, 401 North 11th Street Suite 520, Richmond, VA 23219, USA
e-mail: jnunley@vcu.edu

Physiology/Pathogenesis

Uremic frost is caused by the evaporation of sweat containing high levels of urea and other nitrogenous waste products [2, 4]. In individuals with renal failure the clearance of urea and other waste products from the blood is significantly decreased, and thus the blood urea nitrogen levels rise [2]. When the blood urea nitrogen levels reach a very high level, often greater than or equal to 200 mg/100 mL, the concentration of urea in the sweat consequently has increased significantly as well [6]. As the sweat containing high levels of urea and other nitrogenous waste products evaporates, the urea crystallizes and is deposited on the skin as a whitish crystalline coating [1–3, 5, 6, 8].

Clinical Findings

Uremic frost, as its name implies, is often described as a "frosted" appearance of the skin [1, 5, 6]. A white, or sometimes yellowish, coating of urea crystals forms on the skin due to eccrine deposition of urea, as described above [1, 2]. This friable white-yellowish crystalline material on the skin is most commonly seen on the face, particularly in the beard area. However, it is also seen on the neck, arms, and trunk [1, 2]. As previously mentioned, this cutaneous manifestation is seen in patients with severe azotemia, often with a pre-dialysis blood urea level greater than 200 mg/100 mL, but can be seen at lower levels as well [1] (Fig. 16.1).

J.R. Nunley and E.V. Lerma (eds.), *Dermatological Manifestations of Kidney Disease*,
DOI 10.1007/978-1-4939-2395-3_16, © Springer Science+Business Media New York 2015

Differential Diagnosis

Uremic frost should be distinguished from other possible diagnosis such as psoriasis, eczema, retention keratosis, atopic dermatitis, and postinflammatory desquamation [2, 4].

Diagnosis

Uremic frost is most commonly a clinical diagnosis. In a patient with ESRD and laboratory findings consistent with severe azotemia (often with blood urea nitrogen levels greater than 200 mg/100 mL), the classical dermatological finding of a whitish crystalline coating, or "frost," on the skin can be diagnostic [1, 4].

Laboratory analysis of the frost scrapings is also possible, but is typically not necessary. Verification that the crystals are composed of urea or nitrogenous waste can confirm the diagnosis [2, 4]. This is done by first taking scrapings of the "frost," or crystals deposited on the skin, and diluting them in normal saline [2–5]. The solution is then tested for elevated urea nitrogen levels. If the urea nitrogen level in the solution is elevated and comparable to the blood urea nitrogen level, the test is positive and the diagnosis is supported and confirmed [2–4]. For example, in one case report in the New England Journal of Medicine (NEJM), the laboratory analysis of the white crystalline deposition on the skin of a patient with ESRD found that the urea nitrogen level of the "frost" scrapings diluted in normal saline was 113 mg/dL, while the corresponding serum blood urea nitrogen level was 120 mg/dL [5].

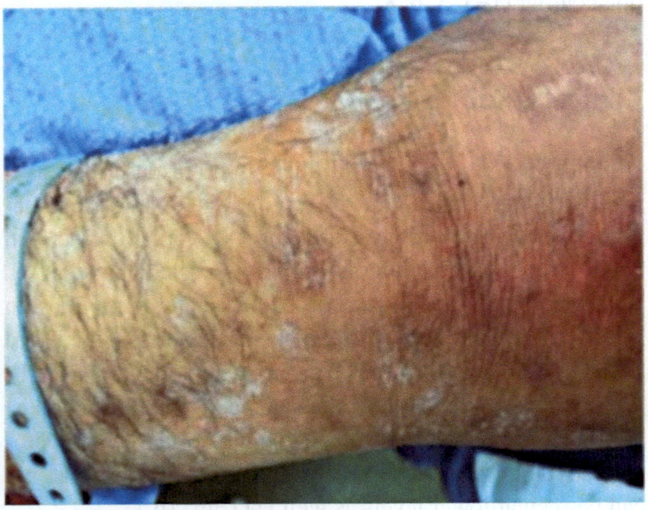

Fig. 16.1 Uremic frost crystalline deposits on the upper extremities. (Reprinted from Mayo Clinic Proceedings, 83 (12), Bhattarai N, Panda M. Uremic Frost, 1309, Copyright 2008, with permission from Elsevier)

Treatment

The treatment of uremic frost is management of the underlying causative condition, the elevated levels of serum blood urea nitrogen levels [1, 2]. HD or other forms of renal replacement therapy are the mainstay of treatment for patients with uremic frost, as this dermatological condition indicates life-threatening kidney failure [2–4, 6]. Typically after the initiation of HD, or other renal replacement therapies, resolution of the crystalline deposition, or "frost," on the skin is noted [2–4, 6]. However, the time to resolution of uremic frost after the initiation of dialysis is unclear, but some case reports recount that the dermatologic finding disappeared after about three to seven days of treatment [3, 4].

Significance/Prognosis

Uremic frost carries a grave prognosis and indicates life-threatening kidney failure [1, 2]. With the initiation of dialysis the prognosis is greatly improved, but is still ominous, as with any patient requiring renal replacement therapy [1, 2].

Summary (Table 16.1)

Table 16.1 Uremic frost summary highlights

Uremic frost	
Current incidence	Unknown, but ~0.8–3 %
Incidence…	• *In the pre-dialysis era* → ESRD patients • *Today* → Undeveloped countries and patients noncompliant with HD
Description	Tiny white crystalline skin deposits
Location(s)	Face (particularly the beard area). Also seen on the neck, arms, and trunk
Pathophysiology	The increased deposition of urea in the sweat which then is left behind and crystallizes when the sweat evaporates
Blood urea nitrogen levels	Often ≥ 200 mg/100 mL
Diagnosis	Clinical
Specific tests	Dilute scrapings of the "frost" in normal saline and test the solution for elevated urea nitrogen levels. The level in the solution should be comparable to the blood level.
Treatment	Dialysis
Preventative measures	Early intervention of regular dialysis

HD hemodialysis, *ESRD* end-stage renal disease

References

1. Udayakumar P, Balasubramanian S, Ramalingam KS, Lakshmi C, Srinivas CR, Mathew AC. Cutaneous manifestations in patients with chronic renal failure on hemodialysis. Indian J Dermatol Venereol Leprol. 2006;72(2):119–25. PubMed PMID: 16707817.
2. Markova A, Lester J, Wang J, Robinson-Bostom L. Diagnosis of common dermopathies in dialysis patients: a review and update. Semin Dial. 2012;25(4):408–18. PubMed PMID: 22809004.
3. Mohan D, Railey M. Uremic frost. Kidney Int. 2012;81(11):1153. PubMed PMID: 22584601.
4. Kuo CC, Hung JB, Tsai CW, Chen YM. Uremic frost. CMAJ. 2010;182(17):E800. PubMed PMID: 20696798. Pubmed Central PMCID: 2988568.
5. Pol-Rodriguez MM, Wanner M, Bhat P, Grossman ME. Uremic frost in a critically ill patient. Kidney Int. 2008;73(6):790. PubMed PMID: 18309352.
6. Bhattarai N, Panda M. Uremic frost. Mayo Clin Proc Mayo Clinic. 2008;83(12):1309. PubMed PMID: 19068538.
7. Falodun O, Ogunbiyi A, Salako B, George AK. Skin changes in patients with chronic renal failure. Saudi J Kidney Dis Transpl. 2011;22(2):268–72. PubMed PMID: 21422624.
8. Walsh SR, Parada NA. Images in clinical medicine. Uremic frost. N Engl J Med. 2005;352(13):e13. PubMed PMID: 15800220.

Infections in the Kidney Transplant Recipient

17

James D. Russell and Calvin O. McCall

Introduction

Overview

Fungal infections in humans can be divided into three main groups based on tissue invasion and host characteristics: superficial cutaneous, subcutaneous, and opportunistic. The superficial cutaneous fungal infections consist of two major types: dermatophytes and nondermatophytes. Dermatophytes are grouped together because of their ability to induce an inflammatory response in an immunocompetent host. Infections of these organisms are referred to as "tinea" followed by the location on the body. Nondermatophytes, on the other hand, typically cause few or no symptoms in hosts. All superficial mycoses are limited to the stratum corneum, hair, and nails.

Subcutaneous fungal infections are those that invade the dermis and subcutis. They are usually introduced via puncture wounds. They can reproduce locally but do not typically spread to distant sites in the body. Opportunistic fungal infections are an extremely diverse group of pathogens that cause a range of disease in those with an altered immune response. This chapter will focus on opportunistic infections with prominent or characteristic skin findings.

J.D. Russell, M.D.
Department of Dermatology, Virginia Commonwealth University Health System, 401 N. 11th Street, Suite 520, Nelson Clinic, Box 980164, Richmond, VA 23298, USA
e-mail: russell.nd@gmail.com

C.O. McCall, M.D. (✉)
Department of Dermatology, Virginia Commonwealth University Health System, 401 N. 11th Street, Suite 520, Nelson Clinic, Box 980164, Richmond, VA 23298, USA

Dermatology Section, VA Medical Center, Richmond, Richmond, VA 23298, USA
e-mail: comccall@gmail.com

Pathogenesis and Immunosuppression

Dermatophytes, unlike other superficial cutaneous mycoses, produce keratinases, which degrade the keratin of the stratum corneum. This allows shallow invasion of the fungi and explains why they cause more symptoms than nondermatophytes. They do not typically invade deeper due to a number of host defense mechanisms, including the expression of defensins and antimicrobial peptides, release of inflammatory cytokines by keratinocytes, activation of complement, and cellular defense by neutrophils and macrophages [1]. Subcutaneous mycoses require a puncture wound or other injury to bypass the defense mechanisms of the epidermis. Once into deeper tissues, these organisms are usually contained, but not eradicated, by the host's cellular immune response. In competent hosts, the primary defense mechanism against most of the organisms that could otherwise cause opportunistic infections is phagocytosis [2].

When a patient is immunosuppressed, new degrees of infection become possible and new potential pathogens arise. For example, candidiasis changes from a skin-limited, easily treatable entity to a widespread and potentially fatal disease. The reasons for this are myriad. First, the use of broad spectrum antibiotics, which is often necessary, may eliminate competing flora and allow fungi to reproduce unchecked. Second, these patients are more likely to have breaks in the skin barrier, such as intravenous (IV) catheters, that allow access to pathogens. Third, phagocytic cells, namely macrophages and neutrophils, may be reduced in number or quality [3]. As the primary defense against dissemination, this can be crippling to the host response. Once the fungi gain access to blood vessels, they can spread to any organ and the results can be catastrophic.

J.R. Nunley and E.V. Lerma (eds.), *Dermatological Manifestations of Kidney Disease*,
DOI 10.1007/978-1-4939-2395-3_17, © Springer Science+Business Media New York 2015

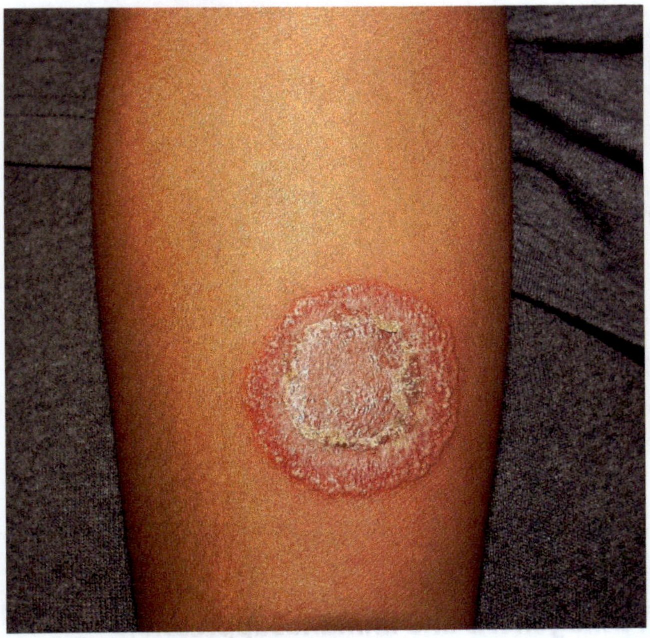

Fig. 17.1 Tinea corporis with the classic appearance of "ringworm"

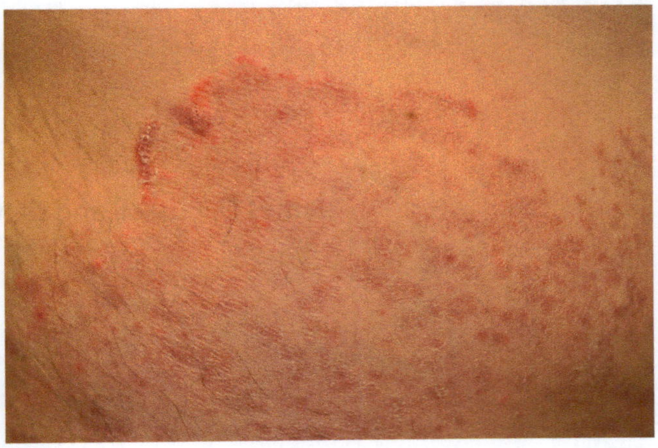

Fig. 17.2 Tinea corporis showing a serpiginous border

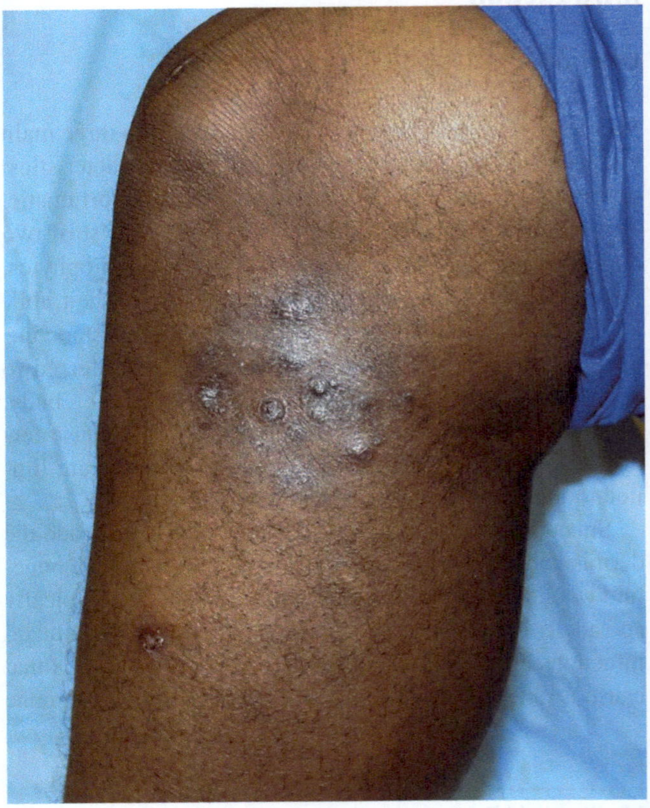

Fig. 17.3 Majocchi granuloma demonstrating follicular-based papules

Dermatophytes

Tinea Corporis

Tinea corporis represents the classic dermatophytosis (Fig. 17.1). It includes infections of the trunk and extremities, excluding the palms, soles, groin, and nails. The most common causative agent in the United States and worldwide is *Trichophyton rubrum*. Other causes include *T. mentagrophytes*, *Microsporum canis*, and *T. tonsurans* [4]. Tinea corporis can be spread in a number of ways including person-to-person, animal-to-person, soil-to-person, and via fomites, such as wrestling mats and locker rooms. It occurs across the globe but is most common in hot and humid climates. While the clinical picture can vary, it typically presents as erythematous, annular thin plaques with peripheral scale (Fig. 17.2). Other clues to the diagnosis can include pustules at the periphery of the lesion, a scalloped or serpiginous border, and the so-called "leading scale," which is due to activity at the edge of a lesion as it advances outward. Application of topical steroids can decrease the amounts of scale and erythema, leading to "tinea incognito," which can be difficult to diagnose without a thorough history.

The differential diagnosis of tinea corporis is extremely broad, but history and a complete physical examination can usually narrow it down considerably. The list includes forms of dermatitis, such as nummular, atopic, seborrheic, and contact; papulosquamous disorders such as psoriasis, parapsoriasis, and pityriasis rosea; infections such as pityriasis (tinea) versicolor and impetigo; and autoimmune/inflammatory conditions like granuloma annulare, erythema annulare centrifugum, and subacute cutaneous lupus erythematosus. The adage, "If it scales, scrape it," is a way to help avoid missing an easily treatable disease that can be confused for so many others.

One notable variant of tinea corporis is Majocchi granuloma, in which the organism invades the hair follicle and surrounding dermis (Fig. 17.3). This leads to the development of nodules and induration, in addition to perifollicular papules and pustules. Majocchi granuloma is most often due to *T. rubrum* and can be seen as a result of shaving, occlusion, or immunosuppression. Mimickers include bacterial folliculitis, eosinophilic folliculitis, acne keloidalis nuchae, Kaposi sarcoma, lymphocytoma cutis, nodular vasculitis, and crusted scabies.

Tinea Cruris

Tinea cruris, commonly known as jock itch, is a dermatophyte infection of the inner thighs and inguinal folds. It primarily affects males. The most common route of infection is local spread from concomitant tinea pedis, via clothing or hand contact. The two most common organisms identified in tinea cruris are *Epidermophyton floccosum* and *T. rubrum* [4]. Clinically, it presents as pruritic red patches or thin plaques in the upper thighs and inguinal folds. Scale may be less obvious due to the local moisture but is most likely to involve the advancing edge of the lesion. Tinea cruris characteristically does not involve the scrotum. It should be noted that cutaneous candidiasis often will involve the scrotum and should be considered in the differential diagnosis when the scrotum is involved.

The differential diagnosis of tinea cruris is rather broad and is similar to that of tinea corporis. Other cutaneous infections like candidiasis and erythrasma can be diagnosed with a potassium hydroxide (KOH) preparation, culture, or Wood lamp examination. Intertrigo is an inflammatory condition of the groin or other skin folds due to friction, occlusion, and other mechanical factors that is commonly colonized or superinfected by fungi, yeast, and bacteria. Psoriasis, seborrheic dermatitis, contact dermatitis, and lichen simplex chronicus can all involve the groin. Finally, less common entities such as mycosis fungoides, Hailey-Hailey disease, pemphigus vegetans, and Langerhans cell histiocytosis can be considered.

Tinea Manuum

Tinea manuum refers to infection of the palmar surface and interdigital areas of the hands. Infections of the dorsal hands behave like tinea corporis and can be treated as such. Tinea manuum is usually associated with tinea pedis and is therefore caused by the same organisms: *E. floccosum*, *T. rubrum*, and *T. mentagrophytes*. However, two nondermatophyte fungi from the genus *Scytalidium* can cause an infection that is identical to tinea manuum [5].

Clinically, tinea manuum presents as diffuse fine scaling of the palm with accentuation of the creases (Fig. 17.4). One or more fingernails may be involved. A classic presentation is known as "one hand, two foot syndrome," in which tinea manuum, usually of the patient's dominant hand, coexists with bilateral tinea pedis (Fig. 17.5). The differential diagnosis includes contact dermatitis, both irritant and allergic; atopic dermatitis; psoriasis; hyperkeratosis; and keratoderma.

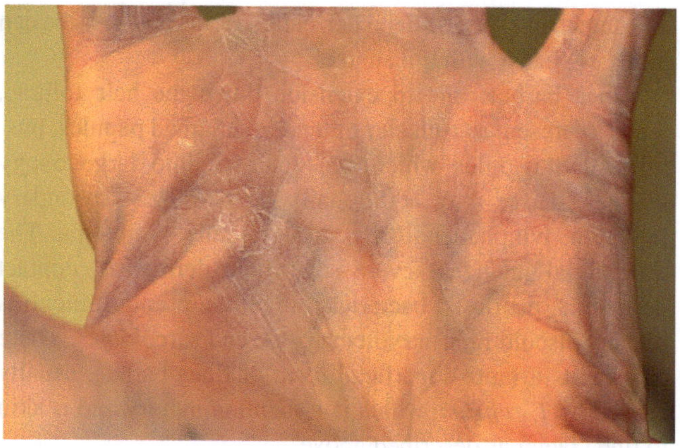

Fig. 17.4 Tinea manuum—note the accentuation of palmar creases

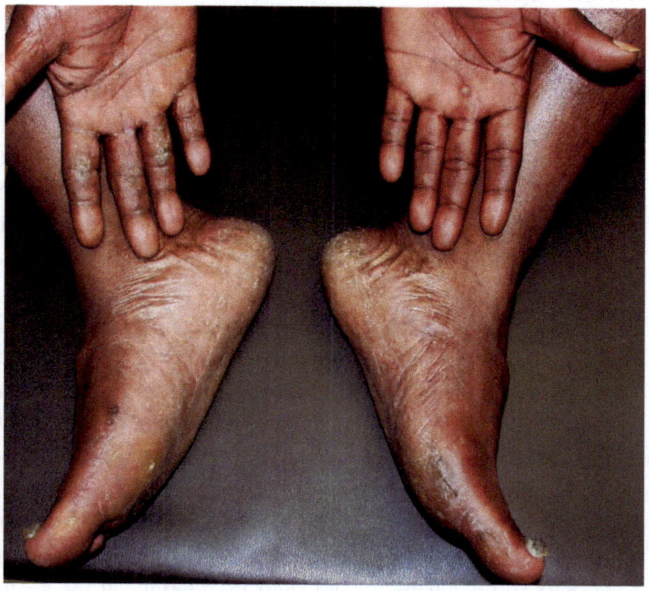

Fig. 17.5 "One hand, two foot" syndrome showing fine scale of the right hand and both feet; the left hand is free of disease

Tinea Faciei

Tinea faciei is a dermatophyte infection of the glabrous, or non-hair-bearing, areas of the face. When a man's beard area is involved, it is referred to as tinea barbae. Tinea faciei and tinea barbae are most commonly acquired from pets but can also be via local spread on the same host or by person-to-person contact. The most common organisms vary by region, but *T. mentagrophytes*, *T. tonsurans*, and *T. verrucosum* have all been implicated.

More so than the other dermatophytoses, tinea faciei is often misdiagnosed, and therefore mistreated, for long periods of time. While it may have the classic annular plaque with a leading scale, these features are often missing due to anatomic variations of the face and frequent use of topical steroids. Contact dermatitis, seborrheic dermatitis, lupus erythematosus, periorificial dermatitis, acne, and rosacea can all be confused with tinea faciei.

Tinea barbae, due to extension down the hair follicle, tends to present as a cluster of tender, inflamed papules, pustules, and nodules which can coalesce into large boggy plaques. There may additionally be hair loss, secondary infection, lymphadenopathy, and systemic symptoms. The differential includes severe seborrheic dermatitis, contact dermatitis, psoriasis, bacterial folliculitis, pseudofolliculitis barbae, discoid lupus erythematosus, and sarcoidosis. There also exists a more superficial form of tinea barbae, usually caused by *T. rubrum*, which is less inflammatory and is akin to tinea faciei as described above.

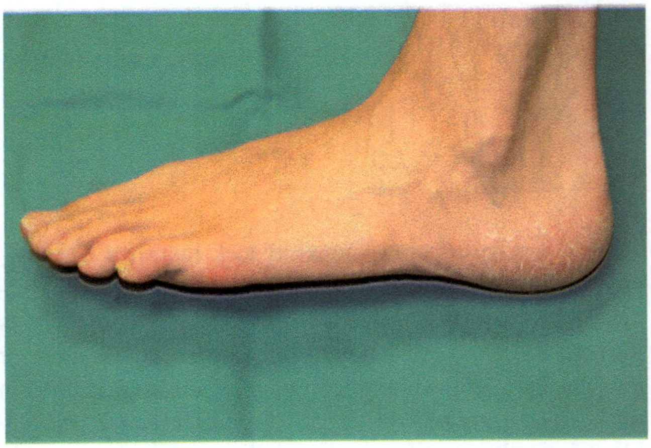

Fig. 17.6 Tinea pedis with a moccasin distribution

Tinea Capitis

Tinea capitis refers to dermatophyte infection of the scalp and hair. While it is common in children, it is rare in the adult population. It can be caused by any *Trichophyton* or *Microsporum* species, but *T. tonsurans* accounts for the vast majority of cases in the United States [6]. The most common route of infection is person-to-person spread, either by direct contact or via fomites such as clothing, combs, and brushes. Animal to human spread exists but is less prevalent.

Tinea capitis can present with a wide range of clinical findings, depending on the organism involved as well as the host immune response. The most common presentation begins with perifollicular red papules that coalesce into scaly plaques. Pustules, crusting, posterior cervical lymphadenopathy, and varying amounts of pruritus may be present. Alopecia is often present and may be the most prominent finding. *T. tonsurans*, an endothrix organism, can invade the hair shaft and weakens it. The shaft then breaks at the scalp surface, leading to the so-called "black dot" tinea capitis. Zoonotic organisms such as *M. canis* tend to cause more of an inflammatory response from the host, which can lead to large boggy plaques called kerions. These are commonly associated with lymphadenopathy and systemic findings, and they tend to heal with scarring and hair loss.

The differential diagnosis of tinea capitis usually includes psoriasis and seborrheic dermatitis, which can both cause significant erythema and scale. If scale is less prominent, alopecia areata and trichotillomania can be considered. Other entities in the differential include lichen planopilaris, discoid lupus, acne keloidalis nuchae, pyoderma, and folliculitis, including folliculitis decalvans and dissecting cellulitis. It is often taught that any child with a scaly scalp deserves a fungal culture to rule out tinea capitis.

Tinea Pedis

Tinea pedis, commonly known as athlete's foot, is a dermatophyte infection of the plantar surface and interdigital spaces of the feet. It is the most common dermatophytosis on the planet. It most often affects adult males, though infection in females is not rare. Risk factors for tinea pedis include hot, humid environments and use of occlusive footwear. Direct contact with communal areas like pools and locker rooms is likely a source of infection. The most common organisms that cause tinea pedis are *T. rubrum* and *E. floccosum* [4].

Tinea pedis usually presents as faint erythema and fine white scale of the toe webs and plantar surface that extends slightly onto the sides of the feet. This presentation is often referred to as "moccasin distribution" (Fig. 17.6). As discussed above, one hand may also be involved in the "one hand, two foot syndrome." Another presentation is bullous tinea pedis, which consists of multiple tense vesicles and bullae on the distal feet and between toes. This is most often caused by *T. mentagrophytes*.

The differential diagnosis of tinea pedis includes infection of nondermatophyte fungi from the genus *Scytalidium*, eczema, contact dermatitis, psoriasis, palmoplantar pustulosis, secondary syphilis, erythrasma, and bacterial infection. Mixed toe web infection is a polymicrobial infection of the distal foot and toe webs that may be a complication of tinea pedis, as this allows a portal of entry. Gram negative organisms, including *Pseudomonas*, are commonly implicated. Clinically this appears as severe maceration of the web spaces with profuse malodorous discharge (Fig. 17.7).

Tinea Unguium

Tinea unguium, or onychomycosis, is an infection of the nail plate. Like tinea pedis, it is very prevalent, and the two are often associated. The most common causative agents in North America and much of Europe are *T. rubrum*, *E. floccosum*, and *T. mentagrophytes*, though any dermatophyte can be involved. Dermatophytes are responsible for up to 90 % of toenail onychomycosis, but *Candida* species commonly cause fingernail infection. Nondermatophyte molds must also be included in the differential diagnosis of nail dystrophy [7].

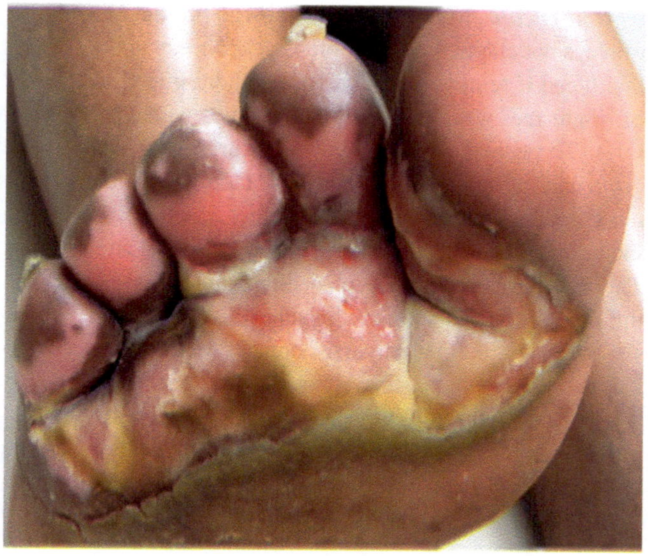

Fig. 17.7 Mixed toe web infection with severe maceration of the toe webs

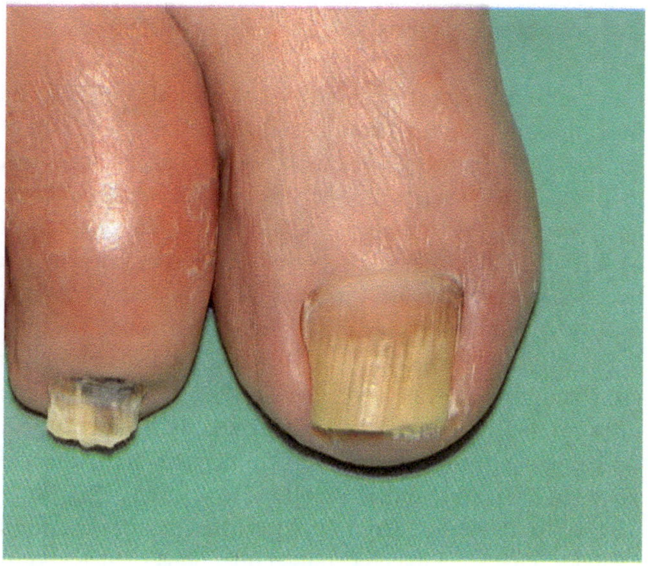

Fig. 17.8 Distal onychomycosis demonstrating onycholysis and subungual debris

The hallmark of onychomycosis is nail dystrophy. This often consists of discoloration of the nail plate, onycholysis (separation of the nail plate from the nail bed), and the presence of chalky subungual debris (Fig. 17.8).

There are two varieties of tinea unguium that have special implications. Proximal subungual onychomycosis, as the name suggests, involves only the proximal portion of the nail plate, and it is frequently associated with human immunodeficiency virus (HIV) infection [8] (Fig. 17.9). Superficial white onychomycosis, which typically stays in the dorsal portion of the nail plate, can be associated with *T. mentagrophytes* and nondermatophytes like *Aspergillus* and *Fusarium*.

The differential diagnosis of tinea unguium includes trauma, psoriasis, atopic dermatitis, subungual tumors, lichen planus, alopecia areata, and contact dermatitis.

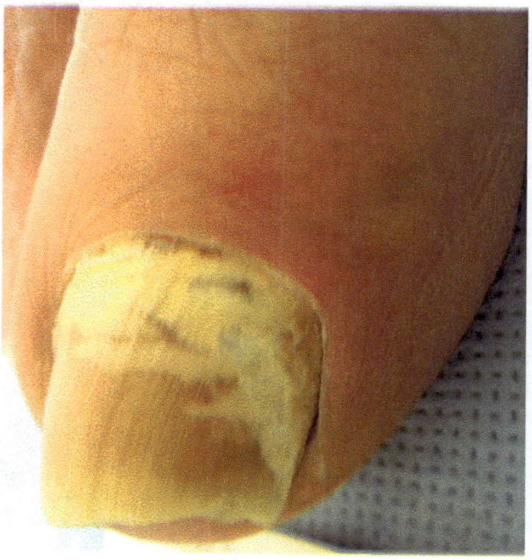

Fig. 17.9 Proximal subungual onychomycosis associated with immunosuppression

Nondermatophytes

Piedra

There are two forms of piedra—white and black—which are both superficial infections of the hair shaft. White piedra, which is common in temperate climates, is primarily caused by *Trichosporon asahii*, formerly known as *Trichosporon beigelii*. White piedra presents as asymptomatic, soft, white or cream colored nodules that are loosely adherent to hair shafts. While this is primarily a self-limited infection, *T. asahii* has been known to cause a systemic infection called trichosporonosis in immunosuppressed patients [9]. This is a multisystem disease that includes fevers, renal failure, pulmonary infiltrates, and skin lesions that range from papules to necrotic nodules.

Black piedra is caused by *Piedraiahortai*, and it occurs only in tropical climates. It presents as tiny, firm black nodules on the hair shafts of the scalp. It is usually asymptomatic but may result in breakage of the hair shafts. Black piedra is not known to cause systemic disease.

The differential of piedra includes pediculosis (lice), hair casts, trichomycosis axillaris, eczema, and psoriasis.

Tinea Nigra

Tinea nigra is a superficial infection caused by *Hortaea werneckii*. It is found in tropical climates, which can include portions of the United States. It is usually found in soil, compost, or decaying wood and vegetation. Infection typically presents as an asymptomatic brown macule or patch on the hand or wrist, though it may also appear in other places on the body. The major item in the differential is acral melanocytic nevus, though malignant melanoma, fixed drug eruption, postinflammatory hyperpigmentation, and external stains can also be considered.

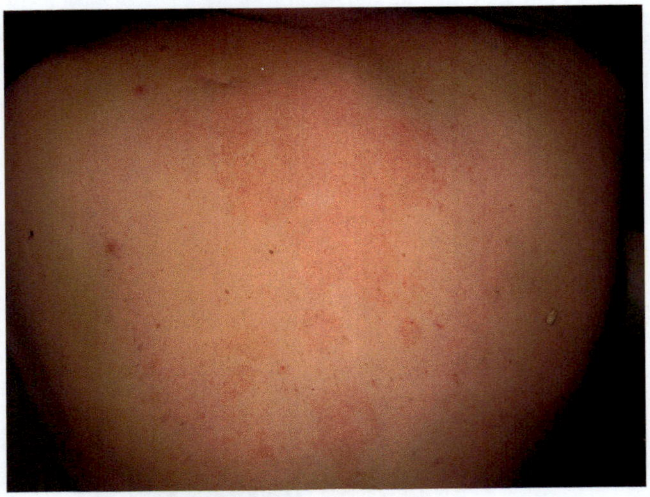

Fig. 17.10 Tinea (pityriasis) versicolor

Tinea Versicolor

Tinea versicolor is caused by lipophilic yeasts in the *Malassezia* genus, including *M. furfur* and *M. globosa*. These are present in small numbers on normal skin, and they cause skin disease only when they proliferate and form hyphae. This is usually stimulated by excessive heat and perspiration, but a number of other factors have been implicated [10]. Tinea versicolor occurs worldwide, with a higher incidence in hot, humid climates.

Clinically, tinea versicolor presents as numerous ovoid patches with fine scale that may coalesce. They can range in color from hypopigmented to red to hyperpigmented, depending on the host. Common areas of involvement are the back, chest, and shoulders (Fig. 17.10). Pruritus is usually absent or minimal. The differential diagnosis includes vitiligo, pityriasis alba, postinflammatory pigment alteration, seborrheic dermatitis, pityriasis rosea, guttate psoriasis, tinea corporis, and secondary syphilis.

M. furfur and *M. globosa* can also invade hair follicles, leading to pityrosporum folliculitis. Common in young men and women, this presents as monomorphic red papules and pustules on the upper trunk and shoulders. It can be pruritic. Pityrosporum folliculitis has also been known to arise in the immunosuppressed and those on chronic antibiotics. The differential commonly includes acne, bacterial folliculitis, and eosinophilic folliculitis.

Mucocutaneous Candidiasis

Mucocutaneous candidal infections can range from benign self-limited infections such as angular cheilitis to chronic and debilitating infections in those with certain immunodeficiencies. *Candida albicans* is the most frequent cause, followed by *C. tropicalis*. Mucosal candidiasis can present in a number of ways but classically resembles thick, cheesy white plaques that bleed if removed. Cutaneous candidal infections consist of bright red, weepy patches and plaques with satellite pustules. These occur most often in flexural areas such as the groin and inframammary areas. Risk factors for mucocutaneous candidal infections include diabetes, immunosuppression including HIV, antibiotic use, corticosteroids, and habitus. The differential for mucocutaneous candidiasis depends on the site(s) involved but includes seborrheic dermatitis, psoriasis, intertrigo, dermatophytosis, contact dermatitis, leukoplakia, and lichen planus, as well as many others.

The term chronic mucocutaneous candidiasis encompasses a number of immunodeficiencies and other disorders whose end result is severe and recalcitrant candidal infection. Invasive candidiasis will be discussed separately.

Subcutaneous Fungal Infections

Chromoblastomycosis

Chromoblastomycosis is caused by a number of dematiaceous fungi that are naturally found in soil and decaying plant matter. *Fonsecaea pedrosoi* is the most common agent, but others in the genera *Fonsecaea*, *Phialophora*, *Cladophialophora*, and *Rhinocladiella* have been identified [11]. These are most often found in tropical and subtropical climates, but they are occasionally seen in the United States. The most common route of infection is local inoculation via trauma. The first lesion is often a small verrucous papule which can slowly grow and spread locally. Over time, large, fungating tumors may develop. These can be complicated by superinfection, regional lymphadenopathy, and loss of function of the affected limb, but they rarely spread distally or to internal organs.

The differential diagnosis for chromoblastomycosis includes other subcutaneous fungal infections such as sporotrichosis and mycetoma, blastomycosis, cutaneous tuberculosis or other atypical mycobacterium, leishmaniasis, tertiary syphilis, warts, and mycosis fungoides.

Sporotrichosis

Sporotrichosis is caused by the dimorphic fungus *Sporothrix schenckii*. It is present in soil and on vegetation such as rose bushes and sphagnum moss. It has a broad geographic distribution which includes portions of the southeastern United States. The organism is introduced to humans almost exclusively through puncture injuries, which are usually occupation related. Sporotrichosis begins as a small red papule or nodule at the site of injury. Within weeks it will exhibit lymphangitic, or "sporotrichoid," spread. This includes the development of

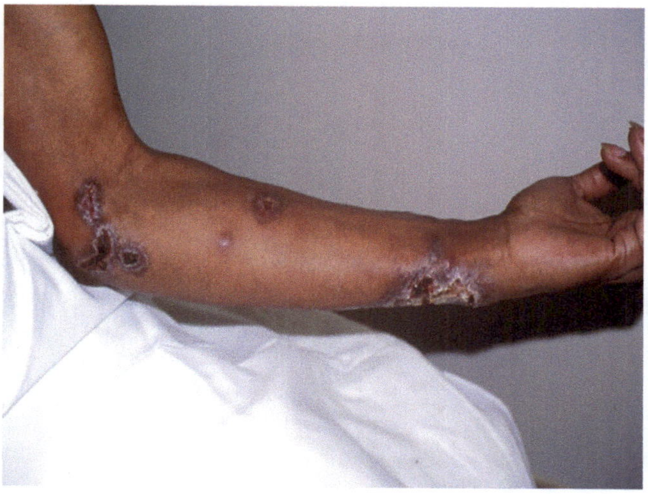

Fig. 17.11 Sporotrichosis. Note the spread of lesions along the local lymphatics

erythematous nodules along the course of lymphatic drainage which may ulcerate (Fig. 17.11). Other forms of sporotrichosis exist, such as a fixed cutaneous form without lymphangitic spread, rosacea-like lesions, and disseminated disease [12]. However, these are the exception to the rule.

The differential diagnosis of sporotrichosis, especially with lymphangitic spread, includes the following: leishmaniasis, atypical mycobacteria, tuberculosis, nocardia, tularemia, lepromatous leprosy, and other deep and subcutaneous fungal infections.

Mycetoma

Mycetoma, or Madura foot, is a phenotype that is caused by two different classes of organisms: true fungi and filamentous bacteria. Eumycetomas, those caused by true fungi, include members of the *Madurella*, *Pseudallescheria*, *Acremonium*, and several other genera [13]. Actinomycetomas are caused by *Nocardia*, *Actinomadura*, *Actinomyces*, and *Streptomyces* species of bacteria. Both kinds of mycetoma are acquired through direct penetration of the organism into the foot or leg from soil. They are also found in similar environments—arid climates near the equator.

Mycetomas, both eumycotic and actinomycotic, are characterized by their draining sinus tracts and profound local edema. The lesions begin as asymptomatic nodules at the site of inoculation, before undergoing a period of steady swelling and growth. They can involve underlying structures such as fascia, muscle, and even bone, while generally remaining painless. The material that drains from the sinuses is composed of characteristic, tightly packed clumps of organisms. While the appearance of mycetoma is fairly characteristic, other subcutaneous and deep infections can be in the differential.

Opportunistic Fungal Infections with Cutaneous Lesions

Systemic Candidiasis

In immunocompromised patients, such as recipients of renal transplants, candidal infections represent the most common systemic fungal infection. The most common pathogen is *C. albicans*, while *C. tropicalis* may be more common in patients with hematologic malignancy. The portal of entry is thought to be the gastrointestinal tract, and long-term IV catheterization is a strong risk factor. The mortality associated with disseminated candidiasis is between 30 and 40 %, so early recognition and initiation of treatment is paramount [14].

Disseminated candidiasis usually presents as fever that is unresponsive to antimicrobials, proximal muscle tenderness, and skin lesions that can range from red macules and papules with a pale center, to purpura, to vesicles and necrotic ulcers. Septic shock and failure of virtually any end organ can occur. Unfortunately blood cultures will not always be positive for yeast, so a high index of suspicion is required. Items in the differential diagnosis include bacterial sepsis or septic shock, as well as other opportunistic infections such as aspergillosis, fusariosis, cryptococcosis, and phaeohyphomycosis.

Aspergillosis

Aspergillosis is an opportunistic fungal infection caused by two *Aspergillus* species, *flavus* and *fumigatus*. Specific risk factors for aspergillosis include neutropenia, burn patients, and high-dose corticosteroids [15]. There are two main ways in which this infection occurs. In the first, the fungus gains entry to the skin and subcutaneous tissue through a burn site, long-standing IV catheter, or compromised wound under occlusion. In an immunocompromised host, it can then invade the local vasculature and become disseminated. The second pathway is via inhalation, which leads to pulmonary infection and dissemination from there.

Cutaneous lesions in aspergillosis usually include purpura, necrotic papules, and ulcers. Disseminated aspergillosis is rapidly fatal, with spread to the lungs, kidneys, heart, and central nervous system (CNS). Septic shock and hemoptysis are frequently present.

Another form of aspergillosis is known as otomycosis, and it represents colonization or infection of the external ear canal. Concomitant infection with bacteria such as *Pseudomonas aeruginosa* is quite common. While this can be perfectly asymptomatic in a healthy host, in the immunocompromised, a progressive and invasive infection may occur that requires prompt parenteral antimicrobial therapy.

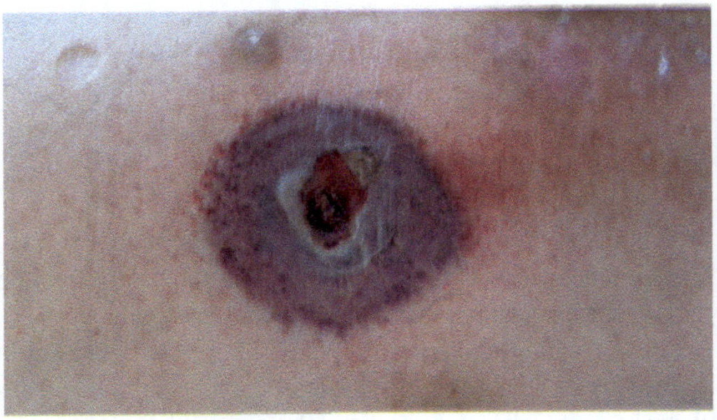

Fig. 17.12 Mucormycosis in an immunocompromised patient—note the sharply demarcated necrotic ulcer. (Courtesy of Alex G. Ortega-Loayza, M.D.)

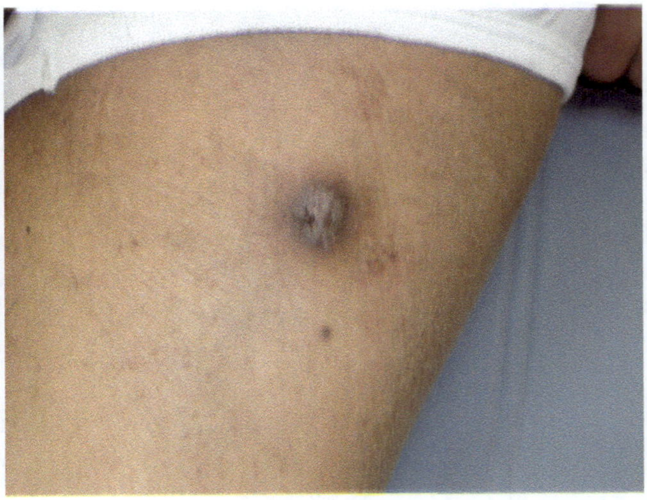

Fig. 17.13 Phaeohyphomycosis. *Exophiala jeanselmei* is a recognized causative agent of mycetoma and phaeohyphomycosis. The clinical presentation can be nonspecific; tissue culture is necessary to make the diagnosis. (Courtesy of Julia R. Nunley, M.D.)

Zygomycosis

Zygomycosis is an opportunistic, angioinvasive infection caused by multiple organisms including *Rhizopus* and *Mucor* species. These fungi are ubiquitous in soil and vegetation but rarely cause disease in immunocompetent hosts. However, they are known to cause rapidly fatal infections in those with leukopenia and acidosis, particularly uncontrolled diabetes [16]. Other predisposing conditions include hematologic malignancy, pharmacologic immunosuppression, solid organ or bone marrow transplantation, burns, trauma, malnutrition, and IV drug use. Of particular interest are infections in patients with iron or aluminum overload, patients undergoing hemodialysis, and those receiving the chelating agent deferoxamine [17]. The classic and most common form of zygomycosis is rhinocerebral, which usually occurs in patients with diabetic ketoacidosis (DKA). Patients may complain of fever and unilateral facial pain, including pain with eye movements. Diffuse erythema and induration will progress to necrotic ulcers with characteristic black centers. A less common form of cutaneous zygomycosis follows trauma and direct inoculation into the skin. This can occur anywhere and usually presents as a sharply demarcated necrotic ulcer with a dark black center (Fig. 17.12). Occasionally these lesions can also occur in various locations on the skin secondary to disseminated disease. Disseminated zygomycosis is a rapidly progressive infection that usually begins in the lungs and spreads to the brain. Patients begin with fever and headaches and soon develop confusion, obtundation, and death. They may or may not have cutaneous findings. In 2008, Reyes et al. [17] reported such a case in a patient with secondary iron overload treated with deferoxamine.

Phaeohyphomycosis

The term phaeohyphomycosis encompasses a large group of dematiaceous fungi with this in common—the production of dark brown or black hyphae in tissue. Most of these organisms are found in soil and plant material, and they are introduced into human hosts via trauma. Phaeohyphomycosis can range from asymptomatic superficial infection, such as tinea nigra, to onychomycosis, to rapidly progressive and fatal systemic infection [18]. Infected puncture wounds can lead to cutaneous papules, subcutaneous cysts, or nodules (Fig. 17.13). In a normal host these lesions typically become walled off but do not spread further. In immunocompromised hosts, these fungi can gain access to the bloodstream and disseminate from there. Common targets of dissemination include the heart valves and central nervous system (CNS), and when present, skin lesions appear as necrotic, dry ulcers and eschars with red borders.

Hyalohyphomycosis

Hyalohyphomycosis includes nondematiaceous fungi that produce tan or white hyphae in tissue. The most important organisms in this group include species of three genera: *Fusarium*, *Penicillium*, and *Paecilomyces*. These organisms are ubiquitous in nature but rarely cause disease in competent hosts. One exception is that *Fusarium* spp. can cause onychomycosis, which is thought to be a possible source of disseminated disease [19]. *Fusarium* spp. are known to affect patients with profound neutropenia, hematologic malignancy, and severe burns. While *Penicillium* species are mostly found in southeast Asia, they have been seen in the United States, primarily in HIV patients [20].

Clinically, patients with disseminated fusariosis will have fevers, severe myalgias, and diffuse targetoid lesions that become necrotic and ulcerated (Figs. 17.14 and 17.15). Skin findings associated with penicilliosis include papules on the

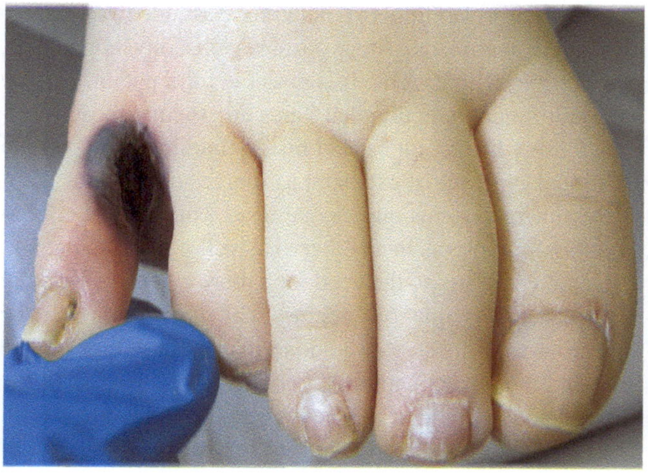

Fig. 17.14 Fusariosis resulting in cutaneous necrosis in an immunocompromised patient. (Courtesy of Alex G. Ortega-Loayza, M.D.)

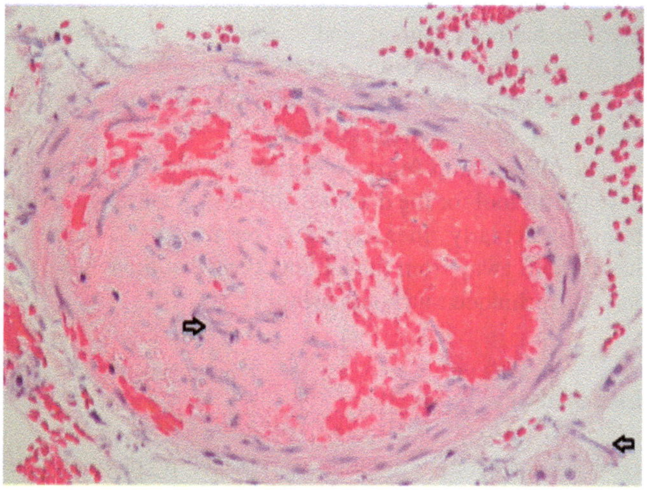

Fig. 17.15 Fusariosis with angioinvasion; *arrows* indicate organisms in and around a blood vessel

forehead and cheeks that resemble acne or molluscum. The differential diagnosis of fusariosis includes other angioinvasive infections like aspergillosis and candidiasis. For penicilliosis, the list is similar but also includes dimorphic fungi like cryptococcosis, blastomycosis, histoplasmosis, and coccidioidomycosis, which can all form molluscum-type lesions in immunocompromised hosts.

Other Opportunistic Fungal Infections

A number of other fungi can cause systemic infections in immunocompromised hosts, but these rarely cause primary cutaneous infection. For this reason, these will be only briefly discussed. *Cryptococcus neoformans* is found in soil and pigeon feces and can cause molluscum-like lesions on the

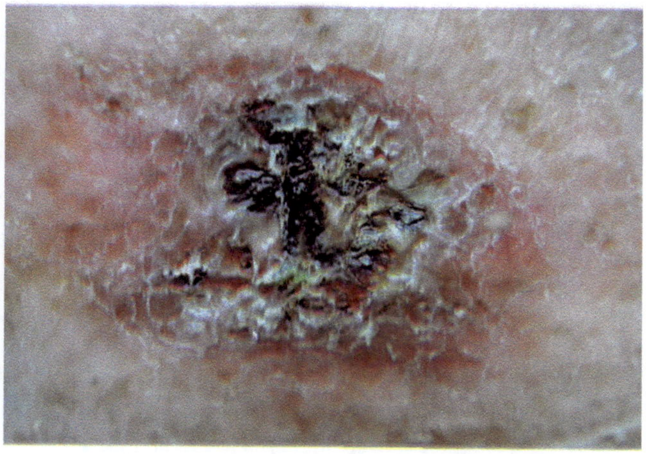

Fig. 17.16 A crusted erosion caused by disseminated blastomycosis

face as part of a disseminated infection. *Histoplasma capsulatum* can be encountered in soil in the Mississippi and Ohio River valleys of the Midwestern United States. The most common form of cutaneous lesions from *H. capsulatum* is oral and other mucosal ulcerations. *Blastomyces dermatitidis*, the cause of North American blastomycosis, is another dimorphic fungus that is present in the eastern United States. Cutaneous involvement secondary to pulmonary or disseminated disease is not uncommon and can range from verrucous plaques and tumors to large ulcerated plaques on exposed skin such as the arm (Fig. 17.16). Primary cutaneous blastomycosis is not common. Coccidioidomycosis is caused by *Coccidioides immitis*, which is found in the southwestern United States as well as parts of Mexico and Central America. A variety of lesions can occur in association with coccidioidomycosis, from papules to nodules to large ulcers and draining tracts. There is a predilection for the face. Of note, pulmonary infection with *C. immitis* in immunocompetent hosts is a known cause of erythema nodosum, and this finding is associated with a good prognosis. Paracoccidioidomycosis, also known as South American blastomycosis, is caused by *Paracoccidioidis brasiliensis*. This organism is known to cause primary mucocutaneous disease after chewing on infected plant matter, which presents as red juicy papules that coalesce into plaques on the lips and perioral skin. Paracoccidioidomycosis can also cause a number of nonspecific cutaneous lesions secondary to disseminated disease.

Mycobacterial Infections

Although relatively rare, mycobacterial infections can cause significant morbidity and mortality in the renal transplant recipient. Whereas *Mycobacterium tuberculosis* remains the most common of these organisms, a wide variety of other atypical mycobacterial organisms have also been reported [21].

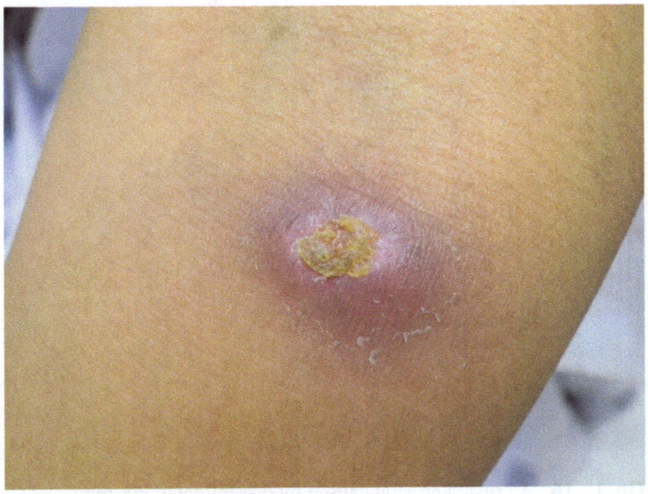

Fig. 17.17 Seen here are the nonspecific changes of a primary cutaneous mycobacterial infection. Diagnosis must be made by biopsy. (Courtesy of Julia R. Nunley, M.D.)

The cutaneous manifestations of these infections are nonspecific (Fig. 17.17), mimic those of subcutaneous fungal infections, and must be differentiated by histology and cultures. Their relative rarity may be partially attributed to clinical oversight or inadequate diagnostic techniques. Furthermore, therapeutic protocols for these infections are complex, and the clinician must be cognizant of confounding drug interactions between these antimicrobial agents and posttransplant immunosuppressive medications.

History and Physical Exam

The approach to the patient with a dermatologic problem is somewhat different from the approach to the patient typically seen by the internist. It begins with a very brief history which is quickly interrupted by the patient showing the provider the lesion or eruption of concern. This rapidly moves the focus to the physical exam. Nonetheless, early attention to the history can be very helpful and timesaving.

Of utmost importance when considering a potential infection is the patient's range of activities and history of exposures. The patient should be asked about the use of public facilities such as gymnasiums, public showers, and group living facilities. The provider should inquire about exposure to individuals with pruritic skin conditions, especially young children. The patient should also be asked about exposure to pets, farm animals, and gardening—all potential sources of fungus. Has the patient traveled recently in areas known for specific infections? It is also essential to ask if the patient has used any form of treatment. Topical steroids, particularly high potency preparations, may mask or change the clinical features of infection. Prescription or over-the-counter antimicrobial medications can dramatically change the physical examination and laboratory findings.

Questions regarding the patient's past medical history may reveal a previous history of tinea pedis, onychomycosis, or other fungal infections. It is possible for a patient to have an occult fungal infection that flares due to immunosuppression. Family history and social history inquires may provide additional evidence of exposure to sources of fungus.

Review of systems may reveal fever, chills, or other constitutional symptoms in an otherwise well-appearing patient. These may be clues to the need for a more extensive workup.

Physical examination begins with inspection of the affected area. This should be done in a room with adequate light and the patient should disrobe sufficiently to show the affected area. Although it is not necessary in all cases, a full body examination is recommended to avoid missing foci of infection or clues to systemic disease that may not be obvious to the patient.

Although frequently neglected, examination of the mucous membranes is especially important in the immunocompromised patient. For example, candidiasis commonly involves the oral, vaginal, and anal mucosa with erythema, white plaques, and satellite pustules. In addition, patients with fungemia may have oral erosions and ulcers in the absence of other cutaneous findings.

The Wood lamp (ultraviolet light, 300 nm) was once a very useful tool for the diagnosis of superficial fungal infections, particularly tinea capitis. Over the years, there has been a shift away from fungal infections that fluoresce making this technique much less useful [22].

Laboratory

Direct microscopic examination ("KOH preparation") of superficial scrapings from skin, mucous membranes, or nails is a common office procedure used by dermatologists for diagnosing superficial fungal infections. Pulled hairs can be examined by the same technique. Occasionally, the same microscopic technique is used in conjunction with skin biopsy [23]. Samples applied to a glass slide are treated with 20 % KOH, a cover slip applied, and examined microscopically. Fungal hyphae, pseudohyphae, or yeast may be seen (Figs. 17.18 and 17.19). These findings are sufficient to make the diagnosis of a superficial fungal infection and begin appropriate treatment. The KOH preparation has the advantage of being quick and relatively sensitive for the diagnosis of fungal infections. It cannot provide information on the type of fungus present beyond the broad categories of probable dermatophyte, probable Candida, tinea versicolor, and the presence of other yeast cells. Also, it is a technique unfamiliar to many internists and not readily available in all practice settings.

Fungal culture is an alternative to the KOH preparation. Scrapings from skin or mucous membranes, toenail

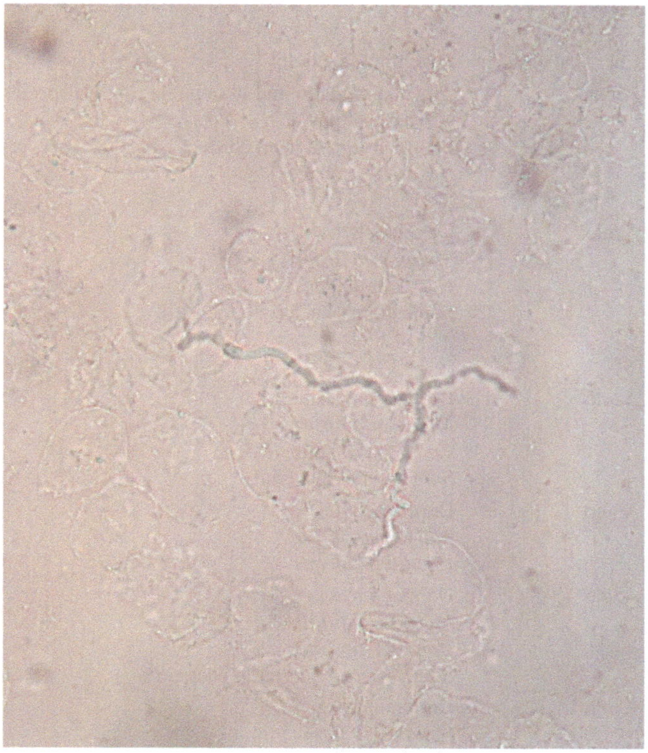

Fig. 17.18 A potassium hydroxide preparation, photomicrograph, showing a branched hypha

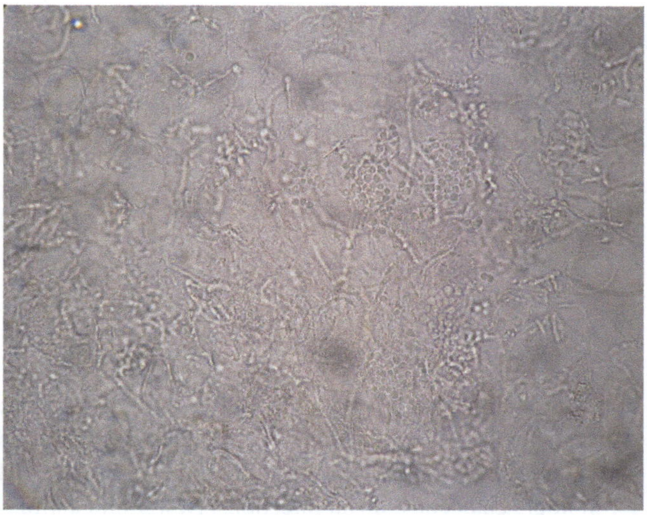

Fig. 17.19 Tinea versicolor, photomicrograph, showing hyphae and spores ("spaghetti and meatballs")

clippings, pulled hairs, or fresh tissue can be submitted in a sterile fashion for culture. These samples are submitted to the laboratory in a sterile container such as a sterile urine cup. In the case of tissue obtained at biopsy, the tissue should be submitted in a sterile container but placed on sterile gauze moistened with saline (without antibacterial agents). In the laboratory, the appropriate media will be selected based on the history provided with the specimen. Laboratory culture offers the advantage of identifying the fungus growing in the culture. This can be very valuable information in selecting appropriate therapy. The disadvantage of all culture techniques is the time required for growth. Results may not be available for 8 weeks or more. In the case of severe infections, empiric therapy may be required prior to obtaining final culture results.

Cutaneous biopsy may occasionally be required for the diagnosis of superficial fungal infections. It is generally required for deeper infections. If a fungal infection is suspected and a biopsy is done, a portion of the tissue should be sent in formalin for histopathology and a portion should be sent in a sterile container, as above, for fungal culture and other cultures as appropriate (bacterial, atypical mycobacterium, viral). A single biopsy may be divided in a sterile manner or two biopsies obtained. The pathologist should be alerted to the possibility of a fungal infection so appropriate stains may be done on the tissue. The biopsy technique employed is usually the punch biopsy. In the case of nodular lesions, particularly in the immunocompromised patient, a more aggressive biopsy may be required—incisional wedge biopsy or excision may be more appropriate. Again, the tissue should be divided with a portion submitted for standard histopathology and a portion for culture.

Other laboratory testing such as complete blood count and chemistry studies are unrevealing in most cutaneous fungal infections. Both should be obtained prior to beginning and for monitoring during the administration of systemic antifungal agents. Screening for antibodies to dimorphic fungi (*Blastomyces*, *Coccidioides*, *Histoplasma*) and cryptococcal, aspergillus, histoplasma, and candida antigens may be useful if these infections are suspected. Imaging studies are not routinely ordered. They are needed if involvement of deeper structures (bones, joints) is suspected in severe infections. Blood cultures are required if systemic infection is suspected.

Treatment

Superficial infections of glabrous skin generally respond well to topical antifungal agents but when extensive or recalcitrant to therapy may require systemic treatment. Infections of the scalp, beard, fingernails, and toenails require administration of oral agents [22]. In the immunocompromised host, superficial infections may require prolonged or repeated treatment but can usually be treated topically [24]. Topical antifungal agents are generally used as monotherapy but can be combined with topical steroids to rapidly reduce inflammation. If combination therapy is used, the topical steroid should be low potency such as hydrocortisone 2.5 % or desonide and only used for several days to control inflammation [25]. Higher potency topical steroids and combination

Table 17.1 Topical therapy [26]

Name	Dosage form	Dose frequency	Chemical class	Spectrum of activity
Nystatin	Cream Ointment Powder Suspension Pastille	BID, skin; QID, suspension or pastille for thrush	Polyene	*Candida albicans* and susceptible candida species Not dermatophytes Poorly absorbed from GI tract
Miconazole	Cream Ointment Spray Powder Solution Gel	BID	Azole	Dermatophytes *Malassezia furfur* *Candida albicans* Some gram+ bacteria[a]
Clotrimazole	Cream Solution/lotion Oral troches	BID, skin; five times daily for oral troches	Azole	Dermatophytes *Malassezia furfur* *Candida albicans* Some gram+ bacteria[a]
Ketoconazole	Cream Foam Shampoo (1–2 %)	Daily to BID	Azole	Dermatophytes *Malassezia furfur* *Candida albicans*
Econazole	Cream	Daily to BID	Azole	Dermatophytes *Malassezia furfur* *Candida albicans* Some gram+ and gram– bacteria[a]
Oxiconazole	Cream Lotion	Daily to BID	Azole	Dermatophytes *Malassezia furfur* *Candida albicans*[b]
Naftifine	Cream Gel	Daily to BID	Allylamine	Dermatophytes
Terbinafine	Cream Spray	Daily to BID	Allylamine	Dermatophytes *Candida albicans*[b]
Butenafine	Cream	Daily	Benzylamine	Dermatophytes *Candida albicans*[b]
Ciclopirox	Cream Gel Lotion/suspension Shampoo Nail lacquer	BID; daily for nail lacquer	Hydroxypyridone	Dermatophytes *Candida albicans* *Malassezia furfur* Saprophytic fungi Some gram+ and gram– bacteria[a]
Selenium sulfide	Lotion (2.5 %) Shampoo (1–2.5 %)	Multiple dosing schedules		*Malassezia furfur*

BID twice daily, *QID* four times daily, *GI* gastrointestinal
[a]Not used as topical antibiotic
[b]Less effective than other agents in azole class

products should be avoided because they may induce fungal folliculitis. Topical agents are usually well tolerated. Potential side effects include skin irritation, erythema, stinging, burning sensation, eczema, contact dermatitis, edema, maceration, urticaria, and rarely hypersensitivity [24]. Topical agents are presented in Table 17.1.

Oral antifungal agents are employed when topical agents fail or in the case of infections not expected to respond to topical therapy. The latter case includes onychomycosis, follicular infection, and widespread infections [22]. Identification of the causative organism is needed prior to initiating oral therapy since the various organisms do not respond uniformly to the available systemic antifungal agents, and numerous noninfectious conditions of the skin, hair, and nails mimic fungal infections. Topical agents are often used in combination with oral therapy and may be continued as maintenance therapy after the oral medication is discontinued. Griseofulvin and ketoconazole are Food and Drug Administration approved for multiple cutaneous fungal infections. Newer oral antifungal agents have more limited approved indications but are often more efficacious and better tolerated [22]. Citing a significant risk of hepatotoxicity, the FDA recently issued an alert that oral ketoconazole should not be first-line therapy for any fungal infection [27]. There is much literature to support the use of the newer systemic antifungal agents beyond their approved indications. These off-label uses are now common and will be included in the discussion below. All of the currently available oral antifungal agents carry some risk for hepatotoxicity. For that reason, the patient's past medical history, liver function testing, and concomitant medications must be considered prior to the administration of these medications. Some systemic antifungal agents administered to women or men may increase the risk for birth defects, and the use of these medications must be weighed against that risk [24]. In addition, the potential adverse events for most of these agents include one or more of the following: cardiac arrhythmias (and Q-T changes), blood dyscrasias, hypersensitivity reactions, and serious skin reactions. Oral medications are presented in Table 17.2.

Surgical and destructive modalities may be employed in localized infections of the dermis and subcutaneous tissues.

Extensive subcutaneous infections, angioinvasive infections, and infections accompanied by systemic symptoms, especially in the immunosuppressed patient, require aggressive therapy. Consultation with infectious disease specialists is needed because these infections, if not already disseminated, may rapidly spread with a lethal outcome. Prolonged oral or IV therapy is often required. Discussion of these more advanced therapies is beyond the scope of this text.

Therapies for more commonly encountered fungal infections are presented below. The suggested treatments are representative—multiple options exist for each disease entity.

Tinea Corporis, Tinea Cruris, Tinea Faciei, and Tinea Manuum

Tinea corporis, tinea cruris, tinea faciei, and tinea manuum can usually be successfully treated with topical antifungal agents once or twice daily, depending on the medication used (see Table 17.1). Treatment duration should be at least 2 weeks. Extensive infection, resistance to topical medication, and coinfection with tinea capitis or onychomycosis may necessitate systemic therapy (Fig. 17.20). Options for oral therapy include griseofulvin, terbinafine, or itraconazole [39].

Tinea Pedis

Tinea pedis is more recalcitrant to therapy. It can be treated topically but usually requires longer periods of treatment than tinea corporis. A topical antifungal should be applied daily or twice daily, depending on the medication used (see Table 17.1). Extensive infection, resistance to topical medication, or the presence of onychomycosis may necessitate systemic therapy with one of the following oral agents: griseofulvin, terbinafine, itraconazole, or fluconazole [39]. Extensive weeping of the toe webs may require concomitant therapy with topical drying agents such as aluminum acetate (Domeboro or Burow solution). Secondary bacterial infection and cellulitis require coadministration of systemic antibiotics (Fig. 17.21). Tinea pedis is a risk factor for cellulitis in the immunocompromised patient—it should be treated aggressively.

Mixed Toe Web Infection

Mixed toe web infection requires bed rest and hospitalization if extensive. Maceration and denudation of the toe webs and plantar surface lead to significant weeping requiring the use of a drying agent, as mentioned above. Econazole is useful topically. In addition to its antifungal activity, it has been shown in clinical trials to decrease both gram positive and gram negative bacteria [26]. Oral ciprofloxacin or other systemic antibiotic may be required. Antibiotic selection should be based on culture results when possible. Blood cultures and empiric antibiotic therapy should be initiated in patients with mixed toe web infection and evidence of septicemia.

Majocchi Granuloma

Majocchi granuloma, a fungal folliculitis, requires systemic therapy due to infection of the hair follicle. Oral terbinafine is usually curative; 6 weeks is suggested when the patient has received a renal transplant [40]. Elimination of exacerbating factors (topical steroids and occlusion) is also required.

Tinea Barbae and Tinea Capitis

Tinea barbae and tinea capitis require systemic therapy. Options for adults include griseofulvin [33] or oral terbinafine [39]. Itraconazole and fluconazole are alternatives. If extensive inflammation is present (kerion), a short course of systemic corticosteroids can reduce the potential for scarring and hair loss.

Onychomycosis

Onychomycosis requires systemic therapy for cure [41]. There are many treatment options. Griseofulvin is currently seldom used due to long treatment courses and low cure rates. Oral terbinafine daily for 6 weeks is administered for dermatophyte infections of the fingernails and 12 weeks for toenails. Alternatively, itraconazole daily may be given for 12 weeks for toenail infection. For fingernails the preferred course of itraconazole is a 1 week pulse each month for a total of two pulse doses. For onychomycosis, itraconazole is approved in immunocompetent patients. Literature also supports the use of fluconazole weekly for 3–6 months for fingernails and 9–12 months for toenails [39]. Onychomycosis, especially of the fingernails, may be caused by *C. albicans* and these infections are poorly responsive to terbinafine. Fluconazole is often effective for these infections. Laboratory monitoring should be performed during these prolonged courses of oral antifungal agents. Topical therapy may be useful as adjunctive therapy.

Table 17.2 Systemic therapy

Name/indications	Dosage route, forms, and comments	Renal adjustment (CrCl in mL/min) [28]	Pregnancy class	Spectrum of in vitro activity	Selected AE, also see text
Terbinafine [29, 30] Indications: dermatophyte onychomycosis of fingernails and toenails	Oral 250 mg tablets Oral granules	CrCl < 50: avoid use	B	*Trichophyton mentagrophytes*, *Trichophyton rubrum*, *Candida albicans*, *Epidermophyton floccosum*, *Scopulariopsis brevicaulis*	Exacerbation of SLE and psoriasis, angioedema, depression, rhabdomyolysis, pancreatitis, photosensitivity, taste/smell disturbance
Itraconazole [31] Indications: Blastomycosis, histoplasmosis, aspergillosis. Onychomycosis in immunocompetent patients[a]	Oral 100 mg tablets, suspension 10 mg/mL Administer with full meal	Caution advised; CrCl < 10: decrease dose 50 %; HD/PD: 100 mg q12-24 hrs	C, avoid pregnancy[b]	*Blastomyces dermatitidis*, *Histoplasma capsulatum*, *Histoplasma duboisii*, *Aspergillus flavus*, *Aspergillus fumigatus*, *Candida albicans*, *Cryptococcus neoformans*[c]	CHF; serious drug interactions; pancreatitis, pulmonary edema, peripheral edema, hearing loss, peripheral neuropathy
Fluconazole [32] Indications: Vaginal candidiasis; oral pharyngeal and esophageal candidiasis; *Candida* urinary tract infections, peritonitis, and systemic *Candida* infections; cryptococcal meningitis	Oral, IV 50, 100, 150, 200 mg tablets, oral suspension (see package insert); IV	CrCl < 50: loading dose x1, then decrease dose 50 %; HD: usual dose after dialysis, no supplement; PD: Decrease dose 50 %, no supplement	C,D	*Candida albicans*, other *Candida* species, not *Candida krusei* Also *Cryptococcus neoformans*	Seizures, angioedema
Griseofulvin [33] (microsize)[d] Indications: dermatophyte infections including skin, hair, and nails	Oral 500 mg tablets; 125/5 mL suspension Give with high fat meal	No adjustment needed	C, avoid pregnancy[b]	*Trichophyton rubrum*, *Trichophyton tonsurans*, multiple other *Trichophyton* species, *Microsporum audouinii*, *Microsporum canis*, *Microsporum gypseum*, *Epidermophyton floccosum*	Paresthesias, fatigue, dizziness, insomnia, mental confusion, proteinuria, SLE exacerbation, photosensitivity
Ketoconazole [34] Indications: systemic blastomycosis, coccidioidomycosis, histoplasmosis, chromomycosis, paracoccidioidomycosis in patients who have failed or who are intolerant to other therapies	Oral 200 mg tablet Food needed for absorption; citrus or cola beverage increases absorption	No adjustment needed	C, see package insert	*Paracoccidioides brasiliensis*, *Histoplasma capsulatum*, *Coccidioides immitis*, *Blastomyces dermatitidis*	Drug interactions; adrenal insufficiency (see text regarding FDA alert)
Voriconazole [35] Indications: invasive aspergillosis, systemic candidiasis; *Scedosporium apiospermum* and *Fusarium* spp. infections if refractory or intolerant of other agents	Oral, IV 50, 200 mg tablet; oral suspension (see package insert); IV	CrCl < 50 avoid IV use	D	*Aspergillus fumigatus*, *Aspergillus flavus*, *Aspergillus niger*, *Aspergillus terreus*, *Candida albicans*, other *Candida* species, *Fusarium* spp., *Scedosporium apiospermum*	Cholestasis, pancreatitis, acute renal failure, sepsis, vision changes, angioedema, drug interactions. Photosensitivity and a possible association with skin cancer are reported [36, 37]
Posaconazole [38] Indications: prophylaxis of invasive *Aspergillus* and *Candida* infections; oropharyngeal candidiasis	Oral 40 mg/mL oral suspension	CrCl ≥ 20 no adjustment; <20 monitor for breakthrough fungal infections	C, see package insert	*Aspergillus fumigatus*, *Candida albicans* (including isolates from patients refractory to itraconazole or fluconazole)	Severe nausea, vomiting, adrenal insufficiency, hemolytic uremic syndrome, acute renal failure, pulmonary embolus, drug interactions

IV intravenous, *HD* hemodialysis, *PD* peritoneal dialysis, *CrCL* creatinine clearance, *AE* adverse effects, *SLE* systemic lupus erythematosus, *CHF* congestive heart failure, *FDA* federal drug administration

[a] In patients with aspergillosis who are intolerant or refractory to amphotericin B

[b] Contraception recommended for males and females

[c] Itraconazole has variable in vitro activity against other *Candida species*, *Soprothrix schenckii*, *Trichophyton* species

[d] Griseofulvin is available in microsize and ultramicrosize formulations. They are not interchangeable

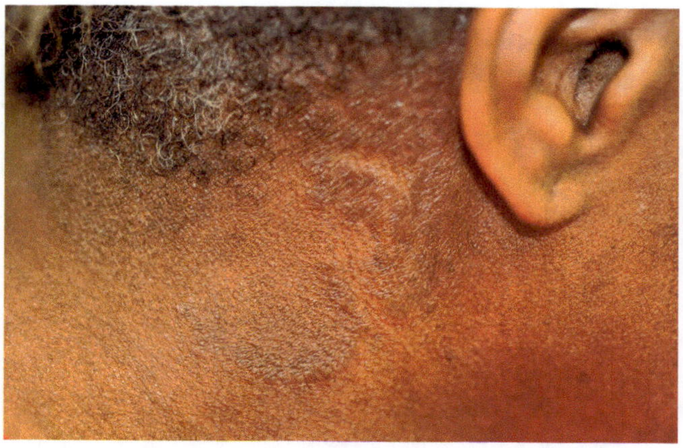

Fig. 17.20 Tinea corporis complicated by tinea capitis

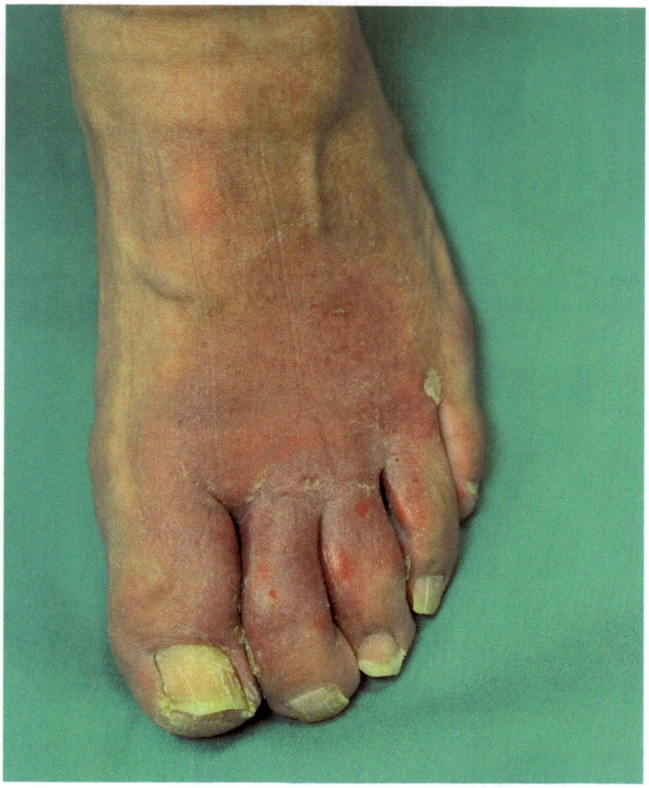

Fig. 17.21 Tinea pedis complicated by cellulitis

Tinea Versicolor

Tinea versicolor, a benign condition usually with few symptoms, should be treated topically in virtually all cases. Only if patients have significant pruritus and have failed topical therapy should oral therapy be considered. Although many therapies clear the skin, none prevent recurrences without continued use. Topical selenium sulfide lotion is widely used. It is applied to the affected areas, left on the skin for 10 min, and then rinsed off thoroughly—this is best done just prior to bath or shower.

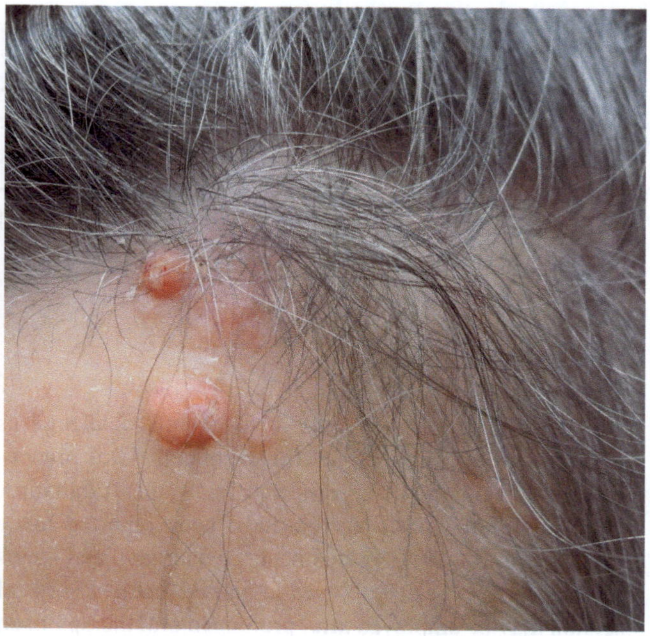

Fig. 17.22 Lesions of molluscum contagiosum are usually small umbilicated papules but can be widely distributed and larger in immune suppressed individuals. (Courtesy of Julia R. Nunley, M.D.)

Longer applications may lead to skin irritation. After daily treatment for 2 weeks the treatment should be repeated once weekly indefinitely. Alternatively, a topical azole can be applied daily for 2 weeks and then weekly. If oral therapy is deemed necessary, fluconazole weekly for 1–4 weeks [35] or itraconazole daily for 7 days can be used [42]. Both are best used in conjunction with topicals and a topical maintenance regimen should be continued to prevent relapse. Ketoconazole orally cannot be recommended based on the new FDA recommendations [27]. Pityrosporum folliculitis may respond to topical agents, but in the setting of immunosuppression will likely require oral therapy.

Mucocutaneous Candidiasis

Mucocutaneous candidiasis therapy is determined by the presentation. Intertrigo and balanitis can be treated with a topical azole or ciclopirox (cream or lotion) twice daily until resolved. For severe cases oral fluconazole or itraconazole may be effective. Oropharyngeal candidiasis can be treated with nystatin solution 100,000 units/mL, 5 mL swish and swallow four times daily. Clotrimazole 10 mg troches can be used five times daily. Oral fluconazole daily continued for 1–2 weeks after clinical symptoms clear is the treatment of choice for immune compromised patients with moderate to severe disease. Chronic mucocutaneous candidiasis requires a prolonged course of fluconazole for eradication and suppression [43].

Sporotrichosis

Sporotrichosis can be treated with daily itraconazole administered for 3–6 months. Potassium iodide, an alternative therapy, is contraindicated in patients with renal impairment [44]. Disseminated disease in adults may respond to itraconazole administered for up to 6 months. Amphotericin B and voriconazole are alternative therapies [43, 44].

Chromoblastomycosis

Chromoblastomycosis presents a therapeutic challenge as there are no uniformly successful treatments. Oral itraconazole daily, sometimes for years, may be useful. Terbinafine, voriconazole, and posaconazole have been reported to be effective also. Locally applied heat, cryosurgery, and surgical excision have been employed in limited disease. Surgical excision may be employed after prolonged oral therapy in an attempt to eradicate residual disease [43–45].

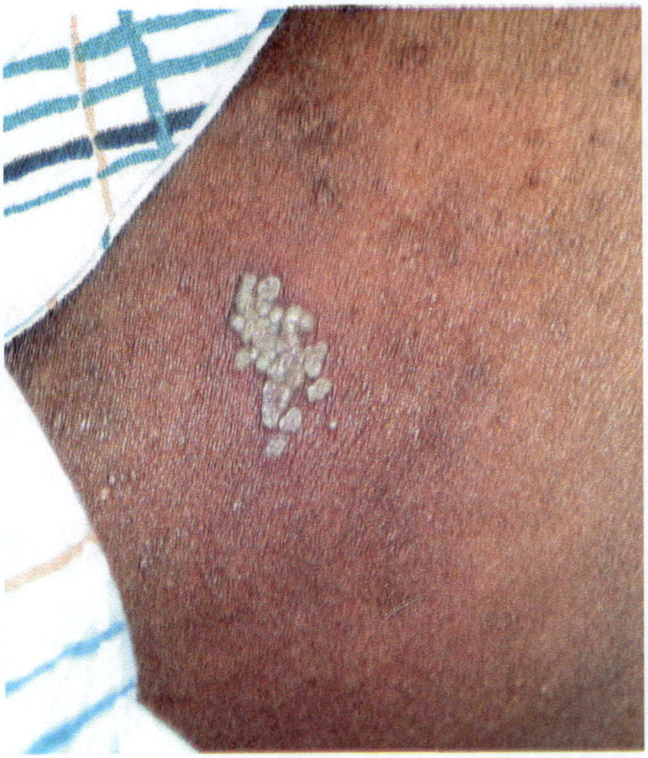

Fig. 17.23 Recurrent herpes simplex type 2 with its classic, geographic pattern of umbilicated pustules. (Courtesy of Julia R. Nunley, M.D.)

Viruses

Viral infections can cause significant mucocutaneous disease or systemic complications in the transplant population. The most important viral pathogens include the human herpesviruses, human papillomaviruses, and molluscum contagiosum (Fig. 17.22) [46]. Of these, herpes simplex (Fig. 17.23) is the most common and can be associated with chronic ulcers (Fig. 17.24) or disseminated disease (Fig. 17.25). Although more problematic in the population infected with the HIV, Kaposi sarcoma (Fig. 17.26) can be seen as a manifestation of the human herpes virus type 8 virus. Human papillomaviruses can cause intractable mucocutaneous warts (Fig. 17.27a, b) and specific subtypes are associated with malignant transformation. Cytomegalovirus and Epstein-Barr virus are known for significant systemic adverse effects. Treatment can involve various systemic antiviral medications and/or the physical destruction of warty lesions, and monitoring for malignant transformation.

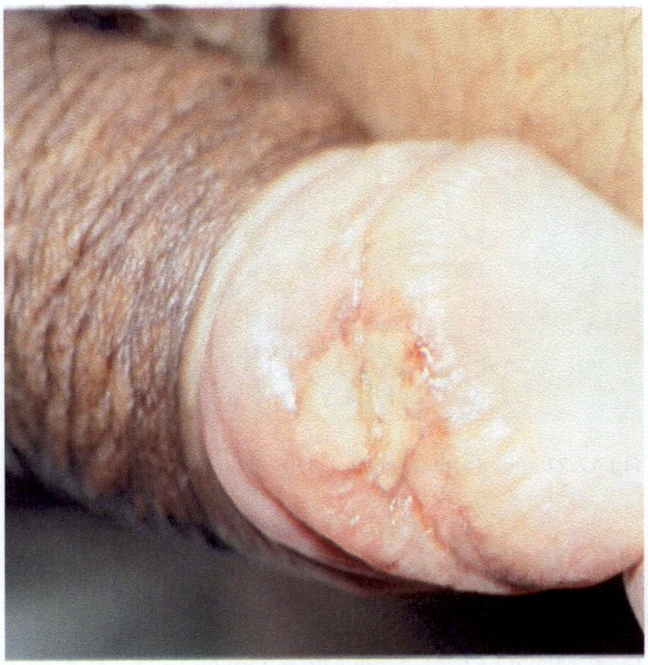

Fig. 17.24 Herpes simplex can cause chronic ulcers in immune suppressed individuals. (Courtesy of Julia R. Nunley, M.D.)

Conclusion

Transplant recipients are prone to various types of infection. Fungal infections are very common and can range from slight scale on the feet to life-threatening multisystem disease. Though less common, mycobacterial infections should be considered for persistent cutaneous lesions or abscesses. Transplant recipients are at higher risk of progressive or disseminated disease, and a high index of suspicion is required in these patients. Viral infections can cause significant mucocutaneous disease or be associated with systemic complications. With proper awareness, the vast majority of infections can be identified and successfully treated.

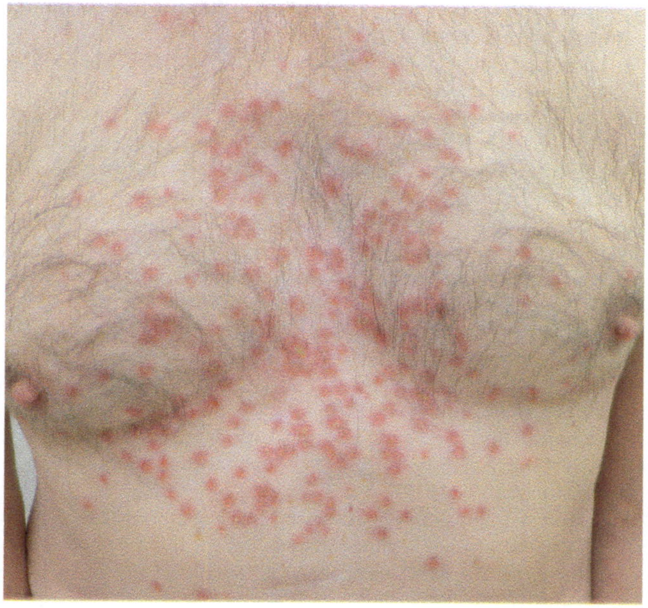

Fig. 17.25 Disseminated herpes simplex as seen here should be treated with intravenous antivirals in the transplant population. (Courtesy of Julia R. Nunley, M.D.)

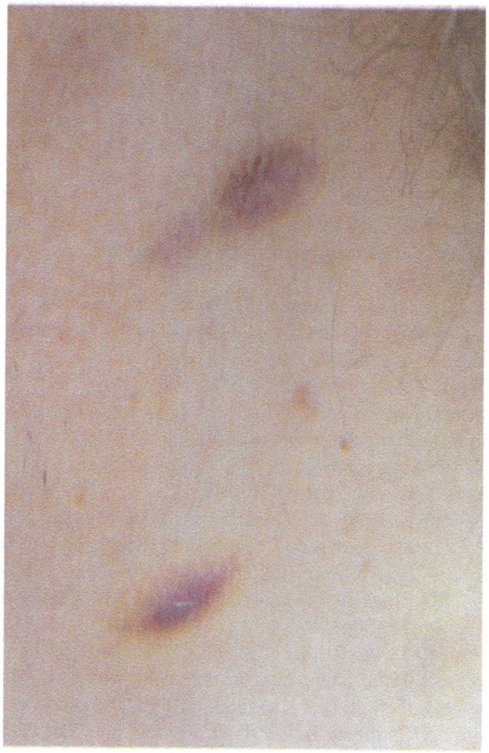

Fig. 17.26 Kaposi sarcoma is due to human herpes type 8. (Courtesy of Julia R. Nunley, M.D.)

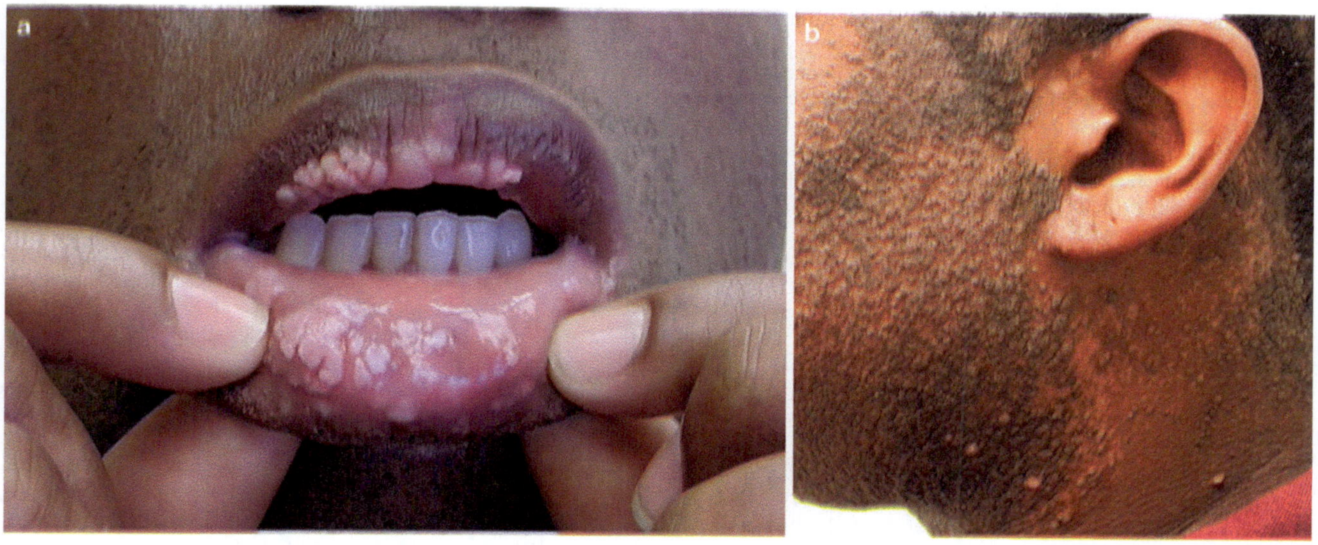

Fig. 17.27 (**a**, **b**) Immune compromised individuals can have extensive mucocutaneous lesions from human papillomaviruses. (Courtesy of Julia R. Nunley, M.D.)

References

1. Brasch J. Current knowledge of host response in human tinea. Mycoses. 2009;52(4):304–12.
2. Chotirmall SH, Al-Alawi M, Mirkovic B, et al. Aspergillus-associated airway disease, inflammation, and the innate immune response. Biomed Res Int. 2013;2013:723129.
3. Mansour MK, Tam JM, Vyas JM. The cell biology of the innate immune response to Aspergillus fumigatus. Ann N Y Acad Sci. 2012;1273:78–84.
4. Foster KW, Ghannoum MA, Elewski BE. Epidemiologic surveillance of cutaneous fungal infection in the united states from 1999 to 2002. J Am Acad Dermatol. 2004;50(5):748–52.
5. Summerbell RC, Kane J, Krajden S. Onychomycosis, tinea pedis and tinea manuum caused by non-dermatophytic filamentous fungi. Mycoses. 1989;32(12):609–19.

6. Kelly BP. Superficial fungal infections. Pediatr Rev. 2012; 33(4):e22–37.
7. Elewski BE. Onychomycosis: pathogenesis, diagnosis, and management. Clin Microbiol Rev. 1998;11(3):415–29.
8. Daniel III CR, Norton LA, Scher RK. The spectrum of nail disease in patients with human immunodeficiency virus infection. J Am Acad Dermatol. 1992;27(1):93–7.
9. Roman AD, Salvana EM, Guzman-Penamora MA, Roxas EA, Leyritana KT, Saniel MC. Invasive trichosporonosis in an AIDS patient: case report and review of the literature. Int J STD AIDS. 2014;25(1):70–5.
10. Brasch J, Morig A, Neumann B. Proksch E. Mycoses: Expression of antimicrobial peptides and toll-like receptors is increased in tinea and pityriasis versicolor; 2013.
11. Correia RT, Valente NY, Criado PR, Martins JE. Chromoblastomycosis: study of 27 cases and review of medical literature. An Bras Dermatol. 2010;85(4):448–54.
12. Bonifaz A, Vazquez-Gonzalez D. Sporotrichosis: an update. G Ital Dermatol Venereol. 2010;145(5):659–73.
13. van Belkum A, Fahal A, van de Sande WW. Mycetoma caused by Madurella mycetomatis: a completely neglected medico-social dilemma. Adv Exp Med Biol. 2013;764:179–89.
14. Pappas PG. Invasive candidiasis. Infect Dis Clin North Am. 2006;20(3):485–506.
15. Ben-Ami R, Lewis RE, Kontoyiannis DP. Enemy of the (immunosuppressed) state: an update on the pathogenesis of Aspergillus fumigatus infection. Br J Haematol. 2010;150(4):406–17.
16. Ibrahim AS, Spellberg B, Walsh TJ, Kontoyiannis DP. Pathogenesis of mucormycosis. Clin Infect Dis. 2012;54 Suppl 1:S16–22.
17. Reyes HM, Tingle EJ, Fenves AZ, Spiegel J, Burton EC. Pulmonary invasive mucormycosis in a patient with secondary iron overload following deferoxamine therapy. Proc (Bayl Univ Med Cent). 2008;21(4):378–81.
18. Revankar SG. Phaeohyphomycosis. Infect Dis Clin North Am. 2006;20(3):609–20.
19. Bourgeois GP, Cafardi JA, Sellheyer K, Andea AA. Disseminated fusarium infection originating from paronychia in a neutropenic patient: a case report and review of the literature. Cutis. 2010;85(4):191–4.
20. Nong S, Liang J. Bone marrow Penicillium marneffei infection in acquired immunodeficiency syndrome patients: report of 35 cases. Trop Biomed. 2013;30(1):89–91.
21. Queipo JA, Broseta E, Santos M, Sanchez-Plumed J, Budia A, Jimenez-Cruz F. Mycobacterial infection in a series of 1261 renal transplant recipients. Clin Microbiol Infect. 2003;9:518–25.
22. Gupta AK, Tu LQ. Dermatophytes: diagnosis and treatment. J Am Acad Dermatol. 2006;54(6):1050–5.
23. Ortega-Loayza AG, McCall CO. Images in clinical medicine. Cutaneous blastomycosis. N Engl J Med. 2013;368(10):e13.
24. Smith EB. The treatment of dermatophytosis: safety considerations. J Am Acad Dermatol. 2000;43(5):S113–9.
25. Lesher JL. Medscape.com [homepage on the Internet]. Elston DM, editor. http://emedicine.medscape.com/article/1091473-treatment.
26. Phillips RM, Rosen T. Topical antifungal agents. In: Wolverton SE, editor. Comprehensive dermatologic drug therapy. 3rd ed. Philadelphia, PA: Elsevier Saunders; 2012.
27. Food and Drug Administration [Internet] Washington, D.C. MedWatch The FDA Safety Information and Adverse Event Reporting Program.Nizoral (ketoconazole): drug safety communication – potentially fatal liver injury, risk of drug interactions and adrenal gland problems [Posted 07/26/2013]. http://www.fda.gov/Safety/MedWatch/SafetyInformation/SafetyAlertsforHumanMedicalProducts/ucm362672.htm.
28. Epocrates Online [homepage on the Internet] San Mateo, CA. https://online.epocrates.com.
29. Lamisil (terbinafine hydrochloride tablet) [package insert] East Hanover, NJ: Novartis Pharmaceuticals Corp.; Revised 6/2013. https://www.pharma.us.novartis.com/product/pi/pdf/Lamisil_tablets.pdf.
30. Lamisil (terbinafine hydrochloride tablet) [package insert] East Hanover, NJ: Novartis Pharmaceuticals Corp.; Revised 6/2013. http://www.pharma.us.novartis.com/product/pi/pdf/Lamisil_Oral_Granules.pdf.
31. Sporanox (itraconazole capsule) [package insert] Raritan, NJ: Ortho-McNeil-Janssen Pharmaceuticals, Inc.; Revised 6/2012. http://dailymed.nlm.nih.gov/dailymed/lookup.cfm?setid=a4d555fa-787c-40fb-bb7d-b0d4f7318fd0.
32. Diflucan (fluconazole tablets) [package insert] New York, NY: Pfizer Inc.; Revised 3/2013. http://labeling.pfizer.com/ShowLabeling.aspx?id=575.
33. Grifulvin V (griseofulvin microsize) [package insert] Los Angles, CA: Ortho Dermatologics; Revised 8/2013. http://dailymed.nlm.nih.gov/dailymed/drugInfo.cfm?setid=6149c044-58bb-402c-a4b5-18b96dd9b3b9.
34. Nizoral (ketoconazole tablet) [package insert] Titusville, NJ: Janssen Pharmaceuticals, Inc.; Revised 7/2013. http://dailymed.nlm.nih.gov/dailymed/lookup.cfm?setid=090660c1-6e6d-457f-adb5-046ddfcd1465.
35. VFEND (voriconazole tablets) [package insert] New York, NY: Pfizer Inc.; Revised 11/2011. http://labeling.pfizer.com/ShowLabeling.aspx?id=618.
36. Miller DD, Cowen EW, Nguyen JC, McCalmont TH, Fox LP. Melanoma associated with long-term voriconazole therapy. Arch Dermatol. 2012;146(3):300–4.
37. Clancy CJ, Nguyen MH. Long-term voriconazole and skin cancer: is there cause for concern? Curr Infect Dis Rep. 2011;13:536–43.
38. Noxafil (posaconazole oral suspension) [package insert] Whitehouse Station, NJ: Merck & Co., Inc.; Revised 12/2012. http://www.merck.com/product/usa/pi_circulars/n/noxafil/noxafil_pi.pdf.
39. Gupta AK. Systemic antifungal agents. In: Wolverton SE, editor. Comprehensive dermatologic drug therapy. 3rd ed. Philadelphia, PA: Elsevier Saunders; 2012.
40. Schwartz RA. Medscape.com [homepage on the Internet]. Majocchi granuloma. Elston DM, editor. http://emedicine.medscape.com/article/1092601-treatment.
41. Moossavi M, Bagheri B, Scher RK. Systemic antifungal therapy. Dermatol Clin. 2001;19(1):35–52.
42. Burkhart CG. Medscape.com [homepage on the Internet]. Tinea versicolor. Elston DM, editor. http://emedicine.medscape.com/article/1091575-treatment.
43. Elewski BE, Hughey LC, Sobera JO, Hay R. Fungal diseases. In: Bolognia JL, Jorizzo JL, Schaffer JV, editors. Dermatology. 3rd ed. Philadelphia, PA: Elsevier Saunders; 2012.
44. James WD, Berger TG, Elston DM. Andrews' diseases of the skin. 11th ed. Philadelphia, PA: Elsevier Saunders; 2011.
45. Schwartz RA. Medscape.com [homepage on the Internet]. Elston DM, editor. http://emedicine.medscape.com/article/1092695-treatment#1.
46. Tan H-H, Goh C-L. Viral infections affecting the skin in organ transplant recipients. Am J Clin Dermatol. 2006;7:13–29.

18 Cutaneous Malignancies

Melinda B. Chu, Brandon T. Beal, and Ian A. Maher

Skin cancer is reaching epidemic proportions in the United States [1]. Currently, an estimated 20 % of the general population will be diagnosed with skin cancer during his/her lifetime [2–4]. It is estimated that greater than 2,000,000 Americans were diagnosed with nonmelanoma skin cancer [4, 5] and greater than 76,250 were diagnosed with melanoma in 2012 [6, 7].

Moreover, the incidence of skin cancer is increasing in the United States and is expected to escalate significantly over the coming years [3]. As such, all health care providers must be aware and have an understanding of skin cancer. Those providers caring for patients on chronic immunosuppression must be particularly aware of cutaneous neoplasms as iatrogenic immunosuppression greatly increases the rate and morbidity of skin cancer [8]. Consequently immunosuppressed patients demand closer and more individualized surveillance than a "normal" patient. The majority of this chapter will focus on the skin cancer-related care of renal allograft recipients.

It is important to remember that patients with chronic kidney disease (CKD) without renal allografts also have risks in regard to skin cancer due to immune system dysfunction, but recommendations for skin cancer follow-up for these patients are the same as the general population [9]. The American Academy of Dermatology (AAD) recommends that patients over 40 years of age start annual full-body skin exams (FBSEs) performed by a dermatologist [10]. Starting annual FBSEs at an earlier age may be recommended for patients with specific risk factors (e.g., history of tanning, sunburns/sun exposure, or family history of melanoma). It is recommended that patients with a history of NMSC have an FBSE every 3–6 months for 2 years, then annually. For patients with a previous diagnosis of melanoma, it is recommend they receive skin cancer screenings every 3 months for 2 years, then every 6 months for 2 years, and then yearly for life.

M.B. Chu, M.D. (✉) • B.T. Beal, B.S. • I.A. Maher, M.D.
Department of Dermatology, Anheuser-Busch Institute,
School of Medicine, Saint Louis University, 1402 S. Grand Blvd., 4th Floor, St. Louis, MO 63104, USA
e-mail: chumb@slu.edu; bealbt@slu.edu; maheria@slu.edu

Epidemiology

Skin cancer is the most common malignancy that occurs after organ transplantation [11]. While skin cancer is common in both the transplanted and nontransplanted US population, the prevalence of different types and clinical behavior of these tumors differs significantly between the two groups.

The blanket term "nonmelanoma skin cancer" (NMSC) comprises a variety of skin cancers, but the overwhelming majority are either basal cell carcinomas (BCCs) or squamous cell carcinomas (SCCs). In the general population BCCs occur more often than SCCs in a 4:1 ratio [12, 13]. Both BCC and SCC favor anatomical locations receiving increased sun exposure, and SCC is the most common NMSC [12, 14, 15]. Melanoma accounts for approximately 4–5 % of all skin cancers diagnosed annually and 75 % of the mortality from skin cancer [6, 7].

In contrast to the general population, SCC is the most common skin cancer in solid organ transplant recipients (SOTRs) accounting for greater than 90 % of all NMSC and occurring at 65–250 times the rate in the general population [15–17]. Thus, the ratio of BCC to SCC of 4:1 for the general population changes to 1:4 in the SOTR [15, 17]. SCC tends to be more aggressive in SOTRs with a higher incidence of invasion and metastatic disease and 5–8 % risk of mortality [15, 18–20]. Skin cancers most often present 5–10 years posttransplant [15, 16]. Risk factors for aggressive behavior in SCCs in SOTRs are the same as in the general population: local recurrence, rapid growth, multiple tumors, histologic

J.R. Nunley and E.V. Lerma (eds.), *Dermatological Manifestations of Kidney Disease*,
DOI 10.1007/978-1-4939-2395-3_18, © Springer Science+Business Media New York 2015

poor differentiation, and invasion as outlined by the American joint committee on cancer (AJCC) and National Comprehensive Cancer Network (NCCN) SCC guidelines [21, 22]. In addition, the type of solid organ transplanted and level of immunosuppression are contributing factors to SCC risk. Heart/lung transplant recipients (which require the highest level of immunosuppression) are thought to be at the highest risk, liver transplant recipients, the lowest, with renal transplant recipients (RTRs) falling somewhere in between with an intermediate risk of developing SCCs [23].

The risk of melanoma in SOTRs is slightly increased at 1.6–3.4 times greater than that of the general population [15]. Melanoma presents ~5 years after organ transplantation [15, 24]. Approximately 27 % of SOTRs also have, or have had, an NMSC at the time of melanoma diagnosis [24]. The occurrence of a melanoma portends almost universal certainty of a future second skin malignancy, usually an NMSC [25].

It has also been suggested that the development of an NMSC in an SOTR indicates an increased risk for an internal solid tumor malignancy. Braconnier et al. found that SOTRs with skin cancers were five times more likely to develop an internal solid tumor compared to SOTRs who did not develop skin cancers [26].

The rest of this chapter will deal primarily with the management of cutaneous cancerous and precancerous lesions in the setting of immunosuppression.

Cutaneous Malignancy in the Setting of Immunosuppression

The etiology of cutaneous carcinogenesis in an RTR is multifactorial. However, immunosuppressive therapy is the strongest associated risk factor for its development [15, 16, 27, 28]. Immunosuppressive therapy decreases immune surveillance that under normal conditions hinders cutaneous carcinogenesis [20, 29–33].

It has been established that skin cancer risk increases with increased immunosuppression and duration of immunosuppressive treatment [15]. It is unclear what the relative role of the total level of immunosuppression has versus the specific immunosuppressive agents used in cutaneous carcinogenesis [34–36]. The fact that patients on a three-drug regimen reportedly have three times more NMSCs than those on a two-drug regimen supports the theory that the total level of immunosuppression contributes significantly to skin cancer risk [35]. In addition to immunosuppressive effects, some medications have drug-specific mechanisms that further promote carcinogenesis [28, 36–39].

Azathioprine (AZA), an antimetabolite that inhibits lymphocyte proliferation, is associated with an increased risk of malignancy, [40] most commonly SCC [41, 42]. 6-thioguanine, a metabolite of AZA, enhances deoxyribonucleic acid (DNA) oxidative damage which is mutagenic [41, 43]. AZA is also known to increase ultraviolet (UV) light photosensitivity, increasing UV-induced damage [29]. In a large case-controlled study, patients who had received AZA any time during therapy had a 5.2-fold increased risk of skin cancer compared to those who had never received AZA [44].

Mycophenolate mofetil (MMF), another antimetabolite, suppresses de novo purine synthesis, thus inhibiting lymphocytes. The malignancy risk associated with MMF is less than with AZA; therefore, MMF has replaced AZA in comparable drug regimens [20, 36, 45].

Calcineurin inhibitors (cyclosporine A and tacrolimus) exert their therapeutic effects in several ways including blockage of T-cell receptor signal transduction and interleukin (IL)-2 and IL-2 receptor upregulation, and by interfering with p53-mediated DNA repair [41, 46]. This decrease in DNA repair after ultraviolet B (UVB) radiations exposure augments calcineurin-induced carcinogenesis [47].

Cyclosporine A (CsA) is associated with a dose-dependent increase in aggressive neoplasms [48–50] with an increased risk of SCC compared to other immunosuppressants [28, 48]. The CsA formulation appears to affect cancer risk, thought to be a result of greater and more consistent bioavailability; Neoral microemulsion demonstrated a fourfold increased risk of Kaposi sarcoma (KS) compared to Sandimmune [51].

Fewer NMSCs result with tacrolimus (TAC)-based immune suppression compared to CsA. This may merely be a function of the lack of long-term patient data available for TAC, since it is a newer drug. However, in vivo studies have demonstrated that despite similar mechanisms of action, TAC and CsA patients respond differently to UV radiation. More NMSCs in CsA patients may be a result of CsA-mediated effects on UV-damaged keratinocytes; CsA appears to inhibit mechanisms that normally control proliferation of UV-induced mutated keratinocytes, perhaps via alterations in mitochondrial permeability transition pore (MPTP) channels as demonstrated by Norman et al. Interestingly, TAC does not inhibit the MPTP channels [52].

Mammalian target of rapamycin (mTOR) inhibitors (e.g., rapamycin, sirolimus, everolimus) comprise a new class of immunosuppressants that possess multiple immunomodulating mechanisms and antineoplastic effects. Immunosuppressive effects result from a decrease in lymphocyte proliferation, mediated by a blockage in the downstream effects of interleukin (IL)-2. The antineoplastic properties result from antiproliferative and antiangiogenic effects, mediated through the regulation of the cell cycle and inhibition of vascular endothelial growth factor (VEGF) production and effect [40, 49]. Posttransplantation mammalian target of rapamycin (mTOR) immunosuppressive therapy has been associated with a reduction in all de novo malignancies [40, 53]. Sirolimus has been shown to significantly decrease NMSCs in RTRs [53–56].

Assessing Risk for Skin Cancer in the Renal Transplant Recipient

If possible, skin cancer risk should be evaluated prior to transplantation in each patient by a dermatologist; assessment includes personal history, family history, and an FBSE. If not feasible prior to transplantation, assessment by a dermatologist should occur as soon as possible after transplantation. Patients at risk for skin cancer, even without organ transplantation (e.g., fair-skinned, history of sunburns, photoexposure), are at an even greater risk of developing skin cancer posttransplantation. Risk factors should direct future intervals of FBSEs posttransplantation; recommendations/details are discussed below.

History

Patients should be queried regarding a number of factors that place them at increased risk of skin cancer posttransplant.

- Prior personal history of skin cancer [57].
- History of actinic keratoses (pre-skin cancers) [58].
- Family history of skin cancer (NMSCs and melanoma).
- History of chronic sun exposure or sunburns [59].
- The duration and intensity of immunosuppression [23].
- Age at transplantation[1].

[1]Patients transplanted at age >55 years have a 12-fold higher risk of developing NMSC compared to those transplanted <34 years of age [60].

Exam

A comprehensive FBSE and lymph node exam are recommended to assess the following: presence of lesions suspicious for skin cancer, presence of premalignant lesions, and other factors that might modulate the risk of development of future malignant and premalignant lesions such as Fitzpatrick skin type (measure of lightness or darkness of skin color), number of nevi, evidence of human papillomavirus (HPV) infection, and evidence of photodamage [61]. A suggested algorithm for follow-up intervals is shown for all patients with renal disease in Fig. 18.1. Further recommendations for RTRs are detailed in Table 18.1.

Diagnosis

At times it can be difficult to distinguish nonmalignant lesions from malignant lesions by visual inspection alone in transplant recipients. Transplant patients frequently develop multiple hyperkeratotic, HPV-related papules that are visually indistinguishable from cutaneous malignancy. Neurological symptoms, specifically pain, may be an indicator for perineural invasion (PNInv) and should prompt concern for a cutaneous SCC [62]. These lesions always warrant a biopsy.

Despite the advent of new devices including the dermatoscope (magnifying glass with polarized light) and digital image analysis systems to aid visual inspection by the clinician, tissue evaluation after biopsy remains the gold standard for the diagnosis of skin cancers.

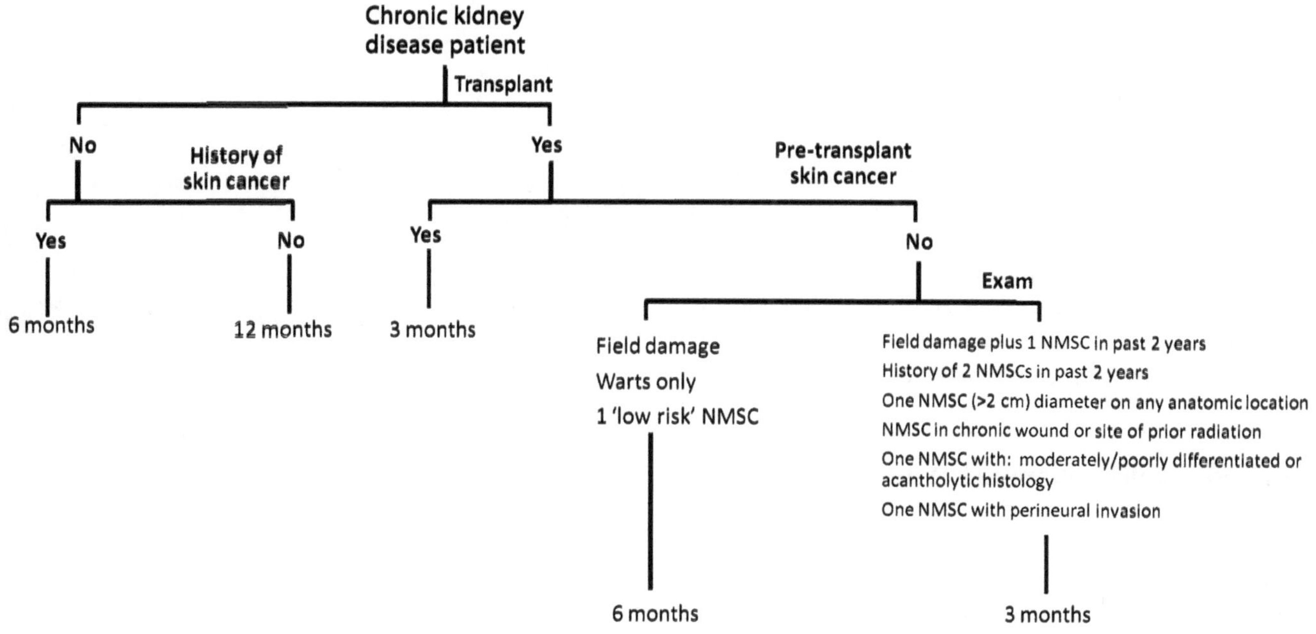

Fig. 18.1 Algorithm for recommended follow-up for patients with chronic kidney disease

Table 18.1 Recommended follow-up intervals for full-body skin exams for renal transplant recipients

Risk factors	Interval between full-body skin exams (no. of months)
Field damage only	6
Warts only	6
One "low-risk" NMSC	6
Field damage plus 1 NMSC in past 2 years	3
History of 2 NMSC in past 2 years	3
One NMSC (>2 cm) diameter on any anatomic location	3
NMSC occurring in chronic wound or site of prior radiation	3
One NMSC skin cancer with: – Moderately/poorly differentiated histology – Acantholytic histology	3
One NMSC with perineural invasion	3

[a]Patients should be referred for dermatologic evaluation sooner if new suspicious lesions or lymphadenopathy is noted
Table adapted from [25, 76]
NMSC nonmelanoma skin cancer

Actinic Keratosis (AK)

AKs are rough scaly pink spots that are typically seen on sun-exposed areas. A sandpaper-like texture allows them to be more easily palpated than seen. They are considered premalignant lesions and if left untreated, 6–25 % may evolve into SCCs [63–65]. It has been suggested that HPV infection may contribute to AK development in RTRs as a co-carcinogen, with UV exposure (see Fig. 18.2).

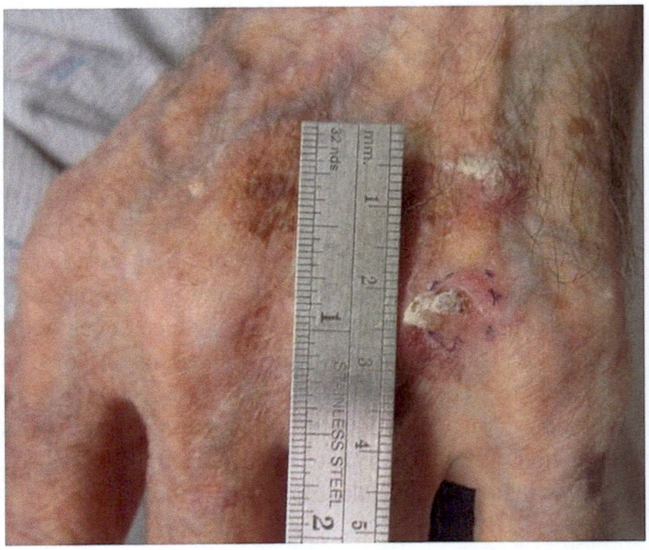

Fig. 18.2 Actinic keratoses (AKs). Two pink papules with sandpaper-like texture: a more sessile lesion proximally and one with overlying cutaneous horn distally. Both morphologies are consistent with actinic keratoses (AKs). Actinic keratoses are premalignant lesions caused by UV damage. If left untreated, they may transform into squamous cell carcinomas (SCCs). Aggressive management of AKs in renal transplant patients is necessary to minimize the development of SCCs

Warts

Warts represent cutaneous HPV infection, which some consider to be premalignant lesions in the setting of immunosuppression due to the potential for HPV-mediated malignant transformation [66]. They may appear as small, rough pink or whitish growths (verruca vulgaris) or flat, smooth lesions (verruca plana) (see Fig. 18.3). In immunosuppressed patients, warts can become large, keratotic, painful nodules and incur significant morbidity [67]. It can be difficult to tell nonmalignant warts from SCCs; a biopsy is recommended for any suspicious verrucous lesion (see Fig. 18.4).

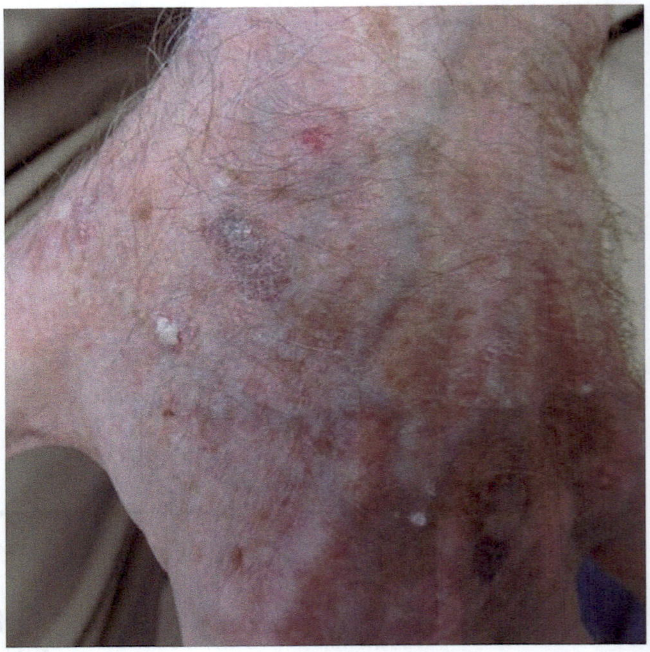

Fig. 18.3 Verruca vulgaris on the hand. A small white keratotic papule characteristic of verruca vulgaris subtype of wart. In most anatomic locations, verrucae are related to non-high-risk human papillomavirus (HPV) subtypes [1–3]. In the genital area, verruca may be associated with high-risk HPV subtypes

Squamous Cell Carcinoma In Situ (SCCIS)

SCCIS present as pink hyperkeratotic papules or plaques, most commonly on sun-exposed areas (see Fig. 18.5). It can be difficult to distinguish between SCCISs and AKs since both are found on sun-exposed areas; SCCIS tends to be thicker and larger with a well-demarcated border [68]. The terms SCCIS and Bowen disease are sometimes used interchangeably. Bowen disease connotes a viral (HPV) etiology. In non-sun-exposed areas, the etiology of SCCIS is invariably HPV-related.

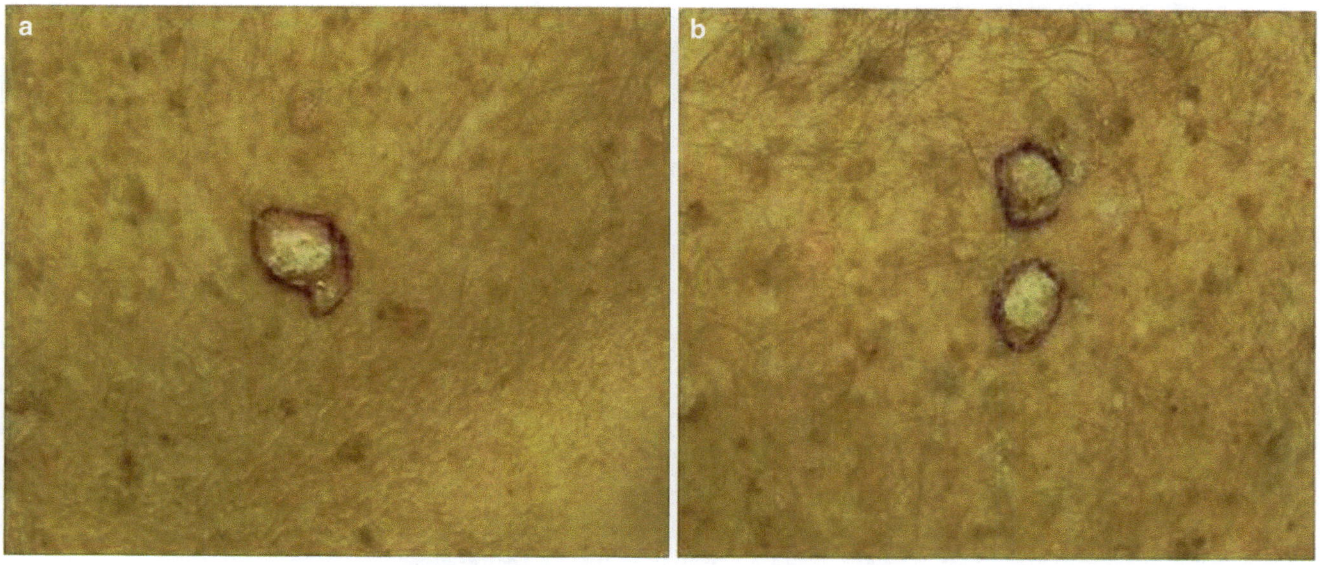

Fig. 18.4 Difficulty distinguishing verruca vulgaris (VV) from squamous cell carcinoma (SCC). Both images show similar appearing pink keratotic papules on the back of a renal transplant patient. Skin biopsy of (**a**) revealed SCC. Pathology of two lesions in (**b**) demonstrated verrucae. Since it can be challenging to distinguish VV (nonmalignant lesion) from SCC (malignant lesion) on clinical presentation alone, it is important to have a low threshold to perform skin biopsy

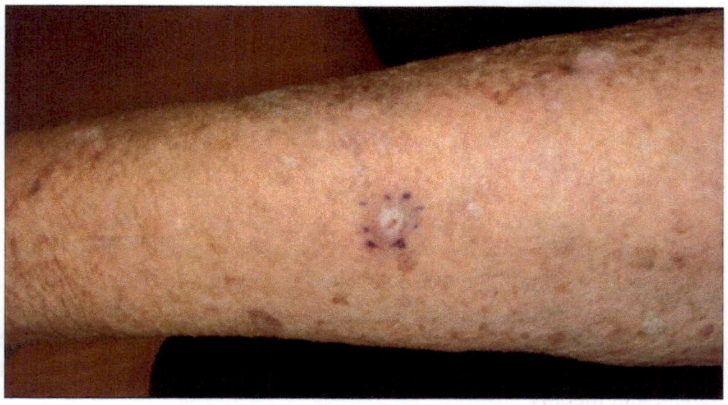

Fig. 18.5 Squamous cell carcinoma in situ (SCCIS). SCCIS presents as pink hyperkeratotic papules or plaques, most commonly on sun-exposed areas. Compared to AKs, SCCIS tends to be thicker and larger with a well-demarcated border. In the non-sun-exposed areas, SCCIS is almost always related to HPV infection

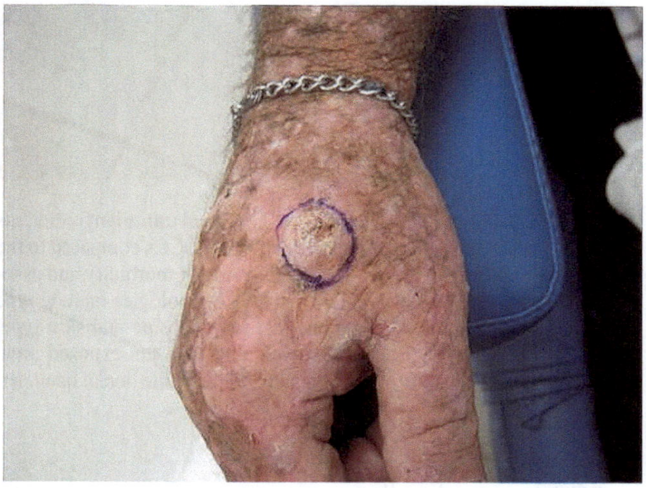

Fig. 18.6 Squamous cell carcinoma developing within an area of field cancerization. Hyperkeratotic pink nodule developing within a field of pink scaly papules and photodamage on the dorsal hand. Field cancerization refers to the development of "dysplastic fields of skin" with differing amounts of genetic abnormalities due to UV damage. Premalignant and malignant lesions can arise within these diffusely photodamaged areas. Vigilant sun protection and cyclical use of field therapies (including topical creams and photodynamic therapy) are essential to the management of field cancerization

Field Cancerization

Some patients with severe photodamage, especially those on long-term immunosuppression, can develop malignant and premalignant lesions that are so numerous that they become confluent and cover large body surface areas such as the dorsal hands and forearms (see Fig. 18.6). This phenomenon, referred to as "field cancerization," describes "dysplastic fields of skin" with varying amounts of genetic abnormalities triggered by UV exposure. These are high-risk areas in which premalignant and malignant lesions frequently develop [69, 70].

Squamous Cell Carcinoma (SCC)

SCCs can vary in presentation but are typically firm, flesh-colored or pink, keratotic papules or plaques or nodules (see Fig. 18.7a–c). They may be smooth or ulcerated. Alternatively, a cutaneous horn may be prominent.

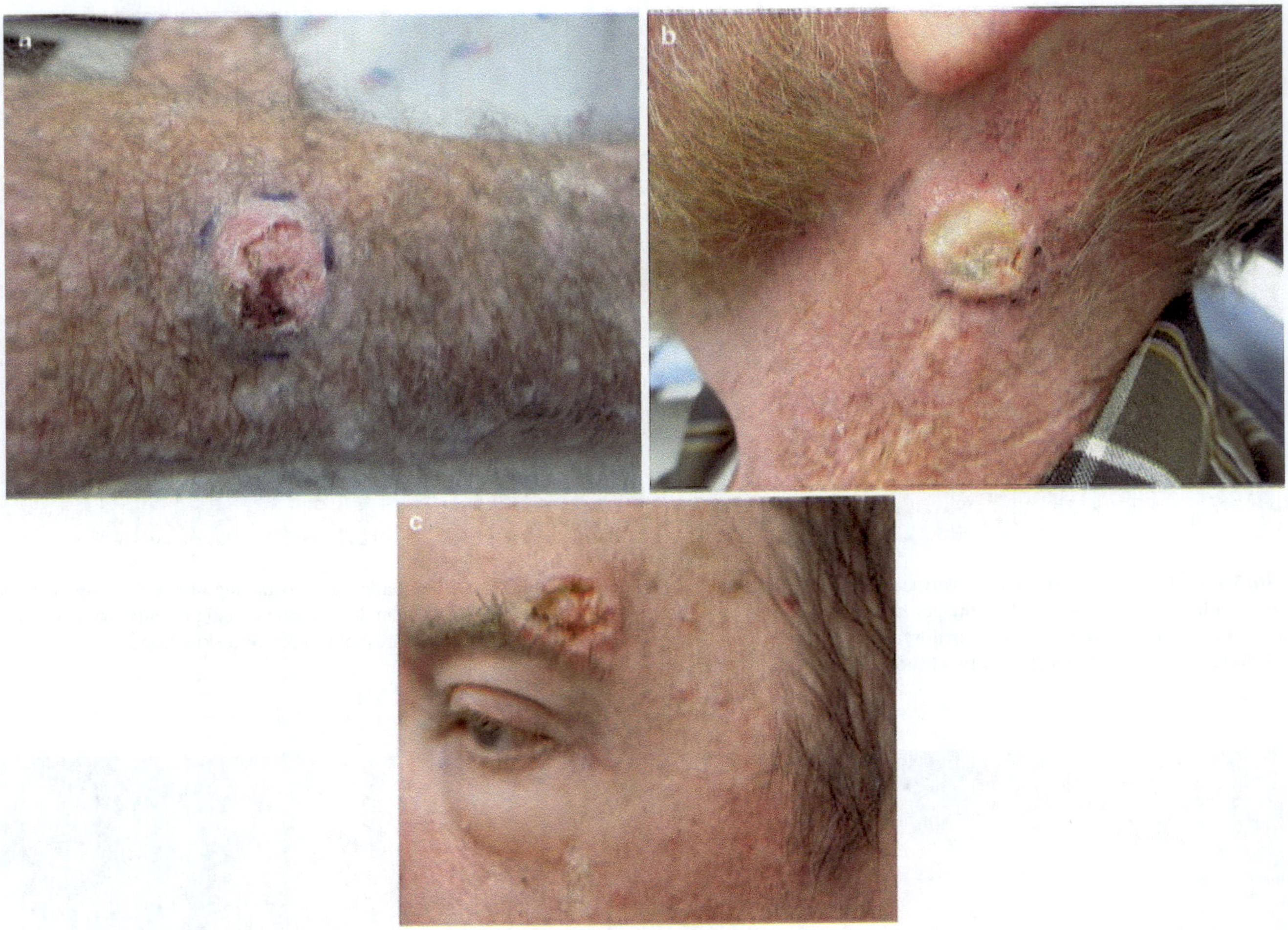

Fig. 18.7 Squamous cell carcinoma (SCC). Renal transplant recipients (RTRs) are at 65 times higher risk of developing SCCs compared to the general population. SCCs are a significant cause of morbidity and associated with a 5–8 % risk of mortality in RTRs. Etiologies include type and duration of immunosuppression, past sun exposure and skin type, and HPV status. (**a**) Typical SCC developing in a sun-exposed area: eroded hyperkeratotic pink dome-shaped nodule on the dorsal hand. (**b**) SCC on the neck: Rapidly growing hyperkeratotic nodule. In this anatomic location, there is a high suspicion for lymph node involvement. (**c**) SCC developing during rapamycin therapy. Though rapamycin-based regimens are the immunosuppression regimen associated with the lowest incidence of SCC, patients may still develop SCCs while on rapamycin therapy

SCCs occur primarily on sun-exposed areas but may be seen in non-sun-exposed areas particularly if HPV-induced. It has been reported that SCCs in immunosuppressed patients have higher rates of both HPV infection overall and with high-risk HPV subtypes compared to the general population [71]. Further studies on the pathogenic role of HPV in skin cancer may have important therapeutic implications in RTRs since prophylactic vaccination could theoretically help to prevent skin cancer development. For now, identifying SCCs at an early stage is particularly important in RTRs as they have a propensity to metastasize and have worse outcome [72–74].

Rapid lesional growth should provoke concern for aggressive behavior and the potential for metastatic spread. SCCs that develop on the ear, lip, scalp, and dorsal hands are at a higher risk for metastatic disease in SOTRs [75–77]. SCCs can be divided into low-risk or high-risk tumors based on overall risk for metastatic spread or local recurrence; risk ultimately determines the definitive treatment. High-risk tumors prompt aggressive surgical management. For low-risk tumors, less aggressive destructive or nonsurgical methods may be indicated.

High-risk features for SCCs in SOTRs are listed in Table 18.2.

Basal Cell Carcinoma (BCC)

BCCs appear as pearly pink papules with telangiectasias (that may resemble a pimple) on sun-exposed areas (see Fig. 18.8). While BCC rates are increased tenfold in SOTRs compared to the immunocompetent population, they are much less frequent than SCCs. Immunosuppression per se is believed to be responsible for the increased number of BCCs; however, the total level of immune suppression is not believed to be relevant to the development of BCC as it is in the development of SCC. The incidence of BCCs in liver/kidney/heart SOTRs was fairly equal, in contrast to the incidence of SCCs previously discussed [16].

Melanoma

Of the four subtypes of melanoma (superficial spreading type (SST), nodular, lentigo maligna, and acral lentiginous), SST melanoma is most common. The characteristic SST melanoma possesses most or all of the following (ABCDE) characteristics for melanoma: asymmetry (A), irregular borders (B), irregular pigment/color (brown, black, whitish, red, and/or blue hues) (C), large diameter (D), central elevation or the lesion is changing or evolving (E) (see Fig. 18.9a, b). While most lesions are pigmented, depigmented, amelanotic (pink or flesh-colored) melanomas (5 %) can be seen [78].

Table 18.2 SCC high-risk features in SOTRs

Anatomic location	Ear, lip, scalp, dorsal hands, eyelid, nose (any size)
Size	>2 cm in any anatomic location >1 cm in intermediate risk area (cheeks, forehead, neck) >0.6 cm in high-risk area ("mask areas of face," genitalia)
Histologic features	Poorly or moderately differentiated subtype Acantholytic subtype Perineural invasion
Clinical characteristics	Recurrent

SCC squamous cell carcinoma, *SOTRs* solid organ transplant recipients

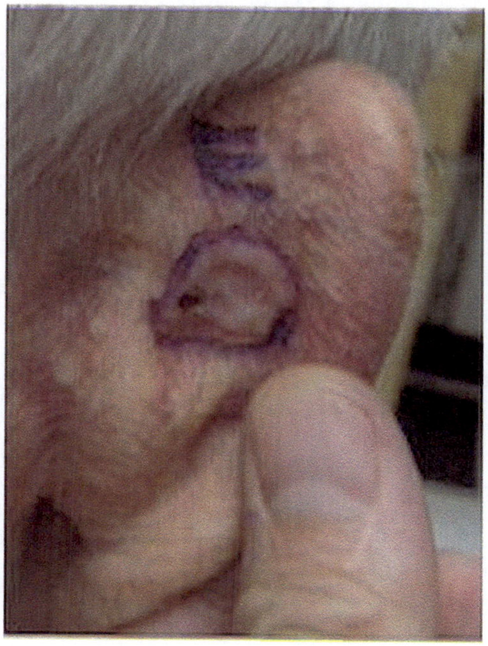

Fig. 18.8 Basal cell carcinoma (BCC). Example of a classic presentation of BCC: pearly ulcerated plaque with rolled border on the posterior ear. BCCs are the most common skin cancer in immunocompetent patients, with 4 BCCs diagnosed for every 1 SCC. In renal transplant recipient (RTRs), the ratio is switched and SCCs are much more common than BCCs (4:1)

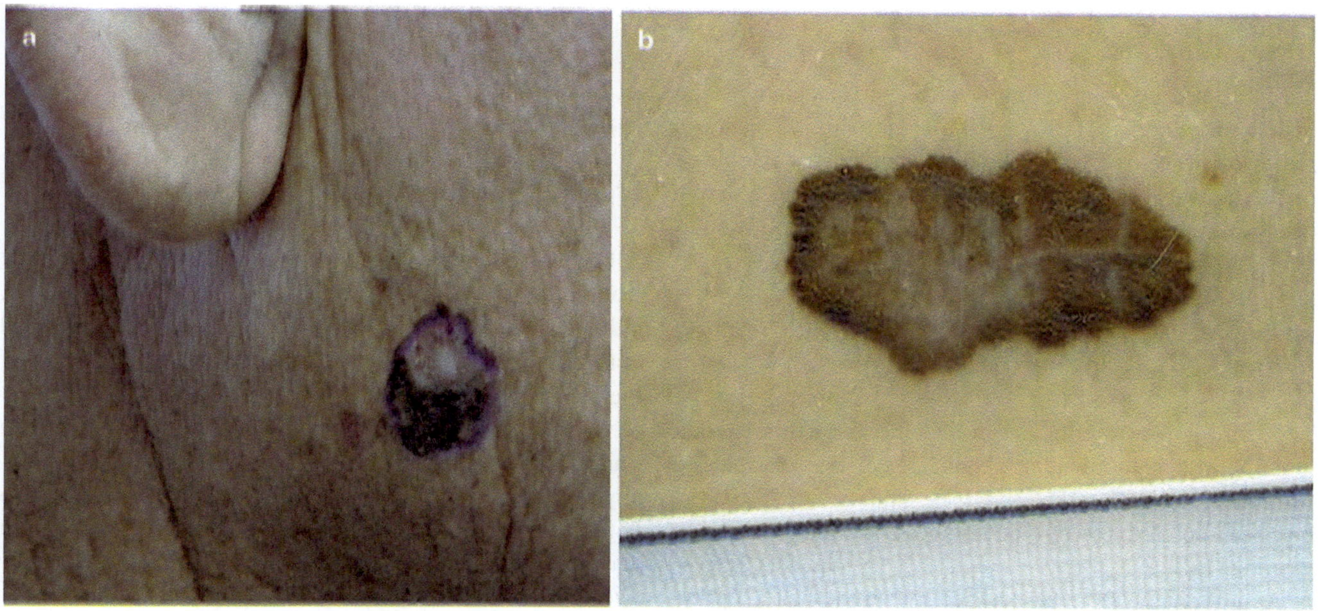

Fig. 18.9 Melanoma. Melanomas in renal transplant recipient (RTRs) have a similar appearance to those in the immunocompetent population with slightly lower survival rates, but overall similar disease course. (**a**) Irregularly colored (*dark brown* and *pink*) irregularly bordered nodule on the cheek. (**b**) Large irregularly pigmented (*brown*, *black*, and *pink*) patch with a scalloped border on the back

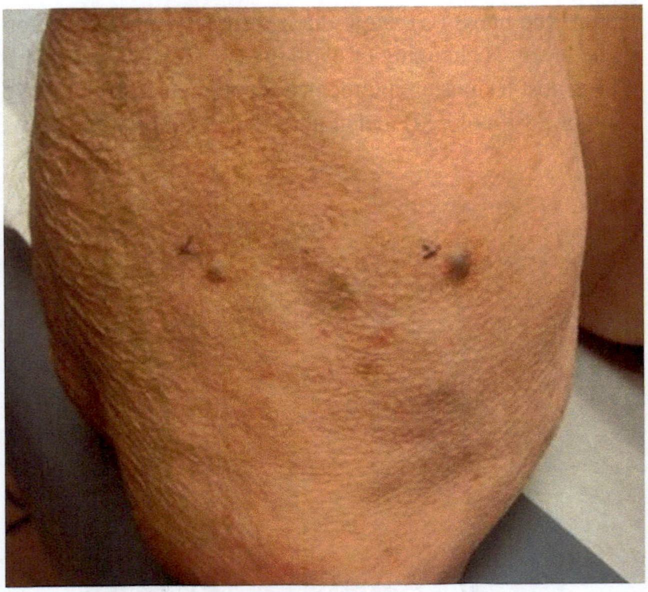

Fig. 18.10 Kaposi sarcoma. Characteristic presentation of Kaposi sarcoma: *Dark blue* papular vascular tumor near the elbow. Kaposi sarcoma is almost exclusively seen in immunosuppressed patients and is caused by reactivation or new human herpesvirus 8 (HHV-8) infection

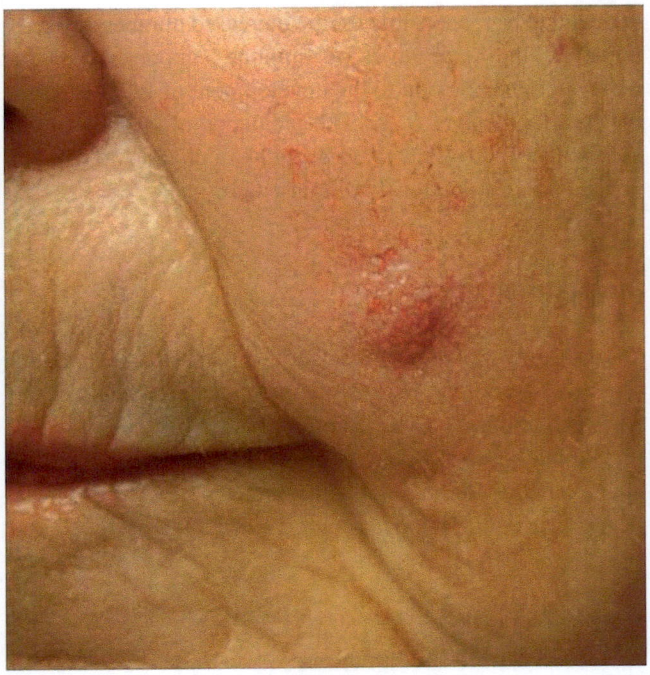

Fig. 18.11 Merkel cell carcinoma (MCC). A common presentation of MCC: rapidly growing asymptomatic nondescript pink nodule on a sun-exposed area. Merkel cell carcinoma pathogenesis has been associated with Merkel cell polyomavirus (MCV) infection. MCC tends to develops at an earlier age in immunosuppressed patients than the immunocompetent population, with lower survival rates. Three-year MCC-specific survival rates are much lower in patients with history of immunosuppression compared to those without (40 % vs. 74 %) [85]

Melanoma is more common in patients with lighter skin types in both immunocompetent and immunocompromised patients. While the prevalence is overall low in RTRs, it is striking that the rate of melanoma in African-American RTR patients is 17.2 times that of the general African-American population [79].

Kaposi Sarcoma (KS)

KS is caused by reactivation of/or recent inoculation with human herpesvirus 8 (HHV-8) and commonly presents as a red-to-purple or dark blue papular or nodular vascular tumor on the legs and arms (see Fig. 18.10). KS is often a systemic disease affecting the gastrointestinal (GI) tract, lymph nodes, liver, and lungs [80, 81].

Merkel Cell Carcinoma (MCC)

Though still rare overall, rates of MCC are 5–10 times higher in immunosuppressed patients than in the general population [82]. MCC usually presents as a firm, painless, rapidly growing, flesh-colored, red or blue nodule, on sun-exposed areas (see Fig. 18.11).

Approximately 80 % are caused by the Merkel cell polyomavirus (MCV); however other contributing factors must be present for malignant transformation since MCV seropositivity is common in the healthy unaffected general population [83].

In SOTRs, MCC occurs ~7–8 years posttransplant, which is a younger than in the immunocompetent population [84] and there appears to be a worse disease-specific survival rate [85].

Management

Preventative Measures

All patients who undergo kidney transplantation will benefit from adhering to sun protective behaviors. Unfortunately, although most SOTR patients are aware of their increased risk of skin cancer, most RTRs do not prioritize reducing their risk among their health concerns [86, 87].

Because immunosuppression is greatest during the acute transplant phase and skin cancer risk correlates with intensity of immunosuppression, it is important for patients to begin avid sun protection immediately after transplantation and to maintain sun protective behaviors throughout their lives. Skin cancer risk appears to be cumulative and continues to increase over time from transplantation [88]. In Queensland, Australia, Ramsay (2002) et al. reported that the cumulative incidence of skin cancer in RTRs after 20 years was 82 % [89].

Table 18.3 Sun protective behavior recommendations

• No indoor tanning
• Avoid prolonged time outside or frequent outdoor activities
• If going outside, avoid peak sunlight hours—10 a.m. until 2 p.m.—when the sun's rays are the strongest
• Sun protective behaviors should become routine to patient and employed daily
– Even when cloudy (as ~70 % of sunrays may still infiltrate) and in the winter
• Apply a "broad-spectrum" sunscreen, one that protects against both UVA and UVB rays with an SPF 30 or higher
– Lotions provide the best coverage, but patients should utilize their preferred formulation (e.g., spray, cream, waxy stick) to increase compliance
– SPF only refers to product's ability to block UVB rays
– Products with zinc oxide or titanium oxide ingredients or "helioplex" or "anthelios" on the label provide UVA protection
– Ideally, two coats of sunscreen should be applied 15–30 min before going outside to provide optimal coverage
– Reapply sunscreen every 1–2 h, especially after swimming of heavy perspiration
• Wear wide-brimmed hats, sunglasses, and clothes with sun protective factors (UPF >50) built into the fabric

UVA ultraviolet A, *UVB* ultraviolet B, *SPF* sun protective factor

The benefits to sun protection are not theoretical; regular sunscreen use has been shown to decrease AK and invasive SCC (and, less so BCC) development in SOTRs [87]. Education is key and repetition is necessary to increase compliance. A list of sun protective recommendations is seen in Table 18.3.

Under no circumstances should SOTRs continue indoor tanning. Patients may engage in normal outdoor activities, but prolonged time outside is ill advised. If outdoor activities (e.g., golf, running, or tennis) are important to patient's quality of life, we recommend that patients avoid going outside from 10 a.m. to 2 p.m. when the sun is the strongest. Wide-brimmed hats or clothes with ultraviolet or sun protective factor (UPF or SPF) >50 built into the fabric are also advised. Sun protective behaviors, especially sunscreen use, should become part of the patient's daily routine and employed even when cloudy (as ~70 % of sunrays may still infiltrate) and in the winter.

As noted above, daily sunscreen use is the cornerstone to effective photoprotection. Lotions provide the best coverage, but patients should utilize their preferred formulation (e.g., spray, gels, cream, wax stick) to increase compliance. The term "broad spectrum" should be on the product label which indicates both ultraviolet A and B (UVA/UVB) protection.

Products with SPF >30 are recommended. SPF refers to the compound's ability to block UVB-induced damage only (not UVA). The SPF calculation is based on the application of one teaspoon to the face or one ounce (golf ball size amount) of lotion to the entire body; application of less decreases the actual SPF in an exponential fashion. A recent study found that most patients typically apply 25–50 % of the recommended amount, which results in an actual SPF of ≤33.3 % of the labeled SPF [90]. Consequently, even a patient who is trying to practice good sun protective behaviors by applying SPF 30 lotion may be inadequately protected if minimal amounts are used, resulting in an effective SPF equivalent to ten or less. Recent studies show that use of higher SPF sunscreen (SPF 70 or SPF 100) may be one way to offset the inadequate amount of sunscreen typically applied [91]. If a patient were to apply 25–50 % of the recommended amount of an SPF 100 sunscreen, in theory the real-life SPF would be approximately 30, the recommended SPF. In 2011, the Food and Drug Administration (FDA) issued more stringent guidelines for the definition of SPF and other terms on sunscreen labels. For now, the FDA classifies sunscreens with SPF 70 or 100 together in one group "SPF 50 or higher" and has yet to decide if SPF 70 or SPF 100 products have any definitive added protective benefit [92].

Terms such as "Helioplex" or "Anthelios" or the ingredients zinc oxide or titanium oxide denote products with UVA coverage. "Helioplex" and "Anthelios" are patented compounds made by Neutrogena and La Roche-Posay, respectively [93, 94]. Aveeno makes a similar compound called "Active Photobarrier Complex" [95]. All of these products contain oxybenzone and avobenzone as well as other chemicals and are formulated to provide both UVA and UVB coverage and to resist photo-degradation. The same ingredients are utilized in most sunscreens and one need not spend a lot of money to ensure adequate protection. As a matter of fact, a recent Consumer Reports analysis found that cheaper generic store brands actually provided better protection than the pricier brands [96].

Unlike oxybenzone or avobenzone, which are organic compounds and UV absorbers, titanium oxide and zinc oxide are physical blockers, which primarily work by reflecting and scattering sunlight particles. Titanium oxide and zinc oxide may bring to mind images of lifeguards with white noses or ghost-like faces, which may make patients hesitant to use them. This should no longer be a concern as the new formulations of titanium and zinc oxide are made of smaller nanoparticles, which blend in and are not as noticeable [92].

There are no "waterproof" sunscreens and almost all products will be inactive within 2 h. In fact, the phrase "waterproof" and other similar terms such as "sunblock," "waterproof," "sweat resistant," and "all day protection" are now prohibited from sunscreen labels as they were deemed inaccurate and misleading by the FDA. In its place, sunscreen labels may have the statements "water resistant (40 min)" and "very water resistant (80 min)" on them. These are terms derived from studies where the SPF was measured before and after subjects were immersed in a whirlpool for 40 min (twice for 20 min) or 80 min (four times for 20 min) [92].

Ideally, two coats of sunscreen should be applied 15–30 min before going outside to provide optimal coverage. Frequent reapplication, every 1–2 h, is necessary for extended periods of time outside.

Many ingredients in sunscreens (in particular oxybenzone) are known to cause allergic contact dermatitis, a delayed-type hypersensitivity reaction in some individuals [97]. If a contact dermatitis is noted after wearing sunscreen, this should not deter the patient from continuing good sun protective behaviors. While patients should discontinue using the offending product, they can continue wearing sunscreen with physical blocker ingredients only (titanium oxide or zinc oxide), which have very minimal to no allergenic potential. Other recommended options include wearing UPF clothing and a wide-brimmed hat as noted above.

It is important to monitor vitamin D levels in SOTRs and supplementation; oral supplementation should be used as necessary. For SOTRs there is a consensus that adequate photoprotection to decrease the risk of skin cancer outweighs the risk of low vitamin D levels since vitamin D can be supplemented [98, 99].

Frequency of Skin Exams

Detection and treatment of existing skin cancers and precancers PRIOR to transplantation is optimal. After transplantation, the frequency of regular skin exams is based on disease burden as depicted in Table 18.2. It is recommended that an FBSE be performed at least every 6 months in patients at risk. Those who develop multiple SCCs may require closer monitoring ever 1–3 months [76].

Management of Actinic Keratoses

Aggressive treatment of AKs or warts with cryotherapy is recommended if there are only a few lesions. For more extensive field damage or numerous AKs, cyclic field therapy is recommended.

Cryotherapy

Cryotherapy involves the application of liquid nitrogen (LN2) onto the skin; duration is determined by anatomic site and lesion type being treated. The LN2 causes rapid cellular freezing, which leads to tissue necrosis. It can be highly efficacious treatment for most AKs and warts. However, for thicker or hyperkeratotic AKs or more diffuse actinic damage, it is not adequate [70].

Field Therapy

Field therapies are employed to treat large photodamaged areas and/or diffuse AKs [70]. Field therapies will not penetrate deep enough to adequately treat skin cancers; one benefit of field therapy is allowing for the visualization of discrete cancerous lesions once the actinic background improves. This may be mistaken for lack of effectiveness but should not dissuade clinicians from continuing field therapy.

Diclofenac

Diclofenac sodium 3 % gel is a topical nonsteroidal anti-inflammatory drug (NSAID) that works via cyclooxygenase 1 and 2 (COX1, COX2) inhibition. It halts AK development by blocking the formation of angiogenic and tumorigenic factors produced from downstream arachidonic acid metabolites.

The recommended regimen for topical 3 % diclofenac is twice daily application for 60–90 days [100, 101]. Relatively low response rates (40 %) are balanced out by increased tolerability compared to other topical therapies. Side effects include mild pruritus, erythema, dry skin, hyper- and paresthesia, and type IV hypersensitivity reactions. Systemic drug interactions similar to that seen with oral NSAIDs are not expected with topical diclofenac therapy. Studies from the rheumatologic literature report that the maximal plasma concentrations following topical application of diclofenac and NSAIDs to body surface areas greater than 100 cm^2, but less than 200–300 cm^2, were less than 15 % of the plasma concentration reported when comparable doses were administered orally [102, 103]. In three clinical trials testing 3 % diclofenac gel to treat AK lesions, serum levels drawn after 105 days of twice daily application to body surface area of up to 75 cm^2 (slightly smaller than area of one's face and typical area of treatment in clinical practice) were extremely low, on average ≤20 ng/mL [104]. By comparison, the area under the curve (a measure of systemic absorption used in pharmacokinetic studies) of a single oral 75 mg dose of diclofenac (Voltaren®) is 1600 ng/h/mL [104]. Topical diclofenac also does not appear to affect renal function. Creatinine elevations were observed in a small fraction of patients (2 of 48) who were treated topical 3 % diclofenac during clinical trials, but this was the same rate as observed in the placebo group (2 of 49) [104].

Topical 5-Fluorouracil

Topical 5-fluorouracil (5-FU) inhibits thymidylate synthetase and subsequently halts DNA synthesis in cutaneous carcinogenesis. Its therapeutic effects were discovered as a fortuitous side effect; patients receiving intravenous 5-FU as a systemic chemotherapy were noted to have inflammation and resolution of AKs. Twice daily application of topical 5-FU for 2–4 weeks is indicated for the treatment of AKs; a longer course consisting of at least 3–6 weeks is needed for superficial BCCs. Response rates of 90 % have been reported in immunocompetent populations [23, 105]. While response rates are higher than observed with diclofenac, adverse effects (AEs) from 5-FU often lead to early discontinuation; thus, the true response rates are difficult to establish. Significant crusting, redness, erosions, and sometimes pain can be seen during topical 5-FU treatment. Eroded skin may become superinfected, with a great concern for infection with methicillin-resistant *Staphylococcus aureus* (MRSA). Pharmacokinetic studies have shown that systemic absorption of 5-FU is minimal (2.4 %) [106].

Topical 5-FU can also be used as part of a "chemowrap," which is a compression bandage that is applied in the office after topical application of 5-FU allowing for prolonged and adequate 5-FU penetration. Chemowraps are commonly employed to treat large areas of skin where it is difficult to apply 5-FU twice daily and/or extensive, severely photodamaged areas amenable to wraps, like the legs. After covering the leg with 5-FU, medicated petrolatum and zinc oxide impregnated gauze are applied. The top layer consists of Coban™, a self-adherent elastic bandage akin to a disposable ACE bandage. "Chemowraps" are replaced every week in the office. Reduction of malignant or premalignant lesions seen 6 weeks following a chemowrap treatment regimen of 4–20 weeks may be maintained for 3 years of follow-up [107, 108]. Chemowraps may also be useful in patients who cannot tolerate surgery.

Imiquimod

Imiquimod is a topical cream that is effective for the treatment of AKs, warts, and superficial BCCs in the RTR as well as in the immune competent patient [109, 110]. Imiquimod is a toll-like receptor (TLR) 7 agonist, which triggers a local immune response through upregulation of numerous cytokines including interferon (IFN)-alpha and IFN-gamma [111, 112]. Though it is generally considered safe, its use in SOTRs was initially limited due to concerns that the immunomodulation it would induce might increase systemic IFN levels causing an increase in graft rejection [113]. However, a large randomized trial demonstrated no increase in graft rejection [112]. The defined treatment area for these studies was 100 m^2, essentially the entire area of a face which is the largest surface area that would be treated in clinical practice at one time [112]. Although imiquimod may be used for field therapy, it is more often used to treat discrete precancerous and cancerous lesions, which limits the possibility of systemic absorption. Efficacy (based on 3–5 times per week application for 16 weeks) is reported to be similar in SOTRs and in nontransplanted populations (~70 %) [112]. Side effects are similar to that of 5-FU (erythema, inflammation, itching, pain) but tend to be milder. Some patients may exhibit exuberant inflammatory response, which may be indicative of good therapeutic effect. Systemic AEs, simulating a flu-like illness, have also been described with imiquimod.

Ingenol Mebutate

Ingenol mebutate is a newer topical medication recently FDA-approved for AK treatment in immunocompetent patients. It is a biologically active compound extracted from a milkweed plant, *Euphorbia peplus*. No studies exist on its effectiveness in SOTRs. Unlike other topical field therapies, ingenol mebutate only requires 2–3 days of treatment as compared to several weeks [114]. While current evidence suggests that it may be less efficacious than other topical field therapies, it can provide durable results in a subset of patients who demonstrate a good initial response [115]. Long-term lesion reduction and sustained lesion clearance (~87 %) at 12 months have been reported in this same subset of superior responders.

Photodynamic Therapy (PDT)

PDT differs from other field cancerization options as it is an in-office procedure. Upon arrival, patients are pretreated with a topical photosensitizer such as aminolevulinic acid (ALA) or its methyl ester methyl aminolevulinate (MAL). After 1–2 h of incubation patients are exposed to a device with either red light (635 nm) or blue light (410 nm) for ~15 min. The combination of oxygen, the absorbed photosensitizer, and the chemical-specific light wavelength causes cell death in rapidly dividing cells via production of reactive oxygen species (ROS) [70, 113, 116]. While more extensively studied as a treatment for AKs, PDT has similarly excellent rates of clearing BCCs, particularly superficial BCC. Complete clearance rates for superficial BCCs are as high 85–93 % at 3 months [117]. Like other topical field cancerization treatments, depth of penetration is a limiting factor in its effectiveness. PDT is most effective on areas with thinner skin such as the face and neck. In areas with thicker skin, such as the hands or arms, PDT is less effective.

As a chemopreventive modality, studies have shown clearance of AKs for up to 3 months in SOTRs after 2 sequential PDT sessions performed 1–2 weeks apart [113, 118]. Cyclical ALA-PDT (every 4–8 weeks) has also been demonstrated to decrease the incidence of new SCCs by 95 % after 2 years of treatment [119, 120]. Side effects include discomfort and burning during treatment and post-treatment swelling (especially periorbitally), infections, and redness; in addition, herpes simplex virus (HSV) reactivation has been reported [121]. Strict sun avoidance for 48 h after each treatment is required because of prolonged photosensitivity. Since PDT is an in-office procedure, patient compliance is not an issue. However, the time commitment (frequent 2–3 h-long visits over 2 years) proposed for SOTR regimens may be difficult to incorporate into a patient's schedule.

During field therapy treatment, it is important to biopsy any "ugly duckling" lesion or any lesion that fails to respond to therapy. While field cancerization is useful for most SOTRs, it is not recommended for SOTRs in whom effective chemoprevention (see below) is necessary.

Systemic Chemoprevention

Systemic chemoprevention may be appropriate in a select population of SOTRs: those with multiple [5–10] SCCs per year or multiple SCCs in high-risk locations, or SOTR with a history of leukemia/lymphoma [76].

Retinoids

Retinoids are vitamin A derivatives that have been used in the treatment and prevention of actinic keratoses and NMSCs. They may also be effective adjuvant therapy following surgery for SCC or in patients who cannot tolerate surgery.

Retinoids may work by altering the keratinocytes' cell cycle and reducing the number of malignant/premalignant lesions while on therapy. Unfortunately, once therapy is discontinued, rebound development of eruptive AKs and SCCs can be observed. Side effects are common and include mucocutaneous dryness, scaling/desquamation, itching, increased cholesterol and triglyceride levels, transaminitis, joint pains, hair loss; side effects may limit dose and duration of therapy. Laboratory monitoring with liver function tests (LFTs) and lipid profiles is recommended every 3 months. Of note, all retinoids are teratogenic; female patients must be counseled to avoid pregnancy during treatment. Acitretin should not be used in women of childbearing potential since its teratogenic effects last 3 years after discontinuation.

In clinical trials, prevention of cancerous lesions was observed with using acitretin 25 mg daily [122]. However, side effects may limit the daily dose to only 10 mg in many patients; this lower dose theoretically has diminished therapeutic effects [123–126].

Oral Capecitabine

Capecitabine, an oral prodrug of 5-FU, has recently been studied for NMSC chemoprophylaxis in SOTRs. It is currently FDA-approved for use in metastatic breast and colon cancers [76, 127]. Capecitabine is metabolized by dihydropyrimidine dehydrogenase (DPD) and pretreatment DPD serum levels should be checked as DPD deficiency may lead to significant toxicity. The efficacy for capecitabine as a chemopreventive measure is based on a relatively small cohort of SOTR patients, with only 15 study patients in the largest report, of whom 80 % were RTRs. Success depended upon lesion type; incidence rates dropped most markedly for AKs (2.45×), with modest decreases in rates of SCCs (0.33) and BCCs (0.04) seen at 12 months [128]. Severe toxicities included fatigue (40 %), hand-foot syndrome (20 %), and diarrhea (20 %) [128].

Treatment of Skin Cancers

Outright NMSCs should be managed by surgical means whenever possible and proceed in concert with ongoing treatment of precancers/field cancerization. The focus of this section is the treatment of NMSCs, primarily SCCs. Management of melanoma, KS, and MCC is discussed briefly.

Melanoma

All melanomas should be treated with wide local excision (WLE) based upon the NCCN or AAD guidelines. The margin of excision and indication for sentinel lymph node biopsy (SLNB) is primarily dependent on the Breslow depth (BD) of tumor; margins recommended for lesional thickness are for in situ: 0.5 cm; for lesions less than or equal to 1 mm BD: 1 cm; for lesions between 1.0 and 2.0 mm BD: 1.0–2.0 cm: for lesions over ≥2.0 mm; 2.0 cm. Survival rates of SOTRs with melanoma are lower than those in non-transplanted patients with similar BD; thus, more aggressive management may be considered for lower risk melanomas in the SOTRs [129].

Kaposi Sarcoma (KS)

Studies report KS lesions limited to the skin have been treated with imiquimod, lasers, surgery, cryotherapy, or radiotherapy [80]. However, radiation for KS has been associated with an increased risk of NMSC [81].

For more extensive cases of KS, decreasing immunosuppressive therapy or switching to rapamycin-based regimen can improve the outcome in RTRs. It is thought that lower immunosuppression is responsible for KS regression, not the antiproliferative effects of sirolimus, as KS recurrence has been reported in sirolimus-based regimens when patients experienced high sirolimus levels [130, 131]. Advanced or systemic KS, unresponsive to the withdrawal of immunosuppression, has been treated somewhat successfully with chemotherapy, particularly with taxols [80].

Merkel Cell Carcinoma

All MCCs in SOTRs should be treated in accordance with NCCN guidelines for immunocompetent patients [132]. MCC treatment involves surgical resection and may involve sentinel lymph node dissection (SLND), adjuvant radiotherapy, and possibly systemic chemotherapy though data is still limited on its effectiveness.

Table 18.4 Treatment options for premalignant and malignant lesions in renal transplant recipients

Discrete AKs or warts	• Cryotherapy (LN2)
Field cancerization (diffuse photodamage)	• Field therapy: 5-FU, imiquimod, or PDT • Chemowraps (w/5-FU) for large surface areas (e.g., legs or scalp)
SCCIS or "low-risk" SCCs ("low-risk" SCC: <1 cm on trunk or extremities of well-differentiated subtype)	• Destructive modalities may be considered: ED&C, 5-FU, or imiquimod • Excision or Mohs may be indicated for SCCIS (depending on anatomic location)
"High-risk" SCCs	• Mohs surgery of standard excision is the gold standard • Slow Mohs (or Staged Excision) may be performed – (For aggressive tumors or those with indistinct borders or PNInv) • XRT as monotherapy if patient is not surgical candidate • Adjuvant XRT if unable to obtain negative margins during surgery or if PNInv • Imaging and/or SLNB if lymphadenopathy or aggressive histologic features (PNInv) during surgery
>5–10 SCCs per year multiple SCCs in "high-risk" locations OTR h/o leukemia lymphoma	• Consider systemic chemoprevention with retinoids or oral capecitabine • Consider revision of immunosuppressive regimen
Metastatic SCCs	• Surgical resection, SLND, and XRT • Consider EGFR inhibitors (cetuximab, erlotinib) or chemotherapy with taxols

SCCIS squamous cell carcinoma in situ, *SCCs* squamous cell carcinomas, *PDT* photodynamic therapy, *FU* fluorouracil, *ED&C* electrodessication and curettage, *XRT* radiation therapy, *SLNB* sentinel lymph node biopsy, *PNInv* perineural invasion, *SLND* sentinel lymph node dissection, *AKs* actinic keratoses, *LN2* liquid nitrogen, *EGFR* epidermal growth factor receptor

Nonmelanoma Skin Cancer

Selection of the treatment modality should be determined by tumor risk factors. For all skin cancers diagnosed in RTR margin control with either Mohs surgery (MMS) or standard excision with documented negative margins is the recommended treatment [76]. In addition, before surgery, high-risk tumors should be evaluated for their metastatic potential to assess if imaging or SLNB or post-op radiation may be indicated. Topical treatments described above and other nonsurgical modalities like electrodessication and curettage (ED&C) may be appropriate for low-risk tumors. A summary of the recommended treatments for premalignant and malignant lesions by severity of disease burden is seen in Table 18.4.

Electrodessication and Curettage

ED&C is a quick (5–10 min), destructive, in-office, nonsurgical procedure used primarily to treat BCCs of superficial histologic subtype and SCCIS. First, the visible tumor or biopsy scar and 4-mm margin of normal skin are anesthetized using subcutaneous lidocaine. A round metal curette (3–4 mm in diameter) and an electrocautery tip are then used to scrape and burn the defined cancerous area. ED&C is generally not used in SCC but has been reported to have good results and low recurrence rates in some low-risk SCCs [76, 133]. It may be also indicated in patients with multiple synchronous tumors or if patients refuse, or are not candidates for, further surgery.

Standard Surgical Resection or Excision

Standard surgical resection or excision is most commonly performed on well-circumscribed low-risk NMSCs on the trunk and extremities that are less than 2 cm in diameter. For such lesions, standard excision can provide 5-year cure rates as high as in 98 % in BCCs and 95 % in SCCs [22, 134, 135]. During standard excision, the visible tumor or biopsy site, rim of surrounding erythema, and a 4–10 mm margin of normal skin are removed together in one procedure [132]. Additional tissue may be removed to provide a surgical closure with an improved cosmetic result. After removal, the tissue is processed as paraffin-embedded permanent sections with vertical sectioning. Approximately 3 % of tissue margins are evaluated after standard surgical resection and vertical sectioning [68]. Though only a small fraction of tissue is examined, it has been demonstrated that margin interpretation, based on this small percentage of tissue, is accurate for these low-risk NMSC tumors.

Mohs Micrographic Surgery (MMS)

MMS is widely accepted as the gold standard treatment for the majority of head-and-neck and high-risk skin cancers due to its superior cure rate [64, 76]. Another benefit is that the MMS technique offers maximal tissue conservation to provide optimal cosmetic outcome [68]. Tumor removal and reconstruction are done in an office setting with local lidocaine anesthesia. During the first stage, the visible tumor and a minimal peripheral margin are taken. The tumor is processed in an on-site lab using a fresh frozen processing technique while the patient is waiting. In contrast to vertical sectioning used during standard excision, during MMS the tissue is processed with horizontal sections. Horizontal sectioning allows the entire (deep and peripheral) margin of the tissue to be examined. If necessary, the Mohs surgeon is able to map out the location of any residual tumor nests and remove these cancerous cells without further disruption of normal skin. Several stages may be needed to ensure complete removal of the tumor.

Due to its superior cure rate with decreased recurrence rates, MMS may be more cost effective relative to standard excision in high-risk areas or high-risk tumors. However it requires a specialized setup (office with surgical suites and in-office lab) that is not universally available.

Slow Mohs (or Staged Excision) Technique

For more aggressive tumors or for those with indistinct borders or PNInv, "Slow Mohs" (or Staged Excision) may be performed [136, 137]. During Slow Mohs, the tumor is removed with 5–10 mm margins and processed on permanent paraffin-embedded sections as performed for standard excisions. In contrast to standard excision, however, excised tissue is processed in horizontal sections and closure is delayed until pathologic review reveals negative margins. A medicated gauze bolster, which may be left in place for 7–14 days, is sewn into place after each stage. Though it takes longer and is likely more expensive, Slow Mohs may provide a superior result, utilizing the horizontal sections of MMS for better margin assessment, along with paraffin-embedded sections of standard excisions, which are free of freeze-artifacts that may affect interpretation in standard MMS.

Reconstruction

Most reconstructions after tumor removal are performed by the Mohs surgeon in the office with local anesthesia. Larger repairs may necessitate coordination with otolaryngology, plastic surgery, oculoplastics, or general surgery in a standard operating suite. A physician's fear of creating a large wound should never prevent or delay the treatment of a potentially deadly skin cancer. It is important to remember that even the most daunting wound can be reconstructed, while our options for treating metastatic SCC or other aggressive tumors are limited.

Sentinel Lymph Node Biopsy (SLNB) in Cutaneous SCC

The role of SLNB in cutaneous SCC management is still being determined. In fact, SLNB is not included in the current NCCN guidelines for the treatment of SCC. Within the literature, however, there is an increasing amount of data supporting the use of SLNB in SCC, especially high-risk tumors. After performing a large systematic review of 11 studies, Ahmed et al. concluded that an SLNB is an accurate and reliable test in SCC with false omission rates of only ~5 %, similar to that of melanoma, a tumor for which it is standard of care [138]. Studies on immunocompetent patients indicate that an SLNB has high specificity in SCC. Reportedly, a positive sentinel lymph node (SLN) can be detected in 21–24 % of patients with high-risk SCC [139]. The identification of subclinical nodal disease in SCC is thought to have important prognostic implications, but because of the limited experience with the technique in SCC, the survival benefits are still uncertain. SLNB should be given special consideration in certain settings in SOTRs since their tumors tend to have an aggressive clinical course with increased rates of metastasis.

Adjuvant Treatments

Adjuvant treatment, radiation or systemic therapy, may be indicated if surgical control of a tumor is not possible. However, there is little evidence to suggest that most adjuvant treatments, except for revision of immunosuppression for certain types of tumors, are useful in improving long-term outcomes in RTRs; therefore energy must be placed on preventing skin cancer and controlling disease at earlier stages.

Radiation Therapy

In both immunocompetent and SOTRs, postoperative radiation therapy is used as adjuvant therapy when negative surgical margins cannot be obtained or when lymph node involvement or PNInv is identified [76]. In addition, radiation is considered first-line therapy for patients who are nonsurgical candidates. To potentially treat localized subclinical spread, wide radiotherapy margins are often employed [140].

Since SCCs commonly occur on head and neck, common side effects of radiation include not only dermatitis but also mucositis and xerostomia which can decrease quality of life and cause considerable morbidity [141]. In addition, though rare, irradiated areas are at increased risk of radiation-induced skin cancer, primarily BCC which develops several years after treatment [142, 143].

Revision of Immunosuppression

Revision of the immunosuppression regimen may be indicated in SOTRs who develop more than 5–10 high-risk SCCs per year [35]. This may be accomplished by reducing doses or by changing the drug regimen. In particular, a change to rapamycin (sirolimus and everolimus) therapy may decrease skin cancer development, as discussed above, as well as cause involution of existing lesions.

The trade-off for a reduction in NMSCs was an increase in other adverse drug-related effects including various skin eruptions and pneumonitis; interestingly, a transition regimen that was slower was better tolerated than a more rapid transition protocol [56, 144].

The decision to change immunosuppressive regimen is always made in concert with the transplant service. Risk of skin cancer must always be balanced with the risk of graft survival and potential AE associated with changing drugs.

Chemotherapy and Molecular-Based Therapies

Fortunately, adjuvant chemotherapy is seldom needed. Consequently, evidence of its effectiveness is scarce and based on case series. Adjuvant chemotherapy utilized since the 1980s have been primarily cisplatin-based. More recently, molecular-based therapies, appropriated from the head and neck literature, have been used in the treatment of metastatic cutaneous SCCs [145]. In particular, the epidermal growth factor (EGFR) inhibitors (e.g., cetuximab, erlotinib) have been utilized with good response [146, 147].

Conclusion

In the past, skin cancer was not considered to be a major health concern for RTR patients. However, because the life expectancy of RTR is becoming increasing longer due to expanding lifesaving medical knowledge and new immunosuppressive regimens, skin cancer is being observed more routinely. It is important for all providers caring for RTRs to be acutely aware of the factors contributing to cutaneous carcinogenesis and to be familiar with the appearance and characteristics of the most common premalignant and malignant lesions in order to facilitate early diagnosis and avoid unnecessary morbidity and mortality. Every effort should be made to educate patients of the risks of skin cancer posttransplantation and to initiate sun protective behaviors as well as encourage clinical follow-up to minimize the negative impact of skin cancer on an RTR's quality of life.

- Skin cancer, the most common malignancy after renal transplantation, is a significant cause of morbidity in RTRs.
- While skin cancer is common in both transplanted and nontransplanted population, the prevalence of different types and clinical behavior differs between the two groups.
- Whereas in the general population the ratio of BCCs to SCCs is 4:1, the ratio is flipped for RTRs with SCCs occurring four times more frequently than BCCs.
- Skin cancers that develop in RTRs are considered to have more aggressive behavior than those that develop in the immunocompetent population with increased rates of recurrence and metastasis.
- The etiology of cutaneous carcinogenesis in renal transplant is multifactorial with immunosuppressive therapy being the strongest associated risk factor for its development.
- The other major contributor to skin cancer development is UV exposure adherence to appropriate sun protective behaviors is important for all RTRs and compliance should be stressed repetitively.
- Every day (even when cloudy and in the winter), RTRs should apply broad-spectrum sunscreen with UVA/UVB coverage with an SPF ≥30, wear wide-brimmed hats or sun protective clothing, and avoid prolonged periods outdoors.
- Close dermatologic follow-up is recommended posttransplantation to identify premalignant lesions (AKs) and NMSCs at earlier stages to decrease morbidity.
- When AKs are identified, they should be managed aggressively with either liquid nitrogen or field therapy to prevent malignant transformation.
- For confirmed skin cancers, MMS and standard surgical excision are the primary treatment modalities, depending on the type of tumor.
- For some patients who continue to develop numerous NMSCs despite sun avoidance and close follow-up, reversal of immunosuppression or systemic chemoprevention with retinoids or capecitabine may be indicated.
- Though much less common than SCCs or BCCs, other cutaneous malignancies (e.g., melanoma, MCC, KS) also occur at increased rates and with poorer outcomes in RTRs compared to the immunocompetent population.
- Skin cancers can have a significant negative impact on an RTR's life posttransplantation, but with a coordinated multidisciplinary approach with patient's nephrologist, transplant surgeon, and dermatologist, the burden can be minimized and the best outcomes achieved.

References

1. Donaldson MR, Coldiron BM. No end in sight: the skin cancer epidemic continues. Semin Cutan Med Surg. 2011;30(1):3–5. PubMed PMID: 21540015.
2. Rigel DS, Friedman RJ, Kopf AW. Lifetime risk for development of skin cancer in the U.S. population: current estimate is now 1 in 5. J Am Acad Dermatol. 1996;35(6):1012–3. PubMed PMID: 8959974.
3. Rogers HW, Weinstock MA, Harris AR, Hinckley MR, Feldman SR, Fleischer AB, et al. Incidence estimate of nonmelanoma skin cancer in the United States, 2006. Arch Dermatol. 2010;146(3):283–7. PubMed PMID: 20231499.
4. Stern RS. Prevalence of a history of skin cancer in 2007: results of an incidence-based model. Arch Dermatol. 2010;146(3):279–82. PubMed PMID: 20231498.
5. "Skin Cancer" The National Cancer Institute website. http://www.cancer.gov/cancertopics/types/skin. Accessed 20 Aug 2013.
6. Siegel R, DeSantis C, Virgo K, Stein K, Mariotto A, Smith T, et al. Cancer treatment and survivorship statistics. CA Cancer J Clin. 2012;62(4):220–41. PubMed PMID: 22700443.
7. Society AC. Cancer facts & figures 2012 2013. http://www.cancer.org/acs/groups/content/@epidemiologysurveilance/documents/document/acspc-031941.pdf. Accessed 20 Aug 2013.
8. DePry JL, Reed KB, Cook-Norris RH, Brewer JD. Iatrogenic immunosuppression and cutaneous malignancy. Clin Dermatol. 2011;29(6):602–13. PubMed PMID: 22014982.
9. Meier P, Dayer E, Blanc E, Wauters JP. Early T cell activation correlates with expression of apoptosis markers in patients with end-stage renal disease. J Am Soc Nephrol. 2002;13(1):204–12. PubMed PMID: 11752039.

10. Jerant AF, Johnson JT, Sheridan CD, Caffrey TJ. Early detection and treatment of skin cancer. Am Fam Physician. 2000;62(2):357. PubMed PMID: 10929700-68, 75-6, 81-2.
11. Vajdic CM, van Leeuwen MT. Cancer incidence and risk factors after solid organ transplantation. Int J Cancer. 2009;125(8):1747–54. PubMed PMID: 19444916.
12. Alam M, Ratner D. Cutaneous squamous-cell carcinoma. New Engl J Med. 2001;344(13):975–83. PubMed PMID: 11274625.
13. Diepgen TL, Mahler V. The epidemiology of skin cancer. Br J Dermatol. 2002;146 Suppl 61:1–6. PubMed PMID: 11966724.
14. Glass AG, Hoover RN. The emerging epidemic of melanoma and squamous cell skin cancer. JAMA. 1989;262(15):2097–100. PubMed PMID: 2795783.
15. Euvrard S, Kanitakis J, Claudy A. Skin cancers after organ transplantation. New Engl J Med. 2003;348(17):1681–91. PubMed PMID: 12711744.
16. Jensen AO, Svaerke C, Farkas D, Pedersen L, Kragballe K, Sorensen HT. Skin cancer risk among solid organ recipients: a nationwide cohort study in Denmark. Acta Derm Venereol. 2010;90(5):474–9. PubMed PMID: 20814621.
17. Webb MC, Compton F, Andrews PA, Koffman CG. Skin tumours posttransplantation: a retrospective analysis of 28 years' experience at a single centre. Transplant Proc. 1997;29(1–2):828–30. PubMed PMID: 9123544.
18. Buell JF, Hanaway MJ, Thomas M, Alloway RR, Woodle ES. Skin cancer following transplantation: the Israel Penn International Transplant Tumor Registry experience. Transplant Proc. 2005;37(2):962–3. PubMed PMID: 15848591.
19. Martinez JC, Otley CC, Stasko T, Euvrard S, Brown C, Schanbacher CF, et al. Defining the clinical course of metastatic skin cancer in organ transplant recipients: a multicenter collaborative study. Arch Dermatol. 2003;139(3):301–6. PubMed PMID: 12622621.
20. Tessari G, Girolomoni G. Nonmelanoma skin cancer in solid organ transplant recipients: update on epidemiology, risk factors, and management. Dermatol Surg. 2012;38(10):1622–30. PubMed PMID: 22805312.
21. Cutaneous squamous cell carcinoma and other cutaneous carcinomas. In: Edge SB, Byrd DR, Compton CC et al., editors. AJCC Cancer staging manual. 7th ed. New York, NY: Springer; 2010. pp. 301–14.
22. Network NCC. Basal and squamous cell skin cancers. NCCN clinical practice guidelines in oncology (NCCN guidelines). 2013. http://www.nccn.org/professionals/physician_gls/pdf/nmsc.pdf. Accessed 5 Aug 2013.
23. Zwald FO, Brown M. Skin cancer in solid organ transplant recipients: advances in therapy and management: part I. Epidemiology of skin cancer in solid organ transplant recipients. J Am Acad Dermatol. 2011;65(2):253–61. quiz 62, PubMed PMID: 21763561.
24. Penn I. Malignant melanoma in organ allograft recipients. Transplantation. 1996;61(2):274–8. PubMed PMID: 8600636.
25. Stasko T, Brown MD, Carucci JA, Euvrard S, Johnson TM, Sengelmann RD, et al. Guidelines for the management of squamous cell carcinoma in organ transplant recipients. Dermatol Surg. 2004;30(4 Pt 2):642–50. PubMed PMID: 15061849.
26. Braconnier P, Del Marmol V, Broeders N, Kianda M, Massart A, Lemy A, et al. Combined introduction of anti-IL2 receptor antibodies, mycophenolic acid and tacrolimus: effect on malignancies after renal transplantation in a single-centre retrospective cohort study. Nephrol Dial Transplant. 2012;27(6):2547–53. PubMed PMID: 22123748.
27. Hiesse C, Rieu P, Kriaa F, Larue JR, Goupy C, Neyrat N, et al. Malignancy after renal transplantation: analysis of incidence and risk factors in 1700 patients followed during a 25-year period. Transplant Proc. 1997;29(1–2):831–3. PubMed PMID: 9123545.
28. Jensen P, Hansen S, Moller B, Leivestad T, Pfeffer P, Geiran O, et al. Skin cancer in kidney and heart transplant recipients and different long-term immunosuppressive therapy regimens. J Am Acad Dermatol. 1999;40(2 Pt 1):177–86. PubMed PMID: 10025742.
29. Hofbauer GF, Bouwes Bavinck JN, Euvrard S. Organ transplantation and skin cancer: basic problems and new perspectives. Exp Dermatol. 2010;19(6):473–82. PubMed PMID: 20482618.
30. Lebwohl MG, Rosen T, Stockfleth E. The role of human papillomavirus in common skin conditions: current viewpoints and therapeutic options. Cutis 2010;86(5):suppl 1–11; quiz suppl 2. PubMed PMID: 21214125.
31. Bindea G, Mlecnik B, Fridman WH, Pages F, Galon J. Natural immunity to cancer in humans. Curr Opin Immunol. 2010;22(2):215–22. PubMed PMID: 20207124.
32. Dunn GP, Old LJ, Schreiber RD. The immunobiology of cancer immunosurveillance and immunoediting. Immunity. 2004;21(2):137–48. PubMed PMID: 15308095.
33. DuPage M, Mazumdar C, Schmidt LM, Cheung AF, Jacks T. Expression of tumour-specific antigens underlies cancer immunoediting. Nature. 2012;482(7385):405–9. PubMed PMID: 22318517, Pubmed Central PMCID: 3288744.
34. Jensen P, Hansen S, Moller B, Leivestad T, Pfeffer P, Fauchald P. Are renal transplant recipients on CsA-based immunosuppressive regimens more likely to develop skin cancer than those on azathioprine and prednisolone? Transplant Proc. 1999;31(1–2):1120. PubMed PMID: 10083500.
35. Otley CC, Maragh SL. Reduction of immunosuppression for transplant-associated skin cancer: rationale and evidence of efficacy. Dermatol Surg. 2005;31(2):163–8. PubMed PMID: 15762208.
36. Robson R, Cecka JM, Opelz G, Budde M, Sacks S. Prospective registry-based observational cohort study of the long-term risk of malignancies in renal transplant patients treated with mycophenolate mofetil. Am J Transplant. 2005;5(12):2954–60. PubMed PMID: 16303010.
37. Marcil I, Stern RS. Squamous-cell cancer of the skin in patients given PUVA and ciclosporin: nested cohort crossover study. Lancet. 2001;358(9287):1042–5. PubMed PMID: 11589933.
38. Wimmer CD, Angele MK, Schwarz B, Pratschke S, Rentsch M, Khandoga A, et al. Impact of cyclosporine versus tacrolimus on the incidence of de novo malignancy following liver transplantation: a single center experience with 609 patients. Transpl Int. 2013;26. PubMed PMID: 23952102.
39. Guba M, Lohe F. Transplantation in cancer disease, and tumors in organ transplantation: current aspects and future prospects. MMW Fortschr Med. 2004;146(24):32–4. PubMed PMID: 15366488. Transplantation bei Tumorerkrankungen – Tumoren nach Organtransplantation. Organ neu, Tumor auch?.
40. Guba M, Graeb C, Jauch KW, Geissler EK. Pro- and anti-cancer effects of immunosuppressive agents used in organ transplantation. Transplantation. 2004;77(12):1777–82. PubMed PMID: 15223891.
41. Gjersvik P, Helsing P, Holdaas H, Bergan S. Immunosuppressive drugs and the development of skin cancer after organ transplantation. Tidsskr Nor Laegeforen. 2012;132(18):2064–8. PubMed PMID: 23038197.
42. Glover MT, Deeks JJ, Raftery MJ, Cunningham J, Leigh IM. Immunosuppression and risk of non-melanoma skin cancer in renal transplant recipients. Lancet. 1997;349(9049):398. PubMed PMID: 9033469.
43. O'Donovan P, Perrett CM, Zhang X, Montaner B, Xu YZ, Harwood CA, et al. Azathioprine and UVA light generate mutagenic oxidative DNA damage. Science. 2005;309(5742):1871–4. PubMed PMID: 16166520, Pubmed Central PMCID: 2426755.
44. Ingvar A, Smedby KE, Lindelof B, Fernberg P, Bellocco R, Tufveson G, et al. Immunosuppressive treatment after solid organ transplantation and risk of post-transplant cutaneous squamous

cell carcinoma. Nephrol Dial Transplant. 2010;25(8):2764–71. PubMed PMID: 19729465.
45. Ho WL, Murphy GM. Update on the pathogenesis of post-transplant skin cancer in renal transplant recipients. Br J Dermatol. 2008;158(2):217–24. PubMed PMID: 18070205.
46. Wu X, Nguyen BC, Dziunycz P, Chang S, Brooks Y, Lefort K, et al. Opposing roles for calcineurin and ATF3 in squamous skin cancer. Nature. 2010;465(7296):368–72. PubMed PMID: 20485437, Pubmed Central PMCID: 3050632.
47. Yarosh DB, Pena AV, Nay SL, Canning MT, Brown DA. Calcineurin inhibitors decrease DNA repair and apoptosis in human keratinocytes following ultraviolet B irradiation. J Invest Dermatol. 2005;125(5):1020–5. PubMed PMID: 16297204.
48. Dantal J, Hourmant M, Cantarovich D, Giral M, Blancho G, Dreno B, et al. Effect of long-term immunosuppression in kidney-graft recipients on cancer incidence: randomised comparison of two cyclosporin regimens. Lancet. 1998;351(9103):623–8. PubMed PMID: 9500317.
49. Guba M, von Breitenbuch P, Steinbauer M, Koehl G, Flegel S, Hornung M, et al. Rapamycin inhibits primary and metastatic tumor growth by antiangiogenesis: involvement of vascular endothelial growth factor. Nat Med. 2002;8(2):128–35. PubMed PMID: 11821896.
50. Hojo M, Morimoto T, Maluccio M, Asano T, Morimoto K, Lagman M, et al. Cyclosporine induces cancer progression by a cell-autonomous mechanism. Nature. 1999;397(6719):530–4. PubMed PMID: 10028970.
51. Cattaneo D, Gotti E, Perico N, Bertolini G, Kainer G, Remuzzi G. Cyclosporine formulation and Kaposi's sarcoma after renal transplantation. Transplantation. 2005;80(6):743–8. PubMed PMID: 16210960.
52. Norman KG, Canter JA, Shi M, Milne GL, Morrow JD, Sligh JE. Cyclosporine A suppresses keratinocyte cell death through MPTP inhibition in a model for skin cancer in organ transplant recipients. Mitochondrion. 2010;10(2):94–101. PubMed PMID: 19836469.
53. Kauffman HM, Cherikh WS, Cheng Y, Hanto DW, Kahan BD. Maintenance immunosuppression with target-of-rapamycin inhibitors is associated with a reduced incidence of de novo malignancies. Transplantation. 2005;80(7):883–9. PubMed PMID: 16249734.
54. Salgo R, Gossmann J, Schofer H, Kachel HG, Kuck J, Geiger H, et al. Switch to a sirolimus-based immunosuppression in long-term renal transplant recipients: reduced rate of (pre-)malignancies and nonmelanoma skin cancer in a prospective, randomized, assessor-blinded, controlled clinical trial. Am J Transplant. 2010;10(6):1385–93. PubMed PMID: 20121752.
55. Campbell SB, Walker R, Tai SS, Jiang Q, Russ GR. Randomized controlled trial of sirolimus for renal transplant recipients at high risk for nonmelanoma skin cancer. Am J Transplant. 2012;12(5):1146–56. PubMed PMID: 22420843.
56. Euvrard S, Morelon E, Rostaing L, Goffin E, Brocard A, Tromme I, et al. Sirolimus and secondary skin-cancer prevention in kidney transplantation. New Engl J Med. 2012;367(4):329–39. PubMed PMID: 22830463.
57. Bouwes Bavinck JN, Euvrard S, Naldi L, Nindl I, Proby CM, Neale R, et al. Keratotic skin lesions and other risk factors are associated with skin cancer in organ-transplant recipients: a case-control study in The Netherlands, United Kingdom, Germany, France, and Italy. J Invest Dermatol. 2007;127(7):1647–56. PubMed PMID: 17380113, Pubmed Central PMCID: 2478722.
58. Taylor AE, Shuster S. Skin cancer after renal transplantation: the causal role of azathioprine. Acta Derm Venereol. 1992;72(2):115–9. PubMed PMID: 1350395.
59. Urwin HR, Jones PW, Harden PN, Ramsay HM, Hawley CM, Nicol DL, et al. Predicting risk of nonmelanoma skin cancer and premalignant skin lesions in renal transplant recipients. Transplantation. 2009;87(11):1667–71. PubMed PMID: 19502958.
60. Otley CC, Cherikh WS, Salasche SJ, McBride MA, Christenson LJ, Kauffman HM. Skin cancer in organ transplant recipients: effect of pretransplant end-organ disease. J Am Acad Dermatol. 2005;53(5):783–90. PubMed PMID: 16243126.
61. Gogia R, Binstock M, Hirose R, Boscardin WJ, Chren MM, Arron ST. Fitzpatrick skin phototype is an independent predictor of squamous cell carcinoma risk after solid organ transplantation. J Am Acad Dermatol. 2013;68(4):585–91. PubMed PMID: 23107311, Pubmed Central PMCID: 3562416.
62. Kwatra SG, Mills KC, Zeitany A, Pearce DJ, Williford PM, D'Agostino Jr RB, et al. Pain and nonmelanoma skin cancer in transplant patients. J Am Acad Dermatol. 2012;67(6):1387–8. PubMed PMID: 23158620.
63. Anwar J, Wrone DA, Kimyai-Asadi A, Alam M. The development of actinic keratosis into invasive squamous cell carcinoma: evidence and evolving classification schemes. Clin Dermatol. 2004;22(3):189–96. PubMed PMID: WOS:000223076700004. English.
64. Wolff KGL, Katz SI, Gilchrest BA, Paller AS, Leffell DJ. Fitzpatrick's dermatology in general medicine. 7th ed. New York, NY: Mcgraw-Hill; 2007.
65. Ratushny V, Gober MD, Hick R, Ridky TW, Seykora JT. From keratinocyte to cancer: the pathogenesis and modeling of cutaneous squamous cell carcinoma. J Clin Invest. 2012;122(2):464–72. PubMed PMID: 22293185, Pubmed Central PMCID: 3266779.
66. Forslund O, Ly H, Reid C, Higgins G. A broad spectrum of human papillomavirus types is present in the skin of Australian patients with non-melanoma skin cancers and solar keratosis. Br J Dermatol. 2003;149(1):64–73. PubMed PMID: 12890196.
67. Joly P, Bastuji-Garin S, Frances C, Lebbe C, Aubin F, Penso-Assathiany D, et al. Squamous cell carcinomas are associated with verrucokeratotic cutaneous lesions but not with common warts in organ-transplant patients. A case-control study. Transplantation. 2010;89(10):1224–30. PubMed PMID: 20559031.
68. Habif T. Clinical dermatology, 5e. St. Louis, MO: Mosby; 2009.
69. Ulrich C. Topical treatment of field cancerization. Canc Treat Res. 2009;146:439–46. PubMed PMID: 19415223.
70. Bangash HK, Colegio OR. Management of non-melanoma skin cancer in immunocompromised solid organ transplant recipients. Curr Treat Options Oncol. 2012;13(3):354–76. PubMed PMID: 22592596.
71. Reuschenbach M, Tran T, Faulstich F, Hartschuh W, Vinokurova S, Kloor M, et al. High-risk human papillomavirus in non-melanoma skin lesions from renal allograft recipients and immunocompetent patients. Br J Cancer. 2011;104(8):1334–41. PubMed PMID: 21427726, Pubmed Central PMCID: 3078602.
72. Rowe DE, Carroll RJ, Day Jr CL. Prognostic factors for local recurrence, metastasis, and survival rates in squamous cell carcinoma of the skin, ear, and lip. Implications for treatment modality selection. J Am Acad Dermatol. 1992;26(6):976–90. PubMed PMID: 1607418.
73. Southwell KE, Chaplin JM, Eisenberg RL, McIvor NP, Morton RP. Effect of immunocompromise on metastatic cutaneous squamous cell carcinoma in the parotid and neck. Head Neck. 2006;28(3):244–8. PubMed PMID: 16395715.
74. Martinez JC, Otley CC, Okuno SH, Foote RL, Kasperbauer JL. Chemotherapy in the management of advanced cutaneous squamous cell carcinoma in organ transplant recipients: theoretical and practical considerations. Dermatol Surg. 2004;30(4 Pt 2):679–86. PubMed PMID: 15061855.
75. Cooper JZ, Brown MD. Special concern about squamous cell carcinoma of the scalp in organ transplant recipients. Arch Dermatol. 2006;142(6):755–8. PubMed PMID: 16785379.

76. Zwald FO, Brown M. Skin cancer in solid organ transplant recipients: advances in therapy and management: part II. Management of skin cancer in solid organ transplant recipients. J Am Acad Dermatol. 2011;65(2):263–79. PubMed PMID: 21763562, quiz 80.
77. Smith KJ, Hamza S, Skelton H. Histologic features in primary cutaneous squamous cell carcinomas in immunocompromised patients focusing on organ transplant patients. Dermatol Surg. 2004;30(4 Pt 2):634–41. PubMed PMID: 15061848.
78. Le Mire L, Hollowood K, Gray D, Bordea C, Wojnarowska F. Melanomas in renal transplant recipients. Br J Dermatol. 2006;154(3):472–7. PubMed PMID: 16445778.
79. Ali FR, Lear JT. Melanoma in organ transplant recipients: incidence, outcomes and management considerations. J Skin Cancer. 2012;2012:404615. PubMed PMID: 23227339, Pubmed Central PMCID: 3512321.
80. Hosseini-Moghaddam SM, Soleimanirahbar A, Mazzulli T, Rotstein C, Husain S. Post renal transplantation Kaposi's sarcoma: a review of its epidemiology, pathogenesis, diagnosis, clinical aspects, and therapy. Transpl Infect Dis. 2012;14(4):338–45. PubMed PMID: 22316356.
81. Zmonarski SC, Boratynska M, Puziewicz-Zmonarska A, Kazimierczak K, Klinger M. Kaposi's sarcoma in renal transplant recipients. Ann Transplant. 2005;10(2):59–65. PubMed PMID: 16218035.
82. Feng H, Shuda M, Chang Y, Moore PS. Clonal integration of a polyomavirus in human Merkel cell carcinoma. Science. 2008;319(5866):1096–100. PubMed PMID: 18202256, Pubmed Central PMCID: 2740911.
83. Kean JM, Rao S, Wang M, Garcea RL. Seroepidemiology of human polyomaviruses. PLoS Pathog. 2009;5(3):e1000363. PubMed PMID: 19325891, Pubmed Central PMCID: 2655709.
84. Poulsen M. Merkel-cell carcinoma of the skin. Lancet Oncol. 2004;5(10):593–9. PubMed PMID: 15465461.
85. Paulson KG, Iyer JG, Blom A, Warton EM, Sokil M, Yelistratova L, et al. Systemic immune suppression predicts diminished Merkel cell carcinoma-specific survival independent of stage. J Invest Dermatol. 2013;133(3):642–6. PubMed PMID: 23190897, Pubmed Central PMCID: 3570636.
86. Skiveren J, Mortensen EL, Haedersdal M. Sun protective behaviour in renal transplant recipients. A qualitative study based on individual interviews and the Health Belief Model. J Dermatolog Treat. 2010;21(6):331–6. PubMed PMID: 20528481.
87. Moloney FJ, Almarzouqi E, O'Kelly P, Conlon P, Murphy GM. Sunscreen use before and after transplantation and assessment of risk factors associated with skin cancer development in renal transplant recipients. Arch Dermatol. 2005;141(8):978–82. PubMed PMID: 16103326.
88. Ramsay HM, Reece SM, Fryer AA, Smith AG, Harden PN. Seven-year prospective study of nonmelanoma skin cancer incidence in U.K. renal transplant recipients. Transplantation. 2007;84(3):437–9. PubMed PMID: 17700173.
89. Ramsay HM, Fryer AA, Hawley CM, Smith AG, Harden PN. Non-melanoma skin cancer risk in the Queensland renal transplant population. Br J Dermatol. 2002;147(5):950–6. PubMed PMID: 12410706.
90. Wang SQ, Dusza SW. Assessment of sunscreen knowledge: a pilot survey. Br J Dermatol. 2009;161 Suppl 3:28–32. PubMed PMID: 19775354.
91. Ou-Yang H, Stanfield J, Cole C, Appa Y, Rigel D. High sun-protection factor sunscreens (>/=70) may provide ultraviolet protection above minimal recommended levels by adequately compensating for lower sunscreen user application amounts. J Am Acad Dermatol. 2013;69(3):481–3. PubMed PMID: 23957971.
92. Jansen R, Osterwalder U, Wang SQ, Burnett M, Lim HW. Photoprotection: part II. Sunscreen: development, efficacy, and controversies. J Am Acad Dermatol. 2013;69(6):867.e1–14. quiz 81–2. PubMed PMID: 24238180.
93. Neutrogena. "Helioplex": Neutrogena. 2014. http://www.neutrogena.com/category/sun/helioplex-+technology.do?sortby=ourPicks&page=all. Accessed 2 Feb 2014.
94. Roche-Posay L. Anthelios 2014. http://www.laroche-posay.us/_us/_en/consumer/catalog/anthelios.aspx. Accessed 2 Feb 2014.
95. Aveeno. Active photobarrier complex. 2014. http://www.aveeno-professional.com/active-photo-barrier. Accessed 2 Feb 2014.
96. Reports C. Sunscreen buying guide. Consumer Reports. May 2013.
97. Landers M, Law S, Storrs FJ. Contact urticaria, allergic contact dermatitis, and photoallergic contact dermatitis from oxybenzone. Am J Contact Dermatitis. 2003;14(1):33–4. PubMed PMID: 14744420.
98. Reichrath J. Dermato-endocrinology remembers Dr. Frank C. Garland: a great scientist who made major contributions to improve our understanding about the importance of vitamin D for human health! Dermatoendocrinology. 2010;2(2):43–5. PubMed PMID: 21547095. Pubmed Central PMCID: 3081683.
99. American Academy of Dermatology. Position statement on vitamin D. 2013. http://www.aad.org/Forms/Policies/Uploads/PS/PS-Vitamin%20D.pdf. Accessed 28 Aug 2013.
100. Nashan D, Meiss F, Muller M. Therapeutic strategies for actinic keratoses – a systematic review. Eur J Dermatol. 2013;23(1):14–32. PubMed PMID: 23477760.
101. Pflugfelder A, Welter AK, Leiter U, Weide B, Held L, Eigentler TK, et al. Open label randomized study comparing 3 months vs. 6 months treatment of actinic keratoses with 3 % diclofenac in 2.5 % hyaluronic acid gel: a trial of the German Dermatologic Cooperative Oncology Group. J Eur Acad Dermatol Venereol. 2012;26(1):48–53. PubMed PMID: 21414035.
102. Roy SD, Manoukian E. Transdermal delivery of ketorolac tromethamine: permeation enhancement, device design, and pharmacokinetics in healthy humans. J Pharm Sci. 1995;84(10):1190–6. PubMed PMID: 8801333.
103. Heyneman CA, Lawless-Liday C, Wall GC. Oral versus topical NSAIDs in rheumatic diseases: a comparison. Drugs. 2000;60(3): 555–74. PubMed PMID: 11030467.
104. Pharmaderm ado FP. Solaraze gel (diclofenac sodium-3 %). [Package insert]. Melville, NY; 2012.
105. Perrett CM, McGregor JM, Warwick J, Karran P, Leigh IM, Proby CM, et al. Treatment of post-transplant premalignant skin disease: a randomized intrapatient comparative study of 5-fluorouracil cream and topical photodynamic therapy. Br J Dermatol. 2007;156(2):320–8. PubMed PMID: 17223873, Pubmed Central PMCID: 2423222.
106. Levy S, Furst K, Chern W. A pharmacokinetic evaluation of 0.5 % and 5 % fluorouracil topical cream in patients with actinic keratosis. Clin Ther. 2001;23(6):908–20. PubMed PMID: 11440290.
107. Mann M, Berk DR, Petersen J. Chemowraps as an adjuvant to surgery for patients with diffuse squamous cell carcinoma of the extremities. J Drugs Dermatol. 2008;7(7):685–8. PubMed PMID: 18664163.
108. Tallon B, Turnbull N. 5 % Fluorouracil chemowraps in the management of widespread lower leg solar keratoses and squamous cell carcinoma. Australas J Dermatol. 2013;8. PubMed PMID: 23651243.
109. Brown VL, Atkins CL, Ghali L, Cerio R, Harwood CA, Proby CM. Safety and efficacy of 5 % imiquimod cream for the treatment of skin dysplasia in high-risk renal transplant recipients: randomized, double-blind, placebo-controlled trial. Arch Dermatol. 2005;141(8):985–93. PubMed PMID: 16103328.
110. Ulrich C, Busch JO, Meyer T, Nindl I, Schmook T, Sterry W, et al. Successful treatment of multiple actinic keratoses in organ transplant patients with topical 5 % imiquimod: a report of six cases. Br J Dermatol. 2006;155(2):451–4. PubMed PMID: 16882188.

111. Trakatelli M, Katsanos G, Ulrich C, Kalabalikis D, Sotiriadis D, Stockfleth E. Efforts to counteract locally the effects of systemic immunosuppression: a review on the use of imiquimod, a topical immunostimulator in organ transplant recipients. Int J Immunopathol Pharmacol. 2010;23(2):387–96. PubMed PMID: 20646334.
112. Ulrich C, Bichel J, Euvrard S, Guidi B, Proby CM, van de Kerkhof PC, et al. Topical immunomodulation under systemic immunosuppression: results of a multicentre, randomized, placebo-controlled safety and efficacy study of imiquimod 5 % cream for the treatment of actinic keratoses in kidney, heart, and liver transplant patients. Br J Dermatol. 2007;157 Suppl 2:25–31. PubMed PMID: 18067628, Pubmed Central PMCID: 2493058.
113. Basset-Seguin N, Baumann Conzett K, Gerritsen MJ, Gonzalez H, Haedersdal M, Hofbauer GF, et al. Photodynamic therapy for actinic keratosis in organ transplant patients. J Eur Acad Dermatol Venereol. 2013;27(1):57–66. PubMed PMID: 22151793.
114. Lebwohl M, Swanson N, Anderson LL, Melgaard A, Xu Z, Berman B. Ingenol mebutate gel for actinic keratosis. New Engl J Med. 2012;366(11):1010–9. PubMed PMID: 22417254.
115. Gupta AK, Paquet M. Network meta-analysis of the outcome "participant complete clearance" in nonimmunosuppressed participants of eight interventions for actinic keratosis: a follow-up on a Cochrane review. Br J Dermatol. 2013;169(2):250–9. PubMed PMID: 23550994.
116. Wlodek C, Ali FR, Lear JT. Use of photodynamic therapy for treatment of actinic keratoses in organ transplant recipients. Biomed Res Int. 2013;2013:349526. PubMed PMID: 23509711, Pubmed Central PMCID: 3591189.
117. Lehmann P. Methyl aminolaevulinate-photodynamic therapy: a review of clinical trials in the treatment of actinic keratoses and nonmelanoma skin cancer. Br J Dermatol. 2007;156(5):793–801. PubMed PMID: 17419691.
118. Bagazgoitia L, Cuevas Santos J, Juarranz A, Jaen P. Photodynamic therapy reduces the histological features of actinic damage and the expression of early oncogenic markers. Br J Dermatol. 2011;165(1):144–51. PubMed PMID: 21615716.
119. Willey A, Mehta S, Lee PK. Reduction in the incidence of squamous cell carcinoma in solid organ transplant recipients treated with cyclic photodynamic therapy. Dermatol Surg. 2010;36(5):652–8. PubMed PMID: 19889154.
120. Wennberg AM, Stenquist B, Stockfleth E, Keohane S, Lear JT, Jemec G, et al. Photodynamic therapy with methyl aminolevulinate for prevention of new skin lesions in transplant recipients: a randomized study. Transplantation. 2008;86(3):423–9. PubMed PMID: 18698246.
121. Nobbe S, Trueb RM, French LE, Hofbauer GF. Herpes simplex virus reactivation as a complication of photodynamic therapy. Photodermatol Photoimmunol Photomed. 2011;27(1):51–2. PubMed PMID: 21198884.
122. George R, Weightman W, Russ GR, Bannister KM, Mathew TH. Acitretin for chemoprevention of non-melanoma skin cancers in renal transplant recipients. Australas J Dermatol. 2002;43(4): 269–73. PubMed PMID: 12423433.
123. Hardin J, Mydlarski PR. Systemic retinoids: chemoprevention of skin cancer in transplant recipients. Skin Therapy Lett. 2010;15(7): 1–4. PubMed PMID: 20700551.
124. Lee JS, Lippman SM, Benner SE, Lee JJ, Ro JY, Lukeman JM, et al. Randomized placebo-controlled trial of isotretinoin in chemoprevention of bronchial squamous metaplasia. J Clin Oncol. 1994;12(5):937–45. PubMed PMID: 8164045.
125. Lippman SM, Lee JJ, Karp DD, Vokes EE, Benner SE, Goodman GE, et al. Randomized phase III intergroup trial of isotretinoin to prevent second primary tumors in stage I non-small-cell lung cancer. J Natl Cancer Inst. 2001;93(8):605–18. PubMed PMID: 11309437.
126. Tangrea JA, Edwards BK, Taylor PR, Hartman AM, Peck GL, Salasche SJ, et al. Long-term therapy with low-dose isotretinoin for prevention of basal cell carcinoma: a multicenter clinical trial. Isotretinoin-Basal Cell Carcinoma Study Group. J Natl Cancer Inst. 1992;84(5):328–32. PubMed PMID: 1738183.
127. Endrizzi B, Ahmed RL, Ray T, Dudek A, Lee P. Capecitabine to reduce nonmelanoma skin carcinoma burden in solid organ transplant recipients. Dermatol Surg. 2013;39(4):634–45. PubMed PMID: 23379978.
128. Jirakulaporn T, Endrizzi B, Lindgren B, Mathew J, Lee PK, Dudek AZ. Capecitabine for skin cancer prevention in solid organ transplant recipients. Clin Transplant. 2011;25(4):541–8. PubMed PMID: 21050273.
129. Brewer JD, Christenson LJ, Weaver AL, Dapprich DC, Weenig RH, Lim KK, et al. Malignant melanoma in solid transplant recipients: collection of database cases and comparison with surveillance, epidemiology, and end results data for outcome analysis. Arch Dermatol. 2011;147(7):790–6. PubMed PMID: 21768478.
130. Babel N, Eibl N, Ulrich C, Bold G, Sefrin A, Hammer MH, et al. Development of Kaposi's sarcoma under sirolimus-based immunosuppression and successful treatment with imiquimod. Transpl Infect Dis. 2008;10(1):59–62. PubMed PMID: 17428275.
131. Boratynska M, Zmonarski SC, Klinger M. Recurrence of Kaposi's sarcoma after increased exposure to sirolimus. Int Immunopharmacol. 2006;6(13–14):2018–22. PubMed PMID: 17161356.
132. Merkel cell carcinoma. NCCN clinical practice guidelines in oncology (NCCN guidelines): National Comprehensive Cancer Network. 2013. http://www.nccn.org/professionals/physician_gls/pdf/mcc.pdf. Accessed 27 Aug 2013.
133. de Graaf YG, Basdew VR, van Zwan-Kralt N, Willemze R, Bavinck JN. The occurrence of residual or recurrent squamous cell carcinomas in organ transplant recipients after curettage and electrodesiccation. Br J Dermatol. 2006;154(3):493–7. PubMed PMID: 16445781.
134. Brodland DG, Zitelli JA. Surgical margins for excision of primary cutaneous squamous cell carcinoma. J Am Acad Dermatol. 1992;27(2 Pt 1):241–8. PubMed PMID: 1430364.
135. Wolf DJ, Zitelli JA. Surgical margins for basal cell carcinoma. Arch Dermatol. 1987;123(3):340–4. PubMed PMID: 3813602.
136. Hilari H, Llorca D, Traves V, Villanueva A, Serra-Guillen C, Requena C, et al. Conventional surgery compared with slow Mohs micrographic surgery in the treatment of lentigo maligna: a retrospective study of 62 cases. Actas Dermosifiliogr. 2012;103(7): 614–23. PubMed PMID: 22572575.
137. Eskiizmir G, Gencoglan G, Temiz P, Hircin Z, Ermertcan A. Staged-surgery with permanent pathology for the management of high-risk nonmelanoma skin cancer of the nose. Eur Arch Otorhinolaryngol. 2011;268(1):117–21. PubMed PMID: 20614128.
138. Ahmed MM, Moore BA, Schmalbach CE. Utility of head and neck cutaneous squamous cell carcinoma sentinel node biopsy: a systematic review. Otolaryngol Head Neck Surg. 2013. PubMed PMID: 24201060.
139. Ross AS, Schmults CD. Sentinel lymph node biopsy in cutaneous squamous cell carcinoma: a systematic review of the English literature. Dermatol Surg. 2006;32(11):1309–21. PubMed PMID: 17083582.
140. Veness MJ, Palme CE, Smith M, Cakir B, Morgan GJ, Kalnins I. Cutaneous head and neck squamous cell carcinoma metastatic to cervical lymph nodes (nonparotid): a better outcome with surgery and adjuvant radiotherapy. Laryngoscope. 2003;113(10): 1827–33. PubMed PMID: 14520114.
141. Radvansky LJ, Pace MB, Siddiqui A. Prevention and management of radiation-induced dermatitis, mucositis, and xerostomia. Am J Health Syst Pharm. 2013;70(12):1025–32. PubMed PMID: 23719879.

142. Marin-Gutzke M, Sanchez-Olaso A, Berenguer B, Gonzalez B, Rodriguez P, De Salamanca JE, et al. Basal cell carcinoma in childhood after radiation therapy: case report and review. Ann Plast Surg. 2004;53(6):593–5. PubMed PMID: 15602259.
143. Meibodi NT, Maleki M, Javidi Z, Nahidi Y. Clinicopathological evaluation of radiation induced basal cell carcinoma. Indian J Dermatol. 2008;53(3):137–9. PubMed PMID: 19882013, Pubmed Central PMCID: 2763736.
144. Hoogendijk-van den Akker JM, Harden PN, Hoitsma AJ, Proby CM, Wolterbeek R, Bouwes Bavinck JN, et al. Two-year randomized controlled prospective trial converting treatment of stable renal transplant recipients with cutaneous invasive squamous cell carcinomas to sirolimus. J Clin Oncol. 2013;31(10):1317–23. PubMed PMID: 23358973.
145. Bonner JA, Keene KS. Is cetuximab active in patients with cisplatin-refractory squamous cell carcinoma of the head and neck? Nat Clin Pract Oncol. 2007;4(12):690–1. PubMed PMID: 17909551.
146. Bauman JE, Eaton KD, Martins RG. Treatment of recurrent squamous cell carcinoma of the skin with cetuximab. Arch Dermatol. 2007;143(7):889–92. PubMed PMID: 17638733.
147. Read WL. Squamous carcinoma of the skin responding to erlotinib: three cases. J Clin Oncol. 2007;25(18S):16519.

Miscellaneous Drug-related Adverse Effects

19

Punam H. Patel and Krista L. Donohoe

Introduction

Immunosuppressants used in renal transplantation have long been associated with a number of drug-related dermatologic adverse effects. Skin and hair changes have been noted with some of the immunosuppressants. The skin complications range in severity and some may be mild in nature and require no additional treatment or they could even be life-threatening and require immediate medical treatment. For some patients the dermatologic conditions associated with the immunosuppressants are considered to be particularly bothersome and patients have discontinued their immunosuppressants, which has resulted in organ rejection and in some cases death. Cutaneous complications of immunosuppression can be managed effectively by periodic evaluations by a dermatologist [1].

Hypertrichosis

Definition/Physiology/Pathogenesis

Hirsutism is characterized by androgen-dependent excessive growth of terminal hair in women in locations that are more typical of male hair growth patterns (e.g., mustache, beard, central chest, shoulders, lower abdomen, back, inner thigh). Hirsutism may be a marker for an underlying hormonal disorder that produces a state of hyperandrogenemia. Hirsutism should be distinguished from hypertrichosis, which is characterized by the presence of excessive amount of hair in a non-androgen-dependent area. Hypertrichosis may involve lanugo hair, vellus hair, and terminal hair and is classified based on age of onset, extent of distribution, and area affected. Hypertrichosis can occur in patients with systemic illnesses, such as hypothyroidism, anorexia nervosa, malnutrition, porphyria, and dermatomyositis, and as a paraneoplastic syndrome. It can also occur in rare familial disorders called congenital hypertrichosis. Often hypertrichosis is caused by medications, examples of which include phenytoin, penicillamine, diazoxide, minoxidil, and cyclosporine [2, 3].

The etiology of hypertrichosis as a side effect of cyclosporine is not fully understood. It is important to note that the stimulatory effect of cyclosporine on hair follicles is not a result of alteration in endocrine status, since hypertrichosis occurs in female patients without introducing virilization and involves non-androgen-stimulated skin sites [4, 5]. Studies speculate cyclosporine-induced hair growth is at least partially attributed to influence on protein kinase C expression and translocation in hair epithelial cells which promotes proliferation, or hair growth, within these cells [6].

Immunosuppressants Associated with Hypertrichosis

An estimate of the frequency of hypertrichosis in patients treated with cyclosporine after organ transplantation varies from 24 to 94 % and is more common in the pediatric population [4, 7].

In trials with cyclosporine, the frequency is estimated to be 21–45 % [8].

Clinical Presentation

Dose-dependent hypertrichosis in patients treated with cyclosporine can develop within the first 6 months of therapy. Cyclosporine's hair growth-stimulating effect is

P.H. Patel, Pharm.D., B.C.P.S. (✉)
Department of Pharmacy, Euclid Hospital, Cleveland Clinic, 18901 Lake Shore Blvd., Euclid, OH 44119, USA
e-mail: patelp7@ccf.org

K.L. Donohoe, Pharm.D., B.C.P.S., C.G.P.
Department of Pharmacotherapy and Outcomes Science, Virginia Commonwealth University School of Pharmacy, 410 North 12th Street, 980533, Richmond, VA 23298-0533, USA

J.R. Nunley and E.V. Lerma (eds.), *Dermatological Manifestations of Kidney Disease*,
DOI 10.1007/978-1-4939-2395-3_19, © Springer Science+Business Media New York 2015

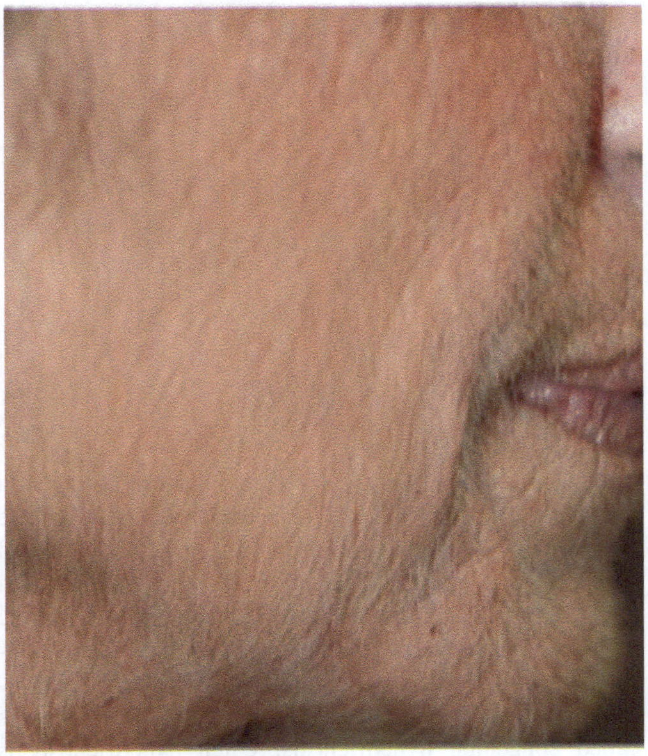

Fig. 19.1 Acquired hypertrichosis lanuginosa. Reprinted from Current Problems in Surgery, 47, Ehst BD, et al. Cutaneous Manifestations of Internal Malignancy, 384–445, 2010, with permission from Elsevier

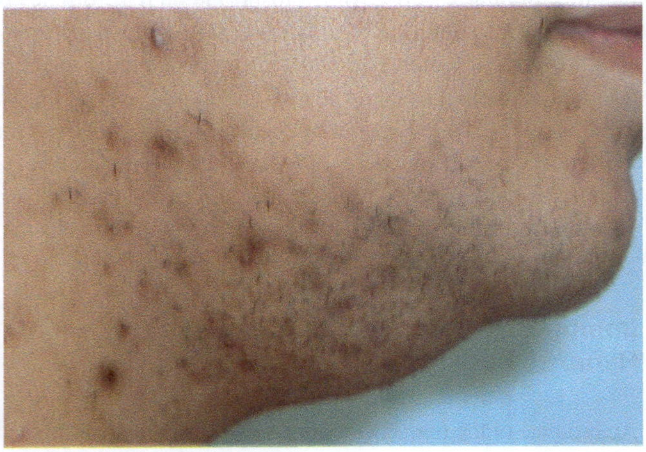

Fig. 19.2 The development of course terminal hairs in a male pattern, in a woman as seen here, is classic for hirsutism. Courtesy of Julia R. Nunley, M.D.

observed not only in normal but also in pathologic conditions of hair growth especially over the face, arms, shoulders, and backs, as seen in Figs. 19.1 and 19.2 [9]. Both male and female patients can develop hypertrichosis with cyclosporine [3, 4, 10–12].

Differential Diagnosis [3]

Acquired Generalized Hypertrichosis:

- Medications
- Malnutrition
- Anorexia nervosa
- Head injury
- Hepatic porphyria
- Hypothyroidism
- Dermatomyositis
- AIDS
- Paraneoplastic hypertrichosis

Workup [13]

An examination of a patient with hypertrichosis should include the following: type of hair involved (e.g., lanugo, vellus, terminal), hair growth pattern, age of onset, history of present or past systemic disorders, medication history, family history, and ethnic and racial background. It must be always kept in mind that hypertrichosis may be a manifestation of a more general medical problem.

Treatment

Hypertrichosis caused by medications, including cyclosporine, is reversible upon discontinuation of the offending agent within several months to 1 year depending on the hair cycling characteristics of the affected site [3]. In the transplant setting, the substitution of a cyclosporine-based regimen with a tacrolimus-based regimen was found to significantly improve hair growth and patient's quality of life without increasing the risk of renal allograft dysfunction or rejection [14–16]. The discontinuation or substitution of cyclosporine with an alternative immunosuppressant should first be discussed with the patient's transplant provider.

In addition, concomitant use of cyclosporine and minoxidil has been reported to augment hypertrichosis and therefore alternate therapy should be considered [17].

There are a number of treatment options for excess hair growth that can be categorized into depilatory or epilatory methods. Depilation is the removal of hair at some point along its shaft, whereas epilation is a process that removes the entire hair shaft. Epilation methods last longer than depilatory methods and may even cause sufficient damage to the follicle to provide long-term or permanent hair removal; however, only destruction of the follicular germ cell will produce permanent hair removal. Individual patient preferences play a role in selecting the most appropriate therapy [3, 18, 19].

Mechanical and chemical depilatory methods are convenient and most widely used, but must repeated often for adequate management of excess hair. Shaving is fast, safe, and effective, but this method is not generally well accepted by adult women for facial hair. Using a pumice stone in the affected area may help remove fine hairs, but can cause irritation and dermatitis with inappropriate use. Two forms of chemical depilatories are available: sulfides of alkali metals and thioglycolate salts. These agents dissolve hair shafts by breaking disulfide bonds. The sulfide preparations are more effective but also more irritating to the skin. Chemical depilatories should be tested on a small area of the skin before widespread use [3, 18, 19].

Epilation, removes hairs down to the hair bulb, and includes tweezing, waxing, and threading. Tweezing or wax epilation of an affected area usually produces good results by removing hairs with the root. Threading is a common technique used in the Middle East which involves a twisted string run rapidly over a hair-bearing area, removing hairs along with it. All of these techniques can cause mild to moderate pain [3, 18, 19].

More permanent methods of hair removal include electrolysis, laser epilation, and photoepilation. Electrolysis, either galvanic or thermal, is painful and time-consuming because each hair follicle needs to be individually targeted. For this reason, electrolysis is a good option only for treating small areas of skin. Laser therapy, which is more expensive, is less painful, faster, and more effective than electrolysis. However, a recent Cochrane review of hair removal methods found little evidence of their effectiveness [20]. Alexandrite and diode lasers reduced hair by approximately 50% up to 6 months after treatment. Less evidence is available for short-term effects of pulsed light, neodymium:yttrium-aluminum-garnet (Nd:YAG), and ruby lasers, and none of these treatments have well-documented long-term outcomes. Laser therapy works best on dark hair but posttreatment hyperpigmentation may occur.

Since most drug-mediated cases of hypertrichosis are not androgen-mediated, antiandrogen therapies may be minimally helpful. Eflornithine (Vaniqa™) is a topical agent that reduces hair growth through inhibition of the enzyme ornithine decarboxylase that is present in hair follicles and important in hair growth. When used for excess facial hair, results are noticed in about 8 weeks. Eflornithine can be used alone or in conjunction with other therapies; side effects include stinging, burning, tingling, and erythema. Hair growth resumes upon discontinuation of eflornithine [21].

Gingival Hyperplasia

Definition/Physiology/Pathogenesis

Gingival hyperplasia is an increase in the size, or growth, of the gingiva. Overgrowth of the gingiva can be caused by a number of factors, including inflammatory conditions and as a side effect of certain medications. Gingival hyperplasia caused by medications is often referred to as drug-induced gingival overgrowth (GO) or gingival enlargement [22]. The use of cyclosporine and calcium channel blockers such as nifedipine, verapamil, amlodipine, and anticonvulsants have been reported to contribute to GO [23].

Though the pathophysiology of drug-induced GO is not completely understood, it is believed to be multifactorial. Studies have shown that the interaction of phenytoin, cyclosporine, and nifedipine with epithelial keratinocytes, fibroblasts, and collagen can lead to GO in susceptible individuals. Both genetic and cellular mechanisms of cyclosporine GO have been proposed. Studies suggest that cyclosporine increases the number of gingival fibroblasts; on the contrary other studies suggest that cyclosporine increases interleukin (IL)-6, a cytokine that inhibits fibroblast proliferation. In fact, IL-6 is known to enhance collagen and glycosaminoglycan synthesis [24, 25]. Additionally, fibroblasts from cyclosporine GO have shown reduced phagocytic activity; therefore an increased rate of synthesis paired with a decreased rate of phagocytosis could result in the increase in connective tissue volume [26]. Recent studies suggest that genetic polymorphisms may also be involved in determining susceptibility to GO caused by this medication [27, 28].

A variety of risk factors may also contribute to the severity of GO caused by cyclosporine. The presence of gingivitis, or gingival inflammation, resulting from poor oral hygiene is a significant factor and can exacerbate the effect of medications [22]. Children and teenagers on cyclosporine are at an increased risk, which suggests a hormonal component. In this population there are higher circulating levels of androgens, and this can have a stimulating effect on gingival fibroblasts to increase collagen synthesis [29]. Males are three times more likely to develop overgrowth compared to females [22]. The relationship between cyclosporine serum concentrations, dosage, and gingival enlargement is controversial. A variety of pharmacokinetic parameters have been investigated with inconsistent findings and, as such, are considered poor prognostic indictors for GO. In spite of these shortcomings, there is a general agreement that an initial, unidentified, threshold serum concentration is required to initiate the overgrowth process [29, 30]. Frequently, patients on cyclosporine are also on concomitant calcium channel blocker therapy that increases the prevalence of GO significantly [30].

Immunosuppressants Associated with Gingival Hyperplasia

GO is a well-documented side effect of cyclosporine. The reported prevalence ranges from 25 to 30 % in transplant recipients. However, these numbers should be interpreted

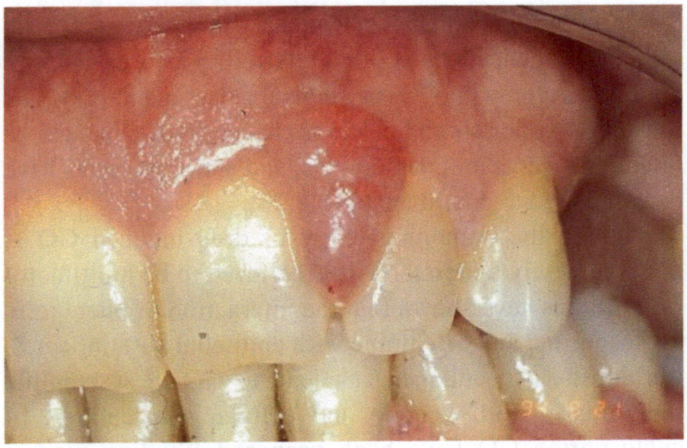

Fig. 19.3 Gingival hyperplasia

with caution as many transplant recipients are also on calcium channel blockers [22, 30].

Clinical Features

The onset of cyclosporine GO generally appears within the first 3 months of drug administration [31]. The growth starts in the interdental papillae and extends to the facial and lingual aspects of the gingival margin, as seen in Fig. 19.3 [32]. The appearance of GO in patients on cyclosporine often presents with a more vascularized, lobulated, inflamed gingiva that bleeds easily compared to GO caused by other medications [33]. The enlargement may become a massive amount of tissue that covers the crowns of the teeth and can interfere with mastication, speech, esthetics, and can lead to shifting of teeth and malocclusion. Gingival enlargement can also complicate the patient's oral hygiene and the patient ability to clean the teeth, thus increasing the inflammatory process and in return further increasing GO [22].

Differential Diagnosis [13]

- Generalized gingivitis
- Pregnancy gingivitis
- Puberty gingivitis
- Pyogenic granuloma
- Leukemia

Workup [34]

Periapical or panorex radiographs are indicated prior to treatment to evaluate the status of the periodontal tissue or any compromised teeth. Complete blood count (CBC) with platelet count is indicated in patients with severe gum bleeding to rule out anemia and leukemia. Culture is recommended to rule out oral candidiasis. Tissue biopsy may be indicated if GO has an unusual clinical presentation or if the patient is not on a medication known to induce GO.

Treatment

Oral hygiene and plaque control combined with the removal of local factors are essential for any patient taking drugs associated with gingival enlargement. While excellent oral hygiene and professional plaque control can potentially prevent or lessen the severity of the condition, they often are insufficient for reversing the process once established [23].

The most effective treatment is the withdrawal of the causative medication and substitution with others. Evidence suggests that GO may resolve in 1–8 weeks in some patients with drug substitution or withdrawal [35]. In the transplant setting, the substitution of a cyclosporine-based regimen with a tacrolimus-based regimen was found to significantly improve gingival hyperplasia without increasing the risk of renal allograft dysfunction or rejection [16]. The discontinuation or substitution of cyclosporine with an alternative immunosuppressant should first be discussed with the patient's transplant provider.

If cyclosporine substitution is not an option, case reports suggest that the gingival hyperplasia can be effectively treated with a 2-week course of metronidazole (750 mg three times per day) while cyclosporine is continued [36, 37]. It is not clear if metronidazole acts in this setting via its antibacterial activity or via another mechanism. Treatment with azithromycin (500 mg per day for 3 consecutive days) may also be effective, particularly among those with mild or early disease [38].

While nonsurgical therapy and, if possible, drug substitutions should be attempted first, surgical or laser gingivectomy may be required. However if the offending agent is not discontinued, recurrence of GO can ensue, requiring additional surgical procedures [39].

Sebaceous Gland Hyperplasia

Definition/Physiology/Pathogenesis

Sebaceous hyperplasia (SH) is an enlargement of sebaceous glands surrounding a follicle.

In general SH is a well-recognized benign condition in older adults. The causative factors include intrinsic and photoaging, accompanied by reduced androgen levels leading to decreased cellular turnover in sebaceous glands, resulting in hyperplasia [40, 41].

Sebaceous hyperplasia is also possible in other populations, though less common. Premature or familial cases of SH have been reported in younger individuals, suggesting a genetic predisposition [42–44]. Muir-Torre syndrome (MTS) is a rare autosomal dominant disorder in which sebaceous neoplasms have been reported in association with a visceral malignancy, usually gastrointestinal or genitourinary carcinomas [45]. Sebaceous hyperplasia has also been linked to transplant recipients taking cyclosporine, though the mechanism is poorly understood. Since cyclosporine is highly lipophilic, it has been suggested that the sebaceous gland may be the major site of cutaneous accumulation leading to hyperproliferation and arrest of sebocytes causing SH. Genetics and hormones may also influence the development of SH caused by cyclosporine as case reports only include male patients [41, 46, 47].

Immunosuppressants Associated with Sebaceous Hyperplasia

Sebaceous hyperplasia is a common skin finding in aging adults, reported to occur in approximately 1 % of the healthy population. In case reports, however, the prevalence of SH has been reported to be as high as 10–16 % in patients receiving long-term immunosuppression with cyclosporine [46, 48, 49].

Clinical Presentation

Sebaceous hyperplasia consists of asymptomatic, small flesh-colored to yellow papules with central depression from which a very small amount of sebum can sometimes be expressed, as seen in Fig. 19.4 [50]. The nose, cheeks, and forehead are primarily affected; however very rarely SH can occur on the chest, areola, mouth, scrotum, foreskin, penile shaft, and vulva. Sebaceous hyperplasia appears at higher frequencies after 40–50 years of age and increases in prevalence over time. It is important to note that SH alone does not signify a predisposition to cancer or represent a sign of MTS [40, 51–54].

Cyclosporine can induce SH over an expansive time period, with a clinical presentation ranging from 3 to 19 years of cyclosporine use. In case reports those patients with cyclosporine-induced SH were all male, suggesting a possible genetic and hormonal basis to the development of SH after organ transplant [41, 42, 47]. A recent study found 45.7 % of renal transplant patients with SH to have a history of nonmelanoma skin cancer compared to only 7.3 % of patients without SH. This strong association of nonmelanoma skin cancer with SH remained significant after correction of factors such as age, sex, skin type, and duration since the transplantation [55].

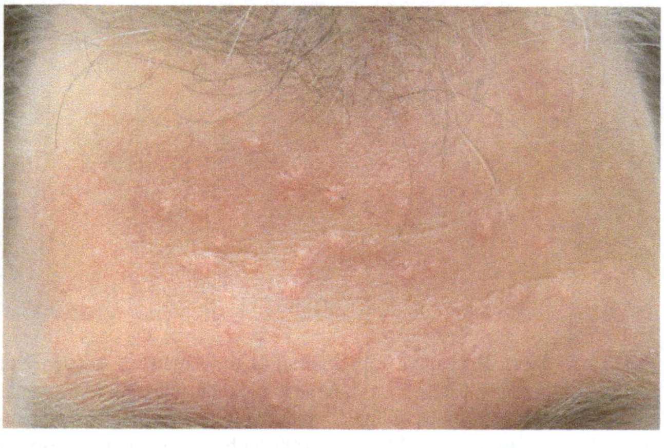

Fig. 19.4 Sebaceous hyperplasia. Courtesy of Julia R. Nunley, M.D.

Differential Diagnosis [2]

- Basal cell carcinoma
- Other sebaceous gland tumors

Workup

Dermoscopy may be useful as a noninvasive tool to aid in the clinical diagnosis and in distinguishing between nodular basal cell carcinoma and sebaceous hyperplasia, reducing unnecessary surgery [56].

Treatment

Sebaceous hyperplasia is completely benign and does not require treatment; however, lesions can be cosmetically bothersome. Treatments are mostly mechanical. Lesions tend to recur unless the entire unit is destroyed or excised. Risk of permanent scarring must be considered when treating benign lesions. The following therapies have been reported to be somewhat effective: photodynamic therapy, cryotherapy, electrodessication, topical chemical treatments (e.g., bichloracetic or trichloroacetic acid), laser treatment (e.g., argon, carbon dioxide, pulse-dye laser), shave excision, and excision [57–60].

Oral isotretinoin can be effective for the treatment of SH because of its ability to temporarily shrink sebaceous glands. Patients with diffuse multiple lesions, including those on cyclosporine therapy, had clearing after 2–6 weeks of treatment. Doses of 10–40 mg every other day can be used. Upon discontinuation of therapy, SH lesions will reoccur. Oral isotretinoin should be taken with extreme caution; this medication is pregnancy category X and is known to cause major fetal abnormalities [43, 46, 61]. In the United States access to this medication is restricted. All patients (male and female), prescribers, wholesalers, and dispensing pharmacists must register and be active in the iPLEDGE™ risk management program, designed to eliminate fetal exposures to isotretinoin. This program covers all isotretinoin products (brand and generic). The iPLEDGE™ program requires that all patients meet qualification criteria and monthly program requirements (e.g., pregnancy testing). Healthcare providers can only prescribe a maximum 30-day supply at each monthly visit and must counsel patients on the iPLEDGE™ program requirements and confirm counseling via the iPLEDGE™ automated system [62].

Acneiform Eruptions/Acne

Definition/Physiology/Pathogenesis

Acne is one of the most common pustular skin conditions [63]. Androgen production after puberty stimulates the release of sebum by the sebaceous glands; if the flow of sebum is impeded due to abnormal keratinization in the pilosebaceous canal, it can lead to the formation of comedones [2, 63]. Inflammation, bacterial overgrowth or infection can result in papules, pustules, and cysts [63, 64].

Sirolimus-induced acne may be due to direct toxic effects on follicles or its chemical toxic modification of sebum [65]. The most likely explanation is that sirolimus inhibits the epidermal growth factor (EGF) pathway which may lead to cutaneous toxicities [65].

Immunosuppressants Associated with Acne

Acne is reported in 2–15 % of organ transplant recipients [66]. It is usually associated with steroid and cyclosporine use; however, it has been reported with several of the immunosuppressants [66]. In a study of 80 patients, the frequency of acne in prednisolone and cyclosporine-treated patients was reported to be 36 % [67].

In sirolimus trials the frequency of acne is estimated to be 15–25 % and is listed at 22 % in the package insert [66, 68]. In a study of cutaneous adverse events in 80 renal transplant patients receiving sirolimus-based therapy, 46 % of patients experienced acne-like eruptions [66]. The skin eruptions occurred soon after initiating sirolimus (median: 1 month); they were more common in men than women, possibly suggesting a hormonal role for this adverse effect [66].

Everolimus has been reported to cause acne in ≥1 to <10 % of kidney and liver transplant patients; however, data in kidney transplant patients includes everolimus in combination with basiliximab, cyclosporine (at reduced doses), and corticosteroids [69]. In a study of everolimus versus placebo in autosomal dominant polycystic kidney disease, acne was reported in 14 % of patients with everolimus compared to 2.8 % of placebo patients [70]. Compared to placebo, basiliximab-treated patients experienced ≥10 % of skin adverse effects, including acne [71].

Two randomized, active-controlled 3-year trials of belatacept in *de novo* kidney transplant patients where belatacept was used in combination with basiliximab induction, mycophenolate mofetil, and corticosteroids reported an 8 % incidence of acne [72]. In clinical trials of patients treated with tacrolimus for either liver, kidney, and/or heart transplant recipients, the incidence of acne was reported to be >3 % and <15 % [73]. In patients treated with mycophenolate mofetil in combination with cyclosporine and corticosteroids, the incidence of acne is reported to be 3 to <20 % [74]. It is difficult to differentiate the true incidence for specific drugs in drug-induced acne when immunosuppressants are studied in combination.

Clinical Features

In the study of 80 sirolimus patients, acne was generally found on the face and trunk and in 21 of the 37 cases combined with scalp folliculitis [65]. Comedones and cysts were present in 21 % of the acneiform eruptions; however, inflammatory components like papules and pustules were observed in 95 % of patients who had acneiform eruptions [65]. Nine patients had painful nodular cervical acne [65]. The lesion locations, clinical, bacteriologic, and histologic features were different in the sirolimus-treated patients from acne vulgaris, as seen in Fig. 19.5 [65].

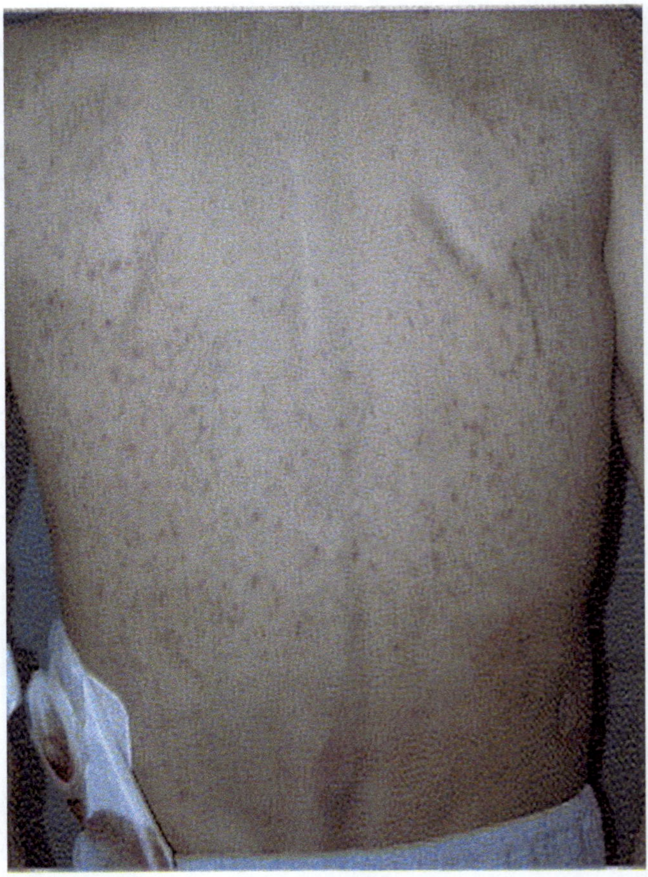

Fig. 19.5 Acne. Reprinted from Journal of the American Academy of Dermatology, 55(1), Mahe E, et al. Acne in recipients of renal transplantation treated with sirolimus: Clinical, microbiologic, histologic, therapeutic, and pathogenic aspects, 139–132, 2006, with permission from Elsevier

Steroid-induced acne may occur 2–5 weeks after starting oral corticosteroids and appears suddenly as follicular pustules and papules. This is different than acne vulgaris as the lesions are uniform in size, symmetric in distribution, and located on the neck, chest, and back. The papules and pustules are usually 1 to 3 mm in size, flesh or pink-to-red in color, and dome shaped [2].

Differential Diagnosis [2, 64]

- Comedonal acne
- Inflammatory acne
- Nodulocystic acne
- Cystic acne
- Pyoderma faciale
- Acne fulminans
- Acne conglobata
- Gram-negative acne
- Acne mechanica
- Acne cosmetic
- Occupational acne
- Excoriated acne
- Senile comedones
- Solid facial edema
- Milia
- Rosacea
- Folliculitis

Workup [64]

The diagnosis of acne is based upon the clinical presentation and examination of the skin. Evaluation of the skin condition should include obtaining a history of current and previous treatments, cosmetics, and all systemic medications.

Treatment

Although drug-induced acne varies from acne vulgaris, therapy management is similar [65]. Mild forms may be treated with topical benzoyl peroxide, a retinoid, or an antibiotic [63, 65]. More severe forms may be treated with an oral antibiotic such as doxycycline [63, 65]. For cystic type acne, isotretinoin may help decrease sebaceous gland size and sebum production, but it is teratogenic and is associated with a possible risk of depression as well as other side effects [63, 65]. In severe treatment-resistant cases of acne, in which medications like isotretinoin fail, discontinuation of the immunosuppressant may be considered [65, 75]. Steroid-induced acne may respond to topical therapy with benzoyl peroxide and/or sulfacetamide/sulfur lotion [2]. The acne should clear up when the steroid is discontinued [2].

Folliculitis

Definition/Physiology/Pathogenesis

Folliculitis is generally caused by a bacterial infection of a hair follicle [2]. It is a superficial inflammation of the epidermis [64, 76]. The most common cause of folliculitis is *Staphylococcus aureus* [2, 75]. *Pseudomonas aeruginosa* folliculitis may be acquired from hot tubs or swimming pools [64].

Immunocompromised individuals, like solid organ transplant patients, are at risk of developing folliculitis due to the inability to fight off infections [63]. Other risk factors include diabetes mellitus and obesity [63].

Immunosuppressants Associated with Folliculitis

Everolimus may cause folliculitis in ≥1 to <10 % of kidney and liver transplant patients; however, data in kidney transplant patients includes everolimus in combination with basiliximab, cyclosporine (at reduced doses), and corticosteroids [69]. Cyclosporine is indicated for use in kidney, liver, and heart transplantation, rheumatoid arthritis, and psoriasis [8]. Folliculitis was reported to occur in 1 to <3 % of patients using cyclosporine for rheumatoid arthritis and psoriasis but not specifically defined in the package insert for transplant patients. In renal transplant patients using Sandimmune® (cyclosporine), there was an incidence of 7 % for wound and skin infections [8]. In a study of 80 renal transplant patients receiving sirolimus, chronic skin folliculitis was reported to occur in 14 % of patients, while 26 % patients developed scalp folliculitis [66]. Scalp folliculitis only developed in male patients who also had acne-like eruptions [66]. Furuncles were reported in 11 % of the transplant patients using sirolimus in the study [66].

Clinical Features

Folliculitis is characterized by erythematous, follicular-based papules, and pustules. Folliculitis is generally asymptomatic but may cause pain or pruritus [64, 77]. Typically, the scalp, thighs, trunk, axilla, and inguinal areas are affected [63]. The infection can extend deeper into the dermis and form a larger erythematous nodule (furuncle) or many (carbuncles) [63]. Rupture of the furuncles may occur and pus and necrotic tissue may be discharged [64].

Differential Diagnosis [63, 76]

- Staphylococcal folliculitis
- Pseudofolliculitis barbae

- Superficial fungal infections
- Cutaneous candidiasis
- Acne
- Keratosis pilaris
- Pseudomonas folliculitis
- Eosinophilic pustular folliculitis
- Pityrosporum folliculitis
- Carbuncles or furuncles

Workup

The diagnosis of folliculitis is based upon the clinical presentation, examination of the skin, and confirmed by culture [64]. Follicular pustules may be cultured by scraping off the pustule with a number 15 blade and placing the entire pustule onto a cotton swab of a transport medium kit [2].

Treatment

Treatment depends upon the type and the severity of folliculitis. In mild cases of folliculitis a topical antibiotic such as clindamycin 1 % or erythromycin 2 % applied two or three times a day to affected areas with an antibacterial soap may be used [63, 64]. A warm compress may be applied three to four times a day for 15–20 minutes if desired [64]. If facial hair is involved, shaving should be avoided until the affected area heals [76]. Antistaphylococcal oral antibiotics, such as cephalexin, may be warranted if there is extensive cutaneous involvement [63]. If the folliculitis is caused by *P. aeruginosa*, ciprofloxacin 500 mg twice daily for 10–14 days will cure the infection [63].

Conclusion

Immunosuppressive therapy with renal transplantation is associated with various skin complications [78]. Quality of life can be significantly impaired in renal transplant recipients especially in patients with visible, infectious or cosmetic skin problems like sebaceous gland hyperplasia and acne [78]. Early referral of patients who experience skin manifestations to a dermatologist may enhance patient's quality of life [78]. If dermatologic manifestations are a concern, then the choice of immunosuppressive agents should also be considered [78].

References

1. Koranda KC, Dehmel EM, Kahn G, Penn I. Cutaneous complications in immunosuppressed renal homograft recipients. JAMA. 1974;229:419–24.
2. Habif TP, editor. Clinical dermatology: a color guide to diagnosis and therapy. 5th ed. Edinburgh: Mosby Elsevier; 2009.
3. Trüeb RM. Causes and management of hypertrichosis. Am J Clin Dermatol. 2002;3(9):617–27.
4. Wysocki GP, Daley TD. Hypertrichosis in patients receiving cyclosporine therapy. Clin Exp Dermatol. 1987;12(3):191–6.
5. Kanitakis J, Thivolet J. Cyclosporine. An immunosuppressant affecting epithelial cell proliferation. Arch Dermatol. 1990;126(3):369–75.
6. Takahashi T, Kamimura A. Cyclosporin A promotes hair epithelial cell proliferation and modulates protein kinase C expression and translocation in hair epithelial cells. J Invest Dermatol. 2001;117(3):605–11.
7. Ghio L, Tarantino A, Edefonti A, Mocciaro A, Giani M, Guerra L, Berardinelli L, Vegeto A. Advantages of cyclosporine as sole immunosuppressive agent in children with transplanted kidneys. Transplantation. 1992;54(5):834–8.
8. Neoral [package insert]. East Hanover, New Jersey: Novartis Pharmaceuticals Corporation; 2013. T2013-38.
9. Silva JA, Mesquita Kde C, Igreja AC, Lucas IC, Freitas AF, Oliveira SM, Costa IM, Campbell IT. Paraneoplastic cutaneous manifestations: concepts and updates. An Bras Dermatol. 2013; 88(1):9–22.
10. Yamamoto S, Jiang H, Kato R. Stimulation of hair growth by topical application of FK506, a potent immunosuppressive agent. J Invest Dermatol. 1994;102(2):160–4.
11. Kahan BD, Flechner SM, Lorber MI, Golden D, Conley S, Van Buren CT. Complications of cyclosporine-prednisone immunosuppression in 402 renal allograft recipients exclusively followed at a single center for from one to five years. Transplantation. 1987; 43(2):197–204.
12. Bencini PL, Montagnino G, Sala F, De Vecchi A, Crosti C, Tarantino A. Cutaneous lesions in 67 cyclosporin-treated renal transplant recipients. Dermatologica. 1986;172(1):24–30.
13. Valia RG. Hypertrichosis. Indian J Dermatol. 2005;50:119–24.
14. Franke GH, Trampenau C, Reimer J. Switching from cyclosporine to tacrolimus leads to improved disease-specific quality of life in patients after kidney transplantation. Transplant Proc. 2006;38(5):1293–4.
15. Fernando ON, Sweny P, Varghese Z. Elective conversion of patients from cyclosporine to tacrolimus for hypertrichosis. Transplant Proc. 1998;30(4):1243–4.
16. Thorp M, DeMattos A, Bennett W, Barry J, Norman D. The effect of conversion from cyclosporine to tacrolimus on gingival hyperplasia, hirsutism and cholesterol. Transplantation. 2000;69(6): 1218–20.
17. Bennett WM, Serra J, Fischer S, Norman DJ, Barry JM. Cyclosporine in renal transplantation with hirsutism. Am J Kidney Dis. 1985;5(3):214.
18. Wendelin DS, Pope DN, Mallory SB. Hypertrichosis. J Am Acad Dermatol. 2003;48(2):161–79.
19. Bode D, Seehusen DA, Baird D. Hirsutism in women. Am Fam Physician. 2012;85(4):373–80.
20. Haedersdal M, Gøtzsche PC. Laser and photoepilation for unwanted hair growth. Cochrane Database Syst Rev. 2006;4:CD004684.
21. Vaniqa [package insert]. Irvine, California: Allergan, Inc.; 2013.
22. Dongari-Bagtzoglou A. Drug-associated gingival enlargement. J Periodontol. 2004;75(10):1424–31.
23. Hood KA. Drug-induced gingival hyperplasia in transplants recipients. Prog Transplant. 2002;12(1):17–21.
24. Tipton DA, Stricklin GP. Fibroblast heterogeneity in collagenolytic response to cyclosporine. J Cell Biochem. 1991;46:152–65.
25. Morton RS, Dongari-Bagtzoglou AI. Regulation of gingival fibroblast interleukin-6 secretion by cyclosporine A. J Periodontol. 1999;70:1464–71.
26. McCulloch CA, Knowles GC. Deficiencies in collagen phagocytosis by human fibroblasts in vitro: a mechanism for fibrosis? J Cell Physiol. 1993;155:461–71.

27. García M, Macías RM, Cubero JJ, Benítez J, Caravaca F, Gervasini G. ABCB1 polymorphisms are associated with cyclosporine-induced nephrotoxicity and gingival hyperplasia in renal transplant recipients. Eur J Clin Pharmacol. 2013;69(3):385–93.
28. Pernu HE, Knuuttila ML, Huttunen KR, Tiilikainen AS. Drug-induced gingival overgrowth and class II major histocompatibility antigens. Transplantation. 1994;57(12):1811–3.
29. Seymore RA, Jacobs DJ. Cyclosporine and gingival tissues. J Clin Periodontol. 1992;19(1):1–11.
30. Somacarrera ML, Hernandez G, Acero J, Moskow BS. Factors related to the incidence and severity of cyclosporin-induced gingival overgrowth in transplant patients. A longitudinal study. J Periodontol. 1994;65(7):671–5.
31. Hallmon WW, Rossman JA. The role of drugs in the pathogenesis of gingival overgrowth. A collective review of current concepts. Periodontol 2000. 1999;21:176–96.
32. Ballini A, Scattarella A, Crincoli V, Carlaio RG, Papa F, Perillo L, et al. Surgical treatment of gingival overgrowth with 10 years of follow-up. Head Face Med. 2010;6:19. Published online 12, 2010. doi:1186/1746-160X-6-19. PMCID: PMC2931464
33. Seymore RA, Heasman PA. Drugs and the periodontium. J Clin Periodontol. 1988;15(1):1–16.
34. Gonsalves WC, Usatine RP. Gingival hyperplasia. In: Usatine RP, Smith MA, Chumley H, Mayeaux Jr E, Tysinger J, editors. The color atlas of family medicine. New York: McGraw-Hill; 2009. Chapter 39. http://www.accessmedicine.com/content.aspx?aID=8201779. Accessed 22 Aug 2013.
35. Wynn RL. Calcium channel blockers and gingival hyperplasia. Gen Dent. 1991;39(4):240–3.
36. Wong W, Hodge MG, Lewis A, Sharpstone P, Kingswood JC. Resolution of cyclosporin-induced gingival hypertrophy with metronidazole. Lancet. 1994;343(8903):986.
37. Cecchin E, Zanello F, De Marchi S. Treatment of cyclosporine-induced gingival hypertrophy. Ann Intern Med. 1997;126(5):409–10.
38. Gómez E, Sánchez-Nuñez M, Sánchez JE, Corte C, Aguado S, Portal C, et al. Treatment of cyclosporin-induced gingival hyperplasia with azithromycin. Nephrol Dial Transplant. 1997;12:2694–7.
39. Mavrogiannis M, Ellis JS, Thomason JM, Seymour RA. The management of drug-induced gingival overgrowth. J Clin Periodontol. 2006;33(6):434–9.
40. Eisen DB, Michael DJ. Sebaceous lesions and their associated syndromes: part I. J Am Acad Dermatol. 2009;61(4):549–60. quiz 561–2.
41. Pang SM, Chau YP. Cyclosporin-induced sebaceous hyperplasia in renal transplant patients. Ann Acad Med Singapore. 2005;34(5):391–3.
42. Dupre A, Bonafe JL, Lamon P. Functional familial sebaceous hyperplasia of the face and premature sebaceous gland hyperplasia: a new and unique entity. J Am Acad Dermatol. 1983;9(5):768–9.
43. Grimalt R, Ferrando J, Mascaro JM. Premature familial sebaceous hyperplasia: successful response to oral isotretinoin in three patients. J Am Acad Dermatol. 1997;37(6):996–8.
44. Wang Q, Liu JM, Zhang YZ. Premature sebaceous hyperplasia in an adolescent boy. Pediatr Dermatol. 2011;28(2):198–200.
45. Johnson PJ, Heckler F. Muir-Torre syndrome. Ann Plast Surg. 1998;40(6):676–7.
46. McDonald SK, Goh MS, Chong AH. Successful treatment of cyclosporine-induced sebaceous hyperplasia with oral isotretinoin in two renal transplant recipients. Australas J Dermatol. 2011;52(3):227–30.
47. de Berker DA, Taylor AE, Quinn AG, Simpson NB. Sebaceous hyperplasia in organ transplant recipients: shared aspects of hyperplastic and dysplastic processes? J Am Acad Dermatol. 1996;35 (5 Pt 1):696–9.
48. Boschnakow A, May T, Assaf C, Tebbe B, Zouboulis CC. Ciclosporin A-induced sebaceous gland hyperplasia. Br J Dermatol. 2003;149(1):198–200.
49. Engel F, Ellero B, Woehl-Jaegle ML, Cribier B. Diffuse sebaceous hyperplasia of the face induced by cyclosporine. Ann Dermatol Venereol. 2005;132(4):342–5.
50. Zakko L, Finch J, Rothe MJ, Grant-Kels JM. Atlas of dermatological manifestations of gastrointestinal disease. 1st ed. New York: Springer Science + Business Media; 2013.
51. Ma HJ, Zhao G, Wang YX. Sebaceous hyperplasia of the scrotum in an adolescent boy. Pediatr Dermatol. 2007;24(3):340–2.
52. Ena P, Origa D, Massarelli G. Sebaceous gland hyperplasia of the foreskin. Clin Exp Dermatol. 2009;34(3):372–4.
53. Ju HY, Kim HS, Kim HO, Park YM. Sebaceous hyperplasia of the penile shaft. J Eur Acad Dermatol Venereol. 2009;23(4):443–4.
54. Malliah R, Gilhooly P, Lambert WC, Heller DS. Sebaceous hyperplasia of the vulva: case report and review of the literature. J Low Genit Tract Dis. 2006;10(1):55–7.
55. Salim A, Reece SM, Smith AG, Harrison D, Ramsay HM, Harden PN, et al. Sebaceous hyperplasia and skin cancer in patients undergoing renal transplant. J Am Acad Dermatol. 2006;55(5):878–81.
56. Zaballos P, Ara M, Puig S, Malvehy J. Dermoscopy of sebaceous hyperplasia. Arch Dermatol. 2005;141(6):808.
57. Alexiades-Armenakas M. Laser-mediated photodynamic therapy. Clin Dermatol. 2006;24(1):16–25.
58. Horio T, Horio O, Miyauchi-Hashimoto H, Ohnuki M, Isei T. Photodynamic therapy of sebaceous hyperplasia with topical 5-aminolaevulinic acid and slide projector. Br J Dermatol. 2003;148(6):1274–6.
59. Rosian R, Goslen JB, Brodell RT. The treatment of benign sebaceous hyperplasia with the topical application of bichloracetic acid. J Dermatol Surg Oncol. 1991;17(11):876–9.
60. Walther T, Hohenleutner U, Landthaler M. Sebaceous gland hyperplasia as a side effect of cyclosporin A. Treatment with the CO_2 laser. Dtsch Med Wochenschr. 1998;123(25–26):798–800.
61. Yu C, Shahsavari M, Stevens G, Liskanich R, Horowitz D. Isotretinoin as monotherapy for sebaceous hyperplasia. J Drugs Dermatol. 2010;9(6):699–701.
62. ipledgeprogram.com [Internet]. (2005). https://www.ipledgeprogram.com/AboutiPLEDGE.aspx. Accessed 27 Aug 2013
63. Goldman L, Schafer AI. Goldman's cecil medicine. 24th ed. Philadelphia: Saunders; 2012.
64. Cevasco NC, Tomecki KJ. Bacterial infections. In: Cleveland clinic: current clinical medicine. 2nd ed. Philadelphia. 2010; pp 318–9 http://www.clevelandclinicmeded.com/medicalpubs/diseasemanagement/dermatology/common-skin-infections/.
65. Mahe E, Morelon E, Lechaton S, Drappier JC, de Prost Y, Kreis H, et al. Acne in recipients of renal transplantation treated with sirolimus: clinical, microbiologic, histologic, therapeutic, and pathogenic aspects. J Am Acad Dermatol. 2006;55(1):139–42.
66. Mahe E, Morelon E, Lechaton S, Sang KH, Mansouri R, Ducasse MF, et al. Cutaneous adverse events in renal transplant recipients receiving sirolimus-based therapy. Transplantation. 2005;79:476–82.
67. Seckin D, Gulec TO, Demirag A, Bilgin N. Renal transplantation and skin diseases. Transplant Proc. 1998;30:802–4.
68. Rapamune [package insert]. Philadelphia, Pennsylvania: Wyeth Pharmaceuticals; 2011. LAB-0579-1.0.
69. Zortress [package insert]. Stein, Switzerland: Novartis Pharma Stein AG; 2013. T2013-09/T2013-10.
70. Walz G, Budde K, Mannaa M, Nurnberger J, Wanner C, Sommerer C, et al. Everolimus in patients with autosomal dominant polycystic kidney disease. N Engl J Med. 2010;363:830–40.
71. Simulect [package insert]. East Hanover, New Jersey: Novartis; 2005. T2005-28 2027722.
72. Nulojix [package insert]. Princeton, New Jersey: Bristol-Myers Squibb; 2013. 721US13PBS00201.
73. Prograf [package insert]. Northbrook, Illinois: Astellas Pharma US, Inc.; 2012. 12A001-PRG-WPI.

74. CellCept [package insert]. San Francisco, California: Genentech, Inc.; 2012. CTCTIO_1061443_PI/MG_2011_02_K.
75. el-Shahawy MA, Gadallah MF, Massry SG. Acne: a potential side effect of cyclosporine A therapy. Nephron. 1996;72(4):679–82.
76. Stevens DL, Bisno AL, Chambers HF, Everett ED, Dellinger P, Goldstein EJ, et al. Practice guidelines for the diagnosis and management of skin and soft-tissue infections. Clin Infect Dis. 2005;41:1373.
77. http://commons.wikimedia.org/wiki/File:Folliculitis_at_the_back_of_hair_scalp_which_also_spread_to_upper_part_of_the_back_body.jpeg. [IMAGE].
78. Moloney FJ, Keane S, O'Kelly P, Conlon PJ, Murphy GM. The impact of skin disease following renal transplantation on quality of life. Br J Dermatol. 2005;153:574–8.

Drug Dosing in Patients with Chronic Kidney Disease and Dermatological Diseases

20

Ali J. Olyaei and Edgar V. Lerma

Introduction

Chronic kidney disease (CKD) affects approximately 26 million adults in the United States [1]. With the incidence of CKD anticipated to increase in conjunction with growing chronic disease trends, early disease detection, and aggressive management are necessary for improving this public health crisis [2]. According to the National Kidney Foundation (NKF) [1], CKD is defined as the presence of kidney damage or glomerular filtration rate (GFR) less than 60 mL/min/1.73 m^2 for 3 or more months. The two main causes of CKD in adults are diabetes and hypertension, with cardiovascular disease the leading cause of death in the CKD population [3]. Dermatological disorders are common among CKD population and dosage adjustment for systemically administered medications is a challenge. Peripheral edema or any damage to skin and soft tissue may alter absorption of many topical agents.

CKD populations are at greater risk of adverse drug reactions and some drugs such as methotrexate (MTX) may result in susceptibility to adverse drug and disease interactions [4]. The kidney plays important role in the pharmacokinetic properties of most drugs; drug absorption, distribution, metabolism, and excretion processes. Subsequently, medication-related errors (under-dose or over-dose) in patients with CKD have led to increases in morbidity and mortality, as well as rising healthcare cost [5, 6]. Failure to properly adjust medications in patients diagnosed with varying stages of CKD may result in harm [7]. Therefore, healthcare professionals must always review patient medications and assess kidney function prior to initiating or modifying pharmacological therapy to ensure patient safety and appropriately delay disease progression. For some agents such as MTX, laboratory and diagnostic monitoring should be performed routinely to avoid toxicities, and in high-risk patients, or patients with abnormal tests results, health care providers should be mindful more monitoring (Table 20.1).

Renal impairment alters the pharmacokinetics of drugs and metabolites requiring drug dosing adjustments. Decreased clearance has been observed for drugs primarily eliminated by the kidney, but also by drugs eliminated by non-renal pathways [8–10]. Further research is necessary utilizing physiologically based pharmacokinetic modeling (PBPK) to explore these changes in renal impairment [11, 12]. Determination of clinical drug-dosing regimens should take potential pharmacokinetic changes into consideration.

The majority of patients with chronic renal disease (CKD) are elderly with multiple comorbidities such as dermatological disorders requiring systemic therapy which place them at high risk for drug-related problems [13–16]. Most of the research conducted on the development of new oral or topical drugs or effects of established drugs excludes older adults, especially those over 70 years old with skin disease and chronic kidney disease [17]. For this reason, there are many different approaches and not always an evidence-based foundation for the prescribing and monitoring of drugs for the population with CKD [18]. There are few absolute contraindications for use of drugs in CKD; however, for most drugs, dosage adjustment is required to avoid toxic accumulation of drug or metabolites [19].

Absorption

Most drugs are absorbed orally by passive diffusion [20]. The site of absorption will determine a drug's absorption speed and amount. The speed and degree of distribution of a drug will determine the amount of drug available to exert

A.J. Olyaei, Pharm.D. (✉)
Nephrology and Hypertension, Oregon State University/Oregon Health and Sciences University, 3181 SW Sam Jackson Park Road, Mail Code CR-9, Portland, OR 97239, USA
e-mail: olyaeia@ohsu.edu

E.V. Lerma, M.D.
Section of Nephrology, Department of Medicine, Advocate Christ Medical Center, University of Illinois at Chicago, Oak Lawn, IL, USA

J.R. Nunley and E.V. Lerma (eds.), *Dermatological Manifestations of Kidney Disease*,
DOI 10.1007/978-1-4939-2395-3_20, © Springer Science+Business Media New York 2015

Table 20.1 MTX drug–drug interactions

Drug	Mechanism	Effects	Severity	Comments
Anti-folate antibiotics	Additive depletion	Pancytopenia	2	Avoid, monitor MTX level
NSAIDs	Impaired MTX excretion	Renal toxicity	3	Avoid, monitor MTX level
Probenecid	Impaired MTX excretion	Increased MTX level	2	Monitor MTX level
Phenytoin	Displaced protein binding	Increased MTX level	3	Monitor MTX level

MTX monitoring:
Blood: baseline and 2 weekly for 8 weeks after each dose increase then monthly × 4 then 3 monthly (assuming stable and no dose increase). withhold drug and repeat test if: white blood cells (WBC) falls below 4.0, neutrophils fall below 2.0, platelets fall below 140, alt or alkaline phosphatase increase to more than twice the upper limits of normal, monitor more closely if progressive change in these parameters
Chest X-ray: withhold drug and repeat chest X-ray plus pulmonary function tests if pulmonary toxicity suspected (i.e. breathlessness or cough)
MTX methotrexate, *NSAIDs* nonsteroidal anti-inflammatory drugs

pharmacological effects on the body and how much time it will take to eliminate the drug from the body. It is possible that the pH and blood flow of different absorption sites in the body, such as the skin, could be altered by the chronic renal failure and so affect the rate and extent of drug absorption and distribution of a particular agent. For example, compared to patients with normal renal function, absorption of a number of topical agents were reported to be reduced following topical administration, in particular hydrophilic compounds, in patients with CKD. Decreased microcirculation or alternation of skin structure in part may be involved in reduced drug absorption for percutaneous administration [21]. The reduced adipose layer of the skin has been shown to be associated with a decrease in the absorption of testosterone or hydrocortisone formulations.

Distribution

The effects of CKD on drug distribution are related to the degree of hypoalbuminemia exhibited by CKD patients experiencing malnutrition and increased albuminuria [22]. Alterations to albumin binding sites reduce affinity for acidic drugs and promote competition for albumin binding with organic acids that accumulate because of reduced renal excretion. Subsequently, protein binding of acidic drugs may be reduced in CKD. Toxicity may result with higher levels of unbound drug exerting its pharmacologic effect requiring frequent monitoring of blood levels. Maintaining lower levels of total drug or monitoring unbound drug is recommended for CKD. Drugs exhibiting decreased protein binding include theophylline, phenytoin, MTX, diazepam, prazosin, cephalosporins, penicillins, furosemide, and valproic acid [23]. In addition to changes in protein binding, pharmacodynamic properties such as activity and affinity of receptors, signal transduction, and hormonal regulation can be affected by chronic kidney disease [24].

Metabolism

Implications of CKD on pharmacokinetics also influences drug-dosing. First-pass drug metabolism and the enterohepatic cycle facilitate drug absorption and bioavailability, but these processes are disrupted in CKD [9]. Decreased intestinal cytochrome P450 (CYP) enzyme activity as well as limited protein and substrate expression is suggested to promote increased bioavailability of several oral drugs in renal failure patients. Most studies have expressed a reduction in expression of cytochrome P-450 enzymatic system in chronic kidney disease. Although there is very limited information, it seems kidney diseases and uremia may influence drug metabolism. Uremic proteins may alter the expression of messenger RNA (mRNA) of cytochrome P450 enzymes. Calcium and phosphate metabolism are disturbed in moderate to severe CKD. Calcium is commonly low-normal or low in renal failure. High parathyroid hormone (PTH) is a physiological response to low calcium, and to the phosphate retention that occurs in renal failure. During chronic kidney disease, PTH and PTH analogous have shown to reduce drug metabolism and downregulate expression of cytochrome P450 enzymes [25]. Cyclosporine, tacrolimus, propranolol, propoxyphene, human immunodeficiency virus (HIV) protease inhibitors, and immunosuppressive drug availability is increased during decreased intestinal metabolism [26]. In contrast, CKD also leads to decreased bioavailability of drugs as influenced by hepatic metabolism through increased release of uremic factors like PTH and inflammatory cytokines resulting in an alkalytic gastric environment. Medications such as antacids, phosphate binders, proton pump inhibitors, and histamine-receptor blockers enhance an elevated pH thus limiting the absorption of drugs requiring an acidic environment like furosemide and ferrous sulfate. Physical symptoms of edema, vomiting, and diarrhea also limit drug transit time in the intestines resulting in decreased drug absorption.

Renal Elimination

Renal impairment alters the pharmacokinetics of drugs and metabolites requiring drug dosing adjustments. Decreased clearance has been observed for drugs primarily eliminated by the kidney, but also by drugs eliminated by non-renal pathways [11, 12]. It is very important to avoid any drug with potential of nephrotoxicity to be avoided or discontinued temporarily or indefinitely (Table 20.2).

Determination of clinical drug-dosing regimens should ultimately be individualized and based upon kidney function as measured by GFR [19]. Since GFR cannot be measured directly, intrinsic markers such as inulin, iothalamate, or iohexol are the desired standard, but unrealistic for use in clinical practice due to a complicated measurement process and expensive laboratory cost [27]. Thus endogenous filtration markers, typically serum creatinine and urine measures, are used to estimate GFR [28, 29]. It is important to note serum creatinine alone is not an adequate representation of kidney function as the serum level is affected by multiple physiologic processes varying widely among individuals. For instance, older age, female sex, restriction of dietary protein, malnutrition, muscle wasting, and amputation decrease serum creatinine concentrations while African American race, ingesting cooked meats, and muscle mass increases levels. Estimates of GFR are achieved through recommended formulas that account for serum creatinine and other patient characteristics (age, sex, weight, or race). The Cockcroft-Gault (CG) equation [30], the Modification of Diet in Renal Disease (MDRD) [31], and the most recent, Chronic Kidney Disease Epidemiology Collaboration (CKD-EPI) equation [32] assist in identifying patients with CKD and screening for those at high-risk of disease development. Variations in GFR estimates exist among these valid equations and it is uncertain which formula provides the most accurate medication dosing recommendations; therefore clinical judgment must be applied appropriately per patient application. The CG equation and MDRD are recommended for determining clinical drug-dosing regimens in CKD despite equation limitations. See Table 20.3 for a comparison of formulas for estimating kidney function test.

In fact, the most common drug dosing recommendations are based on pharmacokinetic studies that used creatinine clearance as estimated by the CG equation for a measure of kidney function. Now MDRD is most commonly used in the clinic setting to assess kidney health and stage CKD. However, healthcare professionals should proceed cautiously using these equations in special populations like geriatrics where use of a conservative estimate (CG equation) may be desired especially when prescribing drugs with a narrow therapeutic index in order to prevent toxicity and maximize efficacy [28].

Table 20.2 Comparison of formulas estimating GFR for drug dosing

Formula name	Equation	Clinical considerations
CG[a]	Creatinine clearance (mL/min) = (140 − age in years) × actual weight (kg)/serum creatinine (micromol/L); Multiply the result by 1.2 for men	• Estimates creatinine clearance not adjusting for BSA; • Standard for drug dosing despite limitations between pharmacokinetics and clinical practice
MDRD[a]	Estimated GFR (mL/min/1.73 m^2) = 186 × $(S_{Cr})^{-1.154}$ × $(Age)^{-.203}$ × (0.742 if female) × (1.210 if African American) = expanded (5.228 − 1.154 × In(S_{Cr}) − 0.203 × In(Age) − (0.299 if female) + (0.192 if African American)	• Estimates GFR adjusting for BSA; • Used for drug dosing despite limitations between pharmacokinetics and clinical practice; • Valid for specified racial groups (African Americans, Europeans, Asians), patients with diabetes, kidney transplant recipients, and potential kidney donors; • Less accurate in those without CKD; • Invalid in children, pregnant women, elderly, some races, nutritional status and muscle mass variation
CKD-EPI	GFR = 141 × min(S_{Cr}/κ,1)^{α} × max(S_{Cr}/κ,1)$^{-1.209}$ × 0.993^{Age} × 1.018 [if female] × 1.159 [if black]; Where S_{Cr} is serum creatinine (mg/dL), κ is 0.7 for females and 0.9 for males, α is −0.329 for females and −0.411 for males, min indicates the minimum of S_{Cr}/κ or 1, and max indicates the maximum of S_{Cr}/κ or 1	• Estimates GFR adjusting for BSA; • Not recommended for drug dosing; • Valid with higher levels of GFR, young patients with type 1 diabetes, and kidney donation evaluation; • Accurate as MDRD equation in CKD patients having lower GFR levels; • Invalid in children, pregnant women, some races, nutritional status and muscle mass variation

[a]Indicates potential need of 24-h urine collection for creatinine clearance when estimates based on serum creatinine may be inaccurate during the following clinical situations: extremes of age and body size, severe malnutrition or obesity, disease of skeletal muscle, paraplegia or quadriplegia, vegetarian diet, rapidly changing kidney function, and pregnancy

CG cockcroft-gault, *MDRD* modification of diet in renal disease, *CKD-EPI* chronic kidney disease epidemiology collaboration, *GFR* glomerular filtration rate, *BSA* body surface area, *CKD* chronic kidney disease

Table 20.3 These agents must be avoided or to be used with caution in patients with chronic kidney disease

Class	Examples
Antibiotics	Aminoglycosides vancomycin, sulfamethoxazole
Antifungals	Amphotericin B
Antivirals	Foscarnet, indinavir, cidofovir
Anticoagulants	Low molecular weight heparins, warfarin
Cardiac drugs	Digoxin, sotalol, ACE-I, ARB, DRIs
Opioids	Morphine, meperidine, prophoxyphene
Psychotropics/ anticonvulsants	Amisulpride, gabapentin, lithium, levetiracetam, topiramate, vigabatrin
Hypoglycaemic drugs	Metformin, glyburide, insulin
Drugs for gout	Allopurinol, colchicine
Others	Methotrexate, penicillamine, NSAIDs

ACE-I angiotensin-converting enzyme inhibitors, *ARB* angiotensin receptor blocker, *DRIs* dopamine reuptake inhibitors, *NSAIDs* nonsteroidal anti-inflammatory drugs

Drug Dosing in Kidney Disease

Loading Dose

Loading doses are used when reaching therapeutic concentrations of medication promptly is necessary for adequate treatment of the patient. Steady state concentrations of medications in patients with normal renal function are reached after approximately five medications half-lives. Often, decreased dosing recommendations for patients with CKD prolongs the time it takes to reach steady-state. Loading doses may be particularly important in this population. Despite possible reductions in maintenance dosing regimens, loading dose recommendations remain consistent despite reductions in kidney function. A formula may be used to assist in calculating an appropriate loading dose [33].

$$\mathrm{LD} = \mathrm{Vd} \times [\mathrm{Cp}]$$

Vd = volume of distribution in l/kg of ideal body weight in kg and Cp is the desired concentration in the plasma in mg/L [34].

Maintenance Dose

As mentioned above, reductions in renal excretion necessitate dose adjustments for many medications, particularly those excreted unchanged in the urine. Consideration of renally eliminated active metabolites should be considered as well. Dose adjustments are primarily determined based on patient calculated GFR (see Table 20.3). Two primary strategies are used for drug adjustment in decreased renal function, dose reductions and increasing dosing interval. The ideal reduction strategy should be based on individual medication pharmacokinetic characteristics and goals of therapy [10]. Dose reductions allow for more constant drug levels within the body. However, the risk of drug accumulation is higher. Extension of dosing interval may be used for dose adjustment as well. Longer dosing intervals allows for the medication to reach adequate peak concentrations with increased duration between doses to allow for slowed clearance in kidney disease. Based on the extent of kidney disease, likely a combination of dosing reductions and extension of dosing interval are necessary for ideal plasma concentrations [35].

Patients with CKD requiring intermittent hemodialysis (IHD) necessitate further considerations when determining maintenance dose. Protein binding, volume of distribution, and molecular weight of the drug are some factors contributing to extent of drug removal during IHD. Drug removal is primarily through diffusion across the dialysis membrane. Highly protein bound medication will not be removed during dialysis as only free drug will be removed. In addition, medications with a large volume of distribution (>0.7 mL/kg) will have minimal removal due to widespread tissue binding. Molecular weight or size of the molecule passing the membrane influences its ability to be removed. Medications <500 Da are readily removed across dialysis membranes. Finally, frequency, duration and type of membrane may influence the extent of drug removal. Consideration can assist in determining maintenance dosing and potential need for supplemental doses post-dialysis to maintain consistent plasma concentrations [36].

Therapeutic Drug Monitoring

Therapeutic drug monitoring can be beneficial for medications with a narrow therapeutic index as dosage adjustments may not be sufficient to prevent toxicities in patients with CKD (Table 20.3). Despite the benefits, therapeutic drug monitoring is unavailable or expensive for many narrow therapeutic index medications. Medications used for dermatological disease such as tacrolimus, cyclosporine, MTX, and others have plasma concentration assays and are commonly monitored. In addition, these agents are at great risk for drug interactions (Tables 20.4, 20.5, 20.6, 20.7, and 20.8). These levels can assist in predicting both clinical response and potential for toxicity. However, it is important to consider the whole patient when utilizing plasma concentrations to dose medications as toxicity may occur despite therapeutic plasma concentrations. Concomitant nephrotoxic medications or competition for secretion can contribute to toxicity despite previously therapeutic plasma levels (Table 20.3). When medications such as these are added to a patient's medication regimen or if fluctuations in renal function occur, therapeutic drug monitoring should be repeated.

Table 20.4 Therapeutic drug monitoring

Drug name	Therapeutic range	When to draw sample	How often to draw levels
Aminoglycosides (conventional dosing) gentamicin, tobramycin, amikacin	Gentamicin and tobramycin: Trough: 0.5–2 mg/L Peak: 5–8 mg/L Amikacin: Peak: 20–30 mg/L Trough: < 10 mg/L	Trough: Immediately prior to dose Peak: 30 min after a 30–45 min infusion	Check peak and trough with third dose For therapy less than 72 h, levels not necessary. Repeat drug levels weekly or if renal function changes
Aminoglycosides (24-h dosing) gentamicin, tobramycin, amikacin	0.5–3 mg/L	Obtain random drug level 12 h after dose	After initial dose. Repeat drug level in 1 week or if renal function changes
Carbamazepine	4–12 mcg/mL	Trough: Immediately prior to dosing	Check 2–4 days after first dose or change in dose
Cyclosporin	150–400 ng/mL	Trough: Immediately prior to dosing	Daily for first week, then weekly
Digoxin	0.8–2.0 ng/mL	12 h after maintenance dose	5–7 days after first dose for patients with normal renal and hepatic function; 15–20 days in anephric patients
Lidocaine	1–5 mcg/mL	8 h after i.v. infusion started or changed	
Lithium	Acute: 0.8–1.2 mmol/L Chronic: 0.6–0.8 mmol/L	Trough: Before a.m. dose at least 12 h since last dose	
Phenobarbital	15–40 mcg/mL	Trough: Immediately prior to dosing	Check 2 weeks after first dose or change in dose. Follow-up level in 1–2 months.
Phenytoin free phenytoin	10–20 mcg/mL 1–2 mcg/mL	Trough: Immediately prior to dosing	5–7 day after first dose or after change in dose
Procainamide NAPA a procainamide metabolite	4–10 mcg/mL Trough: 4 mcg/mL Peak: 8 mcg/mL 10–30 mcg/mL	Trough: Immediately prior to next dose or 12–18 h after starting or changing an infusion Draw with procainamide sample	
Quinidine	1–5 mcg/mL	Trough: Immediately prior to next dose	
Sirolimus	10–20 ng/dL	Trough: Immediately prior to next dose	
Tacrolimus (FK-506)	10–15 ng/mL	Trough: Immediately prior to next dose	Daily for first week, then weekly
Theophylline p.o. or Aminophylline i.v.	15–20 mcg/mL	Trough: Immediately prior to next dose	
Valproic acid (divalproex sodium)	40–100 mcg/mL	Trough: Immediately prior to next dose	Check 2–4 days after first dose or change in dose
Vancomycin	Trough: 5–15 mg/L Peak: 25–40 mg/L	Trough: Immediately prior to dose Peak: 60 min after a 60 min infusion	With third dose (when initially starting therapy, or after each dosage adjustment). For therapy less than 72 h, levels not necessary. Repeat drug levels if renal function changes

NAPA N-acetylprocainamide, *p.o.* per os, *i.v.* intravenous

Table 20.5 Cyclosporine and tacrolimus drug–drug interactions

Drug	Mechanism	Effects	Severity	Comments
Acetazolamide	Decrease clearance	Increase CSA/FK level	3	May cause acidosis
Acyclovir	Crystallization in renal tubules	Nephrotoxicity	4	Avoid dehydration. Infuse over 1 h
Amikacin	Synergistic nephrotoxicity	Nephrotoxicity	3	Monitor aminoglycoside level very closely. Target amikacin level peak 30–40 and trough less than 10
Amiloride	Decrease K+ secretion	Hyperkalemia	3	Avoid in transplant recipients
Amiodarone	Decrease clearance	Nephrotoxicity	3	Very slow onset and offset
Amlodipine	Decrease clearance	Increase CSA/FK level	4	10–15 % increase in CSA/FK level
Amphotericin B	Synergistic nephrotoxicity	Nephrotoxicity	3	Require hydration and electrolyte monitoring
Atrovastatin	CSA decreases clearance of statins	Myopathy, rhabdomyolysis	3	Monitor CPK carefully
Carbamazepine	Increase clearance	Decrease CSA/FK level	3	Slow onset (may take up to 7 days) Monitoring of CSA/FK level
Carvedilol	Decrease clearance	Increase CSA/FK level	3	Can cause toxicity
Cervastatin	CSA decreases clearance of statins	Myopathy, rhabdomyolysis	3	Require close CPK monitoring
Chloroquine	Decrease clearance	Increase CSA/FK level	3	
Cholestyramine	Increase clearance	Decrease CSA/FK level	4	Separate doses by 3 h
Cimetidine	Inhibit creatinine secretion	Increase serum creatinine	4	Use other H_2 antagonist agents (ranitidine, famotidine and nizatidine)
Ciprofloxacin	Decrease CSA effects on IL-2	Pharmacodynamic antagonism	4	May increase risk of rejection
Cisapride	Decrease gastric emptying time	Increase CSA/FK level	2	Metoclopramide is the preferred agent
Clarithromycin	Decrease clearance	Increase CSA/FK level	2	Azithromycin is the preferred agent
Colchicine		Increase neurotoxicity	3	Gastrointestinal dysfunction and neuromyopathy
Co-trimoxazole	Inhibit creatinine secretion	Increase serum creatinine	4	Preferred agent for PCP
Digoxin	CSA may decreases clearance of digoxin	Increase digoxin level	3	Monitor digoxin level closely
Diltiazem	Decrease clearance	Increase CSA/FK level	3	Monitor CSA/FK level closely
Enalapril	Renal dysfunction in RAS	Increase serum creatinine	3	May cause anemia. Use for treatment of post-transplant erythrocytosis
Erythromycin	Decrease clearance	Increase CSA/FK level	2	Azithromycin is the preferred agent
Fluconazole	Decrease clearance	Increase CSA/FK level	3	Increase LFTs, monitor levels carefully
Fluvoxamine	Decrease clearance	Increase CSA/FK level	2	Monitor levels carefully
Fosinopril	Renal dysfunction in RAS	Nephrotoxicity	3	Can cause elevation of Scr
Fosphenytoin	Increase clearance	Decrease CSA/FK level	3	Monitor levels carefully
Ganciclovir	Synergistic Nephrotoxicity	Nephrotoxicity	3	Avoid dehydration
Gentamicin	Synergistic nephrotoxicity	Nephrotoxicity	3	Monitor blood concentrations very closely
Griseofulvin	Unknown	Decrease CSA/FK level	3	Decreased cyclosporine effectiveness
Itraconazole	Decrease clearance	Increase CSA/FK level	3	Monitor levels carefully, decrease dosage 50–85 %
Ketoconazole	Decrease clearance	Increase CSA/FK level	3	Monitor levels carefully, decrease dosage 25–75 %

(continued)

Table 20.5 (continued)

Drug	Mechanism	Effects	Severity	Comments
Lovastatin	CSA decreases clearance of statins	Myopathy, rhabdomyolysis	3	Require close CPK monitoring
Methy-prednisolone	Decrease clearance	Increase CSA/FK level	3	Only high doses
Methytestosterone	Decreased cyclosporine metabolism	Increase CSA/FK level	3	Can cause toxicity
Metoclopramide	Decrease gastric emptying time	Increase CSA/FK level	3	Increase peak and AUC by 25–50 %
Metronidazole	Decrease clearance	Increase CSA/FK level	4	Monitor CSA/FK levels
Mibefradil	Decrease CSA/FK clearance	Increase CSA/FK level	3	Monitor CSA/FK levels
Nafcillin	Increase CSA/FK clearance	Decrease CSA/FK level	3	Monitor CSA/FK levels
Nefazodone	Decrease CSA/FK clearance	Increase CSA/FK level	3	Monitor CSA/FK levels
Nicardipine	Decrease CSA/FK clearance	Increase CSA/FK level	3	Monitor CSA/FK levels
NSAIDs	Synergistic nephrotoxicity	Nephrotoxicity	3	CSA/FK induced vasoconstriction is influenced by prostaglandins inhibition
Octreotide	Decrease intestinal absorption of CSA/FK	Decrease CSA/FK level	3	Monitor CSA/FK levels
Phenobarbital	Increase CSA/FK clearance	Decrease CSA/FK level	3	Slow onset, slow off-set
Phenytoin	Increase CSA/FK clearance	Decrease CSA/FK level	3	Monitor cyclosporine/FK levels
Pravastatin	CSA decreases clearance of statins	Myopathy, rhabdomyolysis	3	Monitor CPK carefully
Rifabutin	Increase CSA/FK clearance	Decrease CSA/FK level	3	Monitor CSA/FK levels, rifabutin is a less potent hepatic enzyme inducer than rifampin
Rifampin	Increase CSA/FK clearance	Decrease CSA/FK level	2	Monitor cyclosporine/FK levels
Sildenafil	Increase FK level	Decrease CSA/FK level	4	
Simvastatin	CSA decreases clearance of statins	Myopathy, rhabdomyolysis	4	Monitor CPK carefully
Spironolactone	Decrease K+ secretion	Hyperkalemia	3	Avoid
Terbinafine	Decrease CSA/FK clearance	Increase CSA/FK level	3	Monitor CSA/FK levels
Ticlopidine	Increase CSA/FK clearance	Decrease CSA/FK level	3	Monitor CSA/FK levels
Tretinoin	Inhibit tretinoin metabolism	Increase tretinoin toxicity	3	
Triamterine	Decrease K+ secretion	Hyperkalemia	3	Avoid
Troglitazone	Increase CSA/FK clearance	Decrease CSA/FK level	3	Hepatotoxicity
Valacyclovir	Hemolytic anemic syndrome	Renal dysfunction	3	Acyclovir or famciclovir are preferred agents for treatment of HSV and VZV

1. Avoid combination
2. Usually avoid (use only no other alternative agents available)
3. Monitor closely
4. No action needed (the risk of ADR is small)

HSV herpes simplex virus, *VZV* varicella zoster virus

Table 20.6 Sirolimus drug–drug interactions

Drug	Mechanism	Effects	Severity	Comments
ACE-I	Synergestic myelosuppression	Anemia, neutropenia	3	Increase bone marrow toxicity
Amprenavir	Increase plasma level	Hyperlipidmia, anemia, neutropenia	3	Monitor sirolimus level
Bromocriptine	Increase plasma level	Hyperlipidmia, anemia, neutropenia	3	Monitor sirolimus level
Carbamazepine	Decrease intestinal absorption	Decrease sirolimus level	2	Monitor sirolimus level
Cholestyramine	Decrease intestinal absorption	Decrease sirolimus level	3	Monitor sirolimus level

(continued)

Table 20.6 (continued)

Drug	Mechanism	Effects	Severity	Comments
Clarithromycin	Increased plasma level	Hyperlipidmia, anemia, neutropenia	2	Monitor sirolimus level Azithromycin is the preferred agent
Cyclosporine	Increase plasma level when taken at the same	Hyperlipidmia, anemia, neutropenia	3	Monitor sirolimus level, Give 4 h after the dose
Danazol	Decrease intestinal absorption	Decrease sirolimus level	3	Monitor sirolimus level
Diltiazem	Increase plasma level	Hyperlipidmia, anemia, neutropenia	2	Monitor sirolimus level Amlodipine is the preferred agent
Erythromycin	Increase plasma level	Hyperlipidmia, anemia, neutropenia	2	Monitor sirolimus level Azithromycin is the preferred agent
Fluconazole	Increase plasma level	Hyperlipidmia, anemia, neutropenia	2	Monitor sirolimus level
Ganciclovir	Synergestic myelosuppression	Anemia, neutropenia	3	
Indinavir	Increase plasma level	Hyperlipidmia, anemia, neutropenia	2	Monitor sirolimus level
Itraconazole	Increase plasma level	Hyperlipidmia, anemia, neutropenia	2	Monitor sirolimus level
Metoclopramide	Increase plasma level	Hyperlipidmia, anemia, neutropenia	3	Monitor sirolimus level
Nicardipine	Increase plasma level	Hyperlipidmia, anemia, neutropenia	2	Monitor sirolimus level Amlodipine is the preferred agent
Phenobarbital	Increase metabolism	Decrease sirolimus level	2	Monitor sirolimus level
Phenytoin	Increase metabolism	Decrease sirolimus level	2	Monitor sirolimus level
Rifabutin	Increase metabolism	Decrease sirolimus level	2	Monitor sirolimus level
Rifampin	Increase metabolism	Decrease sirolimus level	2	Monitor sirolimus level
Ritonavir	Increase plasma level	Hyperlipidmia, anemia, neutropenia	2	Monitor sirolimus level
TMP/SMX	Synergestic myelosuppression	Anemia, neutropenia	3	
Verapamil	Increase plasma level	Hyperlipidmia, anemia, neutropenia	2	Monitor sirolimus level
Voriconazole	Increase plasma level	Hyperlipidmia, anemia, neutropenia	2	Monitor sirolimus level

1. Avoid combination
2. Usually avoid (use only no other alternative agents available)
3. Monitor closely
4. No action needed (the risk of ADR is small)

ACE-I Angiotensin-converting enzyme inhibitors, *TMP/SMX* trimethoprim/sulfamethoxazole

Table 20.7 Azathioprine and mycophenolate drug–drug interactions

Drug	Mechanism	Effects	Severity	Comments
ACE-I	Synergestic myelosuppression	Anemia, neutropenia	3	Increase bone marrow toxicity
Acyclovir	Increase AUC of MMF	Not significant	4	
Allopurinol	Inhibit xanthene oxidase	Severe neutropenia	2	Decrease azathioprine dose by 75 %
Antacids	Decrease absorption of MMF	Decrease efficacy	3	
Cholestyramine	Decrease absorption of MMF		3	Increase bone marrow toxicity
Ganciclovir	Synergistic myelosuppression	Anemia, neutropenia	3	
TMP/SMX	Synergistic myelosuppression	Anemia, neutropenia	3	

1. Avoid combination
2. Usually avoid (use only no other alternative agents available)
3. Monitor closely
4. No action needed (the risk of ADR is small)

ACE-I Angiotensin-converting enzyme inhibitors, *TMP/SMX* trimethoprim/sulfamethoxazole

Table 20.8 Dosage adjustment for immunosuppressive/modulators drugs

			Dosage adjustment in renal failure			
Immunosuppressant	Normal dosage	% of renal excretion	GFR >50 mL/min	GFR 10–50 mL/min	GFR <10 mL/min	Comments
Cyclosporine	3 mg/kg/day	<5	100 %	100 %	50 %	Nephrotoxicity, HTN
Tacrolimus	0.1 mg/kg/day	<5	100 %	75 %	50 %	Nephrotoxicity, HTN
Azathioprine	2 mg/kg/day	<5 %	100 %	75 %	50 %	Myleosuppression
Mycophenolate	1,000 mg bid	<1 %	100 %	100 %	75 %	Myelosuppression
Prednisone	Varies	<1 %	100 %	75 %	25–50 %	Myelosuppression
D-Penicillamine	250–750 mg day	5–15 %	100 %	Avoid	Avoid	
Hydroxychloroquine	200 mg bid	15–25 %	100 %	75 %	50 %	Retinal toxicity or visual field
Acitretin	25–50 mg	<1 %	100 %	Avoid	Avoid	
Isotretinoin	0.25–0.5 mg/kg q12 h	<1 %	100 %	100 %	100 %	Avoid TCN, Vit A, and MTX
Leflunomide	10–20 mg daily	<1 %	100 %	100 %	75 %	Liver toxicity, active metabolites eliminated through kidney
MTX	10–15 mg day	70–80 %	100 %	Avoid	Avoid	Myelosuppression
Sulfasalazine	1,000 mg BID–TID	50 %	100 %	75 %	50 %	Myelosuppression
Etanercept	50 mg every week	ND	100 %	100 %	100 %	Infection
Infliximab	3 mg/kg every 8 weeks	<1 %	100 %	100 %	100 %	Infection
Adalimumab	40 mg every other week	<1 %	100 %	100 %	100 %	Infection
Certolizumab	400 mg every month	ND	100 %	100 %	100 %	Infection
Golimumab	50 mg every month	ND	100 %	100 %	100 %	Infection
Rituximab	1,000 mg every 2 weeks	<1 %	100 %	100 %	100 %	Infection
Abatacept	500–1,000 mg every 2 weeks	<1 %	100 %	100 %	100 %	Infection
Tocilizumab	4 mg/kg every 4 weeks	ND	100 %	100 %	100 %	Infection

Antimicrobal agents in renal failure

Drugs	Normal dosage	% of renal excretion	Dosage adjustment in renal failure: GFR >50 mL/min	GFR 10–50 mL/min	GFR <10 mL/min	Comments	HD	CAPD	Continuous venovenous hemofiltration
Aminoglycoside antibiotics						Nephrotoxic, ototoxic Toxicity worse when hyperbilirubinemic Measure serum levels for efficacy and toxicity			
						Peritoneal absorption increases with presence of inflammation			
						Vd increases with edema, obesity, and ascites			
Streptomycin	7.5 mg/kg q12 h (1.0 g q24 h for TB)	60 %	q24 h	q24 to 72 h	q72 to 96 h	For the treatment of TB. May be less nephrotoxic than other members of class	1/2 normal dose after dialysis	20–40 mg/L/day	Dose for GFR 10–50 mL/min and measure levels
Kanamycin	7.5 mg/kg q8 h	50–90 %	60–90 % q12 h or 100 % q12 to 24 h	30–70 % q12 to 18 h or 100 % q24 to 48 h	20–30 % q24 to 48 h or 100 % q48 to 72 h	Do not use once-daily dosing in patients with creatinine clearance less than 30–40 mL/min or in patients with acute renal failure or uncertain level of kidney function	1/2 full dose after dialysis	15–20 mg/L/day	Dose for GFR 10–50 mL/min and measure levels
Gentamicin	1.7 mg/kg q8 h	95 %	60–90 % q8 to 12 h or 100 % q12 to 24 h	30–to 70 % q12 h or 100 % q24 to 48 h	20–30 % q24 to 48 h or 100 % q48 to 72 h		1/2 full dose after dialysis	3–4 mg/L/day	Dose for GFR 10–50 mL/min and measure levels
Tobramicin	1.7 mg/kg q8 h	95 %	60–90 % q8 to 12 h or 100 % q12 to 24 h	30–70 % q12 h or 100 % q24 to 48 h	20–30 % q24 to 48 h or 100 % q48 to 72 h		1/2 full dose after dialysis	3 to 4 mg/L/day	Dose for GFR 10–50 mL/min and measure levels
Netilmicin	2 mg/kg q8 h	95 %	50–90 % q8 to 12 h or 100 % q12 to 24 h	20–60 % q12 h or 100 % q24 to 48 h	10–20 % q24 to 48 h or 100 % q48 to 72	May be less ototoxic than other members of class. Peak 6 to 8 Trough <2	1/2 full dose after dialysis	3–4 mg/L/day	Dose for GFR 10–50 mL/min and measure levels
Amikacin	7.5 mg/kg q12 h	95 %	60–90 % q12 h or 100 % q12 to 24 h	30–to 70 % q12 to 18 h or 100 % q24 to 48 h	20–30 % q24 to 48 h or 100 % q48 to 72 h	Monitor levels Peak 20 to 30 Trough <5	1/2 full dose after dialysis	15–20 mg/L/day	Dose for GFR 10–50 mL/min and measure levels
Cephalosporin						Coagulation abnormalities, transitory elevation of BUN, rash and serum sickness-like syndrome			

Oral cephalosporin									
Cefaclor	250–500 mg q8 h	70 %	100 %	100 %	50 %		250 mg bid after dialysis	250 mg q8 to 12 h	N/A
Cefadroxil	500 to 1 g q12 h	80 %	100 %	100 %	50 %		0.5–1.0 g after dialysis	0.5 g/day	N/A
Cefixime	200–400 mg q12 h	85 %	100 %	100 %	50 %		300 mg after dialysis	200 mg/day	Not recommended
Cefpodoxime	200 mg q12 h	30 %	100 %	100 %	100 %		200 mg after dialysis	Dose for GFR <10 mL/min	N/A
Ceftibuten	400 mg q24 h	70 %	100 %	100 %	50 %		300 mg after dialysis	No data: Dose for GFR <10 mL/min	Dose for GFR 10–50 mL/min
Cefuroxime axetil	250–500 mg q8 h	90 %	100 %	100 %	100 %	Malabsorbed in presence of H2 blockers. Absorbed better with food	Dose after dialysis	Dose for GFR <10 mL/min	N/A
Cephalexin	250–500 mg q8 h	95 %	100 %	100 %	100 %	Rare allergic interstitial nephritis. Absorbed well when given intraperitoneally. May cause bleeding from impaired prothrombin biosynthesis	Dose after dialysis	Dose for GFR <10 mL/min	N/A
Cephradine	250–500 mg q8 h	100 %	100 %	100 %	50 %		Dose after dialysis	Dose for GFR <10 mL/min	N/A
IV cephalosporin									
Cefazolin	1–2 g IV q8 h	80 %	q8 h	q12 h	q12 to 24 h		0.5–1.0 g after dialysis	0.5 g q12 h	Dose for GFR 10–50 mL/min
Cefepime	1–2 g IV q8 h	85 %	q8 to 12 h	q12 h	q24 h		1 g after dialysis	Dose for GFR <10 mL/min	Not recommended
Cefmetazole	1–2 g IV q8 h	85 %	q8 h	q12 h	q24 h		Dose after dialysis	Dose for GFR <10 mL/min	Dose for GFR 10–50 mL/min
Cefoperazone	1–2 g IV q12 h	20 %	No renal adjustment is required			Displaced from protein by bilirubin. Reduce dose by 50 % for jaundice. May prolong prothrombin time	1 g after dialysis	None	None
Cefotaxime	1–2 g IV q6 to 8 h	60 %	q8 h	q12 h	q12 to 24 h		1 g after dialysis	1 g/day	1 g q12 h
Cefotetan	1–2 g IV q12 h	75 %	q12 h	q12 to 24 h	q24 h		1 g after dialysis	1 g/day	750 mg q12 h
Cefoxitin	1–2 g IV q6 h	80 %	q6 h	q8 to 12 h	q12 h	May produce false increase in serum creatinine by interference with assay.	1 g after dialysis	1 g/day	Dose for GFR 10–50 mL/min
Ceftazidime	1–2 g IV q8 h	70 %	q8 h	q12 h	q24 h		1 g after dialysis	0.5 g/day	Dose for GFR 10–50 mL/min

(continued)

(continued)

Antimicrobal agents in renal failure

Drugs	Normal dosage	% of renal excretion	Dosage adjustment in renal failure GFR >50 mL/min	GFR 10–50 mL/min	GFR <10 mL/min	Comments	HD	CAPD	Continuous venovenous hemofiltration
Ceftriaxone	1–2 g IV q24 h	50 %	No renal adjustment is required				Dose after dialysis	750 mg q12 h	Dose for GFR 10–50 mL/min
Cefuroxime sodium	0.75–1.5 g IV q8 h	90 %	q8 h	q8 to 12 h	q12 to 24 h		Dose after dialysis	Dose for GFR <10 mL/min	1.0 g q12 h
Penicillin						Bleeding abnormalities, hypersensitivity. Seizures			
Oral Penicillin									
Amoxicillin	500 mg po q8 h	60 %	100 %	100 %	50–75 %		Dose after dialysis	250 mg q12 h	N/A
Ampicillin	500 mg po q6 h	60 %	100 %	100 %	50–75 %		Dose after dialysis	250 mg q12 h	Dose for GFR 10–50 mL/min
Dicloxacillin	250–500 mg po q6 h	50 %	100 %	100 %	50–75 %		None	None	N/A
Penicillin V	250–500 mg po q6 h	70 %	100 %	100 %	50–75 %		Dose after dialysis	Dose for GFR <10 mL/min	N/A
IV Penicillin									
Ampicillin	1–2 g IV q6 h	60 %	q6 h	q8 h	q12 h		Dose after dialysis	250 mg q12 h	Dose for GFR 10–50 mL/min
Nafcillin	1–2 g IV q4 h	35 %	No renal adjustment is required				None	None	Dose for GFR 10–50 mL/min
Penicillin G	2–3 million Units IV q4 h	70 %	q4 to 6 h	q6 h	q8 h		Dose after dialysis	Dose for GFR <10 mL/min	Dose for GFR 10–50 mL/min
Piperacillin	3–4 g IV q4 to 6 h		No renal adjustment is required			Sodium, 1.9 mEq/g	Dose after dialysis	Dose for GFR <10 mL/min	Dose for GFR 10–50 mL/min
Ticarcillin/clavulanate	3.1 g IV q4 to 6 h	85 %	1–2 g q4 h	1–2 g q8 h	1–2 g q12 h	Sodium, 5.2 mEq/g	3.0 g after dialysis	Dose for GFR <10 mL/min	Dose for GFR 10–50 mL/min
Piperacillin/tazobactam	3.375 g IV q6 to 8 h	75–90 %	q4 to 6 h	q6 to 8 h	q8 h	Sodium, 1.9 mEq/g	Dose after dialysis	Dose for GFR <10 mL/min	Dose for GFR 10–50 mL/min
Quinolones						Food, dairy products, tube feeding, and Al(OH)3 may decrease the absorption of quinolones			
Ciprofloxacin	200–400 mg IV q24 h	60 %	q12 h	q12 to 24 h	q24 h	Poorly absorbed with antacids, sucralfate, and phosphate binders. IV dose 1/3 of oral dose. Decreases phenytoin levels	250 mg q12 h (200 mg if IV)	250 mg q8 h (200 mg if IV)	200 mg IV q12 h

Levofloxacin	500 mg po q24 h	70 %	q12 h	250 q12 h	250 q12 h	L-isomer of ofloxacin: appears to have similar pharmacokinetics and toxicities	Dose for GFR <10 mL/min	Dose for GFR <10 mL/min	Dose for GFR 10–50 mL/min
Moxifloxacin	400 mg q24 h	20 %	No renal adjustment is required				No data	No data	No data
Nalidixic acid	1.0 g q6 h	High	100 %	Avoid	Avoid	Agents in this group are malabsorbed in the presence of magnesium, calcium, aluminum, and iron. Theophylline metabolism is impaired. Higher oral doses may be needed to treat CAPD peritonitis	Avoid	Avoid	N/A
Norfloxacin	400 mg po q12 h	30 %	q12 h	q12 to 24 h	q24 h	See above	Dose for GFR <10 mL/min	Dose for GFR <10 mL/min	N/A
Ofloxacin	200–400 mg po q12 h	70 %	q12 h	q12 to 24 h	q24 h	See above	100–200 mg after dialysis	Dose for GFR <10 mL/min	300 mg/day
Miscellaneous agents									
Tetracycline	250–500 mg po q24 h	1 %	No renal adjustment is required			No drug–drug interaction with CSA/KF	None		
Minocycline	100 mg po bid	1 %	No renal adjustment is required				None		
Azithromycin	250–500 mg po q24 h	6 %	No renal adjustment is required			No drug–drug interaction with CSA/KF.	None	None	None
Clarithromycin	500 mg po q12 h		No renal adjustment is required			Increase CSA/FK level	None	None	None
Clindamycin	150–450 mg po q8 h	10 %	No renal adjustment is required				None	None	None
Dirithromycin	500 mg po q24 h		No renal adjustment is required			Nonenzymatically hydro-lyzed to active compound erythomycylamine	None	No data: None	Dose for GFR 10–50 mL/min
Erythromycin	250–500 mg po q6 h	15 %	No renal adjustment is required			Increase CSA/FK level, avoid in transplant patients	None	None	None
Ertapenem	1 g IV q24 h		1 g IV q24 h	0.5 g IV q24 h	0.5 g IV q24 h		Dose after Dialysis	Dose for GFR <10 mL/min	Dose for GFR <30
Imipenem/ cilastatin	250–500 mg IV q6 h	50 %	500 mg q8 h	250–500 q8 to 12 h	250 mg q12 h	Seizures in ESRD. Nonrenal clearance in acute renal failure is less than in chronic renal failure. Administered with cilastin to prevent nephrotoxicity of renal metabolite	Dose after dialysis	Dose for GFR <10 mL/min	Dose for GFR 10–50 mL/min
Meropenem	1 g IV q8 h	65 %	1 g q8 h	0.5–1 g q12 h	0.5–1 g q24 h	Less seizures compared to imipenem	Dose after dialysis	Dose for GFR <10 mL/min	Dose for GFR 10–50 mL/min

(continued)

(continued)

Antimicrobial agents in renal failure

Drugs	Normal dosage	% of renal excretion	Dosage adjustment in renal failure			Comments	HD	CAPD	Continuous venovenous hemofiltration
			GFR >50 mL/min	GFR 10–50 mL/min	GFR <10 mL/min				
Metronidazole	500 mg IV q6 h	20 %	No renal adjustment is required			Peripheral neuropathy, increase LFTs, disulfiram reaction with alcoholic beverages	Dose after dialysis	Dose for GFR <10 mL/min	Dose for GFR 10–50 mL/min
Pentamidine	4 mg/kg/day	5 %	q24 h	q24 h	q48 h	Inhalation may cause bronchospasm, IV administration may cause hypotension, hypoglycemia, and nephrotoxicity	None	None	None
Trimethoprim/ sulfameth-oxazole	800/160 mg po q12 h	70 %	q12 h	q18 h	q24 h	Increase serum creatinine. Can cause hyperkalemia	Dose after dialysis	q24 h	q18 h
Vancomycin	1 g IV q12 h	90 %	q12 h	q24 to 36 h	q48 to 72 h	Nephrotoxic, ototoxic, may prolong the neuromuscular blockade effect of muscle relaxants	500 mg q12 to 24 h (high FLX)	1.0 gm q24 to 96 h	500 mg q12 h
						Peak 30–40. Trough 5–10			
Vancomycin	125–250 mg po q6 h	0 %	100 %	100 %	100 %	Oral vancomycin is indicated only for the treatment of C. diff	100 %	100 %	100 %
Antituberculosis antibiotics									
Rifampin	300–600 mg po q24 h	20 %	No renal adjustment is required			Decrease CSA/FK level. Many drug interactions	None	Dose for GFR <10 mL/min	Dose for GFR <10 mL/min
Antifungal agents									
Amphotericin B	0.5–1.5 mg/kg/day	<1 %	No renal adjustment is required			Nephrotoxic, infusion-related reactions, give 250 cc NS before each dose	q24 h	q24 h	q24 to 36 h
Amphotec	4–6 mg/kg/day	<1 %	No renal adjustment is required						
Abelcet	5 mg/kg/day	<1 %	No renal adjustment is required						
AmBisome	3–5 mg/kg/day	<1 %	No renal adjustment is required						
Azoles and other antifungals						Increase CSA/FK level			
Fluconazole	200–800 mg IV q24 h/q12 h	70 %	100 %	100 %	50 %		200 mg after dialysis	Dose for GFR <10 mL/min	Dose for GFR 10–50 mL/min
Flucytosine	37.5 mg/kg	90 %	q12 h	q16 h	q24 h	Hepatic dysfunction. Marrow suppression more common in azotemic patients	Dose after dialysis	0.5–1.0 g/d	Dose for GFR 10–50 mL/min
Griseofulvin	125–250 mg q6 h	1 %	100 %	100 %	100 %		None	None	None

Itraconazole	200 mg q12 h	35 %	100 %	100 %	50 %	Poor oral absorption	100 mg q12 to 24 h	100 mg q12 to 24 h	100 mg q12 to 24 h
Ketoconazole	200–400 mg po q24 h	15 %	100 %	100 %	100 %	Hepatotoxic	None	None	None
Miconazole	1,200–3,600 mg/day	1 %	100 %	100 %	100 %		None	None	None
Posaconazole	200 mg q6 h	1 %	100 %	100 %	100 %				
Terbinafine	250 mg po q24 h	>1 %	100 %	100 %	100 %				
Voriconaozle	4–6 mg/kg q12 h	1 %	100 %	100 %	100 %	Avoid IV formulation in CKD			
Caspofungin	70 mg LD then 50 mg daily	1 %	100 %	100 %	100 %				
Micofungin	100–150 mg IV daily	1 %	100 %	100 %	100 %				
Anidulafungin	200 mg LD, then 100 mg daily	1 %	100 %	100 %	100 %				
Antiviral agents									
Acyclovir	200–800 mg po 5×/day	50 %	100 %	100 %	50 %	Poor absorption Neurotoxicity in ESRD. IV preparation can cause renal failure if injected rapidly	Dose after dialysis	Dose for GFR <10 mL/min	3.5 mg/kg/d
Adefovir	10 mg q24 h	45 %	100 %	10 mg q48 h	10 mg q72 h	Renal toxicity	10 mg weekly after HD	No data	No data
Amantadine	100–200 mg q12 h	90 %	100 %	50 %	q96 h to 7 days		None	None	Dose for GFR 10–50 mL/min
Cidofovir	5 mg/kg weekly ×2 (induction); 5 mg/kg every 2 weeks	90 %	Avoid in CKD	No data: Avoid	No data: Avoid	Dose-limiting nephrotoxicity with preteinuria, glycosuria, renal insufficiency; nephrotoxicity, and renal clearance reduced with coadministration of probenecid	No data	No data	Avoid
Delavirdine	400 mg q8 h	5 %	No data: 100 %	No data: 100 %	No data: 100 %		No data: None	No data	No data: Dose for GFR 10–50 mL/min
Didanosine	200 mg q12 h (125 mg if <60 kg)	40–69 %	q12 h	q24 h	50 % q24 h	Pancreatitis	Dose after dialysis	Dose for GFR <10 mL/min	Dose for GFR <10 mL/min
Emtricitabine	200 mg q24 h	86 %	q24 h	q48 to 72 h	q 96 h			Dose after dialysis	No data
Entecavir	0.5 mg q24 h	62 %	q24 h	q48 to 72 h	q 96 h			Dose after dialysis	No data
Famciclovir	250–500 mg po q12 to q8 h	60 %	q8 h	q12 h	q24 h	VZV: 500 mg po q8 h HSV: 250 po q12 h. Metabolized to active compound penciclovir	Dose after dialysis	No data	No data: Dose for GFR 10–50 mL/min

(continued)

(continued)

Antimicrobal agents in renal failure

Drugs	Normal dosage	% of renal excretion	Dosage adjustment in renal failure GFR >50 mL/min	GFR 10–50 mL/min	GFR <10 mL/min	Comments	HD	CAPD	Continuous venovenous hemofiltration
Foscarnet	40–80 mg IV q8 h	85 %	40–20 mg q8 to 24 h according to ClCr			Nephrotoxic, neurotoxic, hypocalcemia, hypophosphatemia, hypomagnesemia, and hypokalemia	Dose after dialysis	Dose for GFR <10 mL/min	Dose for GFR 10–50 mL/min
Ganciclovir IV	5 mg/kg q12 h	95 %	q12 h	q24 h	2.5 mg/kg q24 h	Granulocytopenia and thrombocytopenia	Dose after dialysis	Dose for GFR <10 mL/min	2.5 mg/kg q24 h
Ganciclovir	1,000 mg po q8 h	95 %	1,000 mg q8 h	1,000 mg q12 h	1,000 mg q24 h	Oral ganciclovir should be used ONLY for prevention of CMV infection. Always use IV ganciclovir for the treatment of CMV infection	No data: Dose after dialysis	No data: Dose for GFR <10 mL/min	N/A
Indinavir	800 mg q8 h	10 %	No data: 100 %	No data: 100 %	No data: 100 %	Nephrolithiasis; acute renal failure due to crystalluria, tubulointerstitial nephritis.	No data: None	No data: Dose for GFR <10 mL/min	No data
Lamivudine	150 mg po q12 h	80 %	q12 h	q24 h	50 mg q24 h	For hepatitis B	Dose after dialysis	No data: Dose for GFR <10 mL/min	Dose for GFR 10–50 mL/min
Maraviroc	300 mg q12 h	20 %	300 mg q12 h	No data	No data	Drug interaction with CYP III-A	No data	No data	No data
Nelfinavir	750 mg q8 h	No data	No data	No data	No data		No data	No data	No data
Nevirapine	200 mg q24 h × 14 d	<3	No data: 100 %	No data: 100 %	No data: 100 %	May be partially cleared by HD and peritoneal dialysis.	Dose after dialysis	No data: Dose for GFR <10 mL/min	No data: Dose for GFR 10–50 mL/min
Oseltamivir	75 mg q12 h	99 %	75 q12 h	75 mg daily	75 mg q48 h		Dose after dialysis		
Ribavirin	500–600 mg q12 h	30 %	100 %	100 %	50 %	Hemolytic uremic syndrome	Dose after dialysis	Dose for GFR <10 mL/min	Dose for GFR 10–50 mL/min
Rifabutin	300 mg q24 h	5 % to 10 %	100 %	100 %	100 %		None	None	No data: Dose for GFR 10–50 mL/min
Rimantadine	100 mg po q12 h	25 %	100 %	100 %	50 %				
Ritonavir	600 mg q12 h	3.50 %	No data: 100 %	No data: 100 %	No data: 100 %	Many drug interactions	No data: None	No data: Dose for GFR <10 mL/min	No data: Dose for GFR 10–50 mL/min
Saquinavir	600 mg q8 h	<4 %	No data: 100 %	No data: 100 %	No data: 100 %		No data: None	No data: Dose for GFR <10 mL/min	No data: Dose for GFR 10–50 mL/min
Stavudine	30–40 mg q12 h	35–40 %	100 %	50 % q12 to 24 h	50 % q24 h		Dose for GFR <10 mL/min after dialysis	No data	No data: Dose for GFR 10–50 mL/min

Telbivudine	600 mg po daily		100 %	600 mg q48 h	600 mg q96 h		Dose for GFR <10 mL/min after dialysis	No data	No data: Dose for GFR 10–50 mL/min
Tenofovir	300 mg q24 h		100 %	300 mg q48 to 72 h	300 mg q96 h	Nephrotoxic	Dose for GFR <10 mL/min after dialysis	No data	No data: Dose for GFR 10–50 mL/min
Valacyclovir	500–1,000 mg q8 h	50 %	100 %	50 %	25 %	Thrombotic thrombocytopenic purpura/hemolytic uremic syndrome	Dose after dialysis	Dose for GFR <10 mL/min	No data: Dose for GFR 10–50 mL/min
Valganciclovir	900 mg po daily or q12 h		100 %	50 %	25 %	Granulocytopenia and thrombocytopenia	Dose after dialysis	Dose for GFR <10 mL/min	450 mg daily
Vidarabine	15 mg/kg infusion q24 h	50 %	100 %	100 %	75 %		Infuse after dialysis	Dose for GFR <10 mL/min	Dose for GFR 10–50 mL/min
Zanamivir	2 puffs q12 h × 5 days	1 %	100 %	100 %	100 %	Bioavailability from inhalation and systemic exposure to drug is low	None	None	No data
Zalcitabine	0.75 mg q8 h	75 %	100 %	q12 h	q24 h		No data: Dose after dialysis	No data	No data: Dose for GFR 10–50 mL/min
Zidovudine	200 mg q8 h, 300 mg q12 h	8–25 %	100 %	100 %	100 mg q8 h	Enormous interpatient variation. Metabolite renally excreted	Dose for GFR <10 mL/min	Dose for GFR <10 mL/min	100 mg q8 h

Analgesic drug dosing in renal failure

Analgesics	Normal dosage	% of renal excretion	Dosage adjustment in renal failure GFR >50 mL/min	GFR 10–50 mL/min	GFR <10 mL/min	Comments	HD	CAPD	Continuous venovenous hemofiltration
Narcotics and narcotic antagonists									
Alfentanil	Anesthetic induction 8–40 mcg/kg	Hepatic	100 %	100 %	100 %	Titrate the dose regimen	N/A	N/A	N/A
Butorphanol	2 mg q3 to 4 h	Hepatic	100 %	75 %	50 %		No data	No data	N/A
Codeine	30–60 mg q4 to 6 h	Hepatic	100 %	75 %	50 %		No data	No data	Dose for GFR 10–50 mL/min
Fentanyl	Anesthetic induction (individualized)	Hepatic	100 %	75 %	50 %	CRRT-titrate	N/A	N/A	N/A
Meperidine	50–100 mg q3 to 4 h	Hepatic	100 %	75 %	50 %	Normeperidine, an active metabolite, accumulates in ESRD and may cause seizures. Protein binding is reduced in ESRD. 20–25 % excreted unchanged in acidic urine	Avoid	Avoid	Avoid
Methadone	2.5–5 mg q6 to 8 h	Hepatic	100 %	100 %	50–75 %		None	None	N/A
Morphine	20–25 mg q4 h	Hepatic	100 %	75 %	50 %	Increased sensitivity to drug effect in ESRD	None	No data	Dose for GFR 10–50 mL/min
Naloxone	0.4–2 mg IV	Hepatic	100 %	100 %	100 %		N/A	N/A	Dose for GFR 10–50 mL/min
Pentazocine	50 mg q4 h	Hepatic	100 %	75 %	75 %		None	No data	Dose for GFR 10–50 mL/min
Propoxyphene	65 mg po q6 to 8 h	Hepatic	100 %	100 %	Avoid	Active metabolite norpropoxyphene accumulates in ESRD	Avoid	Avoid	N/A
Sufentanil	Anesthetic induction	Hepatic	100 %	100 %	100 %	CRRT-titrate	N/A	N/A	N/A
Non-narcotics									
Acetaminophen	650 mg q4 h	Hepatic	q4 h	q6 h	q8 h	Overdose may be nephrotoxic Drug is major metabolite of phenacetin	None	None	Dose for GFR 10–50 mL/min
Acetylsalicylic acid	650 mg q4 h	Hepatic (renal)	q4 h	q4 to 6 h	Avoid	Nephrotoxic in high doses. May decrease GFR when renal blood flow is prostaglandin dependent. May add to uremic GI and hematologic symptoms. Protein binding reduced in ESRD	Dose after dialysis	None	Dose for GFR 10–50 mL/min

Antihypertensive and cardiovascular agent dosing in renal failure

Antihypertensive and cardiovascular agents	Normal doses			Dosage adjustment in renal failure			Comments	HD	CAPD	Continuous venovenous hemofiltration
	Starting dose	Maximum dose	% of renal excretion	GFR >50 mL/min	GFR 10–50 mL/min	GFR <10 mL/min				
ACE-I							Hyperkalemia, acute renal failure, angioedema, rash, cough, anemia, and liver toxicity			
Benazepril	10 mg q24 h	80 mg q24 h	20 %	100 %	75 %	25–50 %		None	None	Dose for GFR 10–50 mL/min
Captopril	6.25–25 mg po q8 h	100 mg q8 h	35 %	100 %	75 %	50 %	Rare proteinuria, nephrotic syndrome, dysgeusia, granulocytopenia. Increases serum digoxin levels	25–30 %	None	Dose for GFR 10–50 mL/min
Enalapril	5 mg q24 h	20 mg q12 h	45 %	100 %	75 %	50 %	Enalaprilat, the active moiety formed in liver	20–25 %	None	Dose for GFR 10–50 mL/min
Fosinopril	10 mg po q24 h	40 mg q12 h	20 %	100 %	100 %	75 %	Fosinoprilat, the active moiety formed in liver. Drug less likely than other ACE-I to accumulate in renal failure	None	None	Dose for GFR 10–50 mL/min
Lisinopril	2.5 mg q24 h	20 mg q12 h	80 %	100 %	50–75 %	25–50 %	Lysine analog of a pharmacologically active enalapril metabolite	20 %	None	Dose for GFR 10–50 mL/min
Pentopril		125 mg q24 h	80–90 %	100 %	50–75 %	50 %		No data	No data	Dose for GFR 10–50 mL/min
Perindopril		2 mg q24 h	<10 %	100 %	75 %	50 %	Active metabolite is perindoprilat. The clearance of perindoprilat and its metabolites is almost exclusively renal. Approximately 60 % of circulating perindopril is bound to plasma proteins, and only 10–20 % of perindoprilat is bound	25–50 %	No data	Dose for GFR 10–50 mL/min
Quinapril	10 mg q24 h	20 mg q24 h	30 %	100 %	75–100 %	75 %	Active metabolite is quinaprilat. 96 % of quinaprilat is excreted renally	25 %	None	Dose for GFR 10–50 mL/min
Ramipril	2.5 mg q24 h	10 q12 h	15 %	100 %	50–75 %	25–50 %	Active metabolite is ramiprilat. Data are for ramiprilat	20 %	None	Dose for GFR 10–50 mL/min
Trandolapril	1–2 mg q24 h	4 mg q24 h	33 %	100 %	50–100 %	50 %		None	None	Dose for GFR 10–50 mL/min

(continued)

Antihypertensive and cardiovascular agent dosing in renal failure

Antihypertensive and cardiovascular agents	Normal doses: Starting dose	Normal doses: Maximum dose	% of renal excretion	Dosage adjustment in renal failure: GFR >50 mL/min	Dosage adjustment in renal failure: GFR 10–50 mL/min	Dosage adjustment in renal failure: GFR <10 mL/min	Comments	HD	CAPD	Continuous venovenous hemofiltration
Angiotensin-II-receptors antagonists							Hyperkalemia, angioedema (less common than ACE-I)			
Candesartan	16 mg q24 h	32 mg q24 h	33 %	100 %	100 %	50 %	Candesartan cilexetil is rapidly and completely bioactivated by ester hydrolysis during absorption from the GI tract to candesartan	None	None	None
Eprosartan	600 mg q24 h	400–800 mg q24 h	25 %	100 %	100 %	100 %	Eprosartan pharmacokinetics more variable ESRD. Decreased protein binding in uremia	None	None	None
Irbesartan	150 mg q24 h	300 mg q24 h	20 %	100 %	100 %	100 %		None	None	None
Losartan	50 mg q24 h	100 mg q24 h	13 %	100 %	100 %	100 %		No data	No data	Dose for GFR 10–50 mL/min
Telmisartan	20–80 mg q24 h		<5 %	100 %	100 %	100 %		None	None	None
Valsartan	80 mg q24 h	160 mg q12 h	7 %	100 %	100 %	100 %		None	None	None
Beta blockers							Decrease HDL, mask symptoms of hypoglycemia, bronchospasm, fatigue, insomnia, depression, and sexual dysfunction			
Acebutolol	400 mg q24 h or q12 h	600 mg q24 h or q12 h	55 %	100 %	50 %	30–50 %	Active metabolites with long half-life	None	None	Dose for GFR 10–50 mL/min
Atenolol	25 mg q24 h	100 mg q24 h	90 %	100 %	75 %	50 %	Accumulates in ESRD	25–50 mg	None	Dose for GFR 10–50 mL/min
Betaxolol	20 mg q24 h	80–90 %	100 %	100 %	50 %	50 %		None	Dose for GFR 10-50 mL/min	Dose for GFR 10–50 mL/min
Bopindolol	1 mg q24 h	4 mg q24 h	<10 %	100 %	100 %	100 %		None	None	Dose for GFR 10–50 mL/min
Carteolol	0.5 mg q24 h	10 mg q24 h	<50 %	100 %	50 %	25 %		No data	None	Dose for GFR 10–50 mL/min
Carvedilol	3.125 mg po q8 h	25 mg q8 h	2 %	100 %	100 %	100 %	Kinetics are dose dependent. Plasma concentrations of carvedilol have been reported to be increased in patients with renal impairment	None	None	Dose for GFR 10–50 mL/min
Celiprolol		200 mg q24 h	10 %	100 %	100 %	75 %		No data	None	Dose for GFR 10–50 mL/min
Dilevalol	200 mg q12 h	400 mg q12 h	<5 %	100 %	100 %	100 %		None	None	No data

Esmolol (IV only)	50 mcg/kg/min	300 mcg/kg/min	10 %	100 %	100 %	100 %	Active metabolite retained in renal failure	None	None	No data
Labetalol	50 mg po q12 h	400 mg q12 h	5 %	100 %	100 %	100 %	For IV use: 20 mg slow IV injection over a 2-min period. Additional injections of 40 mg or 80 mg can be given at 10-min intervals until a total of 300 mg or continuous infusion of 2 mg/min	None	None	Dose for GFR 10–50 mL/min
Metoprolol		50 mg q12 h	100 mg q12 h	<5 %	100 %	100 %		None	None	None
Nadolol	80 mg q24 h	160 mg q12 h	90 %	100 %	50 %	25 %	Start with prolonged interval and titrate	40 mg	None	Dose for GFR 10–50 mL/min
Penbutolol	10 mg q24 h	40 mg q24 h	<10	100 %	100 %	100 %		None	None	Dose for GFR 10–50 mL/min
Pindolol	10 mg q12 h	40 mg q12 h	40 %	100 %	100 %	100 %		None	None	Dose for GFR 10–50 mL/min
Propranolol	40 % to 160 mg q8 h	320 mg/day	<5 %	100 %	100 %	100 %	Bioavailability may increase in ESRD. Metabolites may cause increased bilirubin by assay interference in ESRD. Hypoglycemia reported in ESRD	None	None	Dose for GFR 10–50 mL/min
Sotalol	80 q12 h	160 mg q12 h	70 %	100 %	50 %	25–50 %	Extreme caution should be exercised in the use of sotalol in patients with renal failure undergoing HD. To minimize the risk of induced arrhythmia, patients initiated or re-initiated on sotalol should be placed for a minimum of 3 days (on their maintenance dose) in a facility that can provide cardiac resuscitation and continuous electrocardiographic monitoring	80 mg	None	Dose for GFR 10–50 mL/min
Timolol	10 mg q12 h	20 mg q12 h	15 %	100 %	100 %	100 %		None	None	Dose for GFR 10–50 mL/min
Calcium channel blockers							Dihydropyridine: headache, ankle edema, gingival hyperplasia, and flushing			
							Non-dihydropyridine: bradycardia, constipation, gingival hyperplasia, and AV block			
Amlodipine	2.5 po q24 h	10 mg q24 h	10 %	100 %	100 %	100 %	May increase digoxin and cyclosporine levels	None	None	Dose for GFR 10–50 mL/min
Bepridil	No data	<1 %	No data	No data	No data	Weak vasodilator and antihypertensive		None	No data	No data

(continued)

(continued)

Antihypertensive and cardiovascular agent dosing in renal failure

Antihypertensive and cardiovascular agents	Normal doses: Starting dose	Normal doses: Maximum dose	% of renal excretion	Dosage adjustment in renal failure: GFR >50 mL/min	Dosage adjustment in renal failure: GFR 10–50 mL/min	Dosage adjustment in renal failure: GFR <10 mL/min	Comments	HD	CAPD	Continuous venovenous hemofiltration
Diltiazem	30 mg q8 h	90 mg q8 h	10 %	100 %	100 %	100 %	Acute renal dysfunction. May exacerbate hyperkalemia. May increase digoxin and cyclosporine levels	None	None	Dose for GFR 10–50 mL/min
Felodipine	5 mg po q12 h	20 mg q24 h	1 %	100 %	100 %	100 %	May increase digoxin levels	None	None	Dose for GFR 10–50 mL/min
Isradipine	5 mg po q12 h	10 mg q12 h	<5 %	100 %	100 %	100 %	May increase digoxin levels	None	None	Dose for GFR 10–50 mL/min
Nicardipine	20 mg po q8 h	30 mg po q8 h	<1 %	100 %	100 %		Uremia inhibits hepatic metabolism. May increase digoxin levels	None	None	None
Nifedipine XL	30 q24 h	90 mg q12 h	10 %	100 %	100 %	100 %	Avoid short-acting nifedipine formulation	None	None	None
Nimodipine	30 mg q8 h	10 %	100 %	100 %	100 %		May lower blood pressure	None	None	Dose for GFR 10–50 mL/min
Nisoldipine	20 mg q24 h	30 mg q12 h	10 %	100 %	100 %	100 %	May increase digoxin levels	None	None	Dose for GFR 10–50 mL/min
Verapamil	40 mg q8 h	240 mg/day	10 %	100 %	100 %	100 %	Acute renal dysfunction. Active metabolites accumulate particularly with sustained-release forms	None	None	Dose for GFR 10–50 mL/min
Diuretics							Hypokalemia/hyperkalemia (potassium sparing agents), hyperuricemia, hyperglycemia, hypomagnesemia, increase serum cholesterol			
Acetazolamide	125 mg po q8 h	500 mg po q8 h	90 %	100 %	50 %	Avoid	May potentiate acidosis. Ineffective as diuretic in ESRD. May cause neurologic side effects in dialysis patients	No data	No data	Avoid
Amiloride	5 mg po q24 h	10 mg po q24 h	50 %	100 %	100 %	Avoid	Hyperkalemia with GFR <30 mL/min, especially in diabetics. Hyperchloremic metabolic acidosis	N/A	N/A	N/A
Bumetanide	1–2 mg po q24 h	2–4 mg po q24 h	35 %	100 %	100 %	100 %	Ototoxicity increased in ESRD in combination with aminoglycosides. High doses effective in ESRD. Muscle pain, gynecomastia	None	None	N/A

Chlorthalidone	25 mg q24 h	50 %	q24 h	q24 h	Avoid	Ineffective with low GFR		N/A	N/A	N/A
Ethacrynic alcid	50 mg po q24 h	100 mg po q12 h	20 %	100 %	100 %	100 %	Ototoxicity increased in ESRD in combination with aminoglycosides	None	None	N/A
Furosemide	40–80 mg po q24 h	120 mg po q8 h	70 %	100 %	100 %	100 %	Ototoxicity increased in ESRD, especially in combination with aminoglycosides. High doses effective in ESRD	None	None	N/A
Indapamide	2.5 mg q24 h	<5 %	100 %	100 %	Avoid	Ineffective in ESRD		None	N/A	None
Metolazone	2.5 mg po q24 h	10 mg po q12 h	70 %	100 %	100 %		High doses effective in ESRD. Gynecomastia, impotence	None	None	None
Eplerenone	25 mg daily	200 mg daily	100 %	100 %	100 %					
Spironolactone	100 mg po q24 h	300 mg po q24 h	25 %	100 %	100 %	Avoid	Active metabolites with long half-life. Hyperkalemia common when GFR <30, especially in diabetics. Gynecomastia, hyperchloremic acidosis. Increases serum by immunoassay interference	N/A	N/A	Avoid
Thiazides	25 mg q12 h	50 mg q12 h	>95 %	100 %	100 %	Avoid	Usually ineffective with GFR <30 mL/min. Effective at low GFR in combination with loop diuretic. Hyperuricemia		N/A	N/A
Torasemide	5 mg po q12 h	20 mg q24 h	25 %	100 %	100 %	100 %	High doses effective in ESRD. Ototoxicity	None	None	N/A
Triamterene	25 mg q12 h	50 mg q12 h	5–10 %	q12 h	q12 h	Avoid	Hyperkalemia common when GFR <30, especially in diabetics. Active metabolite with long half-life in ESRD. Folic acid antagonist. Urolithiasis. Crystalluria in acid urine. May cause acute renal failure	Avoid	Avoid	Avoid
Miscellaneous agents										
Amrinone	5 mg/kg/min daily dose <10 mg/kg	10 mg/kg/min daily dose <10 mg/kg	10–40 %	100 %	100 %	100 %	Thrombocytopenia. Nausea, vomiting in ESRD	No data	No data	Dose for GFR 10–50 mL/min
Clonidine	0.1 po q12 h/q8 h	1.2 mg/day	45 %	100 %	100 %	100 %	Sexual dysfunction, dizziness, postal hypotension	None	None	Dose for GFR 10–50 mL/min

(continued)

(continued)

Antihypertensive and cardiovascular agent dosing in renal failure

Antihypertensive and cardiovascular agents	Normal doses			Dosage adjustment in renal failure			Comments	HD	CAPD	Continuous venovenous hemofiltration
	Starting dose	Maximum dose	% of renal excretion	GFR >50 mL/min	GFR 10–50 mL/min	GFR <10 mL/min				
Digoxin	0.125 mg qod/q24 h	0.25 mg po q24 h	25 %	100 %	100 %	100 %	Decrease LD by 50 % in ESRD. Radioimmunoassay may overestimate serum levels in uremia. Clearance decreased by amiodarone, spironolactone, quinidine, verapamil. Hypokalemia, hypomagnesemia enhance toxicity. Vd and total body clearance decreased in ESRD. Serum level 12 h after dose is best guide in ESRD. Digoxin immune antibodies can treat severe toxicity in ESRD	None	None	Dose for GFR 10–50 mL/min
Hydralazine	10 mg po q6 h	100 mg po q6 h	25 %	100 %	100 %	100 %	Lupus-like reaction	None	None	Dose for GFR 10–50 mL/min
Midodrine	No data	No data	75–80 %	5–10 mg q8 h	5–10 mg q8 h	No data	Increased blood pressure	5 mg q8 h	No data	Dose for GFR 10–50 mL/min
Minoxidil	2.5 mg po q12 h	10 mg po q12 h	20 %	100 %	100 %	100 %	Pericardial effusion, fluid retention, hypertrichosis, and tachycardia	None	None	Dose for GFR 10–50 mL/min
Nitroprusside	1 mcg/kg/min	10 mcg/kg/min	<10 %	100 %	100 %	100 %	Cyanide toxicity	None	None	Dose for GFR 10–50 mL/min
Amrinone	5 mcg/kg/min	10 mcg/kg/min	25 %	100 %	100 %	100 %	Thrombocytopenia. Nausea, vomiting in ESRD	No data	No data	Dose for GFR 10–50 mL/min
Dobutamine	2.5 mcg/kg/min	15 mcg/kg/min	10 %	100 %	100 %	100 %		No data	No data	Dose for GFR 10–50 mL/min
Milrinone	0.375 mcg/kg/min	0.75 mcg/kg/min	100 %	100 %	100 %			No data	No data	Dose for GFR 10–50 mL/min

Hypoglycemic agents dosing in renal failure

Hypoglycemic agents	Normal doses: Starting dose	Normal doses: Maximum dose	Normal doses: % of renal excretion	Dosage adjustment in renal failure: GFR >50 mL/min	Dosage adjustment in renal failure: GFR 10–50 mL/min	Dosage adjustment in renal failure: GFR <10 mL/min	Comments	HD	CAPD	Continuous venovenous hemofiltration
							Avoid all oral hypoglycemic agents on CRRT			
Acarbose	25 mg q8 h	100 mg q8 h	35 %	100 %	50 %	Avoid	Abdominal pain, N/V, and flatulence	No data	No data	Avoid
Acetohexamide	250 mg q24 h	1,500 mg q24 h	None	Avoid	Avoid	Avoid	Diuretic effect. May falsely elevate serum creatinine. Active metabolite has $T_{1/2}$ of 5–8 h in healthy subjects and is eliminated by the kidney. Prolonged hypoglycemia in azotemic patients	No data	None	Avoid
Chlorpropamide	100 mg q24 h	500 mg q24 h	47 %	50 %	Avoid	Avoid	Impairs water excretion. Prolonged hypoglycemia in azotemic patients	No data	None	Avoid
Exenatide	5 mcg q12 h	10 mcg q12 h	No data	100 %	Use with caution	Avoid				
Glibornuride	12.5 mg q24 h	100 mg q14 h	No data	No data	No data	No data		No data	No data	Avoid
Gliclazide	80 mg q24 h	320 mg q24 h	<20 %	50–100 %	Avoid	Avoid		No data	No data	Avoid
Glipizide	5 mg q24 h	20 mg q12 h	5 %	100 %	50 %	50 %		No data	No data	Avoid
Glyburide	2.5 mg q24 h	10 mg q12 h	50 %	100 %	50 %	Avoid		None	None	Avoid
Liragutide	0.6 mg daily	1.8 mg daily	6 %	100 %	100 %	Avoid	No data on dialysis			
Metformin	500 mg q12 h	2,550 mg/day (q12 h or q8 h)	95 %	100 %	Avoid	Avoid	Lactic acidosis	No data	No data	Avoid
Piogkitazone	15 mg q24 h	45 mg q24 h	3 %	100 %	100 %	100 %	Drug interactions	None	None	NA
Pramlintide	15 mcg	60 mcg daily	No data	100 %	No data	No data				
Repaglinide	0.5–1 mg	4 mg q8 h								
Rosiglitazone	2 mg q24 h	8 mg q24 h	3 %	100 %	100 %	100 %	Increases LDL	None	None	NA
Sitaglipitin	25 mg	100 mg	79 %	100 %	50 %	25 %				
Tolazamide	100 mg q24 h	250 mg q24 h	7 %	100 %	100 %	100 %	Diuretic effects	Avoid	Avoid	Avoid
Tolbutamide	1 g q24 h	2 g q24 h	None	100 %	100 %	100 %	May impair water excretion	None	None	Avoid
Parenteral agents							Dosage guided by blood glucose levels			
Insulin		Variable	None	100 %	75 %	50 %	Renal metabolism of insulin decreases with azotemia	None	None	Dose for GFR 10–50 mL/min
Lispro insulin		Variable	No data	100 %	75 %	50 %	Avoid all oral hypoglycemic agents on CRRT	None	None	None

Hyperlipidemic agents dosing in renal failure

	Normal doses			Dosage adjustment in renal failure						
Hypoglycemic agents	Starting dose	Maximum dose	% of renal excretion	GFR >50	GFR 10–50 mL/min	GFR <10 mL/min	Comments	HD	CAPD	Continuous venovenous hemofiltration
		400 mg SR q24 h								
Atorvastatin	10 mg/day	80 mg/day	<2 %	100 %	100 %	100 %	Liver dysfunction, myalgia, and rhabdomyolysis with CSA/FK	No data	No data	No data
Bezafibrate		200 mg q12 to q6 h	50 %	50–100 %	25–50 %	Avoid	No data	No data	No data	
Cholestyramine	4 g q12 h	24 g/day	None	100 %	100 %	100 %		No data	No data	No data
Clofibrate	500 mg q12 h	1,000 mg q12 h	40–70 %	q6 to 12 h	q12 to 18 h	Avoid		No data	No data	No data
Colestipol	5 g q12 h	30 g/day	None	100 %	100 %	100 %		No data	No data	No data
Fenofibrate	48 mg daily	145 mg daily	30 %	100 %	100 %	50 %				
Fluvastatin	20 mg daily	80 mg/day	<1 %	100 %	100 %	100 %		No data	No data	No data
Gemfibrozil	600 q12 h	600 q12 h	None	100 %	100 %	100 %		No data	No data	No data
Lovastatin	5 mg daily	20 mg/day	None	100 %	100 %	100 %		No data	No data	No data
Nicotinic acid	1 g q8 h	2 g q8 h	None	100 %	50 %	25 %		No data	No data	No data
Pravastatin	10–40 mg daily	80 mg/day	<10 %	100 %	100 %	100 %		No data	No data	No data
Probucol		500 mg q12 h	<2 %	100 %	100 %	100 %		No data	No data	No data
Rosuvastatin	5 mg daily	20 mg daily	<5 %	100 %	100 %	50 %				
Simvastatin	5–20 mg daily	20 mg/day	13 %	100 %	100 %	100 %		No data	No data	No data

Antithyroid dosing in renal failure

			Dosage adjustment in renal failure					
Antithyroid drugs	Normal dosage	% of renal excretion	GFR >50	GFR 10–50 mL/min	GFR <10 mL/min	HD	CAPD	Continuous venovenous hemofiltration
Methimazole	5–20 mg q8 h	7	100 %	100 %	100 %	No data	No data	Dose for GFR 10–50 mL/min
Propylthiouracil	100 mg q8 h	<10	100 %	100 %	100 %	No data	No data	Dose for GFR 10–50 mL/min

GI agents dosing in renal failure

	Normal doses			Dosage adjustment in renal failure			
GI agents	Starting dose	Maximum dose	% of renal excretion	GFR >50 mL/min	GFR 10–50 mL/min	GFR <10 mL/min	Comments
Anti-ulcer agents							
Cimetidine	300 mg po q8 h	800 mg po q12 h	60 %	100 %	75 %	25 %	Multiple drug-drug interactions; beta blockers, sulfonylurea, theophylline, warfarin, etc
Famotidine	20 mg po q12 h	40 mg po q12 h	70 %	100 %	75 %	25 %	Headache, fatigue, thrombocytopenia, alopecia
Lansoprazole	15 mg po q24 h	30 mg q12 h	None	100 %	100 %	100 %	Headache, diarrhea
Nizatidine	150 mg po q12 h	300 mg po q12 h	20 %	100 %	75 %	25 %	Headache, fatigue, thrombocytopenia, alopecia
Omeprazole	20 mg po q24 h	40 mg po q12 h	None	100 %	100 %	100 %	Headache, diarrhea
Rabeprazole	20 mg po q24 h	40 mg po q12 h	None	100 %	100 %	100 %	Headache, diarrhea
Pantoprazole	40 mg po q24 h	80 mg po q12 h	None	100 %	100 %	100 %	Headache, diarrhea
Ranitidine	150 mg po q12 h	300 mg po q12 h	80 %	100 %	75 %	25 %	Headache, fatigue, thrombocytopenia, alopecia
Metoclopramide	10 mg po q8 h	30 mg po q6 h	15 %	100 %	100 %	50–75 %	Increase cyclosporine/tacrolimus level. Neurotoxic
Misoprostol	100 mcg po q12 h	200 mcg po q6 h		100 %	100 %	100 %	Diarrhea, N/V, abortifacient agent
Sucralfate	1 g po q6 h	1g po q6 h	None	100 %	100 %	100 %	Constipation, decrease absorption of MMF

	Normal doses			Dosage adjustment in renal failure			
Anticonvulsants	Starting dose	Maximum dose	% of renal excretion	GFR>50 mL/min	GFR 10–50 mL/min	GFR <10 mL/min	Comments
Carbamazapine	2–8 mg/kg/day; adjust for side effect and TDM		2 %	100 %	100 %	100 %	Plasma concentration: 4–12, double vision, fluid retention, mylosuppression
Clonazepam	0.5 mg q8 h	2 mg q8 h	1 %	100 %	100 %	100 %	Although no dose reduction is recommended, the drug has not been studied in patients with renal impairment. Recommendations are based on known drug characteristics not clinical trials data
Ethosuximide	5 mg/kg/day; adjust for side effect and TDM		20 %	100 %	100 %	100 %	Plasma concentration: 40–100, headache
Felbamate	400 mg/q8 h	1,200 mg/q8 h	90 %	100 %	50 %	25 %	Anorexia, vomiting, insomnia, nausea
Gabapentin	150 mg q8 h	900 mg q8 h	77 %	100 %	50 %	25 %	Less CNS side effects compared to other agents
Lamotrigine	25–50 mg/day	150 mg/day	1 %	100 %	100 %	100 %	Autoinduction, major drug–drug interaction with valproate
Levetiracetam	500 mg q12 h	1,500 mg q12 h	66 %	100 %	50 %	50 %	
Oxcarbazepine	300 mg q12 h	600 mg q12 h	1 %	100 %	100 %	100 %	Less effect on P450 compared to carbamazapine
Phenobarbital	20 mg/kg/day; adjust for side effect and TDM		1 %	100 %	100 %	100 %	Plasma concentration: 15–40, insomnia
Phenytoin	20 mg/kg/day; adjust for side effect and TDM		1 %	Adjust for renal failure and low albumin			Plasma concentration: 10–20, nystagmus, check free phenytoin level
Primidone	50 mg	100 mg	1 %	100 %	100 %	100 %	Plasma concentration: 5–20
Sodium valproate	7.5–15 mg/kg/day; adjust for side effect and TDM		1 %	100 %	100 %	100 %	Plasma concentration: 50–150, weight gain, hepatitis, check free valproate level
Tiagabine	4 mg q24 h, increase 4 mg/day, titrate weekly		2 %	100 %	100 %	100 %	Total daily dose may be increased by 4–8 mg at weekly intervals until clinical response is achieved or up to 32 mg/day. The total daily dose should be given in divided doses two to four times daily.
Topiramate	50 mg/day	200 mg q12 h	70 %	100 %	50 %	Avoid	
Trimethadione	300 mg q8 to q6 h	600 mg q8 to q6 h	None	q8 h	q8 to 12 h	q12 to 24 h	Active metabolites with long half-life in ESRD. Nephrotic syndrome
Vigabatrin	1 g q12 h	2 g q12 h	70 %	100 %	50 %	25 %	Encephalopathy with drug accumulation
Zonisamide	100 mg q24 h	100–300 mg q24 to q12 h	30 %	100 %	75 %	50 %	Manufacturer recommends that Zonisamide should not be used in patients with renal failure (estimated GFR <50 mL/min) as there has been insufficient experience concerning drug dosing and toxicity. Zonisamide doses of 100–600 mg/day are effective for normal renal function. Dose recommendations for renal impairment based on clearance ratios

Sedatives	Normal dosage	% of renal excretion	Dosage adjustment in renal failure GFR >50 mL/min	GFR 10–50 mL/min	GFR <10 mL/min	Comments
Barbiturates						May cause excessive sedation, increase osteomalacia in ESRD. Charcoal hemoperfusion and HD more effective than peritoneal dialysis for poisoning
Pentobarbital	30 mg q6 to 8 h	Hepatic	100 %	100 %	100 %	
Phenobarbital	50–100 mg q8 to 12 h	Hepatic (renal)	q8 to 12 h	q8 to 12 h	q12 to 16 h	Up to 50 % unchanged drug excreted with urine with alkaline diuresis
Secobarbital	30–50 mg q6 to 8 h	Hepatic	100 %	100 %	100 %	
Thiopental	Anesthesia induction (individualized)	Hepatic	100 %	100 %	100 %	
Benzodiazepines						May cause excessive sedation and encephalopathy in ESRD
Alprazolam	0.25–5.0 mg q8 h	Hepatic	100 %	100 %	100 %	
Clorazepate	15–60 mg q24 h	Hepatic (renal)	100 %	100 %	100 %	
Chlordiazepoxide	15–100 mg q24 h	Hepatic	100 %	100 %	50 %	
Clonazepam	1.5 mg q24 h	Hepatic	100 %	100 %	100 %	Although no dose reduction is recommended, the drug has not been studied in patients with renal impairment. Recommendations are based on known drug characteristics not clinical trials data
Diazepam	5–40 mg q24 h	Hepatic	100 %	100 %	100 %	Active metabolites, desmethyldiazepam, and oxazepam may accumulate in renal failure. Dose should be reduced if given longer than a few days. Protein binding decreases in uremia
Estazolam	1 mg qhs	Hepatic	100 %	100 %	100 %	
Flurazepam	15–30 mg qhs	Hepatic	100 %	100 %	100 %	
Lorazepam	1–2 mg q8 to 12 h	Hepatic	100 %	100 %	100 %	
Midazolam	Individualized	Hepatic	100 %	100 %	50 %	
Oxazepam	30–120 mg q24 h	Hepatic	100 %	100 %	100 %	
Quazepam	15 mg qhs	Hepatic	No data	No data	No data	
Temazepam	30 mg qhs	Hepatic	100 %	100 %	100 %	
Triazolam	0.25–0.50 mg qhs	Hepatic	100 %	100 %	100 %	Protein binding correlates with alpha-1 acid glycoprotein concentration
Benzodiazepines						
Benzodiazepine						
Antagonist						May cause excessive sedation and encephalopathy in ESRD
Flumazenil	0.2 mg IV over 15 s	Hepatic	100 %	100 %	100 %	

Miscellaneous sedative agents						
Buspirone	5 mg q8 h	Hepatic	100 %	100 %	100 %	
Ethchlorvynol	500 mg qhs	Hepatic	100 %	Avoid	Avoid	Removed by hemoperfusion. Escessive sedation
Haloperidol	1–2 mg q8 to 12 h	Hepatic	100 %	100 %	100 %	HTN, excessive sedation
Lithium carbonate	0.9–1.2 g q24 h	Renal	100 %	50–75 %	25–50 %	Nephrotoxic. Nephrogenic diabetes insipidus. Nephrotic syndrome. Renal tubular acidosis. Interstitial fibrosis. Acute toxicity when serum levels >1.2 mEq/L. Serum levels should be measure periodically 12 h after dose. $T_{1/2}$ does not reflect extensive tissue accumulation. Plasma levels rebound after dialysis. Toxicity enhanced by volume depletion, NSAIDs, and diuretics
Meprobamate	1.2–1.6 g q24 h	Hepatic (renal)	q6 h	q9 to 12 h	q12 to 18 h	Excessive sedation. Excretion enhanced by forced diuresis

			Dosage adjustment in renal failure			
Antiparkinson agents	Normal dosage	% of renal excretion	GFR >50 mL/min	GFR 10–50 mL/min	GFR <10 mL/min	Comments
Carbidopa	1 tab q8 h to 6 tabs daily	30	100 %	100 %	100 %	Require careful titration of dose according to clinical response
Levodopa	25–500 mg q12 h to 8 g q24 h	None	100 %	50–100 %	50–100 %	Active and inactive metabolites excreted in urine. Active metabolites with long $T_{1/2}$ in ESRD

			Dosage adjustment in renal failure			
Antipsychotics	Normal dosage	% of renal excretion	GFR >50 mL/min	GFR 10–50 mL/min	GFR <10 mL/min	Comments
Phenothiazines						Orthostatic hypotension, extrapyramidal symptoms, and confusion can occur
Chlorpromazine	300–800 mg q24 h	Hepatic	100 %	100 %	100 %	
Promethazine	20–100 mg q24 h	Hepatic	100 %	100 %	100 %	Excessive sedation may occur in ESRD
Thioridazine	50–100 mg po q8 h. Increase gradually. Maximum of 800 mg/day					
Trifluoperazine	1–2 mg q12 h. Increase to no more than 6 mg					
Perphenazine	8–16 mg po q12 h, q8 h, or q6 h. Increase to 64 mg daily					
Thiothixene	2 mg po q8 h. Increase gradually to 15 mg daily					
Haloperidol	1–2 mg q8 to 12 h	Hepatic	100 %	100 %	100 %	Hypotension, excessive sedation
Loxapine	12.5–50 mg IM q4 to 6 h					Do not administer drug IV
Clozapine	12.5 mg po. 25–50 daily to 300–450 by end of 2 weeks					
Maximum: 900 mg daily	Metabolism nearly complete					
Risperidone	1 mg po q12 h. Increase to 3 mg q12 h					
Olanzapine	5–10 mg	Hepatic				Potential hypotensive effects
Quetiapine	25 mg po q12 h. Increase in increments of 25–50 q12 h or q8 h. 300–400 mg daily by day 4	Hepatic				
Ziprasidone	20–100 mg q12 h	Hepatic				

			Dosage adjustment in renal failure			
Corticosteroids	Normal dosage	% of renal excretion	GFR >50 mL/min	GFR 10–50 mL/min	GFR <10 mL/min	Comments
Betamethasone	0.5–9.0 mg q24 h	5	100 %	100 %	100 %	May aggravate azotemia, Na^+ retention, glucose intolerance, and HTN
Budesonide	No data	None	100 %	100 %	100 %	Same as above
Cortisone	25–500 mg q24 h	None	100 %	100 %	100 %	Same as above
Dexamethasone	0.75–9.0 mg q24 h	8	100 %	100 %	100 %	Same as above
Hydrocortisone	20–500 mg q24 h	None	100 %	100 %	100 %	Same as above
Methylprednisolone	4–48 mg q24 h	<10	100 %	100 %	100 %	Same as above
Prednisolone	5–60 mg q24 h	34	100 %	100 %	100 %	Same as above
Prednisone	5–60 mg q24 h	34	100 %	100 %	100 %	Same as above
Triamcinolone	4–48 mg q24 h	No data	100 %	100 %	100 %	Same as above

Anticoagulants	Normal doses			Dosage adjustment in renal failure			
	Starting dose	Maximum dose	% of renal excretion	GFR >50	GFR 10–50 mL/min	GFR < 10 mL/min	Comments
Alteplase	60 mg over 1 h then 20 mg/h for 2 h		No data	100 %	100 %	100 %	tPa
Anistreplase	30 U over 2–5 min		No data	100 %	100 %	100 %	
Aspirin	81 mg/day	325 mg/day	10 %	100 %	100 %	100 %	GI irritation and bleeding tendency
Clopidogrel	75 mg/day	75 mg/day	50 %	100 %	100 %	100 %	
Dabigatran	150 mg po q12 h	150 mg po q12 h	7 %	100 %	50 %	No data	
Dalteparin	2,500 U Sq/day	5,000 U Sq/day	Unknown	100 %	100 %	100 %	
Dipyridamole	50 mg q8 h		No data	100 %	100 %	100 %	
Enoxaparin	20 mg/day	30 mg q12 h	8 %	100 %	75–50 %	50 %	1 mg/kg q12 h for treatment of DVT. Check anti-factor Xa activity 4 h after second dose in patients with renal dysfunction. Some evidence of drug accumulation in renal failure
Fondaparinux	2.5–10 mg daily		77 %	100 %	Avoid	Avoid	
Heparin	75 U/kg load then 15 U/kg/h		None	100 %	100 %	100 %	Half-life increases with dose
Iloprost	0.5–2.0 ng/kg/min for 5–12 h		No data	100 %	100 %	50 %	
Indobufen	100 mg q12 h	200 mg q12 h	<15 %	100 %	50 %	25 %	
Rivaroxaban	20 mg q24 h	20 mg q24 h		100 %	75 %	Avoid	
Streptokinase	25,0000 U load then 10,0000 U/h		None	100 %	100 %	100 %	
Sulfinpyrazone	200 mg q12 h		25–50 %	100 %	100 %	Avoid	Acute renal failure. Uricosuric effect at low GFR
Sulotroban	No data		52–62 %	50 %	30 %	10 %	
Ticlopidine	250 mg q12 h	250 mg q12 h	2 %	100 %	100 %	100 %	Decrease CSA level and may cause severe neutropenia and thrombocytopenia
Tranexamic acid	25 mg/kg q8 to q6 h		90 %	50 %	25 %	10 %	
Urokinase	4,400 U/kg load then 4,400 U/kg qh		No data	No data	No data	No data	
Warfarin	5 mg/day	Adjust per INR	<1 %	100 %	100 %	100 %	Monitor INR very closely. Start at 5 mg/day. 1 mg Vit. K IV over 30 min or 2.5–5 mg po can be used to normalize INR

MTX methotrexate, *BID* twice daily, *TID* three times a day, *GFR* glomerular filtration rate, *TCN* tetracycline, *HTN* hypertension, *TB* tuberculosis, *BUN* blood urea nitrogen, *CAPD* continuous ambulatory peritoneal dialysis, *ESRD* end-stage renal disease, *AV* atrioventricular, *IV* intravenous, *NS* normal saline, *CKD* chronic kidney disease, *LD* loading dose, *PO* per os, *HD* hemodialysis, *VZV* varicella zoster virus, *HSV* herpes simplex virus, *CMV* cytomegalovirus, *CYP* cytochrome P450, *CRRT* continuous renal replacement therapy, *GI* gastrointestinal, *ACE-I* angiotensin-converting enzyme inhibitors, HDL high-density lipoprotein, *Vd* volume of distribution, *LDL* low-density lipoprotein, *N/V* nausea/vomiting, *TDM* therapeutic drug monitoring, *CNS* central nervous system, *qhs* before bed, *NSAIDs* nonsteroidal anti-inflammatory drugs, *tPa* tissue-type plasminogen activator, *DVT* deep vein thrombosis, *INR* international normalized ratio

Conclusion

As the incidence of CKD is on the rise, understanding pharmacokinetic and pharmacodynamics changes in patients with CKD has become increasingly important. Optimizing medication dosing to reduce toxicities while maintaining therapeutic effects can be difficult. Many patients with CKD have multiple comorbid disorders including dermatologic disease that put them at higher risk for medication-related adverse effects. The principles discussed above will assist in determining optimal medication dosing when initiating new therapies in these complex patient populations.

References

1. National Institutes of Health, National Institute of Diabetes and Digestive and Kidney Diseases. U.S. renal Data System. USRDS 2009 annual data report: atlas of end-stage renal disease in the United States. National Institutes of Health, National Institute of Diabetes and Digestive and Kidney Diseases, Bethesda, MD, 2009. 2014. Ref Type: Generic.
2. Hossain MP, Goyder EC, Rigby JE, El Nahas M. CKD and poverty: a growing global challenge. Am J Kidney Dis. 2009;53(1):166–74.
3. Burt VL, Cutler JA, Higgins M, et al. Trends in the prevalence, awareness, treatment, and control of hypertension in the adult US population. Data from the health examination surveys, 1960 to 1991. Hypertension. 1995;26(1):60–9.
4. Yarlagadda SG, Perazella MA. Drug-induced crystal nephropathy: an update. Expert Opin Drug Saf. 2008;7(2):147–58.
5. Olyaei AJ, Steffl JL. A quantitative approach to drug dosing in chronic kidney disease. Blood Purif. 2011;31(1–3):138–45.
6. Olyaei AJ, Bennett WM. Drug dosing in the elderly patients with chronic kidney disease. Clin Geriatr Med. 2009;25(3):459–527.
7. Farag A, Garg AX, Li L, Jain AK. Dosing errors in prescribed antibiotics for older persons with CKD: a retrospective time series analysis. Am J Kidney Dis. 2014;63(3):422–8.
8. Wooten JM. Adverse drug reactions: part I. South Med J. 2010;103(10):1025–8.
9. Philips BJ, Lane K, Dixon J, Macphee I. The effects of acute renal failure on drug metabolism. Expert Opin Drug Metab Toxicol. 2014;10(1):11–23.
10. Rifkin DE, Winkelmayer WC. Medication issues in older individuals with CKD. Adv Chronic Kidney Dis. 2010;17(4):320–8.
11. Zhao P, Vieira ML, Grillo JA, et al. Evaluation of exposure change of nonrenally eliminated drugs in patients with chronic kidney disease using physiologically based pharmacokinetic modeling and simulation. J Clin Pharmacol. 2012;52(1 Suppl):91S–108.
12. Zhang L, Xu N, Xiao S, et al. Regulatory perspectives on designing pharmacokinetic studies and optimizing labeling recommendations for patients with chronic kidney disease. J Clin Pharmacol. 2012;52(1 Suppl):79S–90.
13. McLean AJ, Le Couteur DG. Aging biology and geriatric clinical pharmacology. Pharmacol Rev. 2004;56(2):163–84.
14. Zhou XJ, Rakheja D, Yu X, Saxena R, Vaziri ND, Silva FG. The aging kidney. Kidney Int. 2008;74(6):710–20.
15. McDonald M, Hertz RP, Unger AN, Lustik MB. Prevalence, awareness, and management of hypertension, dyslipidemia, and diabetes among United States adults aged 65 and older. J Gerontol A Biol Sci Med Sci. 2009;64(2):256–63.
16. Turnheim K. Pharmacokinetic dosage guidelines for elderly subjects. Expert Opin Drug Metab Toxicol. 2005;1(1):33–48.
17. Ng BL, Anpalahan M. Management of chronic kidney disease in the elderly. Intern Med J. 2011;41(11):761–8.
18. U.S. Department of Health and Human Services. Food and Drug Administration. Center for Drug Evaluation and Research (CDER). Guidance for industry pharmacokinetics in patients with impaired renal function — study design, data analysis, and impact on dosing and labeling. March 2010. http://www.fda.gov/downloads/Drugs/…/Guidances/UCM204959.pdf. Accessed 23 Sept, 2013.
19. Matzke GR, Aronoff GR, Atkinson Jr AJ, et al. Drug dosing consideration in patients with acute and chronic kidney disease-a clinical update from Kidney Disease: Improving Global Outcomes (KDIGO). Kidney Int. 2011;80(11):1122–37.
20. Lassiter J, Bennett WM, Olyaei AJ. Drug dosing in elderly patients with chronic kidney disease. Clin Geriatr Med. 2013;29(3):657–705.
21. Bosomworth MP, Sandoe JA. Drug dosing and estimates of kidney function. Ann Clin Biochem. 2013;50(Pt 6):520–2.
22. Keller F, Maiga M, Neumayer HH, Lode H, Distler A. Pharmacokinetic effects of altered plasma protein binding of drugs in renal disease. Eur J Drug Metab Pharmacokinet. 1984;9(3):275–82.
23. Naud J, Nolin TD, Leblond FA, Pichette V. Current understanding of drug disposition in kidney disease. J Clin Pharmacol. 2012;52(1 Suppl):10S–22.
24. Lalande L, Charpiat B, Leboucher G, Tod M. Consequences of renal failure on non-renal clearance of drugs. Clin Pharmacokinet. 2014;53(6):521–32.
25. Michaud J, Naud J, Chouinard J, et al. Role of parathyroid hormone in the downregulation of liver cytochrome P450 in chronic renal failure. J Am Soc Nephrol. 2006;17(11):3041–8.
26. Nolin TD, Naud J, Leblond FA, Pichette V. Emerging evidence of the impact of kidney disease on drug metabolism and transport. Clin Pharmacol Ther. 2008;83(6):898–903.
27. Lessard BA, Zaiken K. Comparison of equations for dosing of medications requiring renal adjustment. J Am Pharm Assoc. 2013; 53(1):54–7.
28. Nyman HA, Dowling TC, Hudson JQ, Peter WL, Joy MS, Nolin TD. Comparative evaluation of the Cockcroft-Gault Equation and the Modification of Diet in Renal Disease (MDRD) study equation for drug dosing: an opinion of the Nephrology Practice and Research Network of the American College of Clinical Pharmacy. Pharmacotherapy. 2011;31(11):1130–44.
29. Steffl JL, Bennett W, Olyaei AJ. The old and new methods of assessing kidney function. J Clin Pharmacol. 2012;52(1 Suppl):63S–71.
30. Cockcroft DW, Gault MH. Prediction of creatinine clearance from serum creatinine. Nephron. 1976;16(1):31–41.
31. Levey AS, Bosch JP, Lewis JB, Greene T, Rogers N, Roth D. A more accurate method to estimate glomerular filtration rate from serum creatinine: a new prediction equation. Modification of Diet in Renal Disease Study Group. Ann Intern Med. 1999;130(6):461–70.
32. Levey AS, Stevens LA. Estimating GFR using the CKD Epidemiology Collaboration (CKD-EPI) creatinine equation: more accurate GFR estimates, lower CKD prevalence estimates, and better risk predictions. Am J Kidney Dis. 2010;55(4):622–7.
33. Munar MY, Singh H. Drug dosing adjustments in patients with chronic kidney disease. Am Fam Physician. 2007;75(10):1487–96.
34. Papaioannou A, Clarke JA, Campbell G, Bedard M. Assessment of adherence to renal dosing guidelines in long-term care facilities. J Am Geriatr Soc. 2000;48(11):1470–3.
35. ElDesoky ES. Pharmacokinetic-pharmacodynamic crisis in the elderly. Am J Ther. 2007;14(5):488–98.
36. Choi G, Gomersall CD, Tian Q, Joynt GM, Freebairn R, Lipman J. Principles of antibacterial dosing in continuous renal replacement therapy. Crit Care Med. 2009;37(7):2268–82.

Index

J.R. Nunley and E.V. Lerma (eds.), *Dermatological Manifestations of Kidney Disease*,
DOI 10.1007/978-1-4939-2395-3, © Springer Science+Business Media New York 2015

I

T

MIX
Papier aus verantwortungsvollen Quellen
Paper from responsible sources
FSC® C105338

If you have any concerns about our products,
you can contact us on
ProductSafety@springernature.com

In case Publisher is established outside the EU,
the EU authorized representative is:
Springer Nature Customer Service Center GmbH
Europaplatz 3, 69115 Heidelberg, Germany

Printed by Libri Plureos GmbH
in Hamburg, Germany